SpringerWienNewYork

Frank A. Granderath
Thomas Kamolz
Rudolph Pointner (Eds.)

Gastroesophageal Reflux Disease

Principles of Disease, Diagnosis, and Treatment

SpringerWienNewYork

Dr. Frank A. Granderath
Mag. Dr. Thomas Kamolz
Univ.-Prof. Dr. Rudolph Pointner
Allgemein öffentliches Krankenhaus, Zell am See, Austria

Printed in Austria

SpringerWienNewYork is part of Springer Science + Business Media
springeronline.com

Typesetting: Thomson Press Ltd., Chennai, India
Printing: Holzhausen Druck und Medien GmbH, 1140 Wien, Austria

Printed on acid-free and chlorine-free bleached paper
SPIN: 11339267

With 130 (partly coloured) Figures

Library of Congress Control Number: 2005933709

ISBN-10 3-211-23589-2 SpringerWienNewYork
ISBN-13 978-3-211-23589-8 SpringerWienNewYork

*This book is dedicated to my parents – Rolf and Wiltrud,
who supported me all over the years with all their love.
Special thanks for all to my wife Ursula Maria
and my teacher Rudolph Pointner.*

F. A. Granderath

*To the loves of my life – Uli, Max and Sophie – my parents,
family, friends and all staff members.
Thank you all for the support during all the years.*

T. Kamolz

PREFACE

Gastroesophageal reflux disease (GERD) is one of the most common gastrointestinal disorders in the Western world. In recent years, there have been many developments in the field of GERD. At least, all these developments have helped to find new diagnostic procedures and different treatment concepts. As well known, GERD affects patients quality of life and leads to a significant economic burden on society. Therefore, all further investigations should primary aim in an improvement of patients daily life.

The challenge of this book is to critically evaluate the currently available literature and to present for all you who are interested in the field of GERD the basic principles of disease, diagnostic and treatment. We, the editors, are more than proud that a large number of the world wide leading experts have accepted our invitation to contribute on this book.

In the first part of the book, the authors discuss aspects of epidemiology, pathophysiology, GERD in relation to age and gender, the progression of GERD to Barrett's esophagus, GERD and hiatal hernia or the role of *Helicobacter pylori*.

The second part addresses specific areas of medical and endoscopic management as well as general diagnostics and presurgical evaluation: the role of endoscopy, esophageal manometry and pH monitoring or radiology.

The third part includes all relevant aspects of surgical treatment including a historical review of surgical history in GERD. The chapters present aspects such as surgical techniques, outcomes, failures of surgery and their management as well as new trends in surgery such as robotic antireflux surgery or the use of prosthetic material for hiatal closure.

In contrast to other books, we have finally included a fourth block of chapters describing primary the patients view of disease. Therefore, aspects such as patients quality of life before and after different concepts of treatment, psychological aspects of GERD but also the socio-economic view are included.

We all hope that this book will help provide further guidance for all those of you who work in the field of GERD – independently if they work as a general practitioner, a gastroenterologist, a surgeon or a nurse – and that you will find the material helpful for your work.

Zell am See, October 2005

Frank A. Granderath
Thomas Kamolz
Rudolph Pointner

CONTENTS

LIST OF CONTRIBUTORS

Editors

Dr. **F. A. Granderath**, Department of General Surgery, General Hospital Zell am See, 5700 Zell am See, Austria (E-mail: fagzellamsee@yahoo.com)

Dr. **T. Kamolz**, Siedlungsstr. 12, A-5700 Zell am See, Austria (E-mail: kamolz@utanet.at)

Prof. Dr. **R. Pointner**, Department of General Surgery, Public Hospital of Zell am See, Paracelsusstr. 8, 5700 Zell am See, Austria (E-mail: rudolph.pointner@kh-zellamsee.at)

Authors

A. Bansal, MD, Assistant Professor of Medicine, University of Kansas School of Medicine and Veteran Affairs Medical Center, 4801 E. Linwood Blvd, Kansas City, MO 64128-2295, USA (E-mail: a-bansal@rocketmail.com)

G. Bianchi Porro, *see* Dr. F. Pace

W. Breithaupt, *see* Prof. Dr. K.-H. Fuchs

G. B. Cadière, MD, PhD, Service de Chirurgie Digestive, Centre Hospitalier Universitaire Saint-Pierre, 322 Rue Haute, 1000 Bruxelles, Belgium (E-mail: coelio@resulb.ulb.ac.be)

M. A. Carlson, Department of Surgery, University of Nebraska Medical Center, Omaha, USA (E-mail: macarlso@unmc.edu)

D. O. Castell, MD, Professor of Medicine, Director Esophageal Disorders Program, Division of Gastroenterology/Hepatology, Medical University of South Carolina, 96 Jonathan Lucas Street, 210 CSB, Charleston, SC 29425, USA (E-mail: castell@musc.edu)

B. Dallemagne, MD, Département de Chirurgie Digestive, CHC-Les Cliniques Saint Joseph, rue de Hesbaye 75, 4000 Liege, Belgium (E-mail: bernard.dallemagne@chc.be)

G. Dapri, *see* G. B. Cadière

R. Dickman, *see* R. Fass

Prof. Dr. **Ch. Ell**, Klinik Innere Medizin II, HSK Wiesbaden, Ludwig Erhardtstraße 100, 65199 Wiesbaden, Germany (E-mail: christian.ell@hsk-wiesbaden.de)

R. Fass, MD, Southern Arizona VA Health Care System, GI Section (1-111G-1), 3601 South 6th Avenue, Tucson, AZ 85723-0001, USA (E-mail: ronnie.fass@med.VA.gov)

M. Fein, Department of Surgery, University of Würzburg, Joseph-Schneider-Str. 2, 97080 Würzburg, Germany (E-mail: chik211@mail.uni-wuerzburg.de)

C. T. Frantzides, Minimally Invasive Surgery Center, Evanston Northwestern Healthcare, Evanston, USA (E-mail: cfrantzides@enh.org)

Prof. Dr. med. **K.-H. Fuchs**, Department of Surgery Markus-Krankenhaus, Frankfurter Diakonie-Kliniken, Wilhelm-Epstein-Straße 2, 60431 Frankfurt am Main, Germany (E-mail: karl-hermann.fuchs@fdk.info)

N. Guda, *see* N. Vakil

Dr. **E. Güenter**, Klinik Innere Medizin II, HSK Wiesbaden, Ludwig Erhardtstraße 100, 65199 Wiesbaden, Germany

I. Hammer, *see* Prof. Dr. K.-H. Fuchs

J. Himpens, *see* G. B. Cadière

R. A. Hinder, Department of Surgery, Mayo Clinic, 4500 San Pablo Road, Jacksonville, Florida 32224, USA (E-mail: hinder.ronald@mayo.edu)

B. Hugl, *see* R. A. Hinder

P. J. Kahrilas, MD, Northwestern University Medical School, Division of Gastroenterology, Department of Medicine, 676 N. St. Clair St., Suite 1400, Chicago, Illinois 60611, USA (E-mail: p-kahrilas@northwestern.edu)

C. Knippig, *see* P. Malfertheiner

Prof. Dr. **H. Koop**, II. Innere Klinik, HELIOS Klinikum Berlin-Buch, Hobrechtsfelder Chaussee 100, 13122 Berlin, Germany (E-mail: hkoop@berlin.helios-kliniken.de)

D. Korolija, MD, PhD, University Surgical Clinic, Clinical Hospital Center Zagreb, Zagreb Kispaticeva 12, 10 000 Zagreb, Croatia

M. S. Levine, MD, Department of Radiology, Hospital of the University of Pennsylvania, 3400 Spruce Street, Philadelphia, PA 19104, USA (E-mail: marc.levine@uphs.upenn.edu)

Alex G. Little, MD, Professor and Chairman, Clinical Professor and Director Undergraduate Surgical Education, Department of Surgery, Wright State University School of Medicine, 1 Wyoming St., Suite 7000 WCHE, Dayton, OH 45409, USA (E-mail: alex.little@wright.edu)

L. Lundell, MD, PhD, Department of Surgery, Karolinska University Hospital, Huddinge, 141 86 Stockholm, Sweden (E-mail: lars.lundell@karolinska.se)

Prof. Dr. med. **P. Malfertheiner**, Universitätsklinikum, Leipziger Straße 44, 39120 Magdeburg, Germany (E-mail: peter.malfertheiner@medizin.uni-magdeburg.de)

J. Maroske, *see* M. Fein

G. Nilsson, Dr. med. vet./RNT, PhD, Department of Health and Behavioural Sciences, Institute för Hälso- och Beteendevetenskap, University of Kalmar, 391 82 Kalmar, Sweden (E-mail: gunilla.nilsson@hik.se)

S. R. Orenstein, MD, Division of Pediatric Gastroenterology, University of Pittsburgh School of Medicine, Children's Hospital of Pittsburgh, 3705 Fifth Avenue, Pittsburgh, PA 15213, USA (E-mail: sro@pitt.edu)

Dr. **F. Pace**, Department of Gastroenterology, "L. Sacco" University Hospital – Via G.B. Grassi, 74, 20157 Milan, Italy (E-mail: cn.fapac@tin.it)

J. E. Pandolfino, Northwestern University Medical School, Division of Gastroenterology, Department of Medicine, 676 N. St. Clair St., Suite 1400, Chicago, Illinois 60611, USA (E-mail: j-pandolfino@northwestern.edu)

E. M. M. Quigley, MD, FRCP, FACP, FACG, FRCPI, Department of Medicine, Clinical Sciences Building, Cork University Hospital, Cork, Ireland (E-mail: e.quigley@ucc.ie)

R. E. Sampliner, MD, Southern Arizona VA Health Care System, 3601 S. 6th Avenue (111G-1), Tucson, AZ 85723, USA (E-mail: samplinr@email.arizona.edu)

Seema Khan, MD, Division of Pediatric Gastroenterology, University of Pittsburgh School of Medicine, Children's Hospital of Pittsburgh, 3705 Fifth Avenue, Pittsburgh, PA 15213, USA (E-mail: susan.orenstein@chp.edu)

P. Sharma, MD, Associate Professor of Medicine, University of Kansas School of Medicine and Veteran Affairs Medical Center, 4801 E. Linwood Blvd, Kansas City, MO 64128-2295, USA (E-mail: psharma@kumc.edu)

J. Swoger, *see* M. F. Vaezi

R. P. Turk, MD, Clinical Professor and Director Undergraduate Surgical Education, Department of Surgery, Wright State University School of Medicine, 1 Wyoming St., Suite 7000 WCHE, Dayton, OH 45409, USA

R. Tutuian, MD, Division of Gastroenterology/Hepatology, Medical University of South Carolina, 96 Jonathan Lucas Street, 210 CSB, Charleston, SC 29425, USA (E-mail: tutuianr@musc.edu)

M. F. Vaezi, M.D., PhD, Msepi, Professor of Medicine, GI Clinical Director, Director Swallowing and Esophageal Disorders, Director Clinical Research, 1501 TVC, 1301-22nd Ave. South Nashville, TN 37232-5280, USA (E-mail: michael.vaezi@vanderbilt.edu)

Prof. **N. Vakil**, MD, Aurora Sinai Medical Center, 945 North 12th Street, Milwaukee, WI 53212, USA (E-mail: nvakil@wisc.edu)

V. Velanovich, MD, Division of General Surgery, Henry Ford Hospital, 2799 West Grand Blvd., Detroit, Michigan 48202, USA (E-mail: vvelanol@hfhs.org)

Prof. **D. I. Watson**, Flinders University Department of Surgery, Room 3D211, Flinders Medical Centre, Bedford Park, South Australia 5042, Australia (E-mail: david.watson@flinders.edu.au)

Prof. **S. Wood-Dauphinee**, PhD PT, School of Physical and Occupational Therapy, Department of Epidemiology and Biostatistics, Department of Medicine, McGill University, 3654 Promenade Sir-William-Osler, Montreal, Quebec, Canada H3G 1Y5 (E-mail: sharon.wood.dauphinee@mcgill.ca)

C. Zornig, Department of Surgery, Israelitisches Krankenhaus Hamburg, Orchideenstiege 14, 22297 Hamburg, Germany

Chapter 1

CLINICAL SPECTRUM, NATURAL HISTORY AND EPIDEMIOLOGY OF GERD

F. Pace and G. Bianchi Porro

Chair and Department of Gastroenterology, "L. Sacco" University Hospital, Milan, Italy

Summary

GERD is a spectrum disease, i.e., a disease composed by many patient subgroups, ranging from symptomatic disease without mucosal lesions (or NERD) to the complications of erosive esophagitis, such as esophageal stricture, ulceration or Barrett's esophagus. Almost all the transitions are possible amongst groups, even if the progression from one stage to the other has been described mainly based upon retrospective data.

The natural history of the disease is poorly investigated: available data would suggest that symptoms of GERD tend to persist and to worsen with time, independently from the presence and severity of mucosal lesions or the severity of esophageal acid exposure at presentation.

As far as the epidemiological features are concerned, the prevalence of at least monthly GERD symptoms ranges between 26% to 44% in western countries, whereas the prevalence of endoscopic esophagitis at open access endoscopy or in symptomatic patients seem to be very high, up to 20%, with an incidence rate in the general population about hundred time lower.

The principal complication, e.g., Barrett's esophagus, has a prevalence of 15–20% of the GERD population, with a rate of adenocarcinoma development of about 0.5% per patient year of follow up. Mortality for uncomplicated GERD is negligible.

Introduction

The backward flow of gastric content into the esophagus, that is, gastroesophageal reflux (GER), is up to a certain extent a physiological phenomenon, in particular during the early postprandial phase [1]. When the threshold of normality is surpassed, GER may induce inflammatory changes of the esophageal mucosa, different esophageal and extra-esophageal symptoms (even in the absence of detectable lesions), and macroscopic lesions such as erosive or ulcerative esophagitis or so-called atypical manifestations (laringytis, faringytis, dental erosions, and many others).

From this brief introduction is already clear that GER disease (GERD) is a broad disease, with a large clinical spectrum of signs and symptoms, interesting not only the esophageal area but many other regions of the body, including the mouth, lungs, ear, nose and throat, and which can be accompanied or not by esophageal lesions. It is therefore evident that the epidemiology of GERD is difficult to assess because this disease encompasses at least three broad groups of patients: (a) those with typical symptoms, such as heartburn and regurgitation but without reflux esophagits, so called non erosive reflux disease (NERD) patients; (b) patients with reflux esophagitis, and with or without complication, such as stricture, specialized intestinal metaplasia; (c) patients with atypical manifestations (Table 1).

In this chapter, we will address the topic of the clinical spectrum of the disease as well as its natural history, and review the epidemiological data available in the literature.

Clinical spectrum

Compared to relatively few years ago, the concept of GERD clinical spectrum has deeply changed during the last decade. During the last years, in fact, it has been increasingly recognized that the GERD patient population is indeed a multifaceted one; the schematic representation of the entire population of patients, previously presented as an iceberg [2] (see

Fig. 1) has been modified to take into account, as an example, the changing epidemiology of Helicobacter pylori infection (*Fig. 2*), a factor believed to be linked in some way to GERD [3] and it has been revisited up to a point that it has been suggested by Fass [5] that the original iceberg may in fact break into three smaller icebergs (or populations), completely separated and not communicating each other anymore (*Fig. 3*). The latter schematization does in fact represent a new conceptual framework, in that it categorize GERD patients into 3 unique groups of patients: non-erosive reflux disease, erosive esophagitis and Barrett's esophagus; we disagree with this model, for various reasons, but basically we think that the principal conceptual mistake lies in the fact that the Fass' view mix together the concept of natural

Table 1. Atypical (or extraesophageal, or supraesohageal) GERD manifestations

Pulmonary	Ear, nose and throat	Others
- Asthma (non seasonal, non allergic)	- Chronic cough	- Non-cardiac chest pain
- Chronic bronchitis	- Laryngitis	- Dental erosion
- Aspiration pneumonia	- Hoarseness	- Sleep apnea
- Bronchiectasis	- Globus	
- Pulmonary fibrosis	- Pharyngitis	
- Chronic obstructive disease	- Sinusitis	
- Pneumonia	- Vocal cord granuloma	
	- Laryngeal carcinoma (possible)	

Table 2. Epidemiology of GERD

Epidemiologic factor		Reference
Incidence and prevalence of reflux symptoms		
- Symptoms of reflux in USA healthy subjects (at least monthly)	36%	[40]
- Symptoms of reflux in the USA adult population (at least monthly)	44%	[41]
- Symptoms of reflux in the Italian adult population (at least monthly)	26%	[42]
- Symptoms of reflux in the ingaporean population (at least monthly)	$< 2\%$	[43]
Prevalence of esophagitis		
- in symptomatic patients (Europe)	$\approx 30\%$	[37], [38]
- in symptomatic patients (Japan)	15%	[39]
- open access endoscopy	20%	[35]
Incidence of esophagitis		
- in general populations	120/100,000	[34]
Complications of GERD		
- Hemorrhage (% of patients with massive UGI bleeding)	6%	[48]
- Stricture (% of patients seeking medical care)	10%	[50]
- Stricture (% of patients with Barrett's esophagus)	50%	[35]
- Barrett's esophagus (% of patients with symptomatic GERD)	5–20%	[35]
- Adenocarcinoma in Barrett's (incidence per patient year of follow up)	0.5%	
Mortality		
- Death rate per year (general population)	0.10–0.20/100,000	[51], [52]

history, which is the tendency of the disease to progress and to worsen in the absence of therapy, with the concept of clinical spectrum, which simply signifies that many clinical manifestations of a disease are

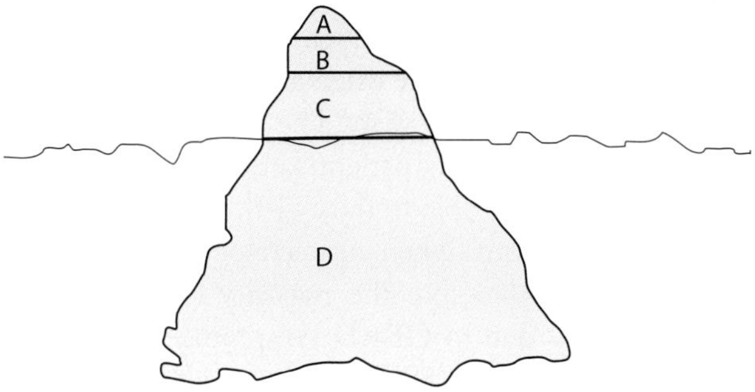

Fig. 1. The iceberg of GERD population (modified from [2]. The "iceberg" represents the populations of patients with gastroesophageal reflux. The largest group are those with mild disease who self medicate with over-the-counter drugs and rarely if ever visit doctors because of their symptoms. The smallest group are those who visit gastroenterologists because of severe disease requiring continuous high-dose therapy. (A) represents those with complications (e.g., symptoms and complications), (B) those with symptoms who seek medical care (e.g., symptoms and complaints), (C) those with symptoms who self medicate and do not seek medical care (e.g., symptoms and no complaints)

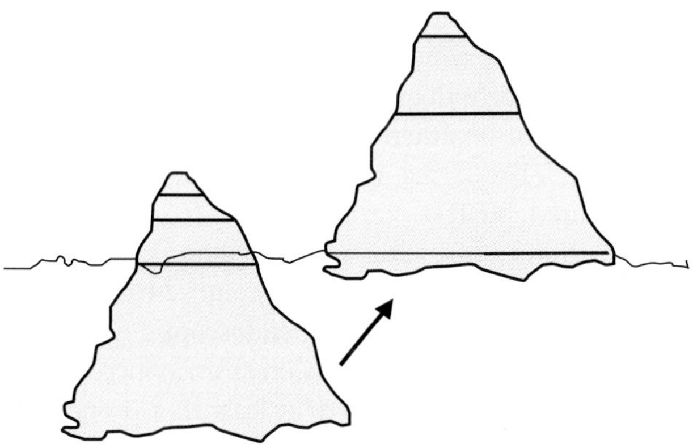

Fig. 2. The "iceberg" of GERD in countries where chronic atrophic gastritis and gastric cancer are common and GERD is rare (from [3]). This illustration depicts the change in the presentation of gastroesophageal reflux associated with the change in the average pattern of gastritis from an atrophic pangastritis to a nonatropic gastritis or normal stomach. Gastric cancer becomes rare, whereas duodenal ulcer and GERD become problems among the populations with *H. Pylori* infection. Thus, the prevalence of GERD is inversely related to that of gastric cancer. This change in patterns occurred during the last part of the 19th and early 20th centuries and is currently ongoing in many countries

clinically possible. We therefore strongly defend the concept of GERD as a disease composed by many patient subgroups with almost all the transitions possible from one group to the other (*Fig. 4*).

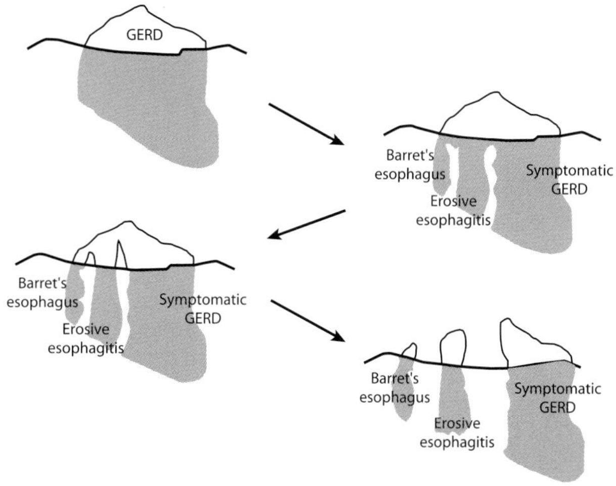

Fig. 3. The GERD iceberg revisited. According to Fass [5] the iceberg of GERD population may in fact be composed by three unique groups of patients: nonerosive reflux disease, erosive esophagitis and Barrett's esophagus, independent from each other and not communicating (modified from [4])

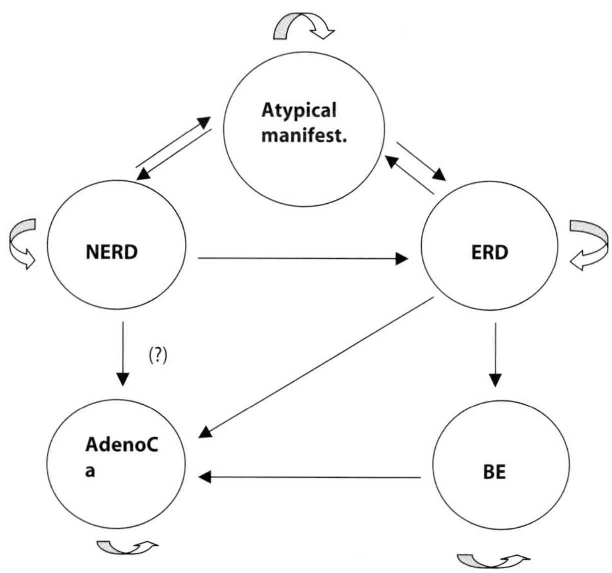

Fig. 4. Natural history of GERD, based on the Markow-state diagram. Each circle indicates a GERD subgroup. In each subgroup is possible to stay (curved arrow) or move into another subgroup (linear arrow). In some cases, data support possibility of reverse movement, whereas in a single instance (transition from NERD to AdenoCa data are insufficient). From [6]

Natural history of GERD

Evaluating the natural history of GERD is useful for a number of reasons, for this knowledge may help to: (a) discern the percentage of the population that will progress from nonerosive to erosive disease and its complications, such as stricture, Barrett's oesophagus, and esophageal adenocarcinoma, or from exclusively esophageal to extraesophageal manifestations; (b) define, assess and validate predictivity of risk factors for such complicated forms of the disease; (c) determine if medical, surgical or endoscopic therapies are able to positively modify the natural course of the disease; and (d) determine the need for maintenance therapy to prevent complications and persistent symptoms.

Others [7], [8] have pointed out that many factors make it difficult to study the natural history of GERD, notably the evolving definition of the disease and the lack of diagnostic standard with an unclear demarcation between physiological reflux and GERD. As a consequence, few studies in the literature have addressed the issue of defining the natural history of erosive GERD, and even less that of nonerosive gastroesophageal reflux disease (NERD), extraesophageal GERD and complications.

Natural history of NERD

Until recently, patients with endoscopic-negative reflux disease (NERD) were considered to suffer from a milder disease [9], i.e., requiring less intensive/prolonged treatment and possibly characterized by a better long-term prognosis. This concept was subsequently proven to be incorrect, since the impairment in disease-related quality of life (HRQoL), for example, appears to be similar in GERD patients with or without endoscopic esophagitis and is related in both instances to symptom severity [10]. Also, the symptomatic acute response to PPI drugs in patients with or without endoscopic mucosal damage seems not to be different, and in fact might be worse in NERD [11], [12]. Finally, after discontinuation of acute treatment, symptomatic relapse within 6 months appears to affect a similarly high proportion of both GERD groups [13].

A study of ours published ten years ago was probably the first reporting the natural history of GERD patients without endoscopic esophagitis but with a pathological esophageal pH-metry [14]. In that study, we showed that 5 of 33 such patients treated with antacids or prokinetc agents developed an endoscopic esophagitis *ex novo* within 6 months, and that the extent of esophageal acid exposure at entry was not predictive of this complication. In a subsequent study [15] we extended the observation of the original patient group up to a median duration of 10 years. The first interesting observation regarding this patient sample is that almost all patients we were able to trace [28], [29] are affected by GERD symptoms when antisecretory drugs are discontinued, and therefore the majority (75%) was on such a therapy due to GERD symptoms. Secondly, a very high proportion (89%) of our patients in whom repeat endoscopy was performed (N = 18) showed an erosive esophagitis. Thus, a considerable proportion of the original patient cohort indeed showed a *progression* from nonerosive to erosive disease.

Schindlbeck et al [16], in a study investigating the fate of GERD patients with and without esophagitis, reported on 16 patients with pH-documented GERD and no esophagitis 3 years after the diagnosis. During this period, four patients (25%) developed reflux esophagitis, while the majority of patient population, which included also patients with esophagitis at entry, was still taking medications on a daily basis because of their GERD symptoms. Symptoms were rated to be equal or worse than at entry by 70% of patients, in the absence of treatment. In the study by Mc Dougall et al [17], 71% of the 17 patients with a pH-metry documented NERD complained of frequent heartburn 3 to 4.5 years after initial diagnosis, 59% were on daily acid suppressive therapy, and 24% of those patients who had repeat endoscopy developed esophagitis. Again, a progression from nonerosive to erosive GERD was observed, at least in a proportion of patients.

These studies, together with our own, seem to indicate that patients with NERD may indeed move from one part of the spectrum to the adjacent one: the model proposed by Fass and colleague appears to be incorrect, since not only is the progression from nonerosive to erosive GERD substantiated by the literature, but also the transition from erosive to Barrett's esophagus does in fact occurr, as shown, for example, in the study by Mc Dougall, in which 11% of patients with erosive esophagitis at entry showed BE at follow up repeat endoscopy [17].

Erosive GERD (ERD)

The above quoted paper by Fass states that "patients with erosive esophagitis tend to remain within this group during their lifetime" and that Barrett's mucosa does not progress or regress over time, and thus patients continue to harbor this type of lesion as long as they live. In fact this is not true, as transition to Barrett's esophagus and to adenocarcinoma has been reported, the latter even in the absence of BE as an intermediate lesion. We have already mentioned the 11% of new developed BE observed in the study by McDougall; Lagergren et al [18] have demonstrated that the risk of adenocarcinoma of the esophagus is much more related to the duration and severity of gastroesophageal reflux disease than to the presence of Barrett's esophagus, and therefore the latter could be considered to be "a common, but not necessary step, in the evolution of esophageal adenocarcinoma" [18]. Similar observations have subsequently been done by Chow et al [19] and by Farrow et al [20].

Conio et al [21], in a retrospective survey, were able to demonstrate that in the Olmsted County many adenocarcinomas of the esophagus occurred in patients without a previous diagnosis of Barrett's esophagus. All these studies represent arguments against the statement that most erosive patients tend to remain in this group, but rather show that a transition from the less to the most advanced segment of the GERD spectrum is possible.

Finally, it has been shown already since many years [22], and has recently been confirmed [23] that, during the course of the erosive-ulcerative disease, the esophagus is involved in a slow but progressive process of "shrinkage" which determines not only a progressive weakness of the anti-reflux mechanism represented by LES length and position, but also the formation of an "endobrachyesophagus", which, to use a more modern terminology, is synonymous with circular long-segment Barrett's esophagus.

Thus, the progression of the disease in this group of patients is not only suggested by epidemiological evidence but is also biologically plausible and clinically confirmed.

Atypical manifestations of GERD

Many extraesophageal (or supraesophageal) manifestations of GERD are now acknowledged as parts of the disease spectrum [24]; we disagree with considering these manifestations as only possible complications of the NERD category, as proposed by Fass and Ofman. If, in fact, it holds true that the majority of such patients do not show esophageal mucosal damage at endoscopy, a definite proportion, between 20% and 30% of such patients do indeed have erosive or ulcerative esophagitis [25]. We too dispute that NERD and "atypical" GERD patients should be regarded as having less severe disease; this is however not based on the absence or presence of mucosal damage, but on the pathogenesis of symptom perception in those patients. NERD patients are in fact possibly at least three groups of different patients (true refluxers, patients with esophageal hyperalgesia and patients with psychological disturbances) [9], and the traditional treatment with antisecretory agents can possibly be more useful in the first group than in the others. Grouping these patients and the "atypical" ones into a single disease entity will only result in greater heterogeneity and less management skill. On the other hand, the diagnostic criterion based on the absence of mucosal damage presently allows only an imperfect, operational diagnosis, which will be rapidly surpassed by new methods of investigating the pathophysiology of GERD (i.e., impedance measurements), similar to what happened some years ago for nonA-nonB hepatitis, which was subsequently positively defined according to virus etiology (hepatitis C virus, delta, E, etc.), when new sierology methods became available.

Barrett's patients

Many studies have shown that the symptom expression in this group of patients is lower than in erosive GERD patients, as a manifestation of a reduced mucosal sensitivity to acid [26], [27]. On the other hand, the presence of a specialized intestinal metaplasia in the distal esophageal mucosa is associated with a small but not negligible risk of developing adenocarcinoma [28]. In any case, the possibility that patients with Barrett's esophagus may subsequently develop adenocarcinoma is seriously considered by guidelines proposed by gastroenterological associations [29], [30], and therefore surveillance is recommended [31], even if the cost-effectiveness of this recommendation is still debated [32].

Epidemiology of GERD

Before revising the existing literature on this topic, we would like to recall the code numbers for GERD and related disorders according to the ninth International Classification of Diseases (ICD-9); overall, the diseases of the esophagus are coded under the ICD code 530 (Table 1): esophagitis in its various forms, including the one induced by GER, is coded as 530.1, ulcer of the esophagus as 530.2, benign stricture as 530.3. Interestingly enough, in the ICD-9 GERD and hiatal hernia are separated conditions, the latter having the code 553.3 (if not complicated); finally, the symptoms of GERD are listed in the code 787 (GI symptoms), where heartburn is coded as 787.1, dysphagia as 787.2, etc.

However, the heterogeneity of this classification does not allow to differentiate, as an example, among esophagitis due to GER or due to other less common causes, such as infection or ingestion of drugs and chemicals. It does also not allow grading of esophagitis severity, as achievable for example by the Los Angeles system or the Savary-Miller classification; finally, the presence of Barrett's esophagus or extra-esophageal complications of GERD are left out from the ICD-9 classification, which is therefore not particularly helpful. It should not be forgotten, also, that GERD is very seldom a cause of death and rarely causes hospital admission. National incidence and prevalence data are therefore mainly estimated from interviews and are subject to over and under-reporting problems. It has also been claimed that, at least for prevalence studies, the external validity of these data is suspected and hardly generalizable worldwide [7].

Incidence and prevalence of esophagitis

Studies concerning the incidence rate of reflux esophagitis (RE) and/or GERD are very rare; historically, the first study on the incidence of (severe) RE was published in 1969 by Brunnen [33], who gave a figure of 4.5 per 100,000 for ulcerative esophagitis or RE complicated by stricture. The study was conducted among residents older than 12 years from the northwestern region of Scotland, and it comprised a total of 200 patients. The occurrence of esophagitis was confirmed by barium studies in all, and endoscopy in most of the patients. The incidence of severe RE showed an almost exponential rise starting at the age of 40 years. Lööf [34] et al published in 1993 an important paper dealing with the incidence of RE; they examined al the reports of upper GI endoscopy performed in patients aged ≥ 16 years and living in a defined catchment area of 226,776 inhabitants during a 2-year period. The incidence of RE was calculated to be 120 per 100,000: in 88% it was a simple, uncomplicated, erosive esophagitis. The incidence of complicated RE and of Barrett's esophagus was 5.6 and 1.7 per 100,000, respectively [34]. In this study, the severity of esophagitis significantly increased with age ($p = 0.003$) and most (75%) of the patients with complicated esophagitis were ≥ 60 years of age. Men had more severe grades of esophagitis than women ($p = 0.003$).

Prevalence

The percentage of patients with reflux symptoms found to have esophagitis at endoscopy varies notably in the published series, from 38% to 75% [35], with an average of 50% or less [36]. Indeed, several recent community-based European studies found even a lower prevalence, of about 30% [37], [38]. In large endoscopic series, reflecting the percentage of patients in general gastroenterological practice, the prevalence of esophagitis is nowadays higher than that of duodenal and gastric ulcer, and ranks first in the upper GI endoscopic diagnosis in Europe and USA, with a figure around 20% [35]. A recent work from Japan [39] investigating the correlation between symptoms and endoscopic finding in RE was conducted in 8031 subjects undergoing upper GI endoscopy for various reasons (and not randomly selected from the community) and who had not taken medication for GI disease; the study found an overall prevalence of 14.9% for RE, with a slight tendency for symptoms to increase in frequency with the increasing severity of esophagitis. Heartburn, as an example, increased from 38% in Los Angeles gr. A to slightly less than 60% in grade D [39].

Incidence and prevalence of GERD symptoms

The first and probably more quoted paper concerning the incidence of GERD symptoms is the study by Nebel et al, published in 1976 [40]; the study was conducted by means of a questionnaire administered to 446 hospitalized and 558 non-hospitalized subjects, as well as in 385 control subjects. In the latter group, daily heartburn occurred in 7%, weekly in 14% and monthly in 15%, giving a total of 36% of subjects having heartburn at least monthly [40]. Data coming from a large national poll [41] about three decade later does confirm the high prevalence of heartburn, with daily heartburn reported by 7%, weekly heartburn by 20% and monthly heartburn by 44%, with an estimated population involved of 13, 27 and 61 millions of adult Americans, respectively. A more recent study conducted in two samples of Italian employees, composed by 424 and 344 subjects, respectively, found a lower figure, with a prevalence rate for monthly heartburn of 21% [42]. Interestingly enough, symptoms of GERD (as well as reflux esophagitis) are much less prevalent in the Asian population; as an example, a monthly occurrence of heartburn is reported by 1.6% of 696 Singaporean subjects participating in a cross-sectional survey using a validate questionnaire [43]. The importance of racial differences in the frequency of symptoms is highlighted by a recent study, conducted in Boston, on 129 out-patients attending general medical clinics and in an Asian community health centre; the study shows that black and white American complain of heartburn by a similar percentage (46% and 35%, respectively) whereas Asian subjects complained much less frequently (3%) ($p < 0.05$) [44]. The similar high prevalence of reflux symptoms among black and white groups in the USA is confirmed by a recent cross-sectional survey conducted by questionnaire on 496 employees at a VA medical centre, who were subsequently submitted to endoscopy [45]. Interestingly, heartburn occurring at least monthly was reported by 40.6% of black subjects and by 35.3% of white ones. Esophagitis however was present in about 50% of white subjects complaining weekly of heartburn, but only in 23% of black patients ($p = 0.02$) [45].

Finally, there is robust evidence that symptom severity is a poor predictor of severity of mucosal damage [36], whereas at least the frequency of symptoms seems to be related to the amount of esophageal acid exposure [46]. Thus, the presence or absence of esophagits, as well as the presence of Barrett's esophagus might not be predicted by the patient'symptom profile, and therefore endoscopic diagnosis is still essential to reliably assess these conditions [47].

Morbidity

The morbidity from GERD arises from both esophageal and extra-esophageal complications. GERD accounts for only approximately 6% of massive upper gastrointestinal hemorrhage [48]. More recent data show that this figure is probably increasing, possibly due to the overall increase of GERD prevalence. For example, Newton et al [49] found that in a inpatient population undergoing upper GI endoscopy at a district general hospital, 58% were referred to gastroscopy for investigation of acute upper gastrointestinal bleeding and esophagitis was found in 33% of them. Stricture complicates reflux disease in approximately 10% of patients seeking medical treatment [50]. It is likely that the incidence of these complications is falling since the introduction and the widespread use of potent antisecretory agents, such as the proton pump inhibitors.

We skip in this chapter the epidemiologic features of Barrett's esophagus, which will be covered in a separate section (cf. Chap. 5).

Mortality

GERD would appear to be associated with a very low adult mortality rate. According to Brunnen et al [33], the annual mortality rate from severe esophagitis was 0.1 per 100,000 from 1951 to 1957. When the operative mortality was considered, this figure rose to 0.16 per 100,000.

Kieser [51] found that there have been 47 deaths in Switzerland (population in 1963, 5.8 million) from 1963 to 1964 in which hiatal hernia had been a basic, a contributing or an immediate cause of death, leading to a mortality rate of about 0.10 per 100,000 per year [51]. More recently, Rantanen et al [52] have analyzed all death certificated due to GERD in Finland, during the period 1990–95; they found that 52 individuals out of the ca. 5 million inhabitants of Finland died of benign GERD treated conservatively during this period, with a mortality rate of about 0.20 per 100,000 inhabitant per year. This figure is even higher than that reported by Brunnen [33] and by Kieser [51], and also higher than the figure reported in Finland during the 1960s, when it was 0.09 per 100,000 [52]. In the study by Newton et al [49], the 30-day mortality of inpatients with esophagitis at endoscopy was significantly higher than in those without (21% vs 10%, $p < 0.04$). However, the most common cause of death was carcinomatosis, and did not differ in patients with or without esophagitis. In conclusion, death from GERD is extremely rare and often due to the concomitant presence of other severe diseases, such as mental disorders, heart diseases, or alcoholism; however, contrary to general opinion, the mortality in conservatively treated GERD patients may not have decreased, possibly due to the overall trend to an increase number of elderly subjects. This is mirrored by an increase in death rate from non-malignant disease of the esophagus (ICD-9 = 530) which has been observed in Europe; as an example, in England and Wales between 1974 and 1988 the number of deaths due to this code trebled in women from 118 to 340 (0.5 to 0.13 per 100,000) and doubled in men, from 131 to 251 (0.55 to 1.0 per 100,000) [53]. The calculation of age specific death rate shows the increase to result from a rise in mortality in those over 75 years and age standardized mortality confirms a rise in overall frequency from 0.29 to 0.70 per 100,000 in men and from 0.52 to 1.31 per 100,000 in women [53].

Risk factors

On the issue of predictive factors for GERD there is a large bulk of literature, which is however rather confusing and of relatively poor quality. Most of the existing studies are retrospective in nature, very few are case-control and can therefore assess the relative risk (RR) or the odds ratio (OR) for individual factors. Among the latter, we would like to recall the study by Nilsson et al [54], which shows a dose-response association between increasing body mass index (BMI) and reflux in both sexes, but more significant in women: the risk of reflux increased among severely obese (BMI > 35) in comparison with those with BMI < 25, with an OR of 3.3 in men and 6.3 in women. The use of postmenopausal hormone therapy increased in the latter the strength of association [54]. In a cross-sectional survey conducted in 4095 Japanese men, it was found that current smoking was significantly associated with GERD (OR vs non smoking 1.35) as it was alcohol consumption [55]. Obesity, the presence of hiatus hernia and male gender were significant independent risk factors for severe erosive esophagitis [56] in the retrospective analysis, by means of a regression model, of the baseline characteristics of patients enrolled in four prospective, multicenter, randomized, double-blind comparative trials of once-daily esomeprazole vs omeprazole for the acute healing of acute esophagitis, involving 6709 *Helicobacter pylori*-negative patients. Hiatus hernia emerged once again as a strong risk factor for development of GERD complications such as stricture, hemorrhage and ulcers in a case-control study involving 1533 patients with and 3428 patients without endoscopically diagnosed reflux esophagits [57].

A retrospective cohort study involving all 172 hospitals of the USA Veterans Administration, involving a total of 194, 527 patients with GERD followed-up for 14 years, found that older age, male sex and white ethnicity were risk factors for the development of severe forms of GERD, i.e., those associated with severe erosive esophagitis, ulcers or strictures [58].

Finally, the risk factors related to the relapse of symptoms and/or esophagitis have been assessed by a few studies: Tytgat et al [59] assessed by means of a Cox proportional hazards regression model the possible influence of a number of clinical demographic data on the duration of endoscopic remission within the frame of two cisapride vs placebo RCTs; it was found that severe symptoms or mucosal lesions at entry were significantly related with a poorer outcome during maintenance treatment. Carlsson et al [60], using a Cox' model regression, meta-analysed 1154 patients included in five individual long-term RCTs comparing the efficacy of different dosage regimens of omeprazole, ranitidine and placebo for the prevention of reflux esophagitis; they found that four factors were associated with a higher relapse rate during placebo and active maintenance therapy: pre-treatment severity of esophagitis, young age, non-smoking, and moderate/severe regurgitation prior to entry into the trials [60].

In a study from Taiwan aiming at assessing the long-term outcome and the specific prognostic indicators in 128 reflux esophagitis patients in a low prevalence GERD area [61], found that the presence of hiatal hernia and the severity of esophagitis at initial endoscopy were independent, significant predictors of those patients requiring long-term acid suppressive therapy.

In conclusions, there is circumstantial evidence that obesity, older age, the presence of a hiatal hernia and the severity of symptoms (and of mucosal damage when found to be present) are factors which may suggest a more aggressive clinical picture and/or the need of long-term potent antisecretory therapy in GERD patients.

Finally, Labenz et al [62] recently investigated the patient-associated risk factors for erosive esophagitis by means of a multivariate stepwise analysis conducted on some 2455 patients, recruited in the ProGERD study. They found that male gender, overweight, regular use of alcohol, a history of GERD > 1 year and smoking were associated with a higher risk of erosive esophagitis, whereas a higher level of education and a positive *Helicobacter pylori* status were predictive of a lower risk.

References

[1] Sifrim D, Holloway R, Silny R et al (2001) Composition of the postprandial refluxate in patients with gastroesophageal reflux disease. Am J Gastroenterol 96: 647–655

[2] Richter JE, Castell DO (1982) Gastroesophageal reflux. Pathogenesis, diagnosis and therapy. Ann Intern Med 97: 93–103

[3] Graham D (2003) The changing epidemiology of GERD: geography and Helicobacter pylori. Am J Gastroenterol 98: 1462–1470

[4] Quigley EMM (2003) Factors that influence therapeutic outcomes in symptomatic gastroesophageal reflux disease. Am J Gastroenterol 98 (Suppl): 24–30

[5] Fass R, Offman JJ (2002) Gastroesophageal reflux disease – should we adopt a new conceptual framework? Am J Gastroenterol 97: 1901–1909

[6] Pace F, Bianchi Porro G (2004) Gastroesophageal reflux disease: a typical spectrum disease (a new conceptual framework is not needed). Am J Gastroenterol 99: 946–949

[7] Eisen G (2001) The epidemiology of gastroesophageal reflux disease: what we know and what we need to know. Am J Gastroenterol 96 (Suppl): S16–S18

[8] Locke GR III, Talley NJ, Fett SL et al (1997) Prevalence and clinical spectrum of gastroesophageal reflux: a populaton-based study in Olmsted County, Minnesota. Gastroenterology 112: 1448–1456

[9] Quigley EMM, DiBaise JK (2001) Non-erosive reflux disease: the real problem in gastro-oesophageal reflux disease. Digest Liver Dis 33: 523–527

[10] Glise H, Hallerback B, Wiklund I (1996) Quality of life: a reflection of symptoms and concerns. Scand J Gastroenterol 31 (Suppl 221): 14–17

[11] Smout AJPM (1997) Endoscopy-negative acid reflux disease. Aliment Pharmacol Ther 11 (Suppl 2): 81–85

[12] Fass R, Fennerty MB, Vakil N (2001) Non-erosive reflux disease-current concepts and dilemmas. Am J Gastroenterol 96: 303–314

[13] Carlsson R, Dent J, Watts R, Riley S, Sheikh R et al (1998) Gastro-oesophageal reflux disease in primary care: an international study of different treatment strategies with omeprazole. Eur J Gastroenterol Hepatol 10: 119–124

[14] Pace F, Santalucia F, Bianchi Porro G (1991) Natural history of gastro-oesophageal reflux disease without oesophagitis. Gut 32: 845–848

[15] Pace F, Bollani S, Molteni P, Bianchi Porro G (2004) Natural history of gastro-oesophageal reflux disease without oesophagitis (NERD) – a reappraisal 10 years after. Digest Liver Dis 36: 111–115

[16] Schindlbeck NE, Klauser AG, Berghammer G, Londong W, Mueller-Lissner SA (1992) Three years follow up of patients with gastroesophageal reflux. Gut 33: 1016–1019

[17] McDougall NI, Johnston BT, Kee F, Collins JSA, McFarland RJ, Love AHG (1998) Three to 4.5 year prospective study of prognostic indicators in gastro-oesophageal reflux disease. Scand J Gastroenterol 33: 1016–1022

[18] LaGERgren J, Bergstrom R, Lindgren A, Nyren O (1999) Symptomatic gastroesophageal reflux as a risk factor for esophageal adenocarcinoma. N Engl J Med 340: 825–831

[19] Chow WH, Finkle WD, McLaughlin JK et al (1995) The relation of gastroesophageal reflux disease and its treatment to adenocarcinomas of the oesophagus and gastric cardia. JAMA 274: 474–477

[20] Farrow DC, Vaughan TL, Sweeney C et al (2000) Gastroesophageal reflux disease, use of H2 receptor antagonists and risk of esophageal and gastric cancer. Cancer Causes Control 11: 231–238

[21] Conio M, Cameron AJ, Romero Y, Branch CD, Schleck CD et al (2001) Secular trends in the epidemiology and outcome of Barrett's oesophagus in Olmsted County, Minnesota. Gut 48: 304–309

[22] Csendes A, Maluenda F, Braghetto I et al (1993) Location of the lower oesophageal shincter and the squamous clumnar mucosal junction in 109 healthy controls and 778 patients with different degrees of endosocpic oesophagitis. Gut 34: 21–27

[23] Mattioli S, D'Ovidio F, Pilotti V et al (2003) Hiatus hernia and intrathoracic migration of esophagogastric junction in gastroesophageal reflux disease. Dig Dis Sci 48: 1823–1831

[24] Jailwala JA, Shaker R (2000) Supra-oesophageal complications of reflux disease. Digest Liver Dis 32: 267–274

[25] Jaspersen D, Kulig M, Labenz J et al (2003) Prevalence of extra-oesophageal manifestations in gastro-oesophageal reflux disease: an alysis based on the Pro-GERD study. Aliment Pharmacol Ther 17: 1515–1520

[26] Johnson DA, Winters C, Spurling TJ et al (1987) Esophageal acid sensitivity in Barrett's oesophagus. J Clin Gastroenterol 9: 23–27

[27] Murphy PP, Johnston BT, Collins JS (1994) Mucosal sensitivity and salivary response to infused acid in patients with columnar-lined oesophagus. Eur J Gastroenterol Hepatol 6: 901–905
[28] Shaheen N, Ransohoff DF (2002) Gastroesophageal reflux, Barrett oesophagus, and esophageal cancer. JAMA 287: 1972–1981
[29] DeVault K, Castell DO (1999) Updated guidelines for the diagnosis and treatment of gastroesophageal reflux disease. Am J Gastroenterol 94: 1434–1442
[30] Sampliner RE (1998) Practice guidelines on the diagnosis, surveillance and therapy of Barrett's esopahgus. Am J Gastroenterol 93: 1028–1032
[31] Cooper GS (2003) Endoscopic screening and surveillance for Barrett's oesophagus: can claims data determine its effectiveness? Gastrointest Endosc 57: 914–917
[32] Baldi F, Crotta S, Penagini R (1998) Guidelines for the diagnostic and therapeutic management of patients with gastro-oesophageal reflux disease. A position statement of *The Italian Association of Hospital Gastroenterologists* (AIGO), *Italian Society of Gastrointestinal Endoscopy* (SIED), and *Italian Society of Gastroenterology* (SIGE). Ital J Gastroenterol Hepatol 30: 107–112
[33] Brunnen PL, Karmody AM, Needham CD (1969) Severe peptic oesophagitis. Gut 10: 831–837
[34] Lööf L, Götell P, Elfberg B (1993) The incidence of reflux oesophagitis. A study of endoscopy reports from a defined catchment area in Sweden. Scand J Gastroenterol 238: 1134–1138
[35] Howard PJ, Heading RC (1992) Epidemiology of gastro-oesophageal reflux disease. World J Surg 16: 288–293
[36] Fass R (2003) Epidemiology and pathophysiology of symptomatic gastroesophageal reflux disease. Am J Gastroenterol 98 (Suppl): 2–7
[37] Lind T, Havelund T, Carlsson R et al (1997) Heartburn without oesophagitis: efficacy of omeprazole therapy and features determining therapeutic response. Scand J Gastroenterol 32: 974–979
[38] Jones RH, Hungin AP, Phillips J et al (1995) Gastro-oesophageal reflux disease in primary care in Europe: clinical presentation and endoscopic findings. Eur J Gen Pract 1: 149–154
[39] Okamoto K, Iwqkiri R, Mori M et al (2003) Clinical symptoms in endoscopic reflux esophagitis: evaluation in 8031 adult subjects. Dig Dis Sci 48: 2237–2241
[40] Nebel OT, Fornes MF, Castell DO (1976) Symptomatic gastroesophageal reflux: incidence and precipitating factors. Dig Dis 21: 953–956
[41] A Gallup Organization National Survey (1988) Heartburn across America. Princeton, NJ: Gallup Organization
[42] Valle C, Broglia F, Pistorio A, Tinelli C, Perego M (1999) Prevalence and impact of symptoms suggestive of gastroesophageal reflux disease. Dig Dis Sci 44: 1848–1852
[43] Ho KY, Kang JY, Seow A (1998) Prevalence of gastrointestinal symptoms in a multiracial Asian population, with particular reference to reflux-type symptoms. Am J Gastroenterol 93: 1816–1822
[44] Spechler SJ, Jain SK, Tendler DA, Parker RA (2002) Racial differences in the frequency of symptoms and complications of gastro-oesophageal reflux. Aliment Pharmacol Ther 16: 1795–1800
[45] El-Serag H, Petersen NJ, Carter J et al (2004) Gastroesopahgeal reflux among different racial groups in the United States. Gastroenterology 126: 1692–1699
[46] Galmiche JP, Bruley des Varannes S (1994) Symptoms and disease severity in gastro-oesophageal reflux disease. Scand J Gastroenterol 29 (Suppl 201): 62–68
[47] Avidan B, Sonnenberg A, Schnell TG, Sontag SJ (2002) There are no reliable symptoms for erosive oesophagitis and Barrett's oesophagus: endoscopic diagnosis is still essential. Almient Pharmacol Ther 16: 735–742
[48] Silverstein FE, Gilbert DA, Tedesco FJ et al (1981) The national ASGE survey on upper gastrointestinal bleeding. Gastrointest Endosc 27: 73–79
[49] Newton M, Burnham WR, Kamm MA (2000) Morbidity, mortality and risk factors for esophagitis in hospital inpatients. J Clin Gastroenterol 30: 264–269
[50] Butt JH (1989) Gastroesophageal reflux disease: recognizing and managing major complications. Postgrad Med 85: 105–109
[51] Kieser C (1967) Untersuchungen über die tödlichen Komplikationen von Hiatushernien. Gastroenterologia 107: 328–336
[52] Rantanen TK, Salo JA (1999) Gastroesophageal reflux disease as a cause of death: analysis of fatal cases under conservative treatment. Scand J Gastroenterol 34: 229–233
[53] Panos MZ, Walt RP, Stevenson C, Langman MJS (1995) Rising death from non-malignant disease of the oesophagus (NMOD) in England and Wales. Gut 36: 488–491
[54] Nilsson M, Johnsen R, Ye W, Hveem K, LaGERgren J (2003) Onbesity and estrogen as risk factors for gastroesophageal symptoms. JAMA 290: 66–72
[55] Watanabe Y, Fujiwara Y, Shiba M et al (2003) Cigarette smoking and alcohol consumption associated with gastro-oesophageal reflux disease in Japanese men. Scand J Gastroenterol 38: 807–811

[56] El-Serag HB, Johanson JF (2002) Risk factors for the severity of erosive esophagitis in *Helicobacter pylori*-negative patients with gastroesophageal reflux disease. Scand J Gastroenterol 37: 899–904

[57] Avidan B, Sonnenberg A, Schnell TG, Sontag SJ (2001) Risk factors for erosive reflux esophagitis: a case-control study. Am J Gastroenterol 96: 41–46

[58] El-Serag HB, Sonnenberg A (1997) Associations between different forms of gastro-oesophageal reflux disease. Gut 41: 594–599

[59] Tytgat GN, Blum AL, Verlinden M (1995) Prognostic factors for relapse andd maintenance treatment with cisapride in gastro-oesophageal reflux disease. Aliment Pharmacol Ther 9: 271–280

[60] Carlsson R, Galmiche JP, Dent J, Lundell L, Frison L (1997) Prognostic factors influencing relapse of oesophagitis during maintenance therapy with antisecretory drugs: a meta-analysis of long-term omeprazole trials. Aliment Pharmacol the 11: 473–482

[61] Chang CS, Yang SS, Ko CW, Yeh HZ, Chen GH (2003) Predictive factors of the long-term outcome in reflux esophagitis in a low-prevalence gastroesopahgeal reflux disease region. Scand J Gastroenterol 38: 1131–1135

[62] Labenz J, Jaspersen D, Kulig M et al (2004) Risk factors for erosive esophagitis: a multivariate analysis based on the Pro-GERD initiative. Am J Gastroenterol 99: 1652–1656

Chapter 2

THE PATHOPHYSIOLOGY OF GERD

R. Dickman and R. Fass

The Neuro-Enteric Clinical Research Group, Section of Gastroenterology, Department of Medicine, Southern Arizona VA Health Care System and University of Arizona School of Medicine, Tucson, AZ, USA

Abbreviations used: GERD – gastroesophageal reflux disease; LES – lower esophageal sphincter; NERD – non-erosive reflux disease; TLESR – transient lower esophageal sphincter relaxation.

Introduction

The understanding of the pathophysiology of gastroesophageal reflux disease (GERD) has evolved in the last decade primarily by recognizing the multitude of factors that contribute to the emergence of the disorder (*Fig. 1*). These factors may overlap in some patients and differ in others. GERD is primarily considered a motility disorder, because dysfunction of the anti-reflux barrier is still considered as a prerequisite for the development of the disease. However, recent investigation into symptom generation in GERD disclosed the important role of altered esophageal sensation. Recent studies have demonstrated that peripheral and central factors are pivotal for the emergence of symptoms after gastroesophageal reflux had occurred; supporting the view that GERD is a sensory-motor disorder rather than motor disorder alone.

The primary pathophysiologic event in GERD is the movement of acid, pepsin, and other injurious substances from the stomach into the esophagus. This event also occurs as part of normal physiology, but results in GERD when symptoms or tissue damage occurs. Esophageal mucosal injury in GERD results when mucosal defensive factors are overwhelmed by refluxate, occurring secondary to compromised anti-reflux barrier, decreased effective esophageal acid clearance, abnormal mucosal defensive factors and so on.

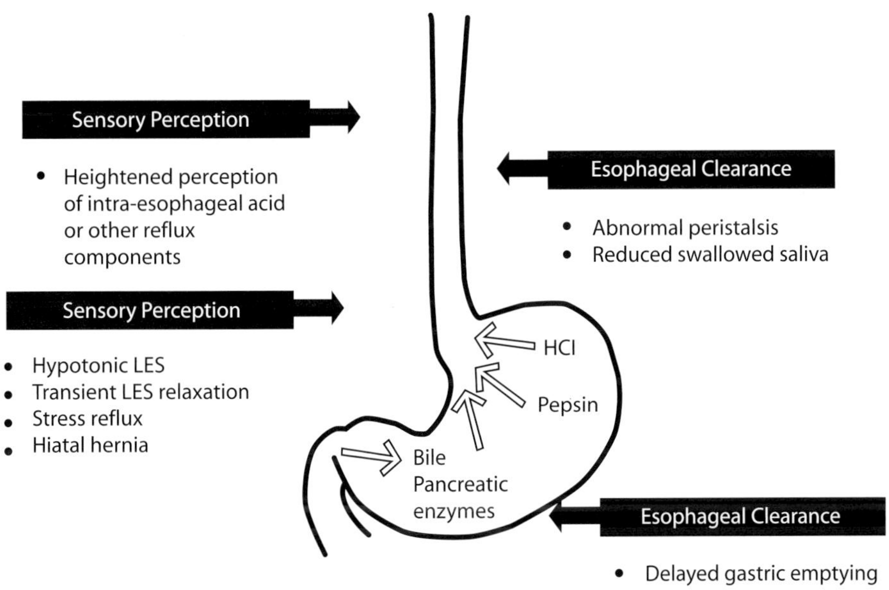

Fig. 1. A summary of the diverse etiological factors that result in gastroesophageal reflux and symptoms

Anti-reflux barrier

Failure of the anti-reflux barrier is considered the most important factor in the pathogenesis of GERD. It is presently accepted that the two major elements that compose the anti-reflux barrier are the lower esophageal sphincter (LES) and the crural diaphragm. The LES is a thickened ring of tonically contracted circular smooth muscle that generates a 2–4 cm high pressure zone at the gastroesophageal junction and serves as a mechanical barrier between the stomach and the esophagus. The right crus of the diaphragm encircles the LES by the phreno-esophageal ligament and thus provides additional mechanical support. Both structures generate a high-pressure zone in the distal esophagus (15 mmHg to 30 mmHg above gastric pressure). Failure of one or both of these complimentary structures may lead to incompetence of the anti-reflux barrier resulting in pathological gastroesophageal reflux. The variations in LES pressure are usually coupled with esophageal and gastric contractions, while the pressure contributed by the crural diaphragm is in response to physical activity such as inspiration, coughing, Valsalva maneuver, abdominal compression and others. Myogenic and neurogenic mechanisms control the LES resting tone during both feeding and resting state.

LES resting pressure exhibits a significant diurnal variation. During daytime, LES pressure is lower in comparison to the postprandial and nighttime periods [1]. Additionally, various substances such as hormones, drugs and foods influence the LES basal pressure. Substances that increase LES pressure include gastrin, motilin, substance P, alfa-adrenergic antagonists, beta-adrenergic agonists, protein, histamine, metoclopramide and prostaglandin F2a. Substances that decrease LES basal pressure include secretin, cholecystokinin, glucagon, somatostatin, progesterone, alfa-adrenergic agonists, beta-adrenergic antagonists, fat, chocolate, ethanol, peppermint, theophylline, prostaglandin E2, serotonin, morphine, calcium channel blockers, diazepam and barbiturates [2].

Originally, gastroesophageal reflux was thought to occur across a hypotensive LES. However, the LES basal pressure is variable in patients with GERD, and in most cases within the normal limits [3]. However, patients with erosive esophagitis or Barrett's esophagus demonstrate a significantly lower mean LES basal pressure than patients with non-erosive reflux disease (NERD) [3]. In patients with NERD, the mean LES basal pressure is similar to normal controls. For most patients with GERD, the predominant mechanism of gastroesophageal reflux is transient lower esophageal sphincter relaxation (TLESR) of an otherwise normal LES (normal resting pressure) [4]. Physiologic reflux occurs mainly in an upright posture, postprandially [5]. This reflux is facilitated by episodes of inappropriate transient LES relaxation. TLESRs are spontaneous, abnormally prolonged episodes of LES relaxation, which are not preceded by a swallow or peristalsis [4], [6]. Transient LES relaxation is a neural reflex, mediated through the brainstem, and the vagus nerve is its efferent pathway [7]. Gastric distension and pharyngeal stimulation have been demonstrated to elicit such relaxation [8]. This is considered the only mechanism of reflux in people without GERD and in most of those with GERD. GERD patients demonstrate prolonged postprandial receptive relaxation of the fundus leading to a delayed emptying of the proximal stomach [9], [10].

TLESRs have been established as the primary mechanism for gastroesophageal reflux in normal subjects and patients with GERD [11]–[13]. They also serve as the underlying mechanism for belching, which may suggest some relationship with gastroesophageal reflux. Although, previous studies suggested that patients with GERD experience more TLESRs than healthy controls, recent trials found no increased rate of TLESRs in patients with GERD. However, TLESR was more likely to be associated with acid reflux in patients with GERD (65%) when compared to healthy controls (35%) [11], [14]. Additionally, it appears that TLESR is the main underlying mechanism responsible for gastroesophageal reflux events in patients with NERD. In NERD patients, who represent the majority of patients seen for reflux symptoms, TLESR rather than hypotensive LES accounts for most gastroesophageal reflux events. In the presence of hiatal hernia, which affects up to 70% of the erosive esophagitis patients, other mechanisms than TLESR play an important role, such as abnormally low LES basal pressure and stress reflux. In NERD patients on the other hand hiatal hernia is relatively uncommon (~30%).

Reduced LES basal pressure and stress reflux are other mechanisms that affect primarily patients with erosive esophagitis. Dent et al [5] evaluated GERD patients with different phenotypic presentations of GERD and found that with increasing severity of esophagitis, absent basal LES pressure became a more common mechanism, accounting for 23% of gastroesophageal reflux episodes in patients with severe erosive esophagitis. Stress reflux is another mechanism responsible for gastroesophageal reflux in which increase in intra-abdominal pressure overwhelms the counter response of the LES and the crural diaphragm resulting in gastroesophageal reflux.

Hiatal hernia is an important factor in the pathogenesis of GERD as it interferes directly with the antireflux barrier. The role of hiatal hernia in aggravating gastroesophageal reflux is discussed in another chapter.

Esophageal dysmotility

Gastroesophageal reflux is the result of transient LES relaxation, stress reflux or an abnormally low LES pressure (free reflux or the common cavity phenomenon) (see *Fig. 2*).

The goal of normal esophageal peristalsis and gravity is to eliminate nearly all of the refluxate from the esophagus, allowing the residual acid to be neutralized effectively by bicarbonate-rich saliva [15]. Impairment of acid clearance can be secondary to either peristaltic dysfunction and/or re-reflux (the to-and-fro movement of the refluxate), which are seen in association with hiatal hernia.

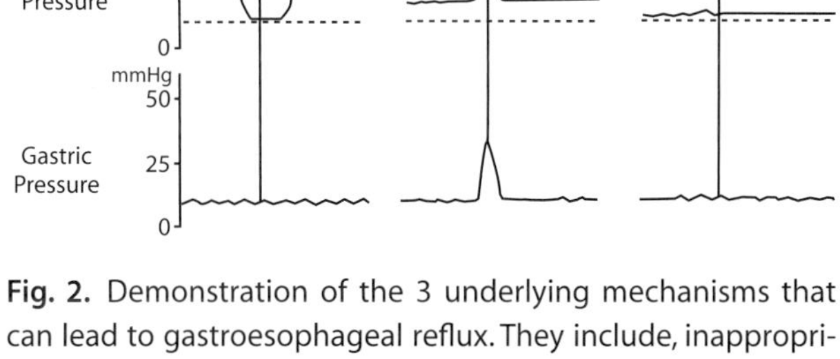

Fig. 2. Demonstration of the 3 underlying mechanisms that can lead to gastroesophageal reflux. They include, inappropriate transient lower esophageal sphincter relaxation, reduced lower esophageal sphincter basal pressure leading to "free reflux" and stress reflux (with permission from [13])

Peristaltic dysfunction of the esophageal body in GERD is well documented [16], [17]. Esophageal peristaltic dysfunction is increasingly observed with more severe grades of erosive esophagitis and particularly in patients with Barrett's esophagus [3]. There has been a long-standing argument as to whether the observed esophageal dysmotility precedes or is caused by GERD [16]. However, studies have demonstrated that elimination of acid reflux and even esophageal mucosal healing do not result in normalization of esophageal body motility.

Impairment of primary esophageal peristalsis has been suggested as the predominant underlying motility abnormality that leads to prolonged acid clearance [13], [18], [19]. Non-transmitted peristalsis, failed contractions and simultaneous esophageal contractions are ineffective in clearing the volume of the refluxate. Ineffective esophageal motility, defined by the presence of abnormally low amplitude (< 30 mmHg) contractions in the distal esophagus (30% or more of wet swallows) were also found to be associated with prolonged esophageal acid clearance in both the upright and recumbent positions. In more advance cases of GERD, absence of distal esophageal peristalsis can be observed. Patients with scleroderma or mixed connective tissue disorder demonstrate involvement of the smooth muscle portion of the esophagus. Deposition of collagen which replaces muscle tissue results in significant reduction of distal esophageal amplitude contractions and in severe cases complete elimination of distal esophageal peristalsis. Additionally, damage to the LES results in reduced mean LES basal pressure and in advanced cases disappearance of the LES high pressure zone. As a result, both disorders may be associated with severe forms of GERD (peptic stricture, Barrett's esophagus and even adenocarcinoma of the esophagus).

Another motor abnormality of GERD patients refers to failed secondary peristalsis of the esophageal body. After a reflux episode, secondary peristalsis is the first motor event involved in acid clearance [14]. In comparison with normal controls, GERD patients exhibit a lower occurrence of secondary peristalsis (18% and 40% of the events, respectively) [20]–[22]. Interestingly, this abnormality does not correlate with defective primary peristalsis [14].

Although previously suggested, salivary gland dysfunction was not found to be an important factor in

GERD patients [23]. However, patients with reduced salivary production like those with Sjörgen's syndrome or active smokers are at higher risk for increased esophageal acid exposure and esophageal mucosal injury. Lastly, some investigators have suggested that the epidermal growth factor content in the saliva of GERD patients may be altered, resulting in reduced rate of esophageal mucosal healing [24].

The refluxate

There is evidence to suggest that both acid and duodenal contents, mainly pepsin (an acid activated proteolytic enzyme) and bile salts (conjugated and deconjugated), are noxious to the esophageal mucosa [25], [26]. However, typically gastric content is acidic, making acid and pepsin the main noxious agents in the refluxate. Original studies reported that deconjugated bile salts and pancreatic enzymes are rendered ineffective at acidic pH (inactivated) [27], [28]. Furthermore, bile salts do not reach cytotoxic concentrations in the refluxate and typical signs of bile acid injury are usually missing [29]. These include intracellular bile salt deposits and membrane microvesiculation [30]–[32]. Moreover, the effectiveness of PPIs in healing esophageal erosions serves as another evidence to support the role of acid as the main mechanism that underlies esophageal mucosal injury.

Presently, we are unable to measure bile reflux directly. Bilirubin, which can be detected in the refluxate by Bilitec 2000 (a spectrophotometric system that measures bilirubin concentration within the esophagus, independent of pH), has been used as a surrogate marker for bile reflux. However, experts elected to use the term duodenogastroesophageal reflux (DGER) instead of bile reflux to denote that Bilitec measures duodenal contents, which may include bile, pancreatic enzymes and pancreatic juice. However, duodenogastroesophageal reflux alone does not appear to cause significant damage to the esophageal mucosa but may act synergistically with acid reflux to produce erosive esophagitis. By using 24-hour esophageal pH monitoring and Bilitec 2000 in patients with GERD, Vaezi et al [33] demonstrated that symptoms or esophageal lesions were relatively uncommon even after partial gastrectomy, where bile reflux is an important component of the refluxate. Furthermore, according to this study, duodenogastroesophageal reflux was usually documented in the esophagus in conjunction with acid reflux. Studies have also demonstrated that simultaneous exposure to acid and duodenogastroesophageal reflux is higher in the more severe presentations of GERD. Barrett's esophagus, for example, exhibited the highest esophageal acid and duodenogastroesophageal reflux exposure [33]–[35]. However, in patients with either long- or short-segment Barrett's esophagus as compared to controls there was no association between history of gastric surgery and the presence of Barrett's esophagus, suggesting that duodenogastroesophageal reflux without acid may not be sufficient to cause Barrett's esophagus [13], [18].

Whilst the concept has been entertained in the past, there is no strong evidence to suggest that hypersecretion of gastric acid plays an important role in the pathogenesis of GERD [11], [12], [14].

Helicobacter pylori

See the chapter *Helicobacter pylori* and GERD.

Gastric dysmotility

Approximately 20%–40% of the patients with GERD may have delayed gastric emptying, but there is no direct correlation between the degree of the delay and the severity of GERD [11], [12], [15]. However, slow proximal gastric emptying in patients with GERD correlated with increase in 24-hour esophageal pH monitoring values, number of reflux episodes per hour and postprandial acid exposure.

Esophageal mucosal defense mechanisms

The esophageal defensive system includes several basic mechanisms. The anti-reflux barrier (LES and the crural diaphragm) and the clearance mechanism that limit the frequency and volume of the refluxate as well as the duration [36]. The third defense mechanism is the esophageal mucosal resistance, which prevents injury by acid, pepsin and other components of the refluxate. Tissue resistance is constituted of structures grouped in three areas: pre-epithelial, epithelial and post-epithelial [36]. The pre-epithelial defense is relatively limited. The esophagus has no well-defined mucus layer and its lumen to surface pH gradient creates only a modest reduction in luminal acidity [36]. The epithelial area consists of cell membranes and intercellular junctional complexes, which block acid and pepsin diffusion, intercellular buffers such as bicarbonate that neutralizes acid and cell membrane ion transporters for cytosolic acid extrusion [36] (*Fig. 3*).

Exchangers at the baso-lateral membrane can restore intracellular pH by exchanging intracellular H^+ for extracellular Na^+ or intracellular Cl^- for extracellular HCO_3^-. The post-epithelial area consists of an adequate mucosal blood flow to remove noxious elements and supply nutrients for maintenance and repair mechanisms [36].

Studies have also shown that GERD patients with or without esophagitis have dilated intracellular spaces (DIS), as documented by transmission electron microscopy, which may lead to increase in esophageal permeability to hydrogen ions [37]. Dilated intercellular spaces and reduced mucin production improve after anti-secretory therapy, suggesting that these abnormalities are caused by gastroesophageal reflux [37], [38].

Mechanisms for heartburn

The mechanisms by which patients with GERD develop symptoms remain incompletely understood. It is postulated that sensitization of esophageal chemoreceptors either directly by exposure to acid reflux or indirectly through release of inflammatory mediators

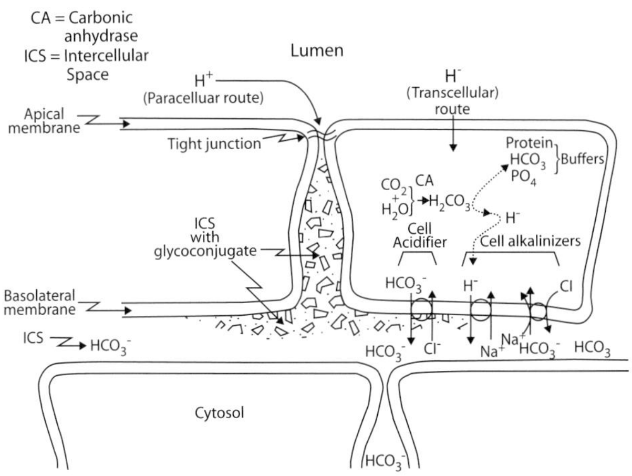

Fig. 3. Epithelial defenses against acid injury that include, cell membrane, intercellular junctional complexes, intracellular buffering and HCO_3 and H^+ extrusion process (with permission from [67])

is responsible for symptom generation in GERD [39]. Reducing acid exposure in patients with GERD appears to normalize the sensitivity to acid [40]. However, the emergence of symptoms in patients with a normal esophageal mucosa and thus without obvious inflammation remains perplexing, particularly among patients with functional heartburn where little or no reflux actually occurs.

Both animal models and human studies have demonstrated dilation of intercellular spaces during or following esophageal mucosal acid exposure [41], [42]. These mucosal findings were evident regardless of the presence or absence of esophageal inflammation [42], [43]. It is assumed that these morphological changes result in an increase in paracellular permeability, allowing acid to reach sensory nerve endings located within the intercellular spaces [44]. However, this altered permeability does not explain symptoms in GERD, specifically in NERD and in functional heartburn as most acid reflux events (> 95%) that occur in these patients are never perceived and symptoms occur even in the absence of acid reflux, suggesting the importance of other factors in modulating esophageal acid perception.

Heartburn symptoms may represent activation of a common pathway in response to different intra-esophageal stimuli. Hypersensitivity to physiological amounts of acid appears to be the underlying mechanism for heartburn in the hypersensitive esophagus subgroup (functional heartburn). This hypersensitivity to acid may stem from peripheral sensitization of esophageal afferents, leading to heightened responses to luminal stimuli or altered modulation of afferent neural function at the level of the spinal dorsal root or the central nervous system [45]. What leads to the development of such hypersensitivity remains an area of controversy. In healthy subjects, Sarkar et al have recently demonstrated that infusion of 0.1 N hydrochloric acid into the distal esophagus for 30 minutes increased the subsequent sensory responses to electrical stimulation in the non-exposed proximal esophagus [46]. In comparison, patients with non-cardiac chest pain already had lower resting esophageal pain thresholds in the proximal esophagus, which fell further and for a longer duration than in healthy subjects after acidification of the distal esophagus. These patients also demonstrated a decrease in pain thresholds in the anterior chest wall. Therefore, this study showed the development of secondary allodynia (visceral hypersensitivity to innocuous stimulus in normal tissue that is in proximity to the site of tissue injury) in healthy subjects and non-cardiac chest pain patients. In the latter group this phenomenon is amplified and lasts longer. The resulting visceral and somatic hypersensitivity is likely due to central sensitization. The increased excitability of spinal cord neurons appears to be the result of activation of nociceptive C fibers due to local tissue injury induced by acid infusion into the distal esophagus. If extrapolated clinically, this study suggests that prior injury to the esophageal mucosa may lead to the development of central sensitization and visceral hyperalgesia in a subset of patients long after the local injury has healed.

To date, only a few studies have attempted to assess the cortical processing of esophageal acid exposure sensation in humans. Kern et al [47] evaluated activation of cerebral cortical responses to esophageal mucosal acid exposure using functional magnetic resonance imaging (fMRI). Ten healthy subjects underwent intra-esophageal perfusion of 0.1 N hydrochloric acid over 10 minutes. None of the study subjects reported GERD symptoms during the acid perfusion. Cerebral cortical activity was concentrated in the posterior cingulate, and the parietal and anteromesial frontal lobes. The superior frontal lobe regions activated in this study corresponded to Brodmann's areas 31, the insula, operculum and the anterior cingulate. Further studies are needed to assess cerebral cortical activation in symptomatic GERD patients undergoing esophageal acid perfusion. In addition, it would be of great interest to determine if there are differences in central processing of an intra-esophageal stimulus between GERD patients and those with NERD or functional heartburn.

Patients with GERD do not perceive most acid reflux events. Many patients and healthy subjects demonstrate multiple acid reflux events on pH testing but often report few, if any, heartburn episodes. It has been estimated that no more than 5% of all acid reflux events ($pH < 4$) produce symptoms, either in patients with or without esophageal mucosal injury [48]. This intriguing observation raises the obvious question of what in a specific acid reflux event leads to its conscious perception. It is not clear if a specific acid reflux event is the determining factor in triggering symptoms or rather the actual hydrogen ion concentration (H^+) of the refluxate, the summation of several short reflux events, or an increased number and/or duration of acid reflux events. However, proximal migration of the acid reflux events has been shown repeatedly to be associated with a higher likelihood of symptom perception.

The most common trigger for GERD symptoms is a meal; in particular if the meal is high in fat. However, the mechanism by which fat exacerbates symptoms in patients with GERD remains controversial. Meyer et al found that fat infusion into the duodenum of subjects with GERD significantly shortened latency to onset of heartburn and intensified the perception of acid induced heartburn [49]. The mechanisms by which luminal fat and potentially other nutrients may modulate the perception of esophageal stimuli remains unclear, but may involve cholecystokinin or other gut neurotransmitters, hormones, and enzymes. While many of these peptides may exert a local action leading to symptoms, it is also conceivable that their action may also involve central neural pathways. It is even possible that other substances in the refluxate (pepsin, bile) or volume per se are the direct cause of symptoms.

Several studies have recently speculated that central and peripheral neural mechanisms modulate esopha-

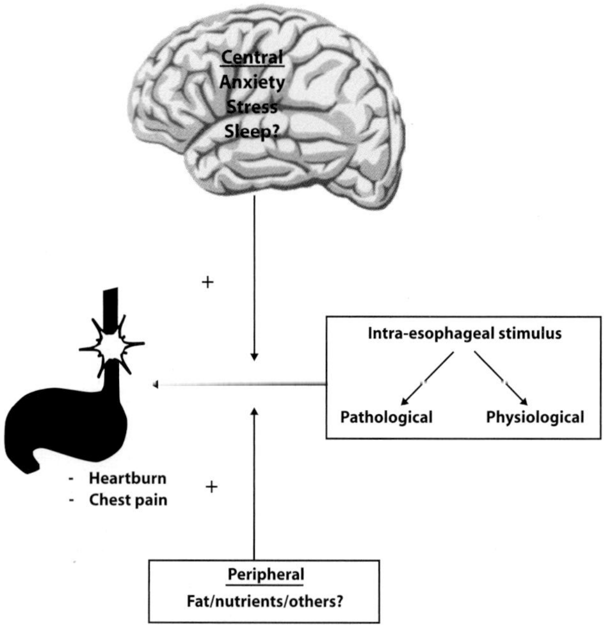

Fig. 4. Proposed conceptual model for esophageal symptom generation. Central and peripheral mechanisms enhance perception of intra-esophageal events (either physiological or pathological), leading to symptom generation [68]

geal perception [50], [51] (*Fig. 4*). Psychological comorbidity (anxiety, stress, depression, etc.) can modulate esophageal perception and cause patients to perceive low intensity esophageal stimuli as being painful [Gut: 27], [52]. These psychological factors seem to be associated with patients paying an excessive attention (hypervigilance) to intra-esophageal events and thus perceiving or interpreting these esophageal events as being painful [53]. Stress has been implicated by 64% of GERD patients as an important cause for symptom exacerbation [54]. However, several studies have failed to demonstrate an increase in acid reflux during stressful stimuli [55]–[57]. Nevertheless, interventions aimed at reducing stress (hypnosis and muscle relaxation) have produced subjective improvement in reflux symptoms ratings [57], [58]. In a study assessing the effect of psychologically induced stress on symptom perception in GERD patients, stress reduced perception thresholds and enhanced the perception of acid during infusion, regardless of the degree of esophageal mucosal injury [59].

A recent study demonstrated that increased basal sympathetic activity and lower vagal activity, as measured by power spectral analysis of heart rate variability, are associated with increased sensitivity to intra-esophageal acid perfusion in patients with non-cardiac chest pain compared with healthy matched controls [60].

These data support the concept of humoral, neural, and psychological factors being associated with an increased susceptibility to symptoms such as heartburn but do not provide at this point a satisfactory mechanistic explanation. However, recent advances in our understanding of the mucosal and esophageal neural response to reflux begin to address this deficiency.

There are mounting data to suggest that the axiom "no acid no heartburn" is obsolete. Non-acid intra-esophageal stimuli may also lead to the development of heartburn. Esophageal balloon distension induces heartburn symptoms in a large subset of normal subjects and reproduces typical heartburn in half of GERD patients [39]. Furthermore, high frequency intra-luminal ultrasonography has demonstrated a close correlation between heartburn episodes and abnormally long durations of longitudinal muscle contractions in the esophagus [61]. These muscle contractions and consequent heartburn episodes can occur in the absence of acid reflux. Thus, both of these studies suggest that mechanical stimuli and motor events may be perceived as heartburn by some patients, even in the absence of actual acid reflux.

Bile reflux has been suggested as a possible cause for heartburn symptoms in patients with NERD, but no study to date has specifically evaluated the role of bile acid in symptom generation in this group. Assessment of bilirubin pigment spectrophotometrically, a proxy indicator for bile reflux, revealed a close correlation between a combination of both acid and duodenogastroesophageal reflux and severity of GERD, as determined by the presence of esophageal mucosal injury and GERD complications [33]. However, symptoms were not specifically examined in this study. The combined reflux was documented in only 50% of NERD patients compared with 79% in erosive esophagitis and 95% in Barrett's esophagus. Others have shown that the mean fasting gastric bile acid concentration in patients with NERD is not significantly elevated compared with healthy controls [51]. Future studies are needed to further determine if bile acid is a contributing factor for symptoms in patients with GERD.

Recent studies using simultaneous intra-esophageal impedance and pH measurement demonstrated non-acidic gastroesophageal reflux (liquid, gas or mixture of gas and liquid) that was similarly frequent in patients with GERD and normal controls [62]. However, more acidic reflux occurred in symptomatic patients with GERD. Vela et al [63] with a similar technique, observed that during treatment of GERD patients with a PPI, postprandial reflux became predominately non-acidic. Although less than acidic reflux, non-acidic reflux was also associated with classic GERD symptoms. It has yet to be determined if the content or volume is responsible for GERD symptoms in the studied subjects. Additionally, as with acid reflux, most of the non-acidic reflux events are not perceived.

Genetic factors

Familial aggregation for GERD, in general, was not demonstrated, but investigators were able to document a significant rate of familial occurrence for both Barrett's esophagus and esophageal adenocarcinoma [64], [65]. Recently, a large twin study has shown an increased concordance for GERD in monozygotic pairs, compared with dizygotic pairs, suggesting that genetic factors accounted for 31% of the liability to

GERD in the U.S. population [11], [66]. Furthermore, a genetic linkage study in pediatric GERD population mapped a locus in chromosome 13q14. Although the importance of this locus was refuted by a subsequent study, it did not completely exclude the possibility of genetic factors in GERD.

References

[1] Storr M, Meining A, Allescher HD (2000) Pathophysiology and pharmacological treatment of gastroesophageal reflux disease. Dig Dis 18: 93–102

[2] Kahrilas PJ (1998) Gastroesophageal reflux disease and its complications. In: Sleisenger and Fordtran's gastrointestinal and liver disease. Pathophysiology/diagnosis/management (Feldman M, Scharschmidt BF, Sleisenger MH, eds), 6th ed. Philadelphia, PA: W. B. Saunders, p 498–516

[3] Kahrilas PJ, Dodds WJ, Hogan WJ, Kern M, Arndorfer RC, Reece A (1986) Esophageal peristaltic dysfunction in peptic esophagitis. Gastroenterology 91: 897–904

[4] Dent J (1997) Patterns of lower esophageal sphincter function associated with gastroesophageal reflux. Am J Med 103: 29S–32S

[5] Dent J, Holloway RH, Toouli J, Dodds WJ (1988) Mechanisms of lower oesophageal sphincter incompetence in patients with symptomatic gastroesophageal reflux. Gut 29: 1020–1028

[6] Holloway RH, Dent J (1990) Pathophysiology of gastroesophageal reflux. Lower esophageal sphincter dysfunction in gastroesophageal reflux disease. Gastroenterol Clin North Am 19: 517–535

[7] Mittal RK, Balaban DH (1997) The esophagogastric junction. N Engl J Med 336: 924–932

[8] Mittal RK, Holloway RH, Penagini R, Blackshaw LA, Dent J (1995) Transient lower esophageal sphincter relaxation. Gastroenterology 109: 601–610

[9] Penagini R, Hebbard G, Horowitz M, Dent J, Bermingham H, Jones K, Holloway RH (1998) Motor function of the proximal stomach and visceral perception in gastro-oesophageal reflux disease. Gut 42: 251–257

[10] Stacher G, Lenglinger J, Bergmann H, Schneider C, Hoffmann M, Wolf G, Stacher-Janotta G (2000) Gastric emptying: a contributory factor in gastro-oesophageal reflux activity? Gut 47: 661–666

[11] Sonnenberg A (2004) Epidemiologic aspects in the occurrence and natural history of gastroesophageal reflux disease. In: Hot topics: GERD/dyspepsia (Fass R, ed). Philadelphia, PA: Hanley & Belfus, p 1–22

[12] Cameron AJ (1999) Barrett's esophagus: prevalence and size of hiatal hernia. Am J Gastroenterol 94: 2054–2059

[13] Dodds WJ, Dent J, Hogan WJ, Helm JF, Hauser R, Patel GK, Egide MS (1982) Mechanisms of gastroesophageal reflux in patients with reflux esophagitis. N Engl J Med 307: 1547–1552

[14] Penagini R, Carmagnola S, Cantu P (2002) Review article: gastro-oesophageal reflux disease – pathophysiological issues of clinical relevance. Aliment Pharmacol Ther 16: 65–71

[15] Helm JF, Dodds WJ, Pelc LR, Palmer DW, Hogan WJ, Teeter BC (1984) Effect of esophageal emptying and saliva on clearance of acid form the esophagus. N Engl J Med 310: 284–288

[16] Singh P, Adamopoulos A, Taylor RH, Colin-Jones DG (1992) Oesophageal motor function before and after healing of oesophagitis. Gut 33: 1590–1596

[17] Lin S, Ke M, Xu J, Kahrilas PJ (1994) Impaired esophageal emptying in reflux disease. Am J Gastroenterol 89: 1003–1006

[18] Locke GR, 3rd, Talley NJ, Fett SL, Zinsmeister AR, Melton LJ, 3rd (1997) Prevalence and clinical spectrum of gastroesophageal reflux: a population-based study in Olmstead County, Minnesota. Gastroenterology 112: 1448–1456

[19] Wong WM, Lam SK, Hui WM, Lai KC, Chan CK, Hui WH, Xia HH, Hu CK, Yuen MF, Chan AO, Wong BC (2002) Long-term prospective follow-up of endoscopic oesophagitis in Southern Chinese – prevalence and spectrum of the disease. Aliment Pharmacol Ther 16: 2037–2042

[20] Penagini R, Schoeman M, Tippett M, Holloway R (1996) Motor event underlying gastroesophageal reflux in ambulant patients with reflux oesophagitis. Neurogastroenterol Motil 8: 131–141

[21] Dodds WJPJK, Dent J, Hogan WJ, Kern MK, Arndorfer RC (1990) Analysis of spontaneous gastroesophageal reflux and esophageal acid clearance in patients with reflux esophagitis. J Gastrointest Motil 2: 79–89

[22] Schoeman M, Tippett M, Akkerman L, Dent J, Holloway R (1995) Mechanism of gastroesophageal reflux in ambulant healthy human subjects. Gastroenterology 108: 83–91

[23] Sonnenberg A (1982) Salivary secretion in reflux esophagitis. Gastroenterology 83: 889–895

[24] Sarosiek J, Scheurich CJ, Marcinkiewicz M, McCallum RW (1996) Enhancement of salivary esophagoprotection: rationale for a physiological approach to gastroesophageal reflux disease. Gastroenterology 110: 675–681

[25] Vaezi MF, Singh S, Richter JE (1995) Role of acid and duodenogastric reflux in esophageal mucosal injury: a review of animal and human studies. Gastroenterology 108
[26] Tobey NA, Hosseini S, Caymaz-Bor C, Wyatt HR, Orlando GS, Orlando RC (2001) The role of pepsin in acid injury to esophageal epithelium. Am J Gastroenterol 96: 3062–3070
[27] Lillemoe KD, Johnson LF, Harmon JW (1983) Alkaline esophagitis: a comparison of the ability of components of gastroduodenal contents to injure the rabbit esophagus. Gastroenterology 85: 621–628
[28] Gotley DC, Morgan AP, Ball D, Owen RW, Cooper MJ (1991) Composition of gastro-oesophageal refluxate. Gut 32: 1093–1099
[29] Salo JA, Lehto VP, Kivilaakso E (1983) Morphological alterations in experimental esophagitis. Light microscopic and scanning and transmission electron microscopic study. Dig Dis Sci 28: 440–448
[30] Bateson MC, Hopwood D, Milne G, Bouchier IA (1981) Oesophageal epithelial ultrastructure after incubation with gastrointestinal fluids and their components. J Pathol 133: 33–51
[31] Salo J, Kivilaakso E (1982) Role of luminal H^+ in the pathogenesis of experimental esophagitis. Surgery 92: 61–68
[32] Schweitzer EJ, Bass BL, Batzri S, Harmon JW (1986) Bile acid accumulation by rabbit esophageal mucosa. Dig Dis Sci 31: 1105–1113
[33] Vaezi MF, Richter JE (1996) Role of acid and duodenogastroesophageal reflux in gastroesophageal reflux disease. Gastroenterology 111: 1192–1199
[34] Kauer WK, Peters JH, DeMeester TR, Ireland AP, Bremner CG, Hagen JA (1995) Mixed reflux of gastric and duodenal juices is more harmful to the esophagus than gastric juice alone. The need for surgical therapy re-emphasized. Ann Surg 222: 525–531; discussion 531–533
[35] Marshall RE, Anggiansah A, Owen WA, Owen WJ (1998) The temporal relationship between oesophageal bile reflux and pH in gastro-oesophageal reflux disease. Eur J Gastroenterol Hepatol 10: 385–392
[36] Orlando RC (2003) Pathogenesis of gastroesophageal reflux disease. Am J Med Sci 326: 274–278
[37] Carlsson R, Fandriks L, Jonsson C, Lundell L, Orlando RC (1999) Is the esophageal squamous epithelial barrier function impaired in patients with gastroesophageal reflux disease? Scand J Gastroenterol 34: 454–458
[38] Namiot Z, Sarosiek J, Marcinkiewicz M, Edmunds MC, McCallum RW (1994) Declined human esophageal mucin secretion in patients with severe reflux esophagitis. Dig Dis Sci 39: 2523–2529
[39] Fass R, Naliboff B, Higa L, Johnson C, Kodner A, Munakata J, Ngo J, Mayer EA (1998) Differential effect of long-term esophageal acid exposure on mechanosensitivity and chemosensitivity in humans. Gastroenterology 115: 1363–1373
[40] Marrero JM, de Caestecker JS, Maxwell JD (1994) Effect of famotidine on oesophageal sensitivity in gastro-oesophageal reflux disease. Gut 35: 447–450
[41] Ferreira KT, Hill BS (1982) The effect of low external pH on properties of the paracellular pathway and junctional structure in isolated frog skin. J Physiol 332: 59–67
[42] Hopwood D, Milne G, Logan KR (1979) Electron microscopic changes in human oesophageal epithelium in oesophagitis. J Pathol 129: 161–167
[43] Tobey NA, Carson JL, Alkiek RA, Orlando RC (1996) Dilated intercellular spaces: a morphological feature of acid reflux – damaged human esophageal epithelium. Gastroenterology 111: 1200–1205
[44] Orlando RC (1999) Pathophysiology of gastroesophageal reflux disease. In: Esophagus (Castell DO, Richter JE, eds.), 3rd ed. Philadelphia: Lippincot Williams & Wilkins, p 409–419
[45] Hollerbach S, Bulat R, May A, Kamath MV, Upton AR, Fallen EL, Tougas G (2000) Abnormal cerebral processing of oesophageal stimuli in patients with noncardiac chest pain (NCCP). Neurogastroenterol Motil 12: 555–565
[46] Sarkar S, Aziz Q, Woolf CJ, Hobson AR, Thompson DG (2000) Contribution of central sensitisation to the development of non-cardiac chest pain. Lancet 356: 1154–1159
[47] Kern MK, Birn RM, Jaradeh S, Jesmanowicz A, Cox RW, Hyde JS, Shaker R (1998) Identification and characterization of cerebral cortical response to esophageal mucosal acid exposure and distention. Gastroenterology 115: 1353–1362
[48] Martinez SD, Malagon I, Garewal HS, Fass R (2001) Abstract: non-erosive reflux disease (NERD) – is it really just a mild form of gastroesophageal reflux disease (GERD)? Gastroenterology 120: A-424, #2163
[49] Meyer JH, Lembo A, Elashoff JD, Fass R, Mayer EA (2001) Duodenal fat intensifies the perception of heartburn. Gut 49: 624–628
[50] Fass R (2001) Focused clinical review: nonerosive reflux disease. Medscape Gastroenterol 3: 1–13
[51] Fass R, Fennerty MB, Vakil N (2001) Nonerosive reflux disease – current concepts and dilemmas. Am J Gastroenterol 96: 303–314
[52] Trimble KC, Pryde A, Heading RC (1995) Lowered oesophageal sensory thresholds in patients with symptomatic but not excess gastro-oesophageal reflux: evidence for a spectrum of visceral sensitivity in GORD. Gut 37: 7–12

[53] Mayer EA (2000) Spinal and supraspinal modulation of visceral sensation. Gut 47: iv69–iv72; discussion iv76
[54] The Gallup Organization (1988) A Gallup survey on heartburn across America. Princeton, NJ
[55] Cook IJ, Collins SM (1986) Does acute emotional stress influence frequency or duration of gastroesophageal reflux in human subjects? Gastroenterology 90: 1380
[56] Bradley LA, Richter JE, Pulliam TJ, Haile JM, Scarinci IC, Schan CA, Dalton CB, Salley AN (1993) The relationship between stress and symptoms of gastroesophageal reflux: the influence of psychological factors. Am J Gastroenterol 88: 11–19
[57] McDonald-Haile J, Bradley LA, Bailey MA, Schan CA, Richter JE (1994) Relaxation training reduces symptom reports and acid exposure in patients with gastroesophageal reflux disease. Gastroenterology 107: 61–69
[58] Richter JE, Bradley LA (1995) Psychophysiological interactions in esophageal diseases. Semin Gastrointest Dis 7: 169–184
[59] Fass R, Malagon I, Naliboff B, Pulliam G, Peleg N, Mayer EA (2000) Abstract: effect of psychologically induced stress on symptom perception & autonomic nervous system response of patients (PTS.) with erosive esophagitis (EE) and non-erosive reflux disease (NERD). Gastroenterology 118: A637, #3250
[60] Tougas G, Spaziani R, Hollerbach S, Djuric V, Pang C, Upton AR, Fallen EL, Kamath MV (2001) Cardiac autonomic function and oesophageal acid sensitivity in patients with non-cardiac chest pain. Gut 49: 706–712
[61] Pehlivanov ND, Liu J, Mittal R (1999) Abstract: sustained esophageal contraction: a motor correlate of heartburn symptom. Gastroenterology 118: A1062, #G4613
[62] Sifrim D, Holloway R, Silney J, Xin Z, Tack J, Lerut A, Janssens J (2001) Acid, nonacid, and gas reflux in patients with gastroesophageal reflux disease during ambulatory 24-hour pH-impedance recordings. Gastroenterology 120: 1588–1598
[63] Vela MF, Camacho-Lobato L, Srinivasan R, Tutuian R, Katz PO, Castell DO (2001) Simultaneous intraesophageal impedance and pH measurement of acid and nonacid gastroesophageal reflux: effect of omeprazole. Gastroenterology 120: 1599–1606
[64] Quigley EM (2003) New developments in the pathophysiology of gastro-oesophageal reflux disease (GERD): implications for patient management. Aliment Pharmacol Ther 17: 43–51
[65] Romero Y, Cameron AJ, Locke GR, 3rd, Schaid DJ, Slezak JM, Branch CD, Melton LJ, 3rd (1997) Familial aggregation of gastroesophageal reflux in patients with Barrett's esophagitis and esophageal adenocarcinoma. Gastroenterology 113: 1449–1456
[66] Cameron AJ, Lagergren J, Henriksson C, Nyren O, Locke GR, 3rd, Pedersen NL (2002) Gastroesophageal reflux disease in monozygotic and dizygotic twins. Gastroenterology 122: 55–59
[67] Orlando RC (1985) Esophageal epithelial resistance. In: Gastroesophageal reflux disease: pathogenesis, diagnosis, therapy (Castell DO, Wu WC, Ott DJ, eds.). Mount Kisco, NY: Futura Publishing Company, p 55
[68] Fass R (2004) Sensory testing of the esophagus. J Clin Gastroenterol 38: 628–641

Chapter 3

GASTROESOPHAGEAL REFLUX DISEASE IN THE ELDERLY

M. F. Vaezi and J. Swoger

Department of Gastroenterology and Hepatology, Center for Swallowing and Esophageal Disorders, Cleveland Clinic Foundation, OH, USA

Introduction

The diagnosis and management of gastroesophageal reflux disease (GERD) in the elderly presents numerous unique challenges to the physician. Between 1980 and 1991, the over 65 year old age group was the fastest growing age group in the US [1]. Projections are that this age group will increase by 66%, to 53.3 million, by 2020 [2]. Additionally, the over 85 year old group will represent the fastest growing group, increasing from 3 to 7 million by year 2020 [2]. Elderly patients are responsible for 47% of hospital days, 60% of health care expenditures, and 35% of hospital discharges [1]. Due to multiple factors, GERD is an under-diagnosed and under-treated condition in the elderly. Older people often under-report and tolerate symptoms that younger people would find less tolerable. Older patients also report less severe reflux symptoms than younger patients, and yet they more often present with more severe complications of reflux disease. Extra-esophageal symptoms are more common in this group, which may cause an additional delay in diagnosis [3]. Comorbid conditions, such as chronic obstructive pulmonary disease and coronary artery disease, can be confused with or exacerbated by GERD, and these are more prevalent in an elderly population. Increased medication usage can also serve to complicate diagnosis and treatment. Acid related disease is associated with high morbidity and mortality in the elderly, and can have a significant effect on an individual's quality of life and health well being. This chapter will review the epidemiology of reflux disease in the elderly, examine age-related changes in the GI tract that may influence the pathogenesis of reflux disease, discuss patient presentation and diagnostic strategy, and explore treatment options for this chronic disease in an elderly population.

Epidemiology

Gastroesophageal reflux disease is defined as an increased frequency or duration of exposure of the distal esophagus to gastric contents. GERD is a chronic disease, that rarely resolves spontaneously, and it is associated with frequent relapses. Several studies have investigated the prevalence of GERD, though few have specifically targeted the elderly. In the 1970's, Locke et al studied the prevalence of reflux symptoms in the general population using a group of hospital workers in Olmsted County. This study found that 7% of subjects had daily symptoms of heartburn and 14% had weekly symptoms [4]. A 1994 Gallup study reported a similar 19% prevalence of weekly GERD among 1000 randomly selected persons, and 44% of subjects had monthly symptoms [5]. In Finland, a study of 1700 patients found daily, weekly, and monthly heartburn in 5%, 15%, and 21% of subjects, and acid regurgitation in 9%, 15%, and 29% [6].

The prevalence of hiatal hernia and esophageal dysfunction increases with age, and since reflux disease is associated with each of these findings, one might expect an increased prevalence of GERD in the elderly (Table 1) [7]. However, the Olmsted study found the classic symptoms of heartburn and acid regurgitation to be present in 20% of patients over 65 at least once/week, and 59% at least once/month, similar rates as those found in studies of younger subjects (18–35% with weekly symptoms) [4]. In the 65–74 year old group, 35% of men and 40% of women reported experiencing heartburn, with 17% and 20% respectively having symptoms at least weekly. The prevalence of heartburn, but not of acid regurgitation, was inversely associated with increasing age in this study. A study of primary care practices in Oklahoma found 14% of the 313 patients older than 62 years old had heartburn once a week [8]. In the subset of subjects with pH data, there was a 20% prevalence of reflux, but only 55% of those with acid reflux reported the symptom of heartburn. Compared to other studies of the prevalence of heartburn in non-elderly populations, these data suggest that older people with GERD may less frequently report heartburn. In a Finnish study of the prevalence of GERD in the elderly, the authors found that 8% of men had symptoms daily, 19% weekly, and 54% experienced symptoms at least monthly [7]. For the female subjects, the rates were 15% daily, 18% weekly, and 66% at least monthly. There was not an age-related trend found in the prevalence of symptoms in this study. Brody and Kleban reported that 34% of their elderly subjects had indigestion or gas in a one-month period [9]. One study found age adjusted prevalence rates not significantly different between three racial groups (white, black, other) for GERD symptoms [5]. In contrast to the above findings, El-Serag et al [5] did find a significant age related increase in the prevalence of at least weekly heartburn and/or regurgitation: 24%, 24%, 30%, 33% for 18–34, 35–44, 45–54, and 55 and older groups. However, the preponderance of available data suggests that the prevalence of classic GERD symptoms is either constant, or slightly declines with age.

Symptoms

The classic symptoms of GERD are heartburn and acid regurgitation, and the presence of these symptoms can be considered diagnostic of the condition, and are sufficient to institute empiric therapy. Elderly patients in a primary care setting commonly report heartburn, with a prevalence of approximately 15% [8]. However, elderly patients often report less severe reflux symptoms, especially in relation to the severity of their disease. Elderly patients also regularly present with various atypical symptoms of reflux disease. Due to the lack of symptoms in many elderly patients, they often present with more severe complications of reflux disease, a consequence of prolonged and untreated GERD [3]. Elderly patients may under-report disease, and physicians may place less emphasis on reflux symptoms when multiple other serious health problems are present, further delaying diagnosis [9].

Table 1. Prevalence of heartburn in the elderly

Author	Ages	Daily	Weekly	Monthly
Locke et al [4]	> 65 – total		20%	59%
	> 65 – male		17%	
	> 65 – female		20%	
Mold et al [8]	> 62		14%	
Raiha et al [7]	> 65 – male	8%	19%	54%
	> 65 – female	15%	18%	66%
El Serag et al [5]	18–34		24%	
	35–44		24%	
	45–54		30%	
	> 55		33%	

Heartburn is classically described as a burning retrosternal pain, although it can also be reported in the epigastrium, neck, throat, and occasionally the back [10]. It usually occurs within 3 hours after a meal, may be worsened by bending over or lying down, and can last up to 2 hours [2]. There is a more variable presentation of reflux disease in the elderly, and heartburn may less commonly be the presenting symptom in this group. In a study of GERD symptoms in the elderly, Triadafilopoulos et al noted heartburn to be the most common symptom reported by subjects with GERD (45%) [11]. Acid regurgitation was present in fewer than 25% of elderly patients with reflux disease. These authors found that 41% and 30% of patients reported non-cardiac chest pain and cough, respectively. Raiha et al studied the prevalence of GERD symptoms in elderly patients referred for endoscopy [12]. They found regurgitation in less than 25%, heartburn in 36%, dysphagia in 20%, and 37% of their subjects reported atypical reflux symptoms. At least two studies have found an increase in dysphagia with increasing age [4], [13]. Those with dysphagia report symptoms for a shorter period of time than those with heartburn, suggesting that dysphagia may be a late manifestation of GERD. Elderly patients tend to have more nocturnal symptoms, which are associated with more severe complications of GERD [3].

The presence of heartburn in the elderly does not correlate as closely with the extent of acid exposure to the esophagus as in younger patients. Several authors have described a poor correlation between pH testing, heartburn as a symptom, and the extent of esophageal damage visualized on endoscopy [3], [12], [14]. Raiha's study found that only 59% of patients with abnormal acid reflux on pH monitoring had GERD symptoms associated with reflux episodes, the rest of the patients having asymptomatic reflux [12]. Symptoms of GERD in this study appeared only when total acid reflux time exceeded 10% in the elderly (compared to 4.2% in younger subjects), suggesting that the threshold for pain perception may be higher in older subjects. Fass et al reported that only 54% of elderly patients with documented GERD complained of heartburn, and also suggested a possible diminished visceral pain perception [15].

Reflux disease in the elderly appears to be more severe for any level of symptom severity than in younger individuals, although controversy does exist in the literature. While some studies have not been able to demonstrate overall differences in symptom severity between elderly and younger patients [11], [14], [16], others have found a decrease in symptom severity in an elderly group [6], [15]. Fass et al found that, among the younger patients, 52% reported "severe" to "very severe" heartburn, while only 18% of elderly patients reported symptoms of this magnitude [15]. The severity of acid regurgitation as a symptom was also significantly higher in the younger group. Several studies have found that elderly patients have more severe disease as demonstrated by the extent of mucosal injury and the frequency of complications of GERD [14]. The elderly tend to have less symptom perception, despite a trend towards increased acid exposure and esophageal mucosal injury [12], [17]. These findings have implications relating to the extent of diagnostic work-up necessary in this population.

Extraesophageal symptoms are frequently encountered in the elderly. This often causes diagnostic difficulties, as these symptoms (such as chest pain and chronic throat symptoms) must be given increased awareness in the elderly patient. This may result in a costly and extensive evaluation. Raiha et al found that 37% of elderly patients with GERD had respiratory symptoms [12]. Furthermore, in those with daily reflux symptoms, 73% also had chronic respiratory symptoms, compared to only 30% of the subjects without reflux symptoms [7].

Asthma due to GERD should be considered in elderly patients with nocturnal cough, in those who developed asthma later in life, and in those whose disease is refractory to standard bronchodilator therapy [18], [19]. Other clues suggesting an association with GERD include worsening of asthma symptoms after eating a large meal, drinking alcohol, or being in the supine position [19]. The estimates of GERD in asthma patients are between 34–89%, and many difficult to treat asthmatics may have clinically silent GERD [19], [20]. Chronic cough is also a common symptom of reflux, with between 4–60% of those with this symptom having acid reflux as the cause [3], [21].

Significant damage to the tracheal mucosa can occur even when the volume of aspirated gastric fluid is too small to cause clinically apparent aspiration pneumonia. Elderly subjects with GERD have shown a restrictive ventilatory defect, in addition to lower vital capacity and forced expiratory flow rates [19]. The supine position, possibly by increasing the likelihood of aspiration of gastric contents into the lung, may lead to pneumonia in patients on mechanical ventilators. Nasogastric tubes augment aspiration of gastric contents by impairing swallowing, causing stagnation of oropharyngeal secretions, and reducing LES tone [22]. Elevating the head of the bed may help to prevent nosocomial pneumonia, a common problem in the elderly population, and one associated with significant mortality.

One of the most difficult symptoms to diagnose and treat in an elderly population is non-cardiac chest pain. Some studies have found that up to 50% of patients with non-cardiac chest pain may have an association with GERD [20], [23]. Esophageal irritation by acid may also cause true angina through a neural reflex, as well as cause tachyarrhythmias [9]. Older patients with chest pain non-responsive to treatment for respiratory or angina-like symptoms, who have had sufficient investigation to rule out serious cardiac causes, should be investigated for GERD [3].

GERD can be found in relation to obstructive sleep apnea (OSA) syndrome in the elderly. Many older patients with OSA complain of sleep-related heartburn and regurgitation of gastric contents into the pharynx. Teramoto and Ouchi noted that nighttime treatment with CPAP can correct the sleep apnea related reflux in patients with OSA [24].

In summary, the presentation of GERD in the elderly population is not "classic", and the severity of reported symptoms does not correlate with the severity of mucosal disease. Due to the variable presentation of this disease in the elderly, GERD should be suspected in patients with atypical angina, difficult-to-manage pulmonary problems, or intractable hoarseness. This is true not only when other factors or diseases (such as coronary artery disease or pulmonary disease) have been ruled out, but also when these conditions are well documented, but are not responsive to treatment or have changed in character [9], [10].

Pathophysiology

Many studies investigated the effect of age on gastrointestinal tract functioning. After multiple conflicting findings, and some drastic paradigm shifts, it is now believed that, in general, many essential aspects of GI function are preserved in old age [1], [25]. Many of the clinically relevant alterations in esophageal function are more likely due to chronic diseases, medications, and lifestyle exposures, than to purely age-related deficits. Comorbid conditions that may influence gastrointestinal function in older adults include coronary disease, diabetes, chronic obstructive pulmonary disease, and neurological conditions such as stroke and Parkinson's disease [1], [3]. For example, a hemispheric stroke will affect the components of swallowing under voluntary control, as well as the pharyngeal and esophageal components such as LES relaxation and pharyngeal peristalsis [26]. The elderly also undergo lifestyle changes that exacerbate reflux, including reduced mobility, increased sedentary lifestyle, and increased recumbency [3], [13]. This section will describe some of the studies and major findings with regard to age-related changes in the GI tract (Table 2), and will show how some of these changes may help explain the pathogenesis of GERD in the elderly.

In general, there are four factors that lead to the development of GERD. These include decreased lower esophageal sphincter (LES) tone, mucosal damage from acid and pepsin, delayed peristalsis and esophageal clearance of refluxed gastric contents, and delayed gastric emptying [27]–[29]. For example, reflux can be due to diminished LES pressure, reduced intra-abdominal esophageal length, inappropriate transient LES relaxations, an altered esophageal mucosal defense barrier, an increased volume of refluxate, or an abnormal composition of the refluxate [27].

A competent LES is essential in protecting the esophagus from the entry of refluxed gastric contents. The primary underlying mechanism of pathologic reflux is a defective LES, either due to anatomical reasons or due to frequent reflux associated TLESR's [23], [30]. TLESR's are responsible for 65–90% of reflux episodes

Table 2. Age-associated changes in the gastrointestinal tract

Lifestyle changes	Increased comorbid diseases – CAD, Diabetes, COPD, CVA, Parkinson's Increased recumbency Increased medication usage
LES tone	No age-related change in resting LES tone Increased hiatal hernia prevalence Diminished LES tone secondary to medications Reduced intra-abdominal esophageal length
Gastric acid secretion	Normal to increased
Esophageal clearance	Impaired clearance Increased duration of acid exposure Decreased mucosal resistance and repair mechanisms
Salivary secretion	Decreased saliva volume Decreased salivary bicarbonate secretion
Esophageal visceral pain tolerance	Increased pain threshold Decreased acid perfusion sensitivity score Decreased symptom perception
Esophageal motility	Decreased amplitude of peristaltic pressures Disordered or absent secondary peristalsis Non-propulsive, repetitive, and synchronous contractions
Pharyngeal defenses	Decreased esophagoglottal closure reflex Higher threshold for triggering pharyngeal swallows Prolonged swallowing
UES tone	Decreased UES tone Delay in UES relaxation after swallow Decrease in UES compliance
Stomach	Possible delayed gastric emptying

[31]. Multiple studies have reported no significant intrinsic difference in resting LES pressure between elderly and young patients [13], [25], [32], [33]. Manometric studies in subjects older than 70 years old do not show a consistent decrease in LES pressure with age [10]. However, LES pressure can be adversely affected by hormones, CNS activity, drugs, and dietary factors [29]. Some medications taken by the elderly can exacerbate GERD, often through a reduction in LES pressure [3]. Drugs that can affect LES tone include anti-cholinergics, nitroglycerine, theophylline, and beta-agonists. Isosorbide and calcium-channel antagonists interfere with calcium uptake by smooth muscle, causing relaxation of the LES and altering the amplitude of the peristaltic contractions.

A hiatal hernia involves the displacement of the LES toward the thoracic cavity, compromising the diaphragmatic component of the LES, and impairing the clearance of refluxate from the esophagus [33], [34]. Although a hiatal hernia is not sufficient to cause GERD, it does contribute to the overall decrease of the LES barrier. Approximately 9% of patients with a hiatal hernia will have reflux disease [31]. Additionally, more patients with proven reflux do have a hiatal hernia (85–95%) [9]. It is well documented that the prevalence of hiatal hernia increases with age, and has been found in 60% of patients over the age of 60 years and in up to 90% of those older than 70 [9], [13], [16]. There is also an increased frequency of esophagitis in patients with a hiatal hernia, and the severity of esophagitis is proportional to the size of the hernia [13], [16]. Several authors have found that although the total length of the LES high-pressure zone is similar in older and younger groups, the elderly tend to have a shorter intra-abdominal segment [32], [33]. This leads to a greater segment the of LES high-pressure zone being above the respiratory pressure inversion point in the elderly, contributing to an increase in reflux and esophageal damage.

Additionally, certain drugs can delay esophageal transport, extending contact time with the esophageal mucosa, and can cause direct mucosal injury [3], [35]. Esophageal tissue resistance may decrease in the elderly as a result of slow cell regeneration, as well as from direct injury by irritant drugs [36]. Medications in this group include doxycycline, quinidine, aspirin, NSAIDs, potassium, tetracycline, and ferrous sulfate [23]. These drugs are taken up by the mucosa, and cause damage after concentrating in the mucosa. Patients with motility disorders may be more prone to esophageal injury from medications. If present, strictures may impede the passage of some pills, leading to further local injury [35]. Alendronate, taken by many elderly patients, is also a cause of drug-induced esophageal ulceration, and must be taken with a large amount of water to avoid prolonged mucosal exposure.

Early studies suggested impaired acid secretion in the elderly, but pure "age-related achlorhydria" has not been found in small studies of healthy subjects [37]. It had initially been suggested that age-related changes in the function of the gastrointestinal tract include a reduction in gastric parietal cell function, leading to impaired acid secretion and an elevation in gastric pH. These early studies found that gastric acid secretion decreased with age in about 25% of elderly people, putting them at less risk of esophageal irritation and symptoms due to regurgitated gastric acid [7]. However, several studies have since challenged these findings, and Hurwitz et al [37] found no age-related increase in achlorhydria or in atrophic gastritis in subjects older than 65 years. The level of hyposecretion in the elderly in this study was similar to that found in a study of healthy young men and women. Additionally, colonization by enteric pathogens and malabsorption of drugs and nutrients – consequences of hypoacidity – have not been shown in the elderly [37]. Most authors now believe that physiologic levels of gastric acid secretion are similar in adults of all ages, in the absence of atrophic gastritis [16], [25], [35], [36]. Although gastric acid secretion does not appear to decrease due to aging alone, older patients with *Helicobacter pylori* and atrophic gastritis may secrete less acid [10]. If atrophic gastritis is present, the composition of the refluxate may be changed to a neutral, or even an alkaline pH. In this case, the refluxate has diminished irritative potential, which causes a delay in activation of the esophageal clearance mechanism [12].

Three factors contribute to the esophageal clearance of refluxate – gravity, peristalsis, and saliva – and an overall decline in esophageal clearance has been noted in the elderly [1], [3], [23], [34]. Elderly patients with GERD have $pH < 4.0$ in distal esophagus for greater percentage of time than younger patients [16]. The amount of time that acid is exposed to the esophageal mucosa is directly related to the risk and extent of mucosal damage [38]. Reduced esophageal clearance during sleep appears to be a major causative factor in serious forms of GERD in all ages [30]. At night, all clearance mechanisms are blunted, and there is a decreased swallowing rate, explaining why nocturnal reflux is associated with severe esophagitis [9], [34]. Sedatives and hypnotics, often used by elderly patients, as well as alcohol, may further depress nocturnal swallowing mechanisms and prolong the duration of nocturnal reflux episodes [7], [9], [12], [34].

Salivary secretion is critical, as it neutralizes the acid that covers the esophageal lining after a reflux episode [39]. Saliva is an effective buffer that helps to re-establish a more alkaline pH in the esophageal lumen. Some studies have found a decline in salivary secretion with age, and Zhu et al found elderly patients to have more severe reflux episodes and compromised clearance of acid compared to younger patients [3], [39], [40]. Several studies have described an age-related decrease in salivary bicarbonate secretion following acid perfusion of the esophagus, which may contribute to increased severity of esophagitis [3], [10], [16], [29]. Some have argued that the age-related decline in salivary secretion may be due to or exacerbated by other comorbid medical conditions in the elderly [26], [41]. For example, several medications used by the elderly can decrease saliva formation, including antihistamines, antidepressants, certain anti-hypertensives, antispasmodics, some neuroleptics, and antiparkinsonian drugs [9], [23].

One well described age-related change in esophageal function is an increase in visceral pain tolerance, which may in part explain the decrease in symptom perception in the elderly. Intraesophageal balloon distention has been used to evaluate the physiological functioning of the esophagus, by using increasing distending volumes to study visceral pain perception. Lasch and Castell found a significant increase in the mean pain threshold of their elderly subjects, and over 50% of their elderly subjects felt no pain at all, even at maximum balloon inflation [42]. These results show a significantly higher pain threshold in the elderly group, corresponding with a dramatic decrease in pain perception. Weusten et al found age-related alterations in cerebral evoked potentials induced by balloon distention, with a decrease in amplitude and an increase in peak latency with age [42]. Fass et al studied chemosensitivity to acid infusion in symptomatic elderly and young patients [15]. The younger patients had a significantly shorter lag time to initial symptom perception, a higher sensory intensity rating, and an acid perfusion sensitivity score that was significantly higher than the older patients. This diminished chemosensitivity was present in the elderly despite increased acid exposure and esophageal mucosal inflammation. Patel et al [15] showed reduced visceral pain perception in the proximal and mid esophagus of normal elderly subjects compared with normal younger subjects using the technique of impedance planimetry. Studies have found an age-related loss of neurons in the myenteric plexus of the esophagus, and have suggested afferent autonomic nerve degeneration as a possible explanation of the greater number of elderly patients who have reflux without symptoms [12], [26], [42]. The reduction in pain perception in the elderly may explain why they often present with complications of reflux rather than with symptoms.

Early studies on esophageal motility in the elderly found significant differences that were thought to be secondary to aging [43]. The term "presbyesophagus" was coined to describe an age related decrease in contractile amplitude and polyphasic waves in the esophageal body, along with incomplete sphincter relaxation and esophageal dilatation [25]. However, the subjects in this study had a high prevalence of diabetes, medication use, and neurological diseases, and the results are now thought to be secondary to these factors, rather than a primary degeneration of esophageal function. Although primary peristalsis may be preserved, secondary peristalsis has been shown to be less frequent, less consistent, and occasionally is totally absent [25], [26], [45], [46]. Secondary esophageal peristalsis is initiated in response to esophageal stimuli, and is thought to play an important role in volume clearance of material remaining in the esophagus after a swallow, such as refluxate [46]. In the elderly, there are more frequent non-propulsive, often repetitive contractions, and even failure of contractions after deglutition in the distal esophagus [10], [13], [25], [47]. Additionally, Hollis and Castell found patients older than 70 years old to have a decrease in the amplitude of peristaltic pressures, but not in the duration or velocity of peristalsis [48]. Ali Kahn et al found the lack of contraction response and relaxation phase of the LES to be 4–6 times more common in an elderly group [43]. This study also described a greater incidence of disordered contractions in the older group, mostly seen as simultaneous contractions.

Using the technique of pharyngeal water stimulation, which can induce complete LES relaxation, investigators have found that the threshold for relaxation is significantly greater in the elderly [26], [33]. Xie et al [33] found that these relaxations were more often associated with reflux events in the elderly group.

Although the frequency of reflux episodes is not thought to vary with age, the duration of individual episodes may be longer in the elderly secondary to defective peristalsis [10], [16]. Ferriolli et al found the duration of reflux episodes to be longer in an older group compared to a younger group [47]. Overall, clearance of the esophagus after reflux episodes in asymptomatic persons older than 70 is impaired, and the reflux episodes in this population last longer than in healthy volunteers younger than 60 years old. These changes further delay esophageal clearance, increasing acid contact time, and leading to more severe reflux disease in the elderly population [47].

Normally, the upper esophageal sphincter (UES) and the supraesophageal region (trachea and esophagoglottal closure reflex) act as additional defense mechanisms to prevent oropharyngeal reflux. Both vocal cord closure and an increase in UES pressure are triggered by an increase in esophageal distention/pressure [32]. Bardan et al along with other authors, found that the esophagoglottal closure reflex can be either absent or less reproducible in the elderly [32]. One study found this protective reflex to be absent in 50% of those subjects over the age of 70 [46]. Shaker et al studied the effect of age, position, and temperature on the threshold volume that triggers pharyngeal swallows [49]. In both the upright and supine positions, spontaneous swallowing was significantly less frequent in the elderly compared with the young. In addition, the threshold volume for swallow initiation in young volunteers was significantly smaller than in the elderly, by 3–5 times. The need in the elderly patients for larger volumes to trigger a pharyngeal swallow may have implications, as the refluxate may have increased risk of being inhaled into the airway.

It has also been reported that the length of UES high pressure zone is shorter in the elderly, and the resting UES pressure is significantly lower than in the younger group [13], [25], [32]. A decreased UES tone may increase the chances of refluxate reaching the larynx, pharynx, and lungs [9]. There is a delay in UES relaxation after swallowing and an increased resistance to flow across the UES as a result of loss of compliance with age [13], [25]. Although there are subtle alterations in the coordination of vocal cord closure and oropharyngeal bolus transit, the overall coordination between airway protection and the transit aspect of the oropharyngeal phase of swallowing is preserved in the elderly [46]. Whether these changes are clinically relevant in the pathogenesis of reflux disease is unclear, and their overall significance may be relatively minor [45].

Most data tend to support the finding that there is a decrease in gastric emptying time with increasing age [13], [23], [29]. While some report impaired emptying of liquids, others have found that 10–15% of patients with GERD may have delayed gastric emptying of solids [23]. Gastric emptying in healthy elderly patients may also be decreased in the presence of atrophic antral gastritis. Emptying is slowed by fatty meals, the supine position, gastric outlet obstruction, anti-cholinergic agents, hormones, and various diseases such as diabetes [9]. Other studies, however, have reported no difference in gastric emptying between young and old volunteers [25], [31], [36].

Diagnosis

There are several factors complicating the diagnosis of GERD in the elderly, and the diagnostic approach in this group should be different than in a younger population. When a healthy young patient presents, with the classic symptoms of heartburn or acid regurgitation, no further testing is needed to diagnose GERD. In this case, the recommendations are to treat first, and reserve diagnostic testing for those with alarming or atypical symptoms, symptoms resistant to medical therapy, those with a sudden onset of symptoms, or patients with chronic relapsing symptoms [3], [13], [44], [50]. Alarm symptoms include GI bleeding, unintentional weight loss, iron deficiency anemia, dysphagia, persistent vomiting, an epigastric mass, or a suspicious barium meal. An improvement in symptoms on acid reduction therapy can be considered diagnostic of GERD [13]. If symptoms show a change in frequency, severity, or periodicity (especially if they become nocturnal), investigation with endoscopy is also warranted [3]. Reflux disease in the elderly, however, may be more difficult to accurately diagnose. Older people may have less severe heartburn, and may underreport their symptoms. They may present with atypical symptoms, and their coexistent illnesses make diagnosis more complex. Potential diagnostic tests for GERD, with an emphasis on the elderly patient, will be discussed in this section (Table 3).

The Bernstein test is a provocative test of mucosal sensitivity to acid and is used to document acid-related symptoms. A positive test is one that reproduces the patient's symptoms following acid infusion. Although this test is more likely to be positive in patients with more severe esophagitis, it has decreased positivity in those with Barrett's [50]. The overall sensitivity of this test is 77% with a specificity of 86% [50]. This test may demonstrate that the symptoms are due to GERD, but it cannot grade the degree of esophagitis. The Bernstein test may be especially useful in the elderly in the evaluation of reflux related non-cardiac chest pain, however, it is no longer commonly used in practice [9].

In general, barium radiography is not a reliable test for diagnosing GERD. Reflux of barium into the esophagus is not specific for GERD, as it can be seen in one-third of patients without GERD [13]. This test has an overall diagnostic accuracy of 24.6% in mild esophagitis, 81.6% in moderate, and 98.7% in severe [50]. However, barium swallow may be more effective in the elderly, as it can characterize anatomy and provide a qualitative determination of esophageal function. Barium esophagrams are most appropriate for those with symptoms of dysphagia for solids or liquids [13], [23]. Dysphagia in the elderly may be related to motility disorders, CNS disease, Zenker's diverticulum, cancer, or a peptic stricture. Barium swallow has a high sensitivity for masses in the esophagus and for

Table 3. Diagnostic testing for GERD in the elderly

Test	Use	Advantages	Disadvantages
Bernstein Test	– Attempt to reproduce reflux symptoms using provocative acid Infusion	– Correlation between infusion and symptoms suggestive of GERD – Useful in evaluating atypical symptoms	– Decreased sensitivity in BE – Cannot grade degree of mucosal damage – Rarely used
Barium Swallow	– Investigate symptoms of dysphagia – Can identify hiatal hernia (non-specific finding)	– Increased accuracy with more severe disease – Characterizes anatomy and structural disease – Qualitative measure of esophageal function – Quantify degree and location of obstruction	– Cannot reliably diagnose GERD – Reduced sensitivity in less severe disease
pH Monitoring	– Identify presence of abnormal reflux – Correlate symptoms and reflux	– Can directly relate symptoms to a reflux event – Useful in diagnosis of atypical reflux – Evaluate optimization of medical management	– Cannot grade degree of mucosal damage – Does not address alkaline or mixed reflux – Cannot perform biopsy
Endoscopy	– Identify erosive esophagitis or Barrett's esophagus – Investigate etiology of upper GI bleeding	– Direct visualization allowing grading of damage – Allows for prognostic Information – Allows for biopsy useful in BE and H. pylori	– Potential for adverse reactions to sedation or procedure – Decreased use in atypical symptoms

strictures, rings, and ulcerations, and can quantify the severity of esophageal obstruction [13], [23]. The use of a solid bolus can assist in the localization of the obstruction [31].

pH monitoring can quantify the degree of reflux in a near-physiological setting, and is able to relate symptoms to a reflux event [10], [13], [20], [51]. This test has the highest sensitivity and specificity for diagnosing reflux disease – up to 88% and 98%, respectively [10], [50]. Six parameters are measured – % total, upright, and supine time with pH less than 4.0, number of reflux episodes, reflux episodes longer than 5 minutes, and longest reflux episode. Patients with atypical symptoms may have a clarification of their syndrome with pH testing – especially those with chest pain, pulmonary symptoms, and chronic hoarseness [2], [13], [50]. This testing is also useful for patients on acid-suppressive therapy who are still experiencing symptoms, to decide if the medical therapy is optimized [31]. pH monitoring should always be performed prior to consideration of anti-reflux surgery. It can also be used in the patient with refractory esophagitis, as a normal study may point towards another etiology, such as pill-induced esophagitis [10], [23]. Patti et al studied the utility of esophageal function tests, including manometry and 24-hour pH monitoring, and concluded that symptoms alone were unreliable in diagnosing GERD [52]. A diagnosis of GERD based on symptoms and endoscopy was incorrect in about 33% of patients, and esophageal function tests were found to be the best way to establish the diagnosis and identify more severe disease. Manometry can measure LES tone, and identify motility problems, but it does not measure reflux. It is reserved for LES localization prior to pH testing and for evaluating peristalsis prior to anti-reflux surgery, as findings can influence the type of procedure done [10], [31].

As early as 1977, Jacobsohn and Levy evaluated and confirmed the safety and feasibility of upper endoscopy in elderly patients [53]. Eshchar et al studied endoscopy in octogenarians, looking at 73 EGD's, and also found it to be a safe and well tolerated procedure [54]. There is no increased morbidity or mortality of endoscopy in the elderly population compared to younger groups [13]. The diagnostic impact of endoscopy is lower in GERD patients < 50 years old, especially in the absence of alarm symptoms [55]. However, endoscopy should be used early as the initial diagnostic test in all elderly patients with heartburn, regardless of the severity or duration of their complaints [10]. This approach is advocated because they often have more severe disease despite milder symptoms. Without endoscopy it is difficult to predict the presence of esophagitis in the elderly, as a correlation between symptoms and severity of disease has not been established [56]. Endoscopy provides direct visualization, with high sensitivity and specificity for the detection of mucosal injury, and biopsy is the most sensitive test for esophagitis and can diagnose H. Pylori [9], [20], [23]. Endoscopy allows the physician to objectively grade GERD severity and gives information on disease prognosis. Although EGD is sensitive and specific for identifying mucosal disease, it may miss 36–50% of patients with GERD found by pH monitoring [13]. Thus, pH testing compliments endoscopy in the diagnosis of GERD when endoscopic findings are apparently normal, or in the presence of atypical symptoms.

Endoscopy should always be performed in the presence of alarm symptoms, such as dysphagia [57]. If a patient has a long history of nicotine and/or alcohol abuse, or regular use of NSAIDs, they should be referred for EGD or barium study to exclude structural disease [29], [57]. Even in elderly patients who are currently asymptomatic, but who have a strong history of reflux symptoms, endoscopy is indicated to rule out Barrett's esophagus (BE) [10]. There is disagreement among physicians concerning the age cut-off for endoscopy in a patient presenting with new-onset reflux symptoms. Recommendations range from 45–65 years old [3], [31], [56], [57]. However, what is agreed upon is that due to the occult severity of disease in the elderly, endoscopy should be done very early in the evaluation [23].

GERD complications

GERD comprises a spectrum of disease, ranging from non-erosive esophagitis, to complications involving increasingly severe esophageal damage. Complications of reflux disease include erosive esophagitis, esophageal ulceration, peptic stricture, BE, and adenocarcinoma of the esophagus. Several studies have shown that complications of GERD tend to occur together. Any GERD complication is 10 times more likely to occur with another GERD complication than without, and this is most often true for strictures and ulcers [39], [58]. In fact, ulcers rarely to never occur as the sole complication. More severe mucosal lesions are usually associated with less spontaneous resolution, lower treatment response and early relapse after the discontinuation of therapy [28], [59].

Several authors have noted that complications of GERD are more common in the elderly, requiring increased vigilance and a more aggressive approach to diagnosis and treatment by physicians. Brunnen et al estimated the overall incidence of severe esophagitis at 4.5 per 100,000 population, with a dramatic increase after the age of 50 [17]. Studies suggest that 50–60% of those with typical reflux symptoms will have erosive esophagitis [31]. Collen et al found that complications such as erosive esophagitis and BE have been reported in up to 81% of patients over 60, compared to 47% younger than 60 [14]. The same study noted that 87% of those 70 years old had mucosal disease. Multiple studies have found that age increases with increasing severity of esophagitis. Authors have reported the mean age of patients with BE to be 61, those with stricture have a mean age of 63–65, and for esophageal ulcer, the mean age is 60–62 [17], [39], [55], [60]. Compared with patients aged > 50 years, the odds ratio of patients aged < 50 years with a major lesion on endoscopy was 0.5 [55]. Reynolds noted that although GERD related ulcerations are rare in younger patients, they occur in up to 20–30% of older individuals [61]. Zhu et al reported grade-III or IV-esophagitis in 20.8% of patients age 65–76 compared to only 3.4% of patients younger than 64 [40].

Age has been shown to be an independent risk factor for esophagitis, with an adjusted odds ratio of 1.18 per 10 year increase [59]. As the severity of esophagitis increases, there is an increase in the proportion of patients with severe heartburn and heartburn > 5 years in duration [62]. Male gender and white race have been noted to be associated with an increased risk for complicated reflux disease [58], [59]. The presence of hiatal hernia increases with increasing severity of mucosal inflammation, and these are more prevalent in an elderly population [60], [62]. Many patients with GERD, especially the elderly, may not seek medical attention until one to three years into their symptoms, which increases the likelihood of developing complications.

Peptic strictures occur in approximately 10–20% of patients with untreated GERD, and they are especially common in elderly men [6], [10], [17], [58]. Patients with strictures tend to demonstrate more frequent disturbances of motility, such as peristalsis, further prolonging acid contact time [58].

Barrett's Esophagus (BE) is a metaplastic condition in which the normal squamous lining of the lower esophagus is replaced by columnar epithelial cells in response to chronic reflux of gastric acid, pepsin, and duodenal contents [64]. Several studies have shown an increase in the prevalence of BE in the elderly, with a mean age of diagnosis of 60 years of age [13], [65]–[69]. However, it is estimated that disease formation itself actually occurs at a mean age of 40–55 [66], [67]. Cameron and Lomboy studied 51,311 patients who underwent endoscopy to further characterize the course of BE [67]. BE was found twice as frequently in men (0.97% vs. 0.49%), and the age distribution was similar in both sexes. The prevalence of disease increased with age to reach a plateau in the seventh to ninth decades. This large study also found no difference in the length of BE segment among different age groups. Patients with BE develop reflux symptoms at an earlier age, have an increased duration of symptoms, increased severity of nocturnal reflux, and increased complications of GERD [28], [65], [70].

Many authors have investigated symptoms of BE, and as many as 25% of patients are asymptomatic at diagnosis [10]. In general, patients with BE report less severe symptoms than those with GERD alone, and among those individuals with BE, elderly patients are less symptomatic that younger patients [16], [65], [69]. In a study of elderly and younger patients with BE, the elderly patients were significantly less symptomatic than the younger subjects, and had symptom scores that were similar to symptomatic controls without GERD [11]. There have been specific studies looking at the relationship between BE, aging, and the presence of symptoms of heartburn and acid regurgitation. Grade et al [69] studied response to acid in elderly compared to young BE patients. They found that all of the young patients had a positive acid perfusion test, but only 58% of elderly patients had a positive test, with 48% of the elderly group having no symptom perception during acid infusion. The mean lag time to initial symptom perception was also significantly longer in elderly patients, and elderly patients had a lower sensory intensity rating at the end of acid perfusion compared with the younger patients. Possible explanations for these findings include "reduced acid sensitivity, the age-related changes in symptom perception, and the presence of columnar epithelium" [58], [65].

Treatment

The medical and surgical treatment of GERD in the elderly population generally follows the same principles as for any adult patient with reflux [10]. The basic goals of treatment are relief of symptoms, early detection of lesions, healing of esophagitis, prevention of relapses, and prevention of complications [28]. Evaluation and management of the elderly patient does require "attention to more subtle, atypical, or non-specific symptoms, recognition of the importance on maintaining function, and patience in the interaction and in the pace of progress" [1]. Education of the patient about the nature of GERD and the factors that may precipitate reflux continues to be the cornerstone of therapy. Characteristics of an ideal agent for the treatment of a chronic condition in an elderly patient include high safety and efficacy, minimal side effects, no need for dose adjustment with age, safety in renal and hepatic insufficiency, a simple dosing regimen, no significant drug interactions, and cost effectiveness [61].

Some physicians assume that the elderly have less severe GERD and reduce the dose of anti-secretory medications because of the belief that basal gastric acid secretion declines with age [14]. However, there is a direct relationship between the degree of 24 hr acid suppression and healing rates. Elderly patients may in fact need higher levels of acid suppression to heal esophagitis and to relieve symptoms than younger patients [25]. While patients with mild reflux symptoms may benefit from a step-up approach to treatment, those with more advanced disease, complications, or atypical presentations of GERD need to be initially started on more potent and aggressive therapy [34].

Conservative therapy

Most guidelines recommend instituting lifestyle changes (Table 4) at the same time as empiric therapy. Lifestyle modifications are considered useful in reducing symptoms, but there are few data to support an impact on healing the esophagus, or any proven long-term benefits [13]. Physiologic studies show that elevation of the head of the bed, decreased fat intake, cessation of smoking, and avoiding recumbency for 3 hours post-prandially decreases distal esophageal acid exposure

Table 4. Lifestyle changes

- Elevation of head of the bed – 6 inches, using a wedge
- Lower fat, higher protein diet
- Eat smaller meals
- Smoking cessation
- Avoidance of recumbency 3 hours post-prandially – avoid late meals
- Weight loss
- Decreased alcohol intake
- Dietary modifications – avoid caffeine, fatty foods, chocolate, spicy foods, peppermint, onions, garlic, tomatoes, and citrus products
- Review medications – increase fluid intake with medications and avoid medications that decrease LES pressure when possible

Table 5. Medications and GERD

Decrease LES tone	Anticholinergics Nitroglycerine Beta-agonists Theophylline Isosorbide Calcium-channel antagonists Hormones Meperidine
Direct mucosal irritant effect	Doxycycline/Tetracycline Quinidine Aspirin Non-steroidal anti-inflammatory Medications Potassium Ferrous sulfate Alendronate
Decreased peristaltic amplitude	Calcium-channel antagonists Isosorbide
Decreased salivary secretion	Antihistamines Antidepressants Antispasmodics Neuroleptics Anti-Parkinsonian medications
Decreased swallowing rate (especially nocturnal effects)	Sedatives Hypnotics Alcohol

[50]. However, this life style modification is being recommended less often given effectiveness of proton pump inhibitors in treating GERD. Other lifestyle changes include weight loss and decreased alcohol intake. Several foods contribute to reflux symptoms, and should be avoided. Foods with an acidic pH can both lower the LES pressure and increase gastric acid secretion, and can precipitate symptoms [30]. Caffeine irritates the esophageal mucosa and increases acid secretion, while fatty foods delay gastric emptying [29]. Additional culprits include chocolate, peppermint, spicy foods, and onions.

Elderly patients are often on multiple medications, which can act through different mechanisms to worsen reflux (Table 5). Medications may reduce saliva production, lower LES pressure, reduce esophageal motility and gastric emptying, and some medications have a direct irritant effect on the esophageal mucosa [9]. An elderly patient's medications should be reviewed, and, especially in the case of the irritant medications, should be taken with plenty of fluids. These conservative measures should be continued throughout all steps of pharmacological therapy, as they help to eliminate factors that inhibit motility-related defense mechanisms. We will next discuss the currently available medical therapies in GERD with emphasis on the advantages and disadvantages of each agent in the elderly (Table 6).

Antacids/Alginic acid

Antacids work locally to increase the pH of the refluxate, neutralizing the acid. The increase in pH-causes pepsin to become inactive, and may also prevent the

Table 6. GERD therapy in the elderly

Medication	Advantages	Disadvantages
Antacids/Alginic acid	– Relief of mild/moderate symptoms (20%) – Over the counter – Rapid effect	– Do not heal mucosal disease – Diarrhea/Constipation – Impaired drug absorption – Must be upright for effect (alginic acid)
Prokinetic agents	– Effectively relieve symptoms – Heal mucosal erosions – Useful for dyspeptic symptoms – nausea, gas, bloating – As effective as H_2B's	– Fatal arrhythmias (Cisapride) – Poor side effect profile – crosses blood-brain barrier (CNS toxicity) – Anti-cholinergic effects (Bethenechol)
Mucosal protective	– Provides symptom relief and esophageal healing	– Dosing four times a day – Affects drug absorption – Drug-drug interactions
Histamine$_2$ receptor blockers	– Symptom relief in $\sim$ 60% – Mucosal healing in $\sim$ 48% – Blocks acid production secondary to multiple stimuli	– Incomplete acid suppression – Tolerance development – Not as effective for erosive esophagitis – May require increased dosing for full effect – Dosage adjustment in renal failure – Short duration of action
Proton pump inhibitors	– Blocks final common pathway of acid secretion – Symptom relief and mucosal healing in up to 95% – Effective in severe disease – Once daily dosing – Effective for maintenance therapy – No dosage adjustments in renal or hepatic failure	– Increased gastrin production – Possible alteration of gastritis pattern in H. Pylori positive patients – Drug-drug interactions are possible – Decreased vitamin B12 levels

injurious effects of certain bile acids [71]. They may increase LES pressure, decreasing the amount of gastroesophageal reflux. Alginic acid forms a foamy barrier on top of the refluxate to protect the esophagus from acid-induced damage. These agents have been shown to be more effective than placebo in providing relief of mild to moderate reflux symptoms [20]. Relief of symptoms can be expected in up to 20% of patients. Antacids and alginic acid are not likely to promote healing of the esophageal mucosa, or any other complications of chronic GERD [2]. There are some adverse effects, which may be of particular concern in the elderly, including constipation with aluminum containing preparations and diarrhea with magnesium containing products. Combination products may lessen these effects. Aluminum containing antacids can cause dialysis encephalopathy and osteomalacia, and should be used with caution in those with renal impairment. Antacids may promote salt overload, induce hypercalcemia, and affect absorption of other drugs, especially antibiotics [10]. In addition, alginic acid requires a patient to be in the upright position to be efficacious, which may be an issue in an elderly population. Antacids should not be use for more than 2 weeks, as this may hide a more severe diagnosis requiring endoscopic evaluation, and more aggressive medical management [72].

Prokinetic agents

This class of agents targets the underlying motility dysfunction that causes GERD. Specifically, they increase lower esophageal sphincter pressure, accelerate gastric clearance, stimulate esophageal peristalsis, and increase the amplitude of esophageal contractions [73]. Each of these agents (bethenechol, metoclopramide, domperidone, and cisapride) is effective in improving symptoms and healing erosions. They are especially useful in the presence of dyspeptic symptoms such as nausea, vomiting, and abdominal bloating [10]. Unfortunately, they have a poor adverse event profile, which is of particular concern in an elderly population, and they should therefore be used sparingly in this population.

Cisapride was removed from the market in 2000, after 80 deaths due to cardiac arrhythmias were reported. It was the most effective promotility agent for the treatment of GERD, both in relieving symptoms (60%) and promoting healing [73]. It was as effective as H_2B's for mild to moderate disease, and may have had a role in maintenance therapy [28]. The combination of cimetidine with a prokinetic agent resulted in improved healing compared to either agent alone [20]. Cisapride not only has prokinetic effects, but it stimulates salivation via a cholinergic mechanism. Orr et al [38] looked at acid clearance with cisapride in patients with symptomatic GERD, and found a significant decrease in the number of swallows required for acid clearance compared to baseline. These authors concluded that the main efficacy of cisapride in treating GERD actually results from its ability to stimulate saliva, not from its relatively weak prokinetic effects. The removal of this medication from the US market was due to a drug interaction with azole antifungals, macrolide antibiotics, and procainamide, resulting in a prolonged QT interval and risk of cardiac arrhythmias. An investigational limited-access program is available for patients whose disease has failed to respond to other standard treatment options and who meet defined eligibility criteria [35].

Bethenachol directly stimulates the parasympathetic nervous system to release acetylcholine. Healing rates with Bethenachol are between 45–52% [73]. It has been shown to decrease the frequency and duration of nocturnal reflux episodes. Bethenachol has significant side effects of abdominal cramping, flushing, blurred vision, fatigue, and increased urinary frequency, which are more common in the elderly. Furthermore, it causes hypotension, bradycardia, worsening of asthma and angina, and worsens Parkinson's disease [9].

Metoclopramide has been found to be as effective as H_2B's in relieving heartburn and other GERD symptoms, but it is not more effective in promoting the healing of erosive esophagitis [73]. Side effects of metoclopramide are a significant drawback. It crosses the blood-brain barrier, and 20–30% of patients have antidopaminergic side effects [13], [73]. These effects are more significant in the elderly, and include drowsiness and lassitude, anxiety, agitation, confusion, hallucinations, extrapyramidal problems, and motor restlessness. The most serious adverse reactions are depression and tardive dyskinesia. Treatment related side effects from metoclopramide have been reported in 25–31% of patients receiving this drug [13]. Domperidone has not been approved by the FDA, and current studies report conflicting results. Domperidone and metoclopramide are not as effective as cisapride in relieving symptoms of GERD [3]. One advantage of domperidone is that it does not cross the blood-brain barrier, and it is therefore better tolerated in an elderly population than metoclopramide [73].

Mucosal-protective agents

The main mucosal protective agent is sucralfate, which works by binding damaged mucosa, and forming a protective barrier against the erosive action of pepsin and bile. Sucralfate may have a comparable rate of symptom relief and healing of erosive esophagitis to H_2B's [2]. The degree of healing with sucralfate correlates inversely with the degree of injury of the mucosa. However, there are significant drawbacks in using this medication for GERD in the elderly. It requires four time a day dosing, and has a potential for drug-drug interactions with digoxin, phenytoin, quinidine, and warfarin. This medication may reduce the absorption of certain drugs, and other medications must be given 2 hours after sucralfate [35]. Due to the increased medication usage in the elderly, this factor makes sucralfate difficult to effectively utilize in this population.

Histamine$_2$-receptor blockers (H_2B's)

This class of medications indirectly suppresses gastric acid and pepsin secretion by occupying Histamine$_2$ receptors. They suppress basal, nocturnal, and pentagastrin secretion, as well as acid secretion induced by insulin, meals, and sham feeding [74]. These medications have no effect on LES pressure or esophageal clearance [31]. Acid suppression is incomplete in response to meals, thus these are less effective in people with advanced reflux disease [35]. The H_2B's reduce nocturnal acid by 85–94% if appropriate doses are determined [74]. Clinical trials have shown that, compared to placebo, H_2B's improve the endoscopic appearance of the esophagus and reflux symptoms in the majority of patients after 6–8 weeks of treatment [27], [73]. In a general population, symptomatic relief can be expected in 32–82% of patients (mean 60%) after a 12 week course, with resolution of endoscopically confirmed esophagitis in 0–82% (mean 48%) [13], [34], [35], [50], [71], [73], [74].

These medications are effective in the management of non-erosive reflux disease and the healing of mild esophagitis [3], [13], [28]. However, esophageal mucosal healing rates are inversely proportional to the severity of esophagitis, and more severe disease may require increased dosages or combination therapy [2], [34], [71]. For grade-II esophagitis, Johnson found 8-week healing rates of 65–83%, which decreased to 15–58% in grade III disease [13]. Another study found that only 17% of patients with grade IV esophagitis achieved complete healing after three-months of high dose therapy [34]. Collen et al [14] treated patients with ranitidine in escalating doses to achieve healing of esophagitis and disappearance of pyrosis. While a majority of patients responded to 300 mg/day, 33% of those healed required a mean dose of 1200 mg/day (range of 600–3000). Fewer patients with esophagitis or BE had healing and symptom resolution at the lower dosages. 34% of elderly patients required increased dosage in this study (mean 1140 mg/day) which was no different from the 38% of < 60 who required increased doses. Others have also reported that the elderly require higher doses for healing, up to 2400 mg/day, to relieve symptoms and heal mucosal lesions [2].

These drugs are generally well tolerated by older adults, however, there are concerns about adverse effects and drug-drug interactions do exist. The overall incidence of adverse events is 3–5%, with most being mild [2]. Cardiovascular events occur most often with cimetidine, and include bradycardia and hypotension. Mental confusion has been reported with cimetidine, with associated factors including high dose, old age, decreased renal function, and cerebral impairment [74]. Other central nervous system effects include delirium, hallucinations, depression, and dyskinesia, seen mostly with the intravenous formulation [31], [74]. Cimetidine causes a reversible decrease in creatinine clearance in 26%, but does not worsen existing renal failure. Cimetidine also causes a transient increase in serum aminotransferases. Other less common effects include rash, myalgia, and neutropenia with cimetidine, and hepatitis, arthralgias, rash, and bone marrow suppression with ranitidine.

Concomitant administration of antacids reduces the bioavailability of most H_2 blockers by 20–25% [35], [74]. Excretion of these drugs occurs through the kidneys, and they are all partially metabolized by the liver, with the degree of liver involvement varying by drug [74]. Cimetidine, and less frequently ranitidine, can alter serum concentrations of drugs using microsomal enzymes, such as phenytoin and theophylline, benzodiazepines, certain beta-blockers, imipramine, ketoconazole, and warfarin [2], [3], [71], [74]. These agents require dosage adjustments in elderly patients with diminished renal function, and cimetidine and ranitidine have prolonged elimination in patients with hepatic dysfunction [2], [23].

Disadvantages of H_2B therapy include short duration of action, incomplete inhibition of acid in response to a meal, and the development of tolerance [73]. Although the addition of a H_2B to twice daily PPI therapy can significantly reduce nocturnal gastric acid reflux, the phenomenon is temporary for most people. Tolerance develops in as short as 1 week, and, after 1 month of continuous therapy, acidity may return to pre-treatment levels [2], [75]. Although an increase in medication dosage can result in improved healing, cost becomes an issue in this case considering the availability of alternate effective medications.

Proton pump inhibitors

Proton Pump Inhibitors (PPI's) offer the optimal defense strategy against GERD in the elderly [35]. The proton pump is the final common pathway for acid secretion in the stomach, and it is located on the luminal surface of gastric parietal cells. The modification of this pump by the drug causes a more consistent and profound inhibition than can be obtained by modifying the basal receptors (Histamine and Acetylcholine) [76].

Proton pump inhibitors produce more frequent and rapid symptom relief and esophageal healing for a greater percentage of patients than do H_2B's [73]. Several studies have examined rates of symptom control and healing. A single daily dose will produce symptom relief and healing of erosive esophagitis in 67–95% after 4–8 weeks of treatment, and continuous therapy will maintain relief and healing for up to 5 years [3], [13], [27]. They also lead to rapid healing, with lansoprazole healing 67% of erosive esophagitis after 2 weeks [2], [36]. PPI's are more effective in healing grades II–IV esophagitis than H_2B's [3], [73]. The PPI's have specific efficacy in patients with severe, refractory reflux disease, non-healing BE ulcers, and peptic strictures [70], [77]. In addition, omeprazole heals between 80–97% of patients with esophagitis who are refractory to H_2B's [2], [34], [71]. Several studies have shown PPI's to be superior to H_2B's in relieving GERD symptoms, including the relief of nocturnal symptoms [71], [76], [77]. PPI's are not associated with development of tolerance, as some H_2B's are [76].

James et al [36] studied H_2B vs. PPI in treatment of reflux esophagitis in an elderly and a young group. After 4 weeks of treatment, 53% of elderly PPI group had complete healing of their lesions, while only 27% of elderly H_2B group had complete healing. After 8 weeks, 70% of elderly PPI group was healed, compared to only 29% of elderly H_2B group. In terms of symptom control, 59% of elderly PPI patients were symptom free after 4 weeks (vs. 33% of H_2B group), which increased to 79% vs. 51% after 8 weeks. At 8 weeks, there were three times as many patients in the H_2B group who remained symptomatic and unhealed. The authors concluded that therapy with omeprazole was superior to H_2B in resolving the lesions of esophagitis as well as relieving the symptoms of GERD in an elderly population.

Adverse events with PPI's are rare, have similar rates as H_2B's, and include headache, diarrhea, nausea, abdominal pain, and flatulence [2], [78]. There is no difference in the frequency or type of adverse events in elderly patients compared to younger patients in clinical trials [36]. However, there are other metabolic and physiologic concerns with long-term PPI therapy. A main concern with long-term PPI therapy is an increase in gastrin production, which was thought to possibly have dangerous trophic effects on the gastric mucosa [50]. There was an increase in the incidence of micronodular hyperplasia, atrophic gastritis (1% to 25%), and there was a strong association between argyrophil cell hyperplasia and degree of corpus gastritis [77]. ECL cell hyperplasia has been shown to occur after long-term exposure to gastrin, and it was hypothesized that this may lead to carcinoid tumor formation. Currently, these potential effects remain theoretical, and there have been no reports of carcinoid tumor formation or any other significant adverse effects from long-term PPI therapy.

Concern was also raised following a study by Kuipers that questioned a possible link between PPI therapy in *H. Pylori* infected individuals leading to gastric atrophy, and eventually to gastric cancer [79]. *H. Pylori* infection causes chronic gastritis, and the persistent inflammation can lead to loss of gastric glands and specialized cells. The resulting atrophic mucosa and intestinal metaplasia increase the risk of dysplasia and gastric cancer. Kuipers found that the activity of corpus gastritis increases in

H. Pylori patients treated with omeprazole. In his *H. Pylori* positive patients, corpus gastritis increased from 59 to 81% ($p = .007$), with atrophic gastritis increasing from 0 to 31%. Signs of atrophy developed in one-third of patients with *H. Pylori* after an average of 5 years of PPI treatment. He concluded that *H. Pylori* patients were at a greater risk for development of atrophic gastritis during profound acid suppression. Therefore, patients requiring long-term PPI therapy, who are infected with *H. Pylori*, should eradicate the infection prior to instituting therapy [79]. However, in this study, the PPI group was older, and glandular atrophy increases with age regardless of PPI treatment [80]. The prevalence of atrophy is twice as high in *H. Pylori* individuals 57–68 years old compared to a younger 46–56 year old group. Lundell et al found no difference in glandular atrophy between a PPI and a surgery group [80]. After further experience, most authors acknowledge that there may be a change in the pattern of *H. Pylori* gastritis during PPI therapy, but this is not thought to be clinically significant [3]. Furthermore, the FDA found that PPI's do not accelerate the development of gastric atrophy, intestinal metaplasia, or cancer, and neither the FDA nor the ACG guidelines recommend a "test and treat" strategy before starting long-term GERD therapy with a PPI [62], [80].

Proton pump inhibitors do have a potential for drug interactions, through the P-450 system [3], although this is mostly confined to omeprazole and lansoprazole. PPI elimination is not significantly affected by renal impairment or hepatic dysfunction, and no dosage adjustments are recommended, giving this medication an advantage in older individuals [2], [61], [71], [76]. There are a few potential drug interactions, including digoxin, metoprolol, calcium-channel blockkers, benzodiazepines, phenytoin, theophylline, and warfarin [3], [61], [71]. These interactions, however, have not been found to have clinical relevance.

These agents alter intragastric pH, and may potentially alter the absorption of medications including ketoconazole, ampicillin, vitamin B12, and iron salts [81]. Studies have found, however, that sufficient gastric acid secretion is produced during PPI therapy to allow for normal protein and carbohydrate digestion, iron and calcium absorption, and for the prevention of bacterial overgrowth [10], [78]. There has been much debate regarding the effects of PPI treatment on B12 levels. In studies of patients with Zollinger-Ellison syndrome, authors found that serum Vitamin B12 levels were significantly lower in patients treated with omeprazole than in patients treated with H_2B's [81]. In elderly patients with acid hyposecretion, low B12 levels can occur because of malabsorption of protein-bound B12. Hypochlorhydria also promotes bacterial overgrowth in the intestine, which may further decrease B12 levels. Many authors agree that it is reasonable to periodically monitor serum B12 levels in patients who require long-term PPI therapy, especially in elderly patients, whose serum vitamin B12 levels may be diminished at baseline [10], [78], [81].

There are several practical advantages to the use of PPI's in an elderly population. Due to the irreversible mechanism of action of these agents, they only require once a day dosing, an important consideration in the elderly [2], [3], [13]. PPI's can be mixed in a water or bicarbonate suspension, and administered by nasogastric tube without a decrease in bioavailability [31]. Omeprazole and lansoprazole caplets can be opened and taken with water, apple or orange juice, applesauce, or yogurt [10]. Pantoprazole is available by infusion, which makes it particularly useful in meeting the special needs of some elderly patients [35]. Finally, due to the chronic nature of the disease, long-term therapy is usually indicated, and medication cost is important in the elderly population [13]. PPI's are cost effective alternatives to H_2B's in patients with GERD, and PPI's as an initial therapy are less costly to treat erosive esophagitis than branded H_2B's [2].

Maintenance therapy

A high percentage of patients with GERD require long-term, possibly lifelong therapy for symptom control. Maintenance therapy keeps the symptoms under control, and prevents development of complications. After complete healing of esophagitis with omeprazole, recurrences occur in up to 82% of patients within 3–6 months if no maintenance therapy is given. Early recurrence has been associated with a hypotensive LES, long-standing symptoms, need for long-term treatment for initial symptom relief and healing, high grade esophagitis, hiatal hernia, and continued symptoms despite esophageal mucosal healing [30]. If ranitidine 150 BID was given, 42% recurred in 6 months. With 20 mg omeprazole/day, only 17% of patients had recurrences at 6 months, and 33% recurred at 2 years [71].

In a study of 5 maintenance regimens, omeprazole alone (20 mg/day) was the most effective regimen, achieving 80% remission [2]. During maintenance therapy with low-dose omeprazole, up to 8% of patients do continue to report occasional mild heartburn [77]. Continuous therapy with a PPI has been shown to maintain complete symptom relief and healing of esophagitis for up to 5 years, even in those patients refractory to H_2B's [10].

Surgery

As life expectancy increases, the number of elderly patients presenting with surgically correctable diseases will increase. However, elderly patients are often medically managed despite refractory symptoms due to fear of surgical morbidity and mortality [27]. There has been reluctance to refer elderly patients for laparoscopic surgery until complications develop, sometimes despite the presence of continued symptoms on appropriate medical therapy [82]. However, many elderly patients are not satisfied with medical therapy due to continued symptoms and the cost of medications. They may also not like the inconvenience of lifestyle modifications or are concerned with the possible effects of long-term medication usage [82].

Underlying chronic diseases are more common in the elderly, increasing their operative risk, and age above 70 is a predictor of increased postoperative complications and in-hospital mortality, as well as longer hospital stay [56]. Laparoscopic procedures have the benefit of shorter hospitalization, earlier ambulation, decreased postoperative pain, lower wound-related morbidity, and more rapid return to normal activities [56], [83]. The healthy elderly patient should not be refused surgery solely based on age but careful preoperative examination is necessary. Endoscopy needs to be performed to exclude BE with dysplasia or early cancer, and manometry can identify a weak esophageal pump. pH monitoring is needed in symptomatic individuals without esophagitis to confirm the diagnosis, and in those with intractable esophagitis to exclude pill-induced esophagitis. In patients with severe bloating, nausea, or vomiting, an emptying study can rule out gastroparesis [10].

Surgery should be considered for patients with a mechanically defective cardia (LES pressure < 6 mm Hg), short overall LES length, or short intraabdominal LES segment [50]. Surgical intervention restores the LES pressure and abolishes acid/alkaline reflux into the esophagus [84]. Other indications for surgery, include failed medical treatment, recurrence of symptoms after stopping treatment, and intolerable side effects from medical therapy [3], [28], [82]. Surgical therapy should also be considered for patients with respiratory complications such as recurrent aspiration pneumonia, laryngitis, or asthma due to GERD [13]. For asthma, around 70% have had improvement of symptoms, and there are also some reports of improvement in chronic cough [18]. The best surgical candidates are those who receive symptom relief with medication, require large doses of medication to control their symptoms, and have poorly responding aspiration symptoms [72].

Several studies have found no significant differences in intraoperative or post-operative complications between elderly and young groups [13], [27], [56], [82]. The laparoscopic procedure has a morbidity rate of 8–20% and a mortality rate of less than 1% [13]. Mortality rate does not differ by age group [82]. The mean hospital stay, reported in several studies, is 2 days in an elderly population [56], [82]. A summary of efficacy by Richardson found an 85–95% success rate, with up to 93% having no heartburn or regurgitation one year post-op [28]. Surgical follow-up studies have claimed symptom resolution in 77–97% of cases and healing of esophagitis in 75–90% [6], [13], [27]. Trus et al found that elderly and young patients were equal with respect to postoperative improvement in symptom scores [82]. Objective measurements of reflux (using 24 h pH probes), were equal in both groups, both preoperatively and postoperatively. Additionally, at 1 year post-op, total time of $\text{pH} < 4$ was similar in the 2 groups. A study with 2 years of follow-up found only 10% of patients were on PPI's after surgery for typical GERD symptoms [83]. An additional 5.7% of the study patients had required repeat fundoplication for heartburn, dysphagia, or bloating. A longer term follow-up study of fundoplication (69 months), showed disappointing recurrences in heartburn, esophagitis, and decreased LES pressure [20]. Quality of life one year after lap surgery is similar to those of normal healthy individuals [28].

Sonnenberg et al showed the cost of a Nissen procedure to be equivalent to 14.5 years of therapy with a PPI, so that medical therapy may be more cost effective [35]. However, other investigators have found that surgery becomes more cost-effective than PPI therapy between 4–10 year of treatment [28]. This will make the option of surgery even more applicable as life expectancy continues to increase.

Worries exists about surgical complications in the elderly due to emergent intervention, presence of comorbid conditions, decreased functional reserve, and severity of the primary disease. However, elective operations with careful pre-op assessment and peri-op management are safe and successful [27], [82]. In the elderly population, anti-reflux surgery is a safe, well tolerated, and efficacious alternative to continued medical therapy [27]. Weber comments on the future role of laparoscopic reflux surgery [56]. As surgeons become more experienced with these procedures, the initial hesitation in offering surgery to elderly patients is decreasing. Based on a decade of experience with laparoscopy, even octogenarians seem to benefit from these procedures. Finally, the proven efficacy and safety of this procedure needs to be communicated to PCP's to prevent delay in referral of elderly patients with persistent reflux symptoms for surgical management.

Conclusion

Gastroesophageal reflux disease is a common condition in the elderly, and will become more prevalent as the population ages. Elderly patients often do not present with the classic symptoms of heartburn and acid regurgitation, which can delay diagnosis and contribute to the development of complications. Atypical symptoms such as chest pain, pulmonary, and laryngeal symptoms are more common in this group, and reflux should be considered early in the work-up if these symptoms are present. Due to an increase in complications of reflux disease in this population, most elderly patients being evaluated for reflux symptoms should have an upper endoscopy early in the diagnostic process. There are some important age related changes in the esophagus, including decreased secondary peristalsis, decreased salivary secretion, and an increased visceral pain threshold. However, many age related changes to motility are not thought to be clinically relevant. More aggressive treatment of reflux disease may be required in the elderly population, as they are more likely to present with complicated disease, despite less severe symptoms. Age alone does not significantly impact the usage of PPI's, and these medications have excellent results in the elderly for symptom relief, healing of esophagitis, and for maintenance therapy. With the advent of laparoscopic surgery, and an increasing life expectancy, this treatment may become more common in the elderly population, as it is associated with excellent results as well as low morbidity and mortality.

References

[1] Barry PP (2000) An overview of special considerations in the evaluation and management of the geriatric patient. Am J Gastro 95: 8–10

[2] Garnett WR, Garabedian-Ruffalo SM (1997) Identification, diagnosis, and treatment of acid-related diseases in the elderly: implications for long-term care. Pharmacotherapy 17: 938–958

[3] Hungin APS, Raghunath A (2004) Managing gastro-oesophageal reflux disease in the older patient. Digestion 69 (Suppl 1): 17–24

[4] Locke GR, Talley NJ, Fett SL et al (1997) Prevalence and clinical spectrum of gastroesophageal reflux: a population-based study in Olmsted County, Minnesota. Gastroenterology 112: 1448–1456

[5] El-Serag HB, Petersen NJ, Carter J et al (2004) Gastroesophageal reflux among different racial groups in the United States. Gastroenterology 126: 1692–1699

[6] Isolauri J, Luostarinen M, Isolauri E et al (1997) Natural course of gastroesophageal reflux disease: 17–22 year follow-up of 60 patients. Am J Gastro 92: 37–41

[7] Raiha IJ, Impivaara O, Seppala M, Sourander LB (1992) Prevalence and characteristics of symptomatic gastroesophageal reflux disease in the elderly. J Am Geriat Soc 40: 1209–1211

[8] Mold JW, Reed LE, Davis AB et al (1991) Prevalence of gastroesophageal reflux in elderly patients in a primary care setting. Am J Gastro 86: 965–970

[9] Mold JW, Rankin RA (1987) Symptomatic gastroesophageal reflux in the elderly. JAGS 35: 649–659

[10] Richter JE (2000) Gastroesophageal reflux disease in the older patient: presentation, treatment, and complications. Am J Gastroenterol 95: 368–373

[11] Triadafilopoulos G, Sharma R (1997) Features of symptomatic gastroesophageal reflux disease in elderly patients. Am J Gastroenterol 92: 2007–2011

[12] Raiha I, Hietanen E, Sourander L (1991) Symptoms of gastro-oesophageal reflux disease in elderly people. Age and Ageing 20: 365–370
[13] Linder JD, Wilcox CM (2001) Acid peptic disease in the elderly. Gastro Clin N Amer 30: 363–376
[14] Collen MJ, Abduliam JD, Chen YK (1995) Gastroesophageal reflux disease in the elderly: more severe disease that requires aggressive therapy. Am J Gastro 90: 1053–1057
[15] Fass R, Pulliam G, Johnson C et al (2000) Symptom severity and oesophageal chemosensitivity to acid in older and young patients with gastro-oesophageal reflux. Age and Ageing 29: 125–130
[16] Johnson DA, Fennerty MB (2004) Heartburn severity underestimates erosive esophagitis severity in elderly patients with gastroesophageal reflux disease. Gastroenterology 126: 660–664
[17] Howard PJ, Heading RC (1992) Epidemiology of gastroesophageal reflux disease. World J Surg 16: 288–293
[18] DeVault KR (2001) Gastroesophageal reflux disease: extraesophageal manifestations and therapy. Seminars in Gastro Disease 12: 46–51
[19] DeVault KR (2003) Extraesophageal symptoms of GERD. Clev Clin J Med 70(S5): S20–S32
[20] DeVault KR, Castell DO (1994) Current diagnosis and treatment of gastroesophageal reflux disease. Mayo Clin Proc 69: 867–876
[21] Glasziou P (1998) Twenty year cough in a non-smoker. BMJ 316: 1660–1661
[22] Yamaya M, Yanai M, Ohrui T et al (2001) Interventions to prevent pneumonia among older adults. J Amer Geriatr Soc 49: 85–90
[23] Vaezi MF, Richter JE (1994) Managing gastroesophageal reflux disease in elderly patients. Clinical Geriatrics 2: 12–28
[24] Teramoto S, Ouchi Y (2000) A possible pathologic link between chronic cough and sleep apnea syndrome through gastroesophageal reflux disease in older people. Chest 117: 1215
[25] Tack J, VanTrappen G (1997) The aging oesophagus. Gut 41: 422–424
[26] Plant RL (1998) Anatomy and physiology of swallowing in adults and geriatrics. Otol Clin N Amer 31: 477–488
[27] Allen R, Rappaport W, Hixson L et al (1991) Referral patterns and the results of antireflux operations in patients more than sixty years of age. Gynecol Obstetrics Surg 173: 359–362
[28] Falk GW, Richter JE (1998) Reflux disease and barrett's esophagus. Endoscopy 30: 61–72
[29] Middlemiss C (1997) Gastroesophageal reflux disease: a common condition in the elderly. Nurse Practitioner 22: 51–59
[30] Kahrilas PJ (2003) GERD pathogenesis, pathophysiology, and clinical manifestations. Clev Clin J Med 70(S5): S4–S19
[31] Katz PO (1998) Gastroesophageal reflux disease. JAGS 46: 1558–1565
[32] Bardan E, Xie P, Brasseur J et al (2000) Effect of ageing on the upper and lower oesophageal sphincters. Euro J Gastroenterol Hepatol 12: 1221–1225
[33] Xie P, Ren J, Bardan E et al (1997) Frequency of gastroesophageal reflux events induced by pharyngeal water stimulation in young and elderly subjects. Am J Physiol Gastro-Liver Physiol 35: G233–G237
[34] Reynolds JC (1996) Influence of pathophysiology, severity, and cost on the medical management of gastroesophageal reflux disease. Am J Health-Syst Pharm 53: S5–S12
[35] Ramirez FC (2000) Diagnosis and treatment of gastroesophageal reflux disease in the elderly. Clev Clin J Med 67: 755–765
[36] James OFW, Parry-Billings KS (1994) Comparison of omeprazole and histamine H_2-receptor antagonists in the treatment of elderly and young patients with reflux oesophagitis. Age and Ageing 23: 121–126
[37] Hurwitz A, Brady DA, Schaal SE et al (1997) Gastric acidity in older adults. JAMA 278: 659–662
[38] Orr WC, Chen CL, Sloan S (2001) The role of age and salivation in acid clearance in symptomatic patients with gastro-oesophageal reflux disease. Aliment Pharmacol Ther 15: 1385–1388
[39] El-Serag HB, Sonnenberg A (1997) Associations between different forms of gastro-oesophageal reflux disease. Gut 41: 594–599
[40] Zhu H, Pace F, Sangaletti O, Bianchi Porro G (1993) Features of symptomatic gastroesophageal reflux in elderly patients. Scand J Gastroenterol 28: 235–238
[41] Sonnenberg A, Steinkamp U, Weise A et al (1982) Salivary secretion in reflux esophagitis. Gastroenterology 83: 889–895
[42] Lasch H, Castell DO, Castell JA (1997) Evidence for diminished visceral pain with aging: studies using graded intraesophageal balloon distension. Amer J Physiol 272: G1–G3
[43] Ali Kahn T, Shragge BW, Crispin JS, Lind JF (1977) Esophageal motility in the elderly. Digestive Dis 22: 1049–1054
[44] Eastwood GL (1984) GI problems in the elderly. Geriatrics 39: 59–60, 64, 69–80 passim
[45] Orr WC, Chen CL (2002) Aging and neural control of the GI tract IV. Clinical and physiological aspects

of gastrointestinal motility and aging. Am J Physiol Gastrointest Liver Physiol 283: G1226–G1231
[46] Shaker R, Staff D (2001) Esophageal disorders in the elderly. Gastroenterol Clin N Amer 30: 335–361
[47] Ferriolli E, Oliveira RB, Matsuda NM et al (1998) Aging, esophageal motility, and gastroesophageal reflux. J Amer Geriat Soc 46: 1534–1537
[48] Hollis JB, Castell DO (1974) Esophageal function in elderly men: a new look at "Presbyesophagus". Ann Intern Med 80: 371–374
[49] Shaker R, Ren J, Zamir Z et al (1994) Effect of aging, position, and temperature on the threshold volume triggering pharyngeal swallows. Gastroenterology 107: 396–402
[50] DeVault KR, Castell DO (1995) Guidelines for the diagnosis and treatment of gastroesophageal reflux disease. Arch Intern Med 155: 2165–2173
[51] Fass R, Sampliner RE, Mackel C et al (1993) Age- and gender-related differences in 24-hour esophageal pH monitoring of normal subjects. Digest Dis Sci 38: 1926–1928
[52] Patti MG, Diener U, Tamburini A et al (2001) Role of esophageal function tests in diagnosis of gastroesophageal reflux disease/Digest Dis Sci 46: 597–602
[53] Jacobsohn WZ, Levy A (1977) Endoscopy of upper gastrointestinal tract is feasible and safe in elderly patients. Geriatrics 32: 80–83
[54] Eshchar J, Pavlotzky MM, Cohen L, Tabac C (1986) Gastrointestinal endoscopy in octagenarians. J Clin Gastroenterol 8: 520–524
[55] Voutilainen M, Sipponen P, Mecklin JP et al (2000) Gastroesophageal reflux disease: prevalence, clinical, endoscopic and histopathological findings in 1,128 consecutive patients referred for endoscopy due to dyspeptic and reflux symptoms. Digestion 61: 6–13
[56] Weber DM (2003) Laparoscopic surgery: an excellent approach in elderly patients. Arch Surg 138: 1083–1088
[57] Talley NJ (1996) Modern management of dyspepsia. Aust Fam Physician 25: 47–52
[58] Fennerty MB (2003) The continuum of GERD complications. Clev Clin J Med 70(S5): S33–S50
[59] El-Serag HB, Johanson JF (2002) Risk factors for the severity of erosive esophagitis in *Helicobacter pylori* negative patients with gastroesophageal reflux disease. Scand J Gastro 8: 899–904
[60] Avidan B, Sonnenber A, Schnell TG, Sontag SJ (2002) Acid reflux is a poor predictor for severity of erosive reflux esophagitis. Digest Dis Sci 47: 2565–2573
[61] Whitaker M (2002) Proton pump inhibitors in the elderly population. Euro J Gastroenterol Hepatol 14 (S1): S5–S9
[62] Falk GW (2001) The possible role of *Helicobacter pylori* in GERD. Sem Gastro Dis 12: 186–195
[63] Marks Rd, Richter JE, Rizzo J et al (1994) Omeprazole versus H_2-receptor antagonists in treating patients with peptic stricture and esophagitis. Gastroenterology 106: 907–915
[64] Lord RVN, Frommer DJ, Inder S et al (2000) Prevalence of helicobacter pylori infection in 160 patients with barrett's oesophagus or barrett's adenocarcinoma. Aust N Z J Surg 70: 26–33
[65] Eloubeidi MA and Provenzale D (2001) Clinical and demographic predictors of barrett's esophagus among patients with gastroesophageal reflux disease. J Clin Gastroenterol 33: 306–309
[66] Cameron AJ (1997) Epidemiology of columnar-lined esophagus and adenocarcinoma. Gastro Clinics N Am 26: 487–494
[67] Cameron AJ, Lomboy CT (1992) Barrett's esophagus: age, prevalence, and extent of columnar epithelium. Gastroenterology 103: 1241–1245
[68] Dixon MF, Neville PM, Mapstone NP et al (2001) Bile reflux gastritis and barrett's oesophagus: further evidence of a role for duodenogastro-oesophageal reflux? Gut 49: 359–363
[69] Grade A, Pulliam G, Johnson C et al (1997) Reduced chemoreceptor sensitivity in patients with barrett's esophagus may be related to age and not to the presence of barrett's epithelium. Am J Gastro 92: 2040–2043
[70] Shaheen N, Ransohoff DF (2002) Gastroesophageal reflux, barrett esophagus, and esophageal cancer. JAMA 287: 1982–1985
[71] Sontag SJ (1990) The medical management of reflux esophagitis – role of antacids and acid inhibition. Gastro Clin N Amer 19: 683–712
[72] Mullick T, Richter JE (2000) Chronic GERD-strategies to relieve symptoms and manage complications. Geriatrics 55: 28–43
[73] Maton PN (2003) Profile and assessment of GERD pharmacotherapy. Clev Clin J Med 70(S5): S51–S70
[74] Lipsy RJ, Fennerty MB, Fagan TC (1990) Clinical review of histamine$_2$ receptor antagonists. Arch Intern Med 150: 745–751
[75] Fackler WK, Ours TM, Vaezi MF, Richter JE (2002) Long-term effect of H_2RA therapy on nocturnal gastric acid breakthrough. Gastroenterololgy 122: 625–632
[76] Avner DL (2000) Clinical experience with pantoprazole in gastroesophageal reflux disease. Clin Therapeut 22: 1169–1185
[77] Klinkenberg-Knol EC, Festen HPM, Jansen JBMJ et al (1994) Long-term treatment with omeprazole for

refractory reflux esophagitis: efficacy and safety. Ann Int Med 121: 161–167

[78] Garnett WR (1998) Considerations for long-term use of proton-pump inhibitors. Am J Health-Syst Pharm 55: 2268–2279

[79] Kuipers EJ, Lundell L, Klinkenberg-Knol EC et al (1996) Atrophic gastritis and *Helicobacter pylori* infection in patients with reflux esophagitis treated with omeprazole or fundoplication. NEJM 334: 1018–1022

[80] Freston JW (2001) Should we eradicate *Heliobacter pylori* before long term antireflux therapy. Gut 2001 (Nov) 49(5): 616–617

[81] Termanini B, Gibril F, Sutliff VE et al (1998) Effect of long-term gastric acid suppressive therapy on serum vitamin B_{12} levels in patients with zollinger-ellison syndrome. Amer J Med 104: 422–430

[82] Trus TL, Laycock WS, Wo JM et al (1998) Laparoscopic antireflux surgery in the elderly. Am J Gastro 93: 351–353

[83] Papasavas PK, Keenan RJ, Yeaney WW et al (2003) Effectiveness of laparoscopic fundoplication in relieving the symptoms of gastroesophageal reflux disease (GERD) and eliminating antireflux medical therapy. Surg Endosc 17: 1200–1205

Chapter 4

GASTROESOPHAGEAL REFLUX DISEASE IN INFANTS AND CHILDREN

Seema Khan and S. R. Orenstein

Division of Pediatric Gastroenterology, University of Pittsburgh School of Medicine, Children's Hospital of Pittsburgh, Pittsburgh, PA, USA

Introduction

Gastroesophageal reflux (GER), represents the retrograde movement of gastric contents into the esophagus, and is a frequently experienced benign but symptomatic condition. At the one end of the spectrum are infants with physiologic reflux, also referred to in the United States as "happy spitters", and at the other end are children with objective pathologic sequelae comprising gastroesophageal reflux disease (GERD). GERD also has come to denote symptoms affecting quality of life even in the absence of objective damage. GERD is the most common pediatric esophageal disorder; although precise data are not available in children, GERD accounts for substantial health care costs in children, as it does in adults [1].

Epidemiology

The epidemiology of GERD in children has been studied to a limited extent due to the challenges posed by the evolving disease spectrum, lack of a diagnostic gold standard, and scarcity of incidence and prevalence data. Estimates of GERD prevalence are based on data analyzed from interviews with patients and parents of children with GERD, and vary according to the symptom frequency and severity queried. The prevalence of GERD symptoms in the general population of infants and children is in the range of 1–10%, in contrast to a prevalence of 15–20% in adults [2], [3]. In a cross sectional study of 798 infants with regurgitation but without neurological or respiratory diseases, pathologic GER was diagnosed in 11% using Rome II criteria [4]. On a cross sectional survey of 566 unselected children aged 3 to 9 years, parents reported heartburn, epigastric pain, and regurgitation in 1.8%, 7.2%, and 2.3% of them, respectively [5]. In the same study, 615 children between 10 and 17 years of age reported the symptoms 5.2%, 5%, and 8.2% of the time, suggesting that parents may underestimate their children's experiences.

Gastroesophageal reflux disease is one of the most prevalent gastrointestinal disorders in children with neurologic and chronic respiratory disorders. This association is thought to arise as a result of the provocations of the mechanisms of reflux. In neuromuscular disorders, spasticity and prolonged recumbency, and in respiratory disorders, increased abdominal to thoracic pressure gradients and decreased tone of the lower esophageal sphincter (LES) due to some of the therapies, are all predispositions to GERD.

Very low birth-weight infants with chronic lung disease are diagnosed and treated for GERD more frequently than those without lung disease [6].

Natural history

Infantile GERD is generally regarded to have a favorable natural history, with persistent symptoms in about 5% of infants by one year of age, following a peak at 4 months, and resolving in the large majority between 12 and 24 months of age [7], [8]. Epidemiological studies of the natural history of GERD and its complications in older children are scarce [9]. Unselected infants with frequent regurgitation may develop feeding problems in the subsequent year of follow-up [10]. Children with chronic respiratory and neurological diseases commonly exhibit recurrent or chronic GERD symptoms. By nine years of age, children with frequent regurgitation during infancy may be more likely to develop persistent reflux symptoms, a phenomenon exacerbated by maternal smoking and maternal reflux symptoms [8]. Children over one year of age without neurological impairment most commonly have "endoscopy-negative GERD", and their esophageal inflammation, even if present, is unlikely to deteriorate during a mean of 28 months of follow-up [11]. However, half of older children with GERD have a chronic relapsing course [12]. Adults with GERD were twice as likely to recall having at least one childhood symptom of GERD as adults without GERD, in a survey of 400 adults [13]. In an uncontrolled study of a cohort of 80 children with GERD followed up as adolescents and young adults at an average of 15 years later, 80% reported monthly reflux symptoms, and at least one third of the individuals reported use of anti-reflux medications [14]. Erosive esophagitis was present in 3 of the 14 individuals who were evaluated by an upper endoscopy.

The increasing diagnosis of GERD in older children and adolescents is a cause for speculating that GERD beginning in infancy or childhood may persist into adult years, thus predisposing to the complications of peptic strictures, Barrett's esophagus, and adenocarcinomas.

Genetics

GERD and its complications are recognized as clustering within families, suggesting a genetic background for GERD phenotypes. A gene mapped for "severe pediatric GERD" with prominent respiratory symptoms in five kindreds was localized to chromosome 13q14 [15]. Later, a genetic linkage for "infantile esophagitis" was identified at a separate locus [16]. A candidate gene approach to screen for mutations that might be causally associated with reflux suggests that a GERD1 gene on chromosome 13q14 might be located within 20 kb of SNP160 or SNP168 [17]. Due to the heterogeneity in GERD phenotypes, more than one genetic locus may be involved and might influence various of the pathophysiologic factors.

Pathophysiology

Understanding of the mechanisms underlying reflux episodes has expanded from the primitive conceptualization of the lower esophageal sphincter (LES) as hypotonic to the more complicated and accurate current model. This current model incorporates dynamic changes at the gastroesophageal junction involving transient LES relaxations (TLESRs) of a sphincter supported actively by hiatal crura which are intricately coordinated with the LES. These motor mechanisms at the gastroesophageal junction are impacted by more distal motor mechanisms, involving gastric volume–pressure relationships promoting TLESRs and reflux, and by more proximal motor mechanisms, involving esophageal clearance of the refluxed material. Sensory phenomena have been appreciated recently, both for their role in the pain symptoms of reflux (with or without esophageal inflammation) and for their role as the gastric afferent limb to the TLESR. Whether reflux produces esophagitis depends not only on the frequency and duration of the reflux episodes produced by the above mechanisms, but also on the balance between the noxiousness of the refluxate and the counteracting esophageal mucosal protective mechanisms. Current attention focuses on the genetic and environmental factors that modulate all of these pathophysiologic mechanisms and thus underlie the determination of who becomes diseased.

Anti-reflux barrier

Transient lower esophageal sphincter relaxation

Very low pressure of the LES is a prerequisite for reflux of gastric contents into the esophagus. Most reflux in infants and children, as in adults, occurs primarily in association with transient lower esophageal sphincter relaxation (TLESR), defined as an abrupt decrease in LES pressure to the level of the intragastric pressure unrelated to swallowing [18]. Premature infants as young as 26 weeks of gestational age who were diagnosed with GERD exhibited more acid reflux during TLESRs, compared with healthy controls [19]. TLESRs may be triggered by gastric distention and by increased intra-abdominal pressure [20], as occurs with straining, obesity, tight clothing, cough, and increased respiratory effort. In infants, extrinsic abdominal compression in semi-seated postures in the post-prandial period is an important factor contributing to the pathogenesis of reflux. Also important are the influences of the meal size, intragastric secretory volume, and osmolarity on the occurrence of TLESRs.

The TLESR is primarily a vagal reflex with neural pathways in the brainstem, and may be triggered by mechanoreceptor afferents upon stretching of the gastric fundus. The neuroenteric mediators responsible for inducing TLESRs include nitric oxide, vasoactive intestinal polypeptide, and cholecystokinin A, while somatostatin, gamma-amino butyric acid B ($GABA_B$), and opiates have the opposite effect. Increasing proximal gastric volumes increases the rate of TLESRs [21].

Hiatal hernia

Hiatal hernia is a fairly common finding in adults, with estimates of its prevalence ranging from 10–80%. Although widely believed to be a predisposition for reflux, it may be also be an incidental finding in asymptomatic persons [22]. Hiatal hernias have affected family members across multiple generations, leading some to suggest an autosomal dominant pattern of inheritance [23]. The diaphragmatic crura normally reinforce the LES as an anti-reflux barrier, and relax when a TLESR occurs. The lack of this reinforcement assumes significance when abrupt changes in abdominal pressure, such as during straining, overcome the LES pressure in a person with a hiatal hernia. Hiatal hernias are more prevalent in severe reflux disease, and have also been reported to be common in conditions associated with severe reflux, such as cystic fibrosis and neurological impairments [24]. Of 718 children with reflux, 6% were identified to have a hiatal hernia, and nearly a fourth of them were neurologically impaired [25]. Severe esophageal damage may occur during the prolonged esophageal acid exposure that can result from the trapping of acid in a hiatal hernia. The risk for reflux is considered to be greater with increasing size of a hiatal hernia, and complications of reflux like Barrett's esophagus are also associated with hiatal hernias [22].

Delayed gastric emptying

Delayed gastric emptying has been associated with more severe GERD in children [26]. Delayed emptying leads to gastric distention, more triggering of TLESRs, and accentuation of the volume and frequency of post-prandial reflux. Gastric emptying is influenced by the volume and osmolarity of the meal consumed; thus overeating and ingestion of fatty foods further provoke reflux. Children with cerebral palsy are considered to be more prone to reflux, due to disturbed motility, particularly gastroparesis. However, gastric emptying, measured by scintigraphy in 28 children with cerebral palsy, was not significantly different from that in a control group, and the emptying times did not correlate with GERD severity on pH monitoring [27]. Gastric fundic accommodation, the increase in gastric fundic volume in response to a meal, measured by barostat or scintigraphically, also likely impacts the occurrence of TLESRs, with greater accommodation allowing acceptance of greater volumes without provoking TLESRs. Other factors affecting intragastric pressure include obesity, tight clothing, provocative postures, straining, coughing, or wheezing.

Gastric sensorimotor aspects

In many patients including children, reflux symptoms of heartburn and chest pain correlate poorly with endoscopy findings. In the absence of erosive esophagitis, these symptoms are referred to as non-erosive reflux disease. In some of these cases, the pain of reflux disease may be associated with histologic esophagitis. In those patients lacking even microscopic inflammation, other potential explanations for the pain sensation include increased sensitivity of esophageal receptors to both nociceptive (painful) and non-painful stimuli, akin to visceral hyperalgesia causing functional pain in irritable bowel syndrome or dyspepsia. Such sensitization is proposed to be due to activation of the prostaglandin (PG) E receptor, and this may be an attractive target for treatment [28]. Studies conducted in adults with reflux demonstrate that acid infusion promotes esophageal pain hypersensitivity that is reduced by proton pump inhibition [29]. Symptoms elicited during acid infusion are also associated with increased esophageal contractility, postulated to be due to peripheral sensitization [30]. In support of a mechanism involving central sensitization of spinal afferents is the report of esophageal hypersensitivity upon duodenal acid exposure [31].

Refluxate

The pathogenicity of the refluxate is determined by the noxiousness of its constituents namely, acid, pepsin, trypsin, and bile salts. Acid in combination with pepsin has been found to be the most injurious to the esophageal mucosa. Most patients with reflux have normal gastric pH, and it has been suggested that volume rather than acidity of the refluxate may be more important in the pathogenesis of reflux. Infants, including premature infants of 24 weeks gestation, maintain that basal gastric pH below 4 from day one of life, but acid secretion is modified by neurocrine, endocrine, and paracrine pathways [32]. Severe reflux, defined by reflux index scores and esophagitis grade, in a small number of children correlated with gastric acid hypersecretion [33]. Pepsin and trypsin, being proteolytic enzymes, are directly damaging to the surface epithelium in their usual milieu, which is pH less than 4 for pepsin, and between 5 and 8 for trypsin. Increased serum pepsinogen values in neonates with upper gastrointestinal bleeding and esophageal lesions further support a pathogenetic role for pepsin [22]. Bile reflux may cause esophageal mucosal damage by rendering the membrane more permeable to acid. Simultaneous pH and bilirubin monitoring demonstrated bile and acid reflux in 9 of 13 children with severe esophagitis as graded by endoscopy [34]. Another report suggests a pathogenetic role for duodenogastric reflux, which was found to be higher in 10 patients with cystic fibrosis compared with 7 healthy controls [35]. Alterations in amino acid metabolism leading to increased esophageal mucosal taurine to serine ratio in patients with increased esophageal mucosal acid exposure may represent adaptive responses to acid reflux, and may precede esophageal inflammation [36]. Polyunsaturated fatty acids, precursors of eicosanoids, are also proposed to have a role in the pathogenesis of esophagitis [37]. In children, increased esophageal mucosal polyunsaturated fatty acids correlate positively with esophageal acid exposure but not with esophageal mucosal damage [37].

Esophageal clearance and mucosal resistance

An important line of defense against reflux is provided by effective peristalsis in coordination with swallowing; sucking appears as an integral part of this complex act in infants as early as 35 weeks of gestation. A disruption of the normal swallowing function particularly threatens the airways of fragile and physiologically immature infants with aspiration, apnea, cyanosis, and bradycardia. In older children, as in adults, upright posture confers an advantage in clearing refluxed material by the action of gravity, but this advantage is lacking in infants, who are generally recumbent in supine and semi-seated positions. Esophageal motor responses were nearly normal in response to infusion of saline in piglets with reflux, including those with esophagitis, but were impaired in response to acid infusion and influenced by acid volumes as well [38]. Primary esophageal peristalsis, initiated by swallowing, comprises 83% of all esophageal responses to reflux in infants [39]. Secondary peristalsis is induced by reflux and esophageal distention, and plays an important role in clearance during active sleep, thereby being crucial to infants who spend a great portion of time asleep. Peristaltic abnormalities may develop secondary to esophagitis; evidence for failed or hypotensive peristalsis is present in 20% of adults with mild, and 50% with severe esophagitis [40], [41]. Long lasting reflux episodes, those greater than 5 minutes, were reported to be more frequent in children with severe reflux than in those with mild reflux and controls [42]. Salivary functions include stimulation of wet swallows and the wash-down and neutralization of refluxed acid secretions. Other protective components proposed in the mucosal defense against acid reflux are prostaglandin E2 and nitric oxide, in low concentrations, but their contributions in children are poorly understood [43].

Helicobacter pylori

The role of H. pylori in relation to GERD symptoms and pathogenesis remains controversial. A recent prospective study compared symptoms before and after H. pylori eradication in 95 children. Symptoms remained unchanged, and were independent of H. pylori status [44]. Another study found that neither the diagnosis nor the severity of peptic esophagitis in H. pylori-infected, neurologically-impaired children was influenced by H. pylori eradication [45].

Clinical presentations

Esophageal presentations attributed to GERD vary according to the age of the patient, and include regurgitation, irritability, arching, and feeding aversion in infants, and vomiting, chest pain, heartburn, and abdominal pain in older children. Circumstantial evidence strongly suggests a relationship between reflux and a variety of extraesophageal presentations. These extraesophageal manifestations involve the airways or dental erosions. The former are best appreciated in light of the intricate coordination of the intimately related human respiratory and the digestive tracts, especially in fragile infants [46]. The relationship between reflux and respiratory symptoms is bi-directional; reflux may precipitate or exacerbate respiratory disease, and vice versa.

Esophageal

Vomiting and regurgitation

Regurgitation and vomiting are the most easily recognizable symptoms of pediatric reflux. Episodes are usually effortless, non-bilious and post-prandial. It is usually the quantity and type of emesis that differentiates physiologic reflux in "happy spitters" from symptomatic reflux in infantile GERD. Some children have persistent or intermittent symptoms beyond the first year of life. Projectile non-bilious emesis in the first few weeks of life may mimic hypertrophic pyloric stenosis but simply represent reflux, whereas bilious emesis mandates evaluation for intestinal obstruction.

Irritability and pain

Irritability coupled with arching in infants is thought to be a nonverbal equivalent of heartburn and chest pain reported by older children with reflux, and strongly believed to be clinical manifestations of esophagitis. However, these symptoms may correlate poorly with gross and microscopic findings in the esophageal mucosa. Infant crying has been demonstrated in association with reflux episodes during video and esophageal pH probe monitoring [47]. In patients with non-erosive reflux disease and normal esophageal histology, these symptoms are speculated to represent heightened sensory perception or visceral hyperalgesia. An important presentation overlapping with GERD, particularly in infants, is cow's milk allergy; studies report the two conditions co-existing in 42–58% children [48], [49]. Generally, in all children with the aforementioned symptoms, other causes of esophagitis, such as eosinophilic or infectious esophagitis, and esophageal motility disorders, warrant consideration.

Failure to thrive

Infants and older children with reflux are frequently reported to suffer from failure to thrive, but preterm infants are relatively protected, probably as a result of special care in intensive care units [50]. In a retrospective review of 295 children with clinical presentations suspicious for reflux, 72.5% (mean age four years) had at least one positive diagnostic test, and these children had a higher frequency of failure to thrive compared to those with negative testing for GERD [51]. Severe reflux may predispose to feeding refusal, and, in turn, to inadequate caloric intake, due to pain provoked by esophageal acid exposure during meals. In addition, loss of nutrients and calories due to emesis may predispose a child to poor growth. As an iatrogenic factor, the use of restricted diets to treat overlapping food sensitivities could also impair oral feeding abilities and contribute to poor growth.

Extra-esophageal

Apnea

Apnea is a frequently cited extraesophageal manifestation of reflux in infants, but the causal relationship is controversial, despite being examined by multiple investigators. Most episodes of apnea of prematurity occur in the post-prandial period, and likely follow bouts of regurgitation, and yet studies using impedance and monitoring cardiorespiratory events have been contradictory [52], [53]. In 21 infants with a history of intermittent reflux and apnea, 81% of apneic events did not follow episodes of reflux [52]. However, using pH and impedance testing in 22 infants with a history of irregular breathing and reflux, 29.7% (49 of 165) apneic episodes were associated with reflux, though only 22.4% of these were related to acid reflux [53], (*Fig. 1*) [54]. Apnea related to reflux has been explained on the basis of a laryngeal chemoreflex causing respiratory pauses and laryngospasm [54], but might also be due to prolongation of normal mechanoreceptor-induced glottic closure [55], or to immaturity of pharyngo-esophageal clearance functions.

Otolaryngologic

Gastroesophageal reflux has been associated with several important otolaryngologic manifestations, including stridor, chronic cough, hoarseness, and "lump in the throat" [56]. Several laryngoscopic and bronchoscopic findings have been described as predictive of reflux. These include post glottic edema, vocal cord edema, nodules, arytenoid edema, tracheal cobblestoning, and sub-glottic stenosis [57]. Significant associations in adults may be limited to posterior commisure erythema (in 76% of GERD, 0% of normals), vocal cord erythema (in 70% of GERD, 2% of normals), and arytenoid medial wall erythema (in 82% of GERD, 30% of normals) [58]. Airway abnormalities such as tracheomalacia and laryngomalacia are often diagnosed in infants and children with stridor, and notably associated with laryngopharyngeal reflux [59], [60], though it is possible that the airway obstruction promotes the reflux. The prevalence of reflux as diagnosed by barium studies and pH metry was 70% in 54 children with laryngotracheomalacia compared with 39% in a control group. Gas reflux episodes with mild acidity have been demonstrated in adults with reflux laryngitis on concurrently performed impedance and pH studies, suggesting a contrast in the quality and quantity of refluxate involved in esophageal and extraesophageal presentations [61]. In 20 adults with laryngitis, a three month open label trial of high dose omeprazole (60 mg/day) resulted in significant improvement in laryngoscopic findings, including in all those patients who had a positive pharyngeal pH study. Symptoms of laryngitis and quality of voice as outcomes did not improve significantly [62]. In 90 of 100 children diagnosed with GERD based on the results of pH metry, the common laryngeal abnormalities were erythema and edema of the posterior laryngeal mucosa, vocal nodules and granulomas. A significant improvement in voice quality and laryngeal status occurred in those with laryngeal abnormalities in response to 12 weeks of anti-reflux therapy [63]. Possible mechanisms underlying these associations are neural reflexes mediated by intraesophageal acid, stimulation of laryngeal chemoreceptors, aspiration, and direct acid related inflammation [64]. Exacerbation of reflux possibly occurs as a consequence of negative intrapleural pressure and altered thoraco-abdominal pressures that allow acid to breach the anti-reflux barrier [65]. In a case-control study, neurologically normal children with GERD were found to be significantly more often affected by sinusitis, laryngitis, asthma, pneumonia, and

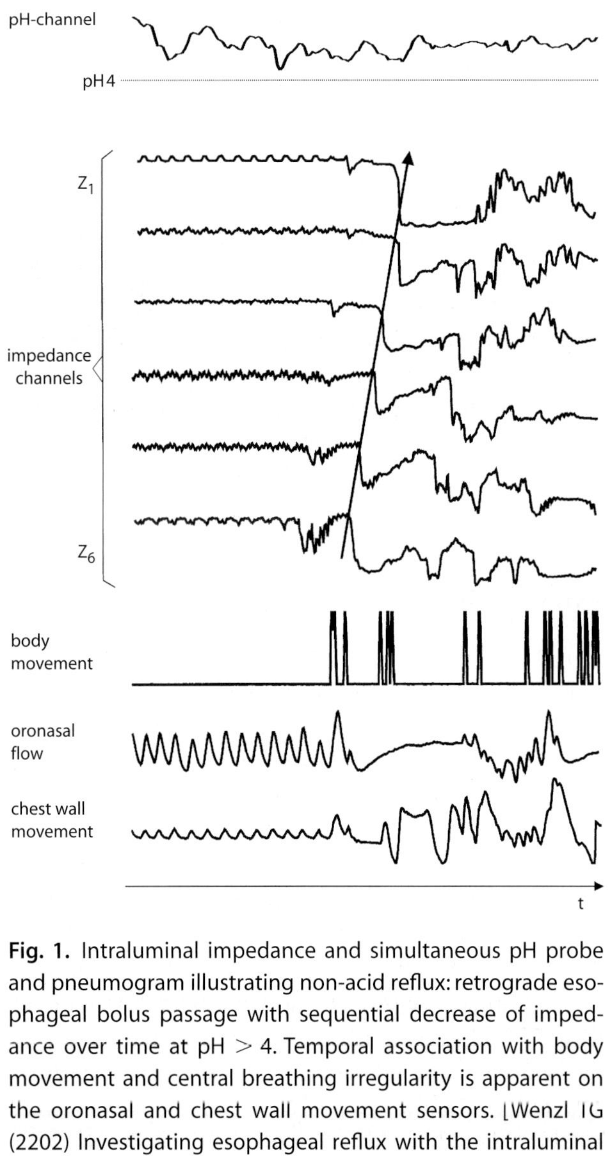

Fig. 1. Intraluminal impedance and simultaneous pH probe and pneumogram illustrating non-acid reflux: retrograde esophageal bolus passage with sequential decrease of impedance over time at pH > 4. Temporal association with body movement and central breathing irregularity is apparent on the oronasal and chest wall movement sensors. [Wenzl TG (2202) Investigating esophageal reflux with the intraluminal impedance technique. J Pediatr Gastroenterol Nutr 34(3): 261–268]

bronchiectasis, but not by otitis media, than those without GERD [66]. Esophageal clearance was significantly delayed in 89 children with chronic respiratory symptoms when compared with those with primarily gastrointestinal symptoms (n = 83) or mixed symptoms (n = 64) in a study determining the severity of acid reflux by pH metry [67].

Asthma

Asthma and reflux commonly co-exist, but the contributions of each to the pathogenesis and symptoms of the other remain debatable, mainly due to differences in the selection criteria of study participants, and outcome measures evaluated [68]. Adult asthmatics report reflux symptoms more frequently than non-asthmatics, and experience more nocturnal awakening in relation to their late eating habits [69]. Children with asthma experience a high prevalence of reflux [70]–[72], but both are common conditions and thus could be associated by a chance in some children. One recent study described a 75% prevalence of reflux in 36 asthmatic children; reflux episodes were more frequent in upright versus supine positioning, but the overall reflux duration was not significantly different between positions [73]. Nuclear scintigraphy, used to detect clinical correlation between reflux symptoms and asthma episodes in asthmatic children, revealed scintigraphic evidence of reflux in 10 of 26 (38.5%) with GER symptoms, compared with 23 of 100 (23%) children without GER symptoms, but did not provide support for a direct causal effect of reflux on asthma [74]. A randomized controlled trial, rare in pediatric reflux-respiratory disease literature, evaluated asthma outcome in 37 children (10–20 years old, mean 14 years), using ranitidine for only four weeks as the intervention. A positive outcome was reported for nocturnal asthma symptoms but not for pulmonary functions [75]. Proposed mechanisms for reflux-induced asthma symptoms are acid-stimulated vagal nerve afferents triggering bronchospasm, or aspiration of gastric contents.

Dental erosions

A limited number of studies have examined the role of acid reflux in producing dental erosions in children [76], [77]. In 37 children evaluated for GERD, 20 of them were identified to have dental erosions, and all of them also had an endoscopic diagnosis of GERD [77]. As in adults, dental erosions in association with acid reflux affect the posterior dentition along the lingual surfaces. Ingestion of acidic (juices) and caffeinated beverages, consumption of ascorbic acid, and poor oral hygiene are other contributory factors.

Sandifer's syndrome

Sandifer's syndrome is characterized by hyperextended posturing involving the head, neck and upper torso. Originally the syndrome was thought to be a manifestation of reflux accompanied by hiatal herniation, but subsequent reports have identified cases in children without a diagnosis of a hiatal hernia [78], [79]. Many of these children are also diagnosed to have a neurological disorder. The majority of children with Sandifer's syndrome respond well to anti-reflux therapy.

Complicated GERD

The important esophageal complications of chronic reflux are strictures, Barrett's esophagus, and adenocarcinoma. Aggressive medical management, preferably with proton pump inhibitors, and close follow-up, using tests to assess symptoms and severity of reflux, are warranted in complicated GERD. Surgical management is contemplated in patients who remain unresponsive to medical therapy.

Strictures

Exposure of the esophagus to acid and perhaps to pepsin is crucial to the pathogenesis of reflux strictures; hiatal hernia and esophageal dysmotility are other risk factors [80]. Reflux strictures are typically located in the distal third of the esophagus, and should be distinguished from congenital esophageal stenosis and other types of strictures: caustic (generally more proximal), eosinophilic, postoperative/anastomotic, following radiation therapy or sclerotherapy, or (rarely in children) malignant. Esophageal mucosal biopsies obtained below the stricture help to confirm the diagnosis of reflux esophagitis and exclude eosinophilic esophagitis, Barrett's esophagus, or malignancy. Reflux strictures are treated with a series of dilations in conjunction with potent antireflux therapy [81]. Surgical resection or strictureplasty are reserved for recalcitrant strictures [82].

Barrett's esophagus
Barrett's esophagus, a rare diagnosis in children, is known to occur with long-standing acid exposure, and in association with cystic fibrosis, severe mental retardation, and repaired esophageal atresia [83], [84]. Genetic predispositions, prolonged duration of esophageal acid exposure, more severe nocturnal symptoms, and a reduced sensitivity to acid are implicated in the causation of Barrett's esophagus. Normal esophageal squamous epithelium is replaced by intestinal columnar metaplasia with goblet cells; the metaplasia is recognized in the distal esophagus as salmon-colored tongues of tissue projecting proximally into the paler pink esophagus. Guidelines for screening and surveillance have been proposed to help identify patients with Barrett's esophagus who may progress to develop dysplasia and adenocarcinoma [85].

Adenocarcinoma
Adenocarcinoma is extremely rare in childhood, but it does occur and should be sought in those with Barrett's esophagus. In an 11 year-old patient, the diagnosis of Barrett's esophagus was reported to progress to adenocarcinoma [86]. The risk of developing esophageal adenocarcinoma increases with hiatal hernia size, Barrett's esophagus length, and acid reflux severity.

Diagnosis

The diagnosis of uncomplicated esophageal reflux is usually established on the basis of a good history, and a thorough examination, with attention to the child's growth, nutritional, respiratory, neurological, and atopic status. A validated questionnaire has been developed for symptom assessment in infants and translated into multiple languages; others designed specifically for older children are now in use in epidemiological studies but must be further tested for reliability and validity [87], [88]. Complicated, unresponsive, and atypical presentations of GERD are indications for specialized investigations such as those discussed in the following section.

Endoscopy
An upper endoscopy, particularly when supplemented by histology, is the most accurate method of demonstrating esophageal damage by reflux, and for differentiating GERD from other diagnostic possibilities (*Fig. 2a–c*). It is performed as an outpatient procedure, and is less cumbersome than a 24-hour pH metry. Histologic abnormalities may be present in biopsies sampled from grossly normal esophageal mucosa. A review of endoscopic evaluation of reflux in 402 neurologically normal children, between 18 months and 25 years of age and without congenital esophageal disease, revealed erosive esophagitis in more than one-third, strictures in 1 to 2%, and suspected Barrett's esophagus (but without histologic confirmation) in nearly 3%.

Histology
A diagnostic upper endoscopy in children is almost always supplemented by distal esophageal biopsies. Biopsies at two levels are important to demonstrate differential eosinophilia in eosinophilic esophagitis. Histologic findings of reflux esophagitis are epithelial hyperplasia (the upper limit of normal basal layer thickness and papillary height in infants is 25% and 53%, respectively [89]), intraepithelial inflammation, vascular dilatation in papillae, balloon cells, and ulceration (*Fig. 3a–c*) [90]. Due to the often superficial, fragmented, and randomly oriented nature of biopsies in children, cellular inflammatory infiltrate may be the only recognizable finding [91]. Neutrophils are seen in about 20% or less of pediatric cases of reflux esophagitis, appearing in the most severe cases, and are hence not a sensitive marker. Eosinophils are not normally present in the epithelium of young children and can be indicators of GERD, but in concentrations greater than 20/high-power field (hpf) are likely to represent eosinophilic esophagitis, making them nonspecific for GERD. A few intraepithelial lymphocytes ("squiggle cells") are normally found, but > 6 squiggle cells/hpf indicate reflux esophagitis [90].

Esophageal pH-probe monitoring
Esophageal pH monitoring (EpHM) is widely accepted as a safe and reliable method for detecting acid reflux. Perhaps its greatest utilities are in clarifying the relationship between reflux and discrete respiratory events such as apnea (with pneumogram), in quantifying acid reflux in extraesophageal GERD, and in assessing the efficacy of antisecretory therapy. In a retrospective analysis of children evaluated for GERD, EpHM detected reflux episodes at a higher rate com-

pared with barium examinations (83% versus 43%), and showed a lower false negative rate (7% versus 48%) [92]. Its utility in infants and children may be limited in the presence of structural upper airway or GI anomalies, and due to the buffering effect of non-acidic infant formula; probe placement, patient positioning, and dietary factors may contribute to day-to-day variability in pH-metry results [93]. Parents of children undergoing pH studies also perceive changes in their child's feeding pattern and activities during EpHM investigations, but the large majority regarded it as a well-tolerated test [94]. The utility of three different formulas to calculate pH probe placement based on patient height has been the subject of recent analyses [95], [96]. Fluoroscopy and, rarely in pediatrics, manometry are also used to verify probe positioning.

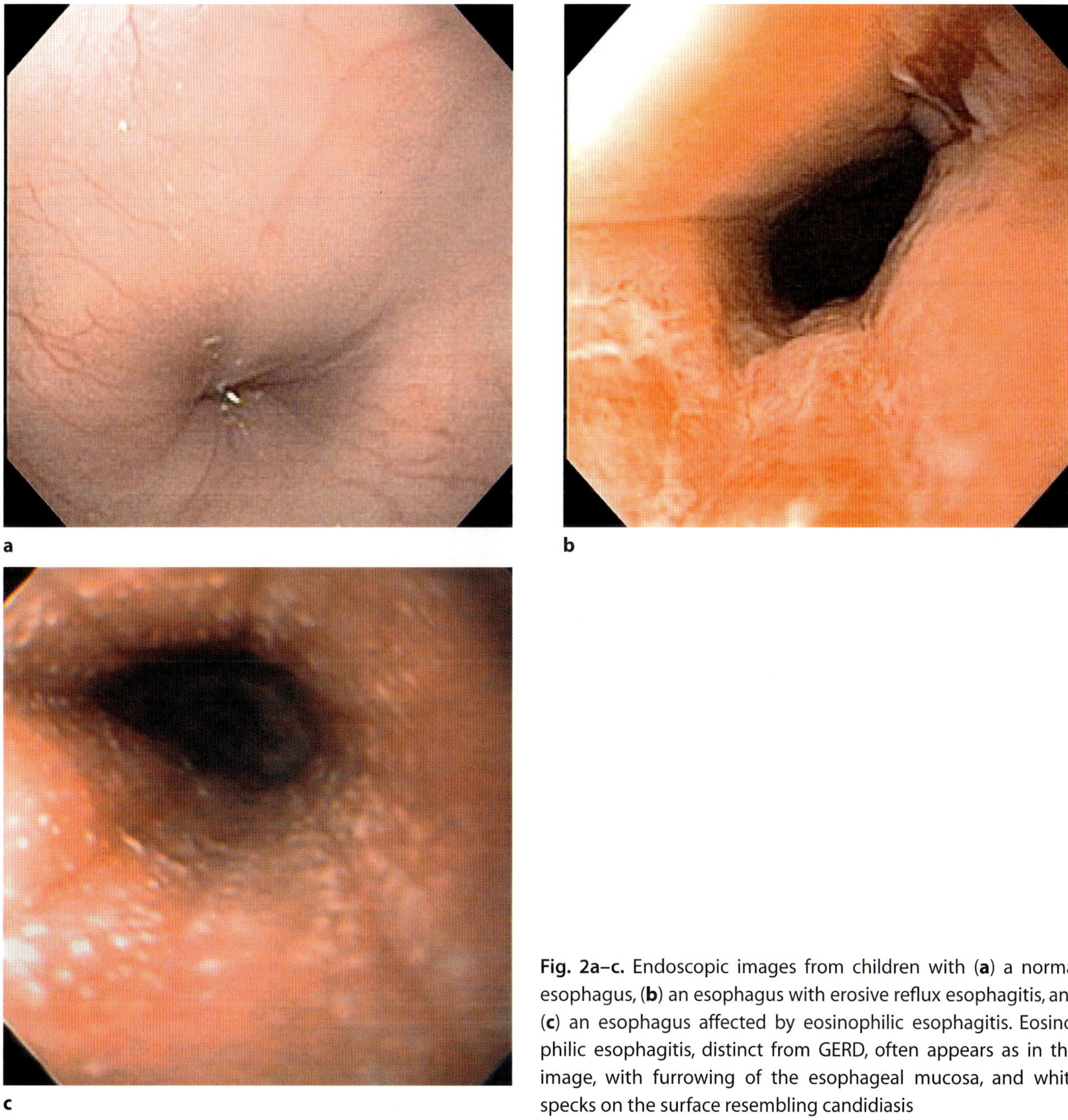

Fig. 2a–c. Endoscopic images from children with (**a**) a normal esophagus, (**b**) an esophagus with erosive reflux esophagitis, and (**c**) an esophagus affected by eosinophilic esophagitis. Eosinophilic esophagitis, distinct from GERD, often appears as in this image, with furrowing of the esophageal mucosa, and white specks on the surface resembling candidiasis

Conventional pH metry normative data includes reflux index (the percentage of time during a 24-hour day that the esophageal pH is <4), number of episodes and number of episodes longer than five minutes. Scores have been developed to associate reflux with respiratory disease, but are not widely used currently [97], [98]. Symptom association with reflux episodes comprises a frequently used function of EpHM [99], [100]. Dual pH monitoring, with the upper probe in upper esophagus, pharynx, or even the airways, is suggested as a potentially useful technique in patients with reflux and airway symptoms, but the limited pediatric data are conflicting and warrant further validation [101], [102]. The value of combining pH metry with impedance to improve the diagnostic yield and to clarify the pathogenetic role of non-acid reflux is now being explored in infants and children. [103], [104]. An exciting development is the application of the Bravo pH capsule system in children with GERD, sparing the patient the discomfort of an indwelling transnasal probe; this technique has the potential for higher quality data acquisition than conventional pH metry [105].

Fluoroscopy

Fluoroscopic evaluation of swallowing and of the upper gastrointestinal tract is often important in the evaluation of the child presenting with obstructive gastrointestinal symptoms or chronic respiratory symptoms. It may also disclose other diagnoses: pyloric stenosis, malrotation, achalasia, and strictures. It has a low sensitivity and specificity for diagnosing reflux and is only a brief snapshot of overall reflux [92]. Barium esophagography or specialized swallowing studies may be useful in identifying abnormalities of pharyngeal, laryngeal, or upper esophageal

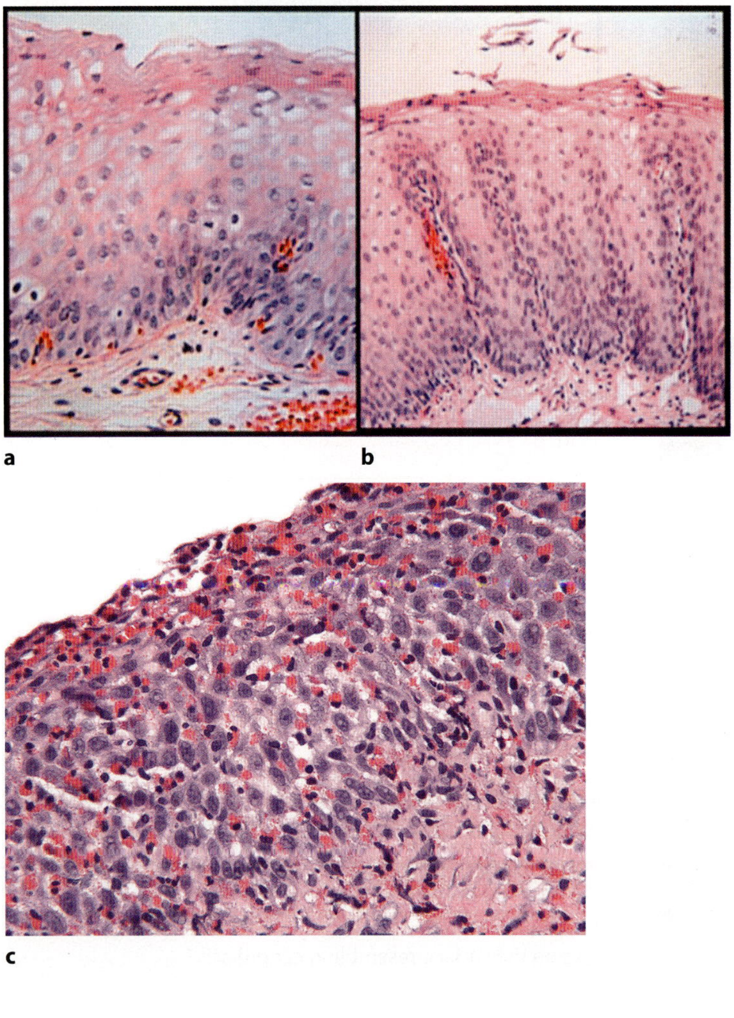

a b c

Fig. 3a–c. Biopsies of the esophagus from children with (**a**) normal histology, (**b**) morphometric changes of reflux manifest in papillary lengthening and basal layer thickening, and (**c**) eosinophilic esophagitis. Extensive esophageal epithelial eosinophilia, as shown in this image (>20eos/hpf), along with papillary elongation and basal layer hyperplasia, constitute the histological features of eosinophilic esophagitis.

function that may prompt aspiration during swallowing and during reflux.

Nuclear scintigraphy
Scintigraphy, also referred to as "a milk scan", is generally performed in infants and children suspected of reflux to gather information regarding reflux-associated aspiration, and to quantify gastric emptying times. The study employs liquid (generally in infants) or solid meals labeled with technetium 99m – for its short (6 hour) half-life and limited radiation burden. It offers the advantage of detecting non-acid reflux in the post-prandial period, but is technically demanding and restrictive for a child. Scintigraphy has a sensitivity of 79% and specificity of 93%, when pH metry is used to define reflux [106]–[108].

Impedance
The multiple intraluminal impedance technique is a valuable tool for diagnosing reflux, and its relationship to respiratory events, particularly in infants, in whom post-prandial reflux is non-acidic (*Fig. 1*) [54]; it also evaluates esophageal clearance and swallowing. In an early report of its use in infants, the sensitivity of impedance was 98.7%, compared with 18.9% for pH metry in identifying all reflux [109]. Despite time-consuming and visually complex analysis, impedance studies are gradually being applied to the evaluation of pediatric GERD, and its therapies [53], [104], [110].

Tests for reflux aspiration
The identification of lipid-laden macrophages in tracheal aspirates is generally considered a useful marker for aspiration but lacks the sensitivity or specificity for it to be considered a highly reliable test [111], [112]. Scores are computed, based on the number of lipid-laden macrophages in a given sample, and used to grade the probability of aspiration. Moderate to large number of macrophages may imply aspiration but does not differentiate between reflux- and swallow-related aspiration. Pepsin in tracheal aspirates, sputum, and saliva has been proposed as a more reliable and specific test of reflux aspiration. A strong association has been reported between positive tracheal pepsin assays in children with reflux or respiratory symptoms, particularly in those with coexisting symptoms [113], [114].

Management

Conservative anti-reflux therapy
Aspects of anti-reflux conservative therapy recommended for adults may also be applied to older children and adolescents with GERD, but must be tailored to infants because of unique developmental and maturational factors.

For infants, who are mostly supine, the gastroesophageal junction is constantly "under water," and accessible to reflux of gastric contents. Although prone position has been shown to reduce reflux compared with supine or seated infant positions, support for instituting such measures has been less than enthusiastic due to the link between prone position and sudden infant death syndrome. Efforts to minimize physically engaging and excitable situations in the post-prandial period may also help in reducing reflux, because of the increase in regurgitant reflux promoted by abdominal contractions [115]. Effective parental reassurance and telephone conversations aimed at educating parents regarding reflux go a long way in symptom resolution for a large number of infants [116]. Thickening of feeds is a first line anti-reflux therapy in infants [104], [117], [118]. Formula viscosity may be increased either by adding rice cereal to feeds or by using commercially available pre-thickened (with rice starch or locust bean gum) anti-regurgitant formulas. This intervention reduces regurgitation, decreases crying, and increases sleep time [118], [119]. Adding 15 mL rice cereal per 30 ml of milk formula increases the caloric density by 50% and may induce constipation. Pre thickened or home thickened formulas are comparable in their anti-regurgitation efficacy, but the former may be better tolerated [119]. Frequent and small volume feedings, as well as lower osmolality feedings, have all been advocated as beneficial to infants with reflux [120].

Pharmacotherapy
Pharmacotherapeutic agents encompass anti-secretory agents, antacids, barrier agents, and prokinetic agents (Table 1). Anti-secretory agents are the first line of pharmacotherapy because they are most efficacious in treating acid related symptoms and complications of reflux. Anti-secretory agents include histamine-2 receptor antagonists (H2RAs) and proton pump inhibitors (PPIs). PPIs have assumed a significant position in management of severe, complicated and extraesoph-

ageal reflux presentations, and have the potential for obviating the need for anti-reflux surgical procedures. Data on the efficacy, safety, tolerability, and dosage for omeprazole and lansoprazole in children are available [121], [122]. Important developments pertaining to the subject include approval of PPIs for pediatric use, as well as the availability of new formulations of both these drugs that are expected to simplify treatment options and compliance. Further information on safety and efficacy of H2RAs is also being gleaned in children, which may prove useful because of their efficacy in fasting and nocturnal reflux, despite their generally lower potency and tendency toward tachyphylaxis [123]. Most studies, at least in older children, have found PPIs to be more efficacious in symptom relief and healing of esophagitis compared with H2RAs, antacids, or barrier agents [121], [122]. The daily doses of PPIs administered to children are higher on a weight basis than the standard adult dosages.

A failure to respond to optimal doses of PPIs should raise considerations of incorrect diagnosis, improper administration (should be given just before

Table 1. Anti-reflux pharmacotherapy, oral dosages, and side-effects. AC = ante-cibum; PC = post-cibum; HS = hour of sleep

Prokinetics		
Metoclopramide	0.1 mg/kg/dose qid: AC, HS	Drowsiness, restlessness, dystonia, gynecomastia, galactorrhea
Erythromycin	3–5 mg/kg/dose qid: AC, HS	Diarrhea,vomiting, cramps, antibiotic effect, pyloric stenosis
Domperidone	Pediatric doses not defined	Hyperprolactinemia, dry mouth, rash, headache, diarrhea, nervousness
Bethanechol	0.1–0.3 mg/kg/dose qid: AC, HS	Hypotension, bronchospasm, salivation, cramps, blurred vision, bradycarida
H2-receptor antagonists		
Cimetidine	10–15 mg/kg/dose qid: AC, HS	Headache, confusion, pancytopenia, gynecomastia
Ranitidine	3–5 mg/kg/dose bid-tid: AC, HS	Headache, rash, constipation, diarrhea, malaise, elevated transaminases, dizziness, thrombocytopenia
Famotidine	0.5 mg/kg/dose bid: AC	Headache, dizziness, constipation, nausea, diarrhea
Nizatidine	Pediatric doses not defined	Headache, dizziness, constipation, diarrhea nausea, anemia, urticaria,
Proton pump inhibitors		
Omeprazole	0.7–3.3 mg/kg/d, 1–2 div doses: AC	Headache, rash, diarrhea, nausea, abdominal pain, vitamin B 12 deficiency
Lansoprazole	15 mg/d (≤ 30 kg); 30 mg/d (>30 kg): AC	Headache, diarrhea, abdominal pain, nausea
Pantoprazole	Pediatric doses not defined	Headache, diarrhea, abdominal pain, nausea, flatulence
Rabeprazole	Pediatric doses not defined	Headache, diarrhea, abdominal pain, nausea
Esomeprazole	Pediatric doses not defined	Headache, diarrhea, nausea, abdominal pain, flatulence, dry mouth, constipation
Barrier agents		
Sucralfate	40–80 mg/kg/d qid: AC, HS	Vertigo, constipation, dry mouth, aluminum toxicity, decreases absorption of concurrently administered drugs
Sodium alginate	0.2–0.5 mL/kg/dose 3–8 times/d PC	Same as antacids
Antacids		
	1 mL/kg/dose, 3–8 times/d	Constipation, seizures, osteomalacia, hypophosphatemia (Al), diarrhea (Mg), fluid retention (Na), milk-alkali syndrome (Ca)

a meal and not in the presence of antacids or H_2RAs), or genetic variation in hepatic cytochrome P-450-2C19, which results in more rapid metabolism of PPIs. For children unable to swallow PPI capsules, granules can be administered orally in a weakly acidic material such as apple juice or yogurt, or in a solution of sodium bicarbonate for administration through jejunal tubes.

Antacids neutralize already-secreted acid, must be given in relatively large doses to compare with anti-secretory therapies, and convey potential side effects. Nonetheless, their immediate neutralization of refluxed acid may be useful for occasional instantaneous relief, and thus also as a rapid diagnostic test for the cause of pain.

Sucralfate is the most widely used barrier agent, and acts by forming a complex with the base of ulcers or erosions. Its main use is in erosive and ulcerative esophagitis.

Prokinetic agents have theoretical benefit in reflux, particularly in young children, but their use has been limited due to lack of objective demonstration of benefit, and due to concerns about serious side effects and toxicity. Bethanechol, a non-selective cholinergic agonist, is without clear benefit and is currently rarely used. Metoclopramide is a dopamine-2 receptor antagonist, 5-HT3 antagonist, 5-HT4 agonist, and a slightly anticholinergic agent that acts by increasing the LES pressure and improving gastric emptying. It has a narrow therapeutic range; extrapyramidal side effects and drowsiness are the most common side effects [124]. Domperidone is a peripheral dopamine-D2 receptor antagonist that has a therapeutic potential for improving gastric emptying and esophageal motility, but clinical efficacy data are lacking [125]. A small number of studies investigating the effects of erythromycin in children with gastroparesis support a role for erythromycin as a prokinetic agent, but it has not been studied in children with reflux [126]. It exerts its prokinetic effects at low doses by direct activation of gastric motilin receptors on cholinergic neurons. Higher doses of erythromycin may stimulate the alternative pathway, activating the *muscular* motilin receptors, and producing prolonged, non-propagated antral contractions which will not improve gastric emptying. Potentially serious side effects are rare with low dose erythromycin; emergence of antimicrobial resistance has not been studied [126]. Cisapride is now generally unavailable for use in United States. A new motilin receptor agonist without antibacterial activity, ABT-229, was shown in a placebo controlled study to significantly reduce mean percentage of time esophageal pH was less than 4, but did not change the results of the esophageal manometry and gastric emptying studies [127].

The potential beneficial effects of baclofen, a GABA type-B receptor agonist, are attributed to its reducing the frequency of reflux episodes by its reduction of TLESRs. Pediatric experience with baclofen in neurologically impaired children was recently reported; administration of baclofen orally or via feeding tube three times daily for one week significantly reduced the frequency of emesis, as well as the pH parameters of total number of reflux episodes, and episodes longer than five minutes. However, baclofen did not positively impact the reflux index [128].

Anti-reflux surgery

Fundoplication remains an important, and perhaps the most definitive, technique for eliminating reflux. The most common indications for performing this surgery in children are GERD refractory to pharmacotherapy and life threatening respiratory complications associated with reflux, such as aspiration. [129]–[131]. The exact role of fundoplication in extraesophageal GERD and in those children with chronic lung diseases is unclear [130]. Symptoms and signs suggestive of reflux may persist or recur after surgery, and may prompt resumption of pharmacotherapy, despite lack of documentation of reflux. In a two-year post fundoplication follow-up of 176 children (two-thirds of whom also had other medical disorders, including neurodevelopmental delay, asthma, and cystic fibrosis), two thirds reported reflux-like symptoms necessitating therapy [132].

Laparoscopic Nissen fundoplication is being increasingly performed in infants and children. Reports cite it as well-tolerated, and associated with favorable early and late outcomes [133]–[135]. Forty-eight children with reflux and symptoms of airway disease had no recurrence of reflux during a one year follow-up post-procedure, and the overwhelming majority of parents perceived the outcome as positive [135]. During a median follow-up of three years after laparoscopic fundoplication in 38 children, 66% were completely asymptomatic and 26% were improved. In comparison with the open surgical technique, children undergoing laparoscopic Nissen fundoplication have a shorter hospital stay and a lower complication rate [136]. The rate of complications in children with and without neurological diseases is reported as 2 and 3.4% in different studies [137], [138]. In one center's experience, almost all of the complications occurred in the first 50% of the cases, underscoring the effects of the learning curve and improved techniques [137].

Esophagogastric separation was performed with favorable results in 10 neurologically impaired children who had failed previous fundoplication; further experience and long-term outcomes with this technique are desirable [139]. Robotic laparoscopic anti-reflux surgery has also been added to the surgical armamentarium, but it has only been performed in a small number of children. The early reports are encouraging, provided instruments appropriate for pediatric cases are made available [140].

Endoscopic treatment

Endoscopic therapies against GERD that have been studied in adults include radiofrequency ablation, gastroplication, and injection of inert biopolymers. Experience with these techniques in children is limited.

Radiofrequency ablation procedure is a novel anti-reflux treatment strategy. A single published pediatric report describes 6 older children with an average age of 18 years, of whom five were asymptomatic at a three month follow-up; at six months follow-up mean GERD symptom scores were significantly better than before the procedure [141]. Endoluminal gastroplication and suturing in adults are reported to improve reflux index and symptom scores. A recent study of children (median age 12.4 years) with refractory GERD undergoing gastroplication reported a significant improvement in symptoms and quality of life scores [142]. At follow-up, 33 months later, 82% remained off anti-reflux medications, and at one year, six of nine patients had improved pH parameters including reflux index on a pH study. This procedure may be complicated by suture perforation, mucosal tear, and bleeding [143]. Early experience with the injection of a biochemically inert and bioabsorable polymer into the muscle of the gastric cardia is encouraging. Further data regarding the efficacy and safety of these three techniques in large controlled studies involving adults are needed before exploration of the precise role and clinical application of these endoluminal therapies can be defined in carefully selected pediatric GERD patients [143].

Conclusion

Gastroesophageal reflux is the most common esophageal disorder in children, and is responsible for heterogeneous presentations ranging from effortless regurgitation in "happy spitters" to complex esophageal and extra-esophageal GERD. The frequency and noxiousness of refluxate in proportion to the various esophageal defense mechanisms, and genetic, physiological and environmental influences ultimately determine the pathogenicity and complications of the disorder. While most children may be confidently diagnosed solely on the basis of a detailed history followed by appropriate response to therapy, diagnostic tools may be useful to clarify the role of reflux in extra-esophageal, and complicated GERD. Prompt identification and intervention for GERD in children is crucial to the prevention of strictures, Barrett's esophagus and adenocarcinoma that are associated with long-standing reflux exposure. The first line of anti-reflux therapy in children is conservative therapy emphasizing thickened feeds, smaller volume meals, proper positioning, and elimination of smoke exposure. Proton pump inhibitor therapy has an established role in the management of those with GERD sequelae, and as empiric therapy in those with extra-esophageal GERD. Fundoplication, reserved for children who are refractory to pharmacotherapy, is being performed successfully; results of laparoscopic surgery in children are favorable with respect to shorter hospital stay, and lower complication rate than open fundoplication.

References

[1] Ashorn M (2003) Gastrointestinal diseases in the paediatric age groups in Europe: epidemiology and impact on healthcare. Aliment Pharmacol Ther 18 (Suppl 3): 80–83

[2] Vandenplas Y, Goyvaerts H, Helven R (1991) Gastroesophageal relfux, as measured by 24-hour pH-monitoring, in 509 healthy infants screened for sudden infant death syndrome. Pediatrics 88: 834–840

[3] Colletti RB, Di Lorenzo C (2003) Overview of pediatric gastroesophageal reflux disease and proton pump inhibitor therapy. J Pediatr Gastroenterol Nutr 37 (Suppl 1): S7–S11

[4] Costa AJ, Silva GA, Gouveia PA et al (2004) Prevalence of pathologic gastroesophageal reflux in regurgitant infants. J Pediatr (Rio J) 80: 291–295

[5] Nelson SP, Chen EH, Syniar GM et al (2000) Prevalence of symptoms of gastroesophageal reflux during childhood: a pediatric practice-based survey. Pediatric Practice Research Group. Arch Pediatr Adolesc Med 154: 150–154

[6] Fuloria M, Hiatt D, Dillard RG et al (2000) Gastroesophageal reflux in very low birth weight infants: association with chronic lung disease and outcomes through 1 year of age. J Perinatol 20: 235–239

[7] Nelson SP, Chen EH, Syniar GM et al (1998) One-year follow-up of symptoms of gastroesophageal reflux during infancy. Pediatric Practice Research Group. Pediatrics 102: E67

[8] Martin AJ, Pratt N, Kennedy JD et al (2002) Natural history and familial relationships of infant spilling to 9 years of age. Pediatrics 109: 1061–1067

[9] Boyle JT, Co J, Davidson G et al (2003) Do children with gastroesophageal reflux become adults with gastroesophageal reflux? What is the role of acid suppression in children? J Pediatr Gastroenterol Nutr 37 (Suppl 1): S65–S68

[10] Rommel N, De Meyer AM, Feenstra L et al (2003) The complexity of feeding problems in 700 infants and young children presenting to a tertiary care institution. J Pediatr Gastroenterol Nutr 37: 75–84

[11] Ashorn M, Ruuska T, Karikoski R et al (2002) The natural course of gastroesophageal reflux disease in children. Scand J Gastroenterol 37: 638–641

[12] Treem WR, Davis PM, Hyams JS (1991) Gastroesophageal reflux in the older child: presentation, response to treatment and long-term follow-up. Clin Pediatr (Phila) 30: 435–440

[13] Waring JP, Feiler MJ, Hunter JG et al (2002) Childhood gastroesophageal reflux symptoms in adult patients. J Pediatr Gastroenterol Nutr 35: 334–338

[14] El-Serag HB, Gilger M, Carter J et al (2004) Childhood GERD is a risk factor for GERD in adolescents and young adults. Am J Gastroenterol 99: 806–812

[15] Hu FZ, Preston RA, Post JC et al (2000) Mapping of a gene for severe pediatric gastroesophageal reflux to chromosome 13q14. JAMA 284: 325–334

[16] Orenstein SR, Shalaby TM, Finch R et al (2002) Autosomal dominant infantile gastroesophageal reflux disease: exclusion of a 13q14 locus in five well characterized families. Am J Gastroenterol 97: 2725–2732

[17] Hu FZ, Donfack J, Ahmed A et al (2004) Fine mapping a gene for pediatric gastroesophageal reflux on human chromosome 13q14. Hum Genet 114: 562–572

[18] Davidson G (2003) The role of lower esophageal sphincter function and dysmotility in gastroesophageal reflux in premature infants and in the first year of life. J Pediatr Gastroenterol Nutr 37 (Suppl 1): S17–S22

[19] Omari TI, Barnett CP, Benninga MA et al (2002) Mechanisms of gastro-oesophageal reflux in preterm and term infants with reflux disease. Gut 51: 475–479

[20] Goldani HA, Fernandes MI, Vicente YA et al (2002) Lower esophageal sphincter reacts against intraabdominal pressure in children with symptoms of gastroesophageal reflux. Dig Dis Sci 47: 2544–2548

[21] Penagini R, Carmagnola S, Cantu P et al (2004) Mechanoreceptors of the proximal stomach: Role in triggering transient lower esophageal sphincter relaxation. Gastroenterology 126: 49–56

[22] Vandenplas Y, Hassall E (2002) Mechanisms of gastroesophageal reflux and gastroesophageal reflux disease. J Pediatr Gastroenterol Nutr 35: 119–136

[23] Carre IJ, Johnston BT, Thomas PS et al (1999) Familial hiatal hernia in a large five generation family confirming true autosomal dominant inheritance. Gut 45: 649–652

[24] Hassall E (1995) Wrap session: is the Nissen slipping? Can medical treatment replace surgery for severe gastroesophageal reflux disease in children? Am J Gastroenterol 90: 1212–1220

[25] Gorenstein A, Cohen AJ, Cordova Z et al (2001) Hiatal hernia in pediatric gastroesophageal reflux. J Pediatr Gastroenterol Nutr 33: 554–557

[26] Hillemeier AC, Lange R, McCallum R et al (1981) Delayed gastric emptying in infants with gastroesophageal reflux. J Pediatr 98: 190–193

[27] Spiroglou K, Xinias I, Karatzas N et al (2004) Gastric emptying in children with cerebral palsy and gastroesophageal reflux. Pediatr Neurol 31: 177–182

[28] Sarkar S, Hobson AR, Hughes A et al (2003) The prostaglandin E2 receptor-1 (EP-1) mediates acid-induced visceral pain hypersensitivity in humans. Gastroenterology 124: 18–25

[29] Sarkar S, Thompson DG, Woolf CJ et al (2004) Patients with chest pain and occult gastroesophageal reflux demonstrate visceral pain hypersensitivity which may be partially responsive to acid suppression. Am J Gastroenterol 99: 1998–2006

[30] Bhalla V, Liu J, Puckett JL et al (2004) Symptom hypersensitivity to acid infusion is associated with hypersensitivity of esophageal contractility. Am J Physiol Gastrointest Liver Physiol 287: G65–G71

[31] Hobson AR, Khan RW, Sarkar S et al (2004) Development of esophageal hypersensitivity following experimental duodenal acidification. Am J Gastroenterol 99: 813–820
[32] Boyle JT (2003) Acid secretion from birth to adulthood. J Pediatr Gastroenterol Nutr 37 (Suppl 1): S12–S16
[33] Kalach N, Badran AM, Jaffray P et al (2003) Correlation between gastric acid secretion and severity of acid reflux in children. Turk J Pediatr 45: 6–10
[34] Orel R, Markovic S (2003) Bile in the esophagus: a factor in the pathogenesis of reflux esophagitis in children. J Pediatr Gastroenterol Nutr 36: 266–273
[35] Hallberg K, Fandriks L, Strandvik B (2004) Duodenogastric bile reflux is common in cystic fibrosis. J Pediatr Gastroenterol Nutr 38: 312–316
[36] D'Eufemia P, Corrado G, Finocchiaro R et al (2001) Increased taurine content in esophageal mucosa of children affected by gastroesophageal reflux. Dig Dis Sci 46: 808–814
[37] D'Eufemia P, Celli M, Finocchiaro R et al (2003) Fatty acid profile of oesophageal mucosa in children with gastro-oesophageal reflux disease. Dig Liver Dis 35: 694–700
[38] Vicente Y, da Rocha C, Perez-Mies B et al (2004) Effect of reflux and esophagitis on esophageal volume and acid clearance in piglets. J Pediatr Gastroenterol Nutr 38: 328–337
[39] Jeffery HE, Ius D, Page M (2000) The role of swallowing during active sleep in the clearance of reflux in term and preterm infants. J Pediatr 137: 545–548
[40] Williams D, Thompson DG, Heggie L et al (1994) Esophageal clearance function following treatment of esophagitis. Gastroenterology 106: 108–116
[41] Kahrilas PJ, Dodds WJ, Hogan WJ et al (1986) Esophageal peristaltic dysfunction in peptic esophagitis. Gastroenterology 91: 897–904
[42] Kostovski A (2003) Long-lasting reflux episodes in gastroesophageal reflux and its complications in children. Hepatogastroenterology 50 (Suppl 2): 309–311
[43] Ransford RA, Jankowski JA (2000) Genetic versus environmental interactions in the oesophagitis-metaplasia-dysplasia-adenocarcinoma sequence (MCS) of Barrett's oesophagus. Acta Gastroenterol Belg 63: 18–21
[44] Levine A, Milo T, Broide E et al (2004) Influence of Helicobacter pylori eradication on gastroesophageal reflux symptoms and epigastric pain in children and adolescents. Pediatrics 113: 54–58
[45] Pollet S, Gottrand F, Vincent P et al (2004) Gastroesophageal reflux disease and Helicobacter pylori infection in neurologically impaired children: inter-relations and therapeutic implications. J Pediatr Gastroenterol Nutr 38: 70–74
[46] Jadcherla SR (2003) Manometric evaluation of esophageal-protective reflexes in infants and children. Am J Med 115 (Suppl 3A): 157S–160S
[47] Feranchak AP, Orenstein SR, Cohn JF (1994) Behaviors associated with onset of gastroesophageal reflux episodes in infants. Prospective study using split-screen video and pH probe. Clin Pediatr (Phila) 33: 654–662
[48] Salvatore S, Vandenplas Y (2002) Gastroesophageal reflux and cow milk allergy: is there a link? Pediatrics 110: 972–984
[49] Nielsen RG, Bindslev-Jensen C, Kruse-Andersen S et al (2004) Severe gastroesophageal reflux disease and cow milk hypersensitivity in infants and children: Disease association and evaluation of a new challenge procedure. J Pediatr Gastroenterol Nutr 39: 383–391
[50] Khalaf MN, Porat R, Brodsky NL et al (2001) Clinical correlations in infants in the neonatal intensive care unit with varying severity of gastroesophageal reflux. J Pediatr Gastroenterol Nutr 32: 45–49
[51] Carr MM, Nguyen A, Nagy M et al (2000) Clinical presentation as a guide to the identification of GERD in children. Int J Pediatr Otorhinolaryngol 54: 27–32
[52] Peter CS, Sprodowski N, Bohnhorst B et al (2002) Gastroesophageal reflux and apnea of prematurity: no temporal relationship. Pediatrics 109: 8–11
[53] Wenzl TG, Schenke S, Peschgens T et al (2001) Association of apnea and nonacid gastroesophageal reflux in infants: Investigations with the intraluminal impedance technique. Pediatr Pulmonol 31: 144–149
[54] Thach BT (1997) Reflux associated apnea in infants: evidence for a laryngeal chemoreflex. Am J Med 103: 120S–124S
[55] Aviv JE, Mohr JP, Blitzer A et al (1997) Restoration of laryngopharyngeal sensation by neural anastomosis. Arch Otolaryngol Head Neck Surg 123: 154–160
[56] Gilger MA (2003) Pediatric otolaryngologic manifestations of gastroesophageal reflux disease. Curr Gastroenterol Rep 5: 247–252
[57] Carr MM, Nguyen A, Poje C et al (2000) Correlation of findings on direct laryngoscopy and bronchoscopy with presence of extraesophageal reflux disease. Laryngoscope 110: 1560–1562
[58] Vaezi MF, Hicks DM, Abelson TI et al (2003) Laryngeal signs and symptoms and gastroesophageal reflux disease (GERD): a critical assessment of cause and effect association. Clin Gastroenterol Hepatol 1: 333–344

[59] Bach KK, McGuirt WF Jr (2002) Postma GN. Pediatric laryngopharyngeal reflux. Ear Nose Throat J 81: 27–31

[60] Yao TC, Chiu CY, Wu KC et al (2004) Failure to thrive caused by the coexistence of vallecular cyst, laryngomalacia and gastroesophageal reflux in an infant. Int J Pediatr Otorhinolaryngol 68: 1459–1464

[61] Kawamura O, Aslam M, Rittmann T et al (2004) Physical and pH properties of gastroesophagopharyngeal refluxate: a 24-hour simultaneous ambulatory impedance and pH-monitoring study. Am J Gastroenterol 99: 1000–1010

[62] Williams RB, Szczesniak MM, Maclean JC et al (2004) Predictors of outcome in an open label, therapeutic trial of high-dose omeprazole in laryngitis. Am J Gastroenterol 99: 777–785

[63] Zalesska-Krecicka M, Krecicki T, Iwanczak B et al (2002) Laryngeal manifestations of gastroesophageal reflux disease in children. Acta Otolaryngol 122: 306–310

[64] Malagelada JR (2004) Review article: supra-oesophageal manifestations of gastro-oesophageal reflux disease. Aliment Pharmacol Ther 19 (Suppl 1): 43–48

[65] Bibi H, Khvolis E, Shoseyov D et al (2001) The prevalence of gastroesophageal reflux in children with tracheomalacia and laryngomalacia. Chest 119: 409–413

[66] El-Serag HB, Gilger M, Kuebeler M et al (2001) Extraesophageal associations of gastroesophageal reflux disease in children without neurologic defects. Gastroenterology 121: 1294–1299

[67] Gorenstein A, Levine A, Boaz M et al (2003) Severity of acid gastroesophageal reflux assessed by pH metry: is it associated with respiratory disease? Pediatr Pulmonol 36: 330–334

[68] Gibson PG, Henry RL, Coughlan JL (2003) Gastrooesophageal reflux treatment for asthma in adults and children. Cochrane Database Sys Rev CD001496

[69] Sontag SJ, O'Connell S, Miller TQ et al (2004) Asthmatics have more nocturnal gasping and reflux symptoms than nonasthmatics, and they are related to bedtime eating. Am J Gastroenterol 99: 789–796

[70] Khoshoo V, Le T, Haydel RM, Jr et al (2003) Role of gastroesophageal reflux in older children with persistent asthma. Chest 123: 1008–1013

[71] Andze GO, Brandt ML, St Vil D et al (1991) Diagnosis and treatment of gastroesophageal reflux in 500 children with respiratory symptoms: the value of pH monitoring. J Pediatr Surg 26: 295–299; discussion 299–300

[72] Tucci F, Resti M, Fontana R et al (1993) Gastroesophageal reflux and bronchial asthma: prevalence and effect of cisapride therapy. J Pediatr Gastroenterol Nutr 17: 265–270

[73] Ay M, Sivasli E, Bayraktaroglu Z et al (2004) Association of asthma with gastroesophageal reflux disease in children. J Chin Med Assoc 67: 63–66

[74] Thomas EJ, Kumar R, Dasan JB et al (2003) Radionuclide scintigraphy in the evaluation of gastro-oesophageal reflux in post-operative oesophageal atresia and tracheo-oesophageal fistula patients. Nucl Med Commun 24: 317–320

[75] Gustafsson PM, Kjellman NI, Tibbling L (1992) A trial of ranitidine in asthmatic children and adolescents with or without pathological gastro-oesophageal reflux. Eur Respir J 5: 201–206

[76] Linnett V, Seow WK, Connor F et al (2002) Oral health of children with gastro-esophageal reflux disease: a controlled study. Aust Dent J 47: 156–162

[77] Dahshan A, Patel H, Delaney J et al (2002) Gastroesophageal reflux disease and dental erosion in children. J Pediatr 140: 474–478

[78] de Ybarrondo L, Mazur JL (2000) Sandifer's syndrome in a child with asthma and cerebral palsy. South Med J 93: 1019–1021

[79] Corrado G, Cavaliere M, D'Eufemia P et al (2000) Sandifer's syndrome in a breast-fed infant. Am J Perinatol 17: 147–150

[80] Pisegna JR (2004) Review article: oesophageal complications and consequences of persistent gastro-oesophageal reflux disease. Aliment Pharmacol Ther 20: 47–56

[81] Marks RD, Richter JE, Rizzo J et al (1994) Omeprazole versus H2-receptor antagonists in treating patients with peptic stricture and esophagitis. Gastroenterology 106: 907–915

[82] al-Bassam A (2003) Surgical management of severe peptic esophageal stricture in children. Hepatogastroenterology 50: 714–717

[83] Hassall E, Weinstein WM, Ament ME (1985) Barrett's esophagus in childhood. Gastroenterology 89: 1331–1337

[84] Hassall E, Israel DM, Davidson AG et al (1993) Barrett's esophagus in children with cystic fibrosis: not a coincidental association. Am J Gastroenterol 88: 1934–1938

[85] Sampliner RE (2002) Updated guidelines for the diagnosis, surveillance, and therapy of Barrett's esophagus. Am J Gastroenterol 97: 1888–1895

[86] Hoeffel JC, Nihoul-Fekete C, Schmitt M (1989) Esophageal adenocarcinoma after gastroesophageal reflux in children. J Pediatr 115: 259–261

[87] Orenstein SR, Cohn JF, Shalaby TM et al (1993) Reliability and validity of an infant gastroesophageal reflux questionnaire. Clin Pediatr (Phila) 32: 472–484

[88] Nelson SP, Chen EH, Syniar GM et al (1997) Prevalence of symptoms of gastroesophageal reflux during infancy. A pediatric practice-based survey. Pediatric Practice Research Group. Arch Pediatr Adolesc Med 151: 569–572

[89] Black DD, Haggitt RC, Orenstein SR et al (1990) Esophagitis in infants. Morphometric histological diagnosis and correlation with measures of gastroesophageal reflux. Gastroenterology 98: 1408–1414

[90] Dahms BB (2004) Reflux esophagitis: sequelae and differential diagnosis in infants and children including eosinophilic esophagitis. Pediatr Dev Pathol 7: 5–16

[91] Brindley N, Sloan JM, McCallion WA (2004) Esophagitis: optimizing diagnostic yield by biopsy orientation. J Pediatr Gastroenterol Nutr 39: 262–264

[92] Al-Khawari HA, Sinan TS, Seymour H (2002) Diagnosis of gastro-oesophageal reflux in children. Comparison between oesophageal pH and barium examinations. Pediatr Radiol 32: 765–770

[93] Nielsen RG, Kruse-Andersen S, Husby S (2003) Low reproducibility of 2×24-hour continuous esophageal pH monitoring in infants and children: a limiting factor for interventional studies. Dig Dis Sci 48: 1495–1502

[94] Arana A, Hauser B, Hegar B et al (2003) Oesophageal pH monitoring in children: how is it perceived by the parents and does the technique change feeding and daily activity? Acta Paediatr 92: 1021–1025

[95] Emmerson AJ, Chant T, May J et al (2002) Assessment of three methods of pH probe positioning in preterm infants. J Pediatr Gastroenterol Nutr 35: 69–72

[96] Day A, Marchant J, Bohane TD (2003) Assessment of three methods of pH probe positioning in preterm infants. J Pediatr Gastroenterol Nutr 36: 292–293; author reply 293

[97] Jolley SG, Halpern CT, Sterling CE et al (1990) The relationship of respiratory complications from gastroesophageal reflux to prematurity in infants. J Pediatr Surg 25: 755–757

[98] Euler AR, Byrne WJ (1981) Twenty-four-hour esophageal intraluminal pH probe testing: a comparative analysis. Gastroenterology 80: 957–961

[99] Shay SS, Johnson LF (1994) Upright refluxers without esophagitis differentiated from bipositional refluxers with esophagitis by simultaneous manometry and pH monitoring conducted in two postures before and after a meal. Am J Gastroenterol 89: 992–1002

[100] Herbst JJ, Minton SD, Book LS (1979) Gastroesophageal reflux causing respiratory distress and apnea in newborn infants. J Pediatr 95: 763–768

[101] Bagucka B, Badriul H, Vandemaele K et al (2000) Normal ranges of continuous pH-monitoring in the proximal esophagus. J Pediatr Gastroenterol Nutr 31: 244–247

[102] Arana A, Bagucka B, Hauser B et al (2001) PH monitoring in the distal and proximal esophagus in symptomatic infants. J Pediatr Gastroenterol Nutr 32: 259–264

[103] Wenzl TG, Moroder C, Trachterna M et al (2002) Esophageal pH monitoring and impedance measurement: a comparison of two diagnostic tests for gastroesophageal reflux. J Pediatr Gastroenterol Nutr 34: 519–523

[104] Wenzl TG, Schneider S, Scheele F et al (2003) Effects of thickened feeding on gastroesophageal reflux in infants: a placebo-controlled crossover study using intraluminal impedance. Pediatrics 111: e355–e359

[105] Bothwell M, Phillips J, Bauer S (2004) Upper esophageal pH monitoring of children with the Bravo pH capsule. Laryngoscope 114: 786–788

[106] Seibert JJ, Byrne WJ, Euler AR et al (1983) Gastroesophageal reflux – the acid test: scintigraphy or the pH probe? AJR Am J Roentgenol 140: 1087–1090

[107] Vandenplas Y, Derde MP, Piepsz A (1992) Evaluation of reflux episodes during simultaneous esophageal pH monitoring and gastroesophageal reflux scintigraphy in children. J Pediatr Gastroenterol Nutr 14: 256–260

[108] Orenstein SR, Klein HA, Rosenthal MS (1993) Scintigraphy versus pH probe for quantification of pediatric gastroesophageal reflux: a study using concurrent multiplexed data and acid feedings. J Nucl Med 34: 1228–1234

[109] Skopnik H, Silny J, Heiber O et al (1996) Gastroesophageal reflux in infants: evaluation of a new intraluminal impedance technique. J Pediatr Gastroenterol Nutr 23: 591–598

[110] Wenzl TG (2003) Evaluation of gastroesophageal reflux events in children using multichannel intraluminal electrical impedance. Am J Med 115 (Suppl 3A): 161S–165S

[111] Collins KA, Geisinger KR, Wagner PH et al (1995) The cytologic evaluation of lipid-laden alveolar macrophages as an indicator of aspiration pneumonia in young children. Arch Pathol Lab Med 119: 229–231

[112] Krishnan U, Mitchell JD, Tobias V et al (2002) Fat laden macrophages in tracheal aspirates as a marker of reflux aspiration: a negative report. J Pediatr Gastroenterol Nutr 35: 309–313

[113] Krishnan U, Mitchell JD, Messina I et al (2002) Assay of tracheal pepsin as a marker of reflux aspiration. J Pediatr Gastroenterol Nutr 35: 303–308

[114] Potluri S, Friedenberg F, Parkman HP et al (2003) Comparison of a salivary/sputum pepsin assay with 24-hour esophageal pH-monitoring for detection of gastric reflux into the proximal esophagus, oropharynx, and lung. Dig Dis Sci 48: 1813–1817

[115] Orenstein SR (1994) Regurgitant reflux, versus non-regurgitant reflux, is preceded by rectus abdominis contraction in infants. Neurogastroenterol Mot 6: 271–277

[116] Shalaby TM, Orenstein SR (2003) Efficacy of telephone teaching of conservative therapy for infants with symptomatic gastroesophageal reflux referred by pediatricians to pediatric gastroenterologists. J Pediatr 142: 57–61

[117] Vanderhoof JA, Moran JR, Harris CL et al (2003) Efficacy of a pre-thickened infant formula: a multicenter, double-blind, randomized, placebo-controlled parallel group trial in 104 infants with symptomatic gastroesophageal reflux. Clin Pediatr (Phila) 42: 483–495

[118] Orenstein SR, Magill HL, Brooks P (1987) Thickening of infant feedings for therapy of gastroesophageal reflux. J Pediatr 110: 181–186

[119] Miyazawa R, Tomomasa T, Kaneko H et al (2004) Effect of locust bean gum in anti-regurgitant milk on the regurgitation in uncomplicated gastroesophageal reflux. J Pediatr Gastroenterol Nutr 38: 479–483

[120] Khoshoo V, Ross G, Brown S et al (2000) Smaller volume, thickened formulas in the management of gastroesophageal reflux in thriving infants. J Pediatr Gastroenterol Nutr 31: 554–556

[121] Hassall E, Israel D, Shepherd R et al (2000) Omeprazole for treatment of chronic erosive esophagitis in children: a multicenter study of efficacy, safety, tolerability and dose requirements. International Pediatric Omeprazole Study Group. J Pediatr 137: 800–807

[122] Scott LJ (2003) Lansoprazole: in the management of gastroesophageal reflux disease in children. Paediatr Drugs 5: 57–61; discussion 62

[123] Abdel-Rahman SM, Johnson FK, Connor JD et al (2004) Developmental pharmacokinetics and pharmacodynamics of nizatidine. J Pediatr Gastroenterol Nutr 38: 442–451

[124] Mejia NI, Jankovic J (2005) Metoclopramide-induced tardive dyskinesia in an infant. Mov Disord 20: 86–89

[125] Barone JA (1999) Domperidone: a peripherally acting dopamine2-receptor antagonist. Ann Pharmacother 33: 429–440

[126] Curry JI, Lander TD, Stringer MD (2001) Review article: erythromycin as a prokinetic agent in infants and children. Aliment Pharmacol Ther 15: 595–603

[127] Netzer P, Schmitt B, Inauen W (2002) Effects of ABT-229, a motilin agonist, on acid reflux, oesophageal motility and gastric emptying in patients with gastro-oesophageal reflux disease. Aliment Pharmacol Ther 16: 1481–1490

[128] Kawai M, Kawahara H, Hirayama S et al (2004) Effect of baclofen on emesis and 24-hour esophageal pH in neurologically impaired children with gastroesophageal reflux disease. J Pediatr Gastroenterol Nutr 38: 317–323

[129] Zeid MA, Kandel T, el-Shobary M et al (2004) Nissen fundoplication in infants and children: a long-term clinical study. Hepatogastroenterology 51: 697–700

[130] Mattioli G, Sacco O, Repetto P et al (2004) Necessity for surgery in children with gastrooesophageal reflux and supraoesophageal symptoms. Eur J Pediatr Surg 14: 7–13

[131] Fonkalsrud EW, Ashcraft KW, Coran AG et al (1998) Surgical treatment of gastroesophageal reflux in children: a combined hospital study of 7467 patients. Pediatrics 101: 419–422

[132] Gilger MA, Yeh C, Chiang J et al (2004) Outcomes of surgical fundoplication in children. Clin Gastroenterol Hepatol 2: 978–984

[133] Esposito C, Van Der Zee DC, Settimi A et al (2003) Risks and benefits of surgical management of gastroesophageal reflux in neurologically impaired children. Surg Endosc 17: 708–710

[134] Lima M, Bertozzi M, Ruggeri G et al (2004) Laparoscopic antireflux surgery in neurologically impaired children. Pediatr Surg Int 20: 114–117

[135] Mattioli G, Sacco O, Gentilino V et al (2004) Outcome of laparoscopic Nissen-Rossetti fundoplication in children with gastroesophageal reflux disease and supraesophageal symptoms. Surg Endosc 18: 463–465

[136] Mattioli G, Repetto P, Carlini C et al (2002) Laparoscopic vs open approach for the treatment of gastroesophageal reflux in children. Surg Endosc 16: 750–752

[137] Allal H, Captier G, Lopez M et al (2001) Evaluation of 142 consecutive laparoscopic fundoplications in children: effects of the learning curve and technical choice. J Pediatr Surg 36: 921–926

[138] Esposito C, Montupet P, Amici G et al (2000) Complications of laparoscopic antireflux surgery in childhood. Surg Endosc 14: 622–624

[139] Islam S, Teitelbaum DH, Buntain WL et al (2004) Esophagogastric separation for failed fundoplication

in neurologically impaired children. J Pediatr Surg 39: 287–291; discussion 287–291

[140] Heller K, Gutt C, Schaeff B et al (2002) Use of the robot system Da Vinci for laparoscopic repair of gastro-oesophageal reflux in children. Eur J Pediatr Surg 12: 239–242

[141] Islam S, Geiger JD, Coran AG et al (2004) Use of radiofrequency ablation of the lower esophageal sphincter to treat recurrent gastroesophageal reflux disease. J Pediatr Surg 39: 282–286; discussion 282–286

[142] Thomson M, Fritscher-Ravens A, Hall S et al (2004) Endoluminal gastroplication in children with significant gastro-oesophageal reflux disease. Gut 53: 1745–1750

[143] Chen YK (2001) Endoscopic treatments for GERD: are they ready for prime time? J Pediatr Gastroenterol Nutr 33: 109–110

Chapter 5

BARRETT'S ESOPHAGUS

R. E. Sampliner

Arizona Health Sciences Center, Chief of Gastroenterology, Southern Arizona VA Health Care System, Tucson, AZ, USA

Introduction

Barrett's esophagus (BE) is defined and the clinical presentation of the disease described. The explosion of information about BE results from the impetus of the continuing increase in the incidence of esophageal adenocarcinoma in the Western world. The lifetime risk for the development of cancer in patients with BE is often overestimated by physicians and patients. The lifetime risk for a patient with BE is 5% or less.

The rationale for screening and surveillance of BE is the potential for the early detection of high grade dysplasia and cancer to enable therapy improving outcome. Better risk stratification for screening and surveillance would result in a major reduction in resource expenditure. Dysplasia is the histologic marker which drives surveillance. Proposed surveillance intervals are presented. Developments in the optical detection of dysplasia and molecular markers are discussed.

The treatment of BE from pharmacologic to surgical and endoscopic is described; proton pump inhibitor therapy, esophageal resection for early cancer and endoscopic ablation therapy for high grade dysplasia.

The criteria and options for managing a patient with high grade dysplasia are detailed. Cancer prevention is the ultimate goal of the management of patients with BE. The role of surveillance and of molecular and optical strategies to improve risk stratification is outlined. Recent developments in chemoprevention with the potential for broader and earlier application are highlighted.

The disease

Barrett's esophagus (BE) is a change in the lining of the distal esophagus from the normal squamous epithelium to a columnar appearing mucosa with intestinal metaplasia demonstrated by biopsy [1]. Endoscopy with biopsy of the abnormal appearing distal esophagus is necessary to meet the current working definition of BE. Intestinal metaplasia (IM) is an epithelium with goblet cells like the small intestine but with a different architecture reflecting the result of an underlying chronic inflammatory condition – GERD. IM is important because it represents the premalignant lesion for esophageal adenocarcinoma (EAC), the most feared complication of BE and the most rapidly rising incidence cancer in the United States and Western Europe since the mid 1970's [2], [3].

At the time of endoscopy the minimal essential evaluation includes measuring the length of and systematically biopsying the BE. The endoscopic landmarks to identify by centimeters from the teeth include the proximally displaced squamocolumnar junction, the esophagogastric junction (EGJ) and the diaphragmatic pinch. The EGJ is equivalent to the "endoscopic lower esophageal sphincter," the location of the change from the tubular esophagus to the saccular stomach and/or the proximal margin of the gastric folds of the commonly present hiatal hernia with minimal air insufflation [4]. Systematic biopsies are necessary to identify IM in what may be a mosaic of metaplastic epithelium in the Barrett's segment. The precise number of biopsies necessary to identify IM is not defined.

The clinical context of Barrett's esophagus

BE is most commonly recognized as part of the endoscopic evaluation of patients with chronic heartburn and/or regurgitation – the most common symptoms of GERD. On a population basis, 5% of adults with chronic GERD have BE [5].

Recently there has been increasing assessment of asymptomatic individuals undergoing colon cancer screening for BE. In a small predominantly male (90%) Veteran study, 25% of subjects lacking reflux symptoms had BE – 7% long segment ($\geq$ 3 cm) [6]. In a larger study of a more diverse population, 60% male, 5.6%

had BE, 0.36% long segment [7]. These patients with presumed asymptomatic BE account for the incidental finding of BE in patients being assessed for upper GI bleeding, ulcers and dyspepsia. The asymptomatic pose a major challenge for screening for BE and cancer prevention and account for a major percent of esophagectomy series for cancer and BE.

The development of neoplasia

Dysplasia is the first step in the neoplastic process. It represents a change in the cytologic characteristics of cells and the glandular architecture detected histologically. The progression of neoplasia can result in cancer – in BE that means EAC. Although the incidence of EAC in BE is controversial, both cohort studies [8] and a funnel analysis of the literature estimate the incidence at 0.5% per year [9]. A more realistic estimate may be the lifetime risk – younger patients do not have a greater risk of developing cancer just because they have a longer life expectancy. An individual patient with BE has an estimated lifetime risk of EAC of 5% or less. This has been documented in a population based study [10] and an accumulation of 10 cohort studies [11]. This is a significantly greater risk than someone with GERD lacking BE or the general population, but less of a risk than perceived by many physicians and patients. What action to take to reduce this risk of EAC will be discussed.

Screening for and surveillance of Barrett's esophagus

Screening is looking for the premalignant disease BE, and surveillance is evaluating the premalignant disease for the early detection of HGD or EAC. The rationale for screening is to detect BE in order to recognize early prevalent HGD and EAC and to appropriately control reflux symptoms. Less than 5% of patients surgically treated for EAC have had BE previously identified [12]. The only opportunity for improved outcome in the highly fatal disease EAC is early detection and effective intervention.

Risk stratification for screening for BE is not evidence based but is de-facto commonly performed in the US as part of the evaluation of GERD patients. The epidemiology of EAC highlights those at risk and provides indirect evidence for who is likely to have BE. The US annual incidence of EAC is 3.6/100,000 in Caucasian men, 0.8 in African American men and 0.3 in Caucasian women [3]. A population based case control study in Sweden documented the relation of frequency – (≥ 3 times per week OR 16.7) and longer duration (≥ 20 years OR 16) of reflux symptoms to the risk of EAC [13]. The longer duration of GERD symptoms have been related to the greater likelihood of finding BE at endoscopy [14], [15].

The likelihood of finding of BE is age related. Under the age of 45 only 1 of 363 patients with dyspepsia lacking alarm symptoms had BE [16]. Based on an epidemiology study, the median age of onset of BE is estimated to be 40 years of age although the first endoscopy diagnosing BE is usually in the 60s [17].

The above data have led to an approach of screening older Caucasian men with chronic GERD symptoms for BE [1]. To be cost effective, the population screened has to include a high prevalence of BE, HGD, and EAC, accurate endoscopic recognition of BE and histologic documentation of intestinal metaplasia and dysplasia, and finally a small drop in health-related quality of life after therapy for HGD/EAC [18]. These criteria are difficult to meet, requiring effective risk stratification.

Surveillance of BE is the current strategy to detect EAC at a treatable stage in patients with BE. There are no prospective randomized trials to determine optimal surveillance intervals. There probably never will be because of the expense of performing such a large trial over many years and the failure to fund such a study by the agencies of 2 countries.

Dysplasia is the biologic marker used in the clinical context for risk stratification. The database culled from 6 prospective series and one registry is seen in Table 1 [11], [19]–[25]. Patients lacking dysplasia or with low grade dysplasia have a low risk of progressing to EAC over the short run. In contrast, patients with HGD have a risk of progressing to EAC greater than 20% over 3 to 7 years.

Table 1. Dysplasia and the development of esophageal adenocarcinoma in prospective cohorts

Dysplasia	n	Cancer (%)
None	382	9 (2.4)
Low grade	145	8 (5.5)
High grade	175	39 (22.3)

From a total of 1077 BE patients followed over 2.9–7.3 years

Based on the limited information on the time course of the progression of dysplasia, recommendations for surveillance intervals based on dysplasia have been made by the *American College of Gastroenterology* [1] (Table 2 – adapted).

Surveillance endoscopy is increasingly supported by retrospective datasets. Initial information was from retrospective surgical experience demonstrating that surveillance detected EAC was earlier stage with greater 5 year survival than patients presenting symptomatically found to have EAC and BE [26], [27]. More recently the survival advantage of endoscopic surveillance has been demonstrated in a community based population study and in the SEER/Medicine database [28], [29]. In the former study the small number of patients with surveillance detected cancer had 73% survival versus none in the EAC patients not undergoing surveillance.

Treatment of Barrett's esophagus – medical

The mainstay of medical therapy of BE is proton pump inhibitor (PPI) therapy for the control of underlying GERD symptoms. Patients with BE tend to have more prolonged esophageal acid exposure as a result of a more defective anti-reflux barrier. Many patients require bid dosing to control reflux symptoms. Even bid PPI therapy fails to normalize esophageal pH < 4 exposure in 25% of BE patients in spite of symptom control [30], [31]. The endpoint of medical therapy is controversial – symptom control versus esophageal pH control. Until more direct data document an effect of esophageal acid control on outcome, this difficult endpoint will unlikely be pursued in practice.

Surgical therapy

The major role of surgery in BE is for curative resection of EAC. Esophagectomy is the only therapy that gives long term cancer free survival. Contemporary results for early stage EAC (T1-tumor limited to the mucosa/submucosa) are impressive with more than 80% 5 year survival [32]–[34].

Table 2. Surveillance intervals for Barrett's esophagus

Dysplasia	How established	Endoscopy
None	2 endoscopies	3–4 years
LGD	Highest grade on 2nd endoscopy	1 year and annual until no dysplasia x2
HGD	Repeat endoscopy: large capacity forceps/ intensive biopsy protocol	3 months

The problem with esophagectomy is the recognition of the relationship of operative mortality to institutional volume [35], [36]. A low volume hospital can have an operative mortality 3 times that of a high volume hospital. Referral to an experienced institution is essential. The role of esophagectomy in the treatment of HGD will be discussed below.

With the widespread application of laparoscopic fundoplication, anti-reflux surgery has been increasingly utilized. Unfortunately, the 5 year results in BE patients, even at an expert center, demonstrate a 20% symptomatic and objective failure rate [37]. Additionally, fundoplication does not prevent the neoplastic progression of BE, both in a meta-analysis of the literature [38] and a randomized trial [39]. A recent collected surgical experience even demonstrated the late occurrence of EAC after fundoplication. Twenty three of 652 patients developed EAC after antireflux surgery – 52% of these 6 or more years after surgery [40].

Endoscopic therapy

Recently, after years of investigation, endoscopic therapy has entered the clinical arena. Endoscopic mucosal resection provides a large specimen, 1 cm or greater in diameter, to better stage early cancers. Additionally, it has been utilized for primary therapy [41] or cotherapy [42]. Photodynamic therapy (PDT) utilizing sodium porfimer as the photosensitizer has been approved in North America for treatment of HGD in patients with BE. In a multicenter randomized trial PDT significantly reduced HGD and the development of EAC after a 2-year follow-up [43]. This is the largest randomized trial to date of any form of therapy in BE and the first to document a reduction in the development of EAC. A long term follow-up of this form of PDT – a mean of 51 months – has been reported with a success rate by intention-to-treat analysis of 93, 78 and 44% for LGD, HGD and early EAC respectively [44].

HGD has been treated with a variety of endoscopic modalities with less deep tissue injury than PDT with porfimer sodium, resulting in lower rates of developing strictures – argon plasma coagulation [45], PDT with

5-aminolevulinic acid [46], and PDT with green light and m-tetrahydroxyphenyl chlorin [47].

The management of high grade dysplasia

HGD poses a special dilemma for both the physician and patient. The factors to be weighed are multiple and not always quantifiable. These include the variable natural history of HGD, interobserver variability in reading HGD, the difficulty of ruling out synchronous EAC, the patient as a surgical candidate, the risk aversion of the patient, and the expertise of the available institution (Table 3). These factors have to be addressed for and with the individual patient to determine an appropriate management strategy. HGD associated with a mass or mucosal irregularity is more likely to have early EAC and even regional nodal involvement [48], [49]. The most recent experience with patients having only HGD prior to esophagectomy demonstrates a lower likelihood of unexpected cancer in the resected specimen – 17% from 1994–2001 versus 43% from 1982–1994 [50]. Once there is cancer below the muscularis mucosa as documented by EMR or endoscopic ultrasound, endoscopic therapy is no longer appropriate as a curative approach. If the patient is elderly and/or has major comorbidity, precluding a substantial duration of life expectancy, then a therapy with major comorbidity or significant mortality may not be appropriate. A patient who values cancer free survival over the short term risk of mortality may well elect surgery. An elderly patient with limited life expectancy may elect local endoscopic therapy.

Cancer prevention

Current efforts at cancer prevention are crude and not documented to be effective. They are focused on surveillance of patients known to have BE in order to detect cancer at an early, curable stage. PDT offers an opportunity for non-surgical reduction of cancer development. Yet only a distinct minority of patients with BE are identified – less than 5% of patients with resected EAC and BE have had previously recognized BE. Better strategies are necessary. A non-endoscopic and less invasive screening method would enable identification of a larger pool of BE patients. Unsedated endoscopy with an ultrathin endoscope lowers the time and cost of the procedure, is accepted by patients, but not widely utilized [51].

Surveillance has to be focused on higher risk patients to be cost-effective [52]. This requires more effective risk stratification. Molecular markers of neoplastic progression have been pursued as the holy grail over a number of decades. Despite the identification of scores of markers, only two have been assessed in a large cohort of patients with BE followed prospectively with an endpoint of development of EAC. Flow cytometric abnormalities of aneuploidy and increased 4N fraction are predictors of the development of EAC. Most importantly, none of 215 patients with no or LGD without flow cytometric abnormalities progressed to EAC over 5 years (95% confidence interval 0–4.7%) [21]. The same group demonstrated that baseline 17p (p53) loss of heterozygosity predicts progression to EAC with a relative risk of 16 [53]. These markers await validation in multicenter studies of BE cohorts.

Techniques to optically detect dysplasia at the time of endoscopy would enable real time stratification of patients as well as the opportunity to apply therapy. These techniques include laser induced fluorescence, photodiagnosis with 5-aminolevulinic acid, light scattering spectroscopy, Raman spectroscopy and optical coherence tomography. Some of these techniques recognize only HGD, others HGD and LGD. These technologies are developmental, expensive and have only preliminary data.

Chemoprevention offers the opportunity for early intervention to prevent the progression of neoplasia in BE. Because of its potential application to many patients it must be safe, inexpensive and effective. Appropriate targets for chemopreventive agents can be gained from advances in the understanding of the molecular biology, cytokines and growth factors and environmental factors leading to carcinogenesis

Table 3. Management of HGD

1. Confirm with therapeutic endoscopy, large capacity biopsy forceps, intensive biopsy protocol
2. Confirm histology interpretation by expert in reading dysplasia
3. EMR for mucosal irregularity
4. Stage with EUS/CT
5. Evaluate patient as operative candidate/risk aversion
6. Expertise at institution
7. Individualize intervention

in BE. A current example of such a targeting is cyclooxyegenase 2 (COX2). COX2 expression increases with the progression of IM to dysplasia and EAC [54]. Both selective and non-selective COX2 inhibition significantly reduced the development of EAC in a rat esophagojejunostomy model of BE [55]. A meta-analysis of epidemiologic case control studies demonstrates a significant reduction of EAC with ASA and NSAID use in patients [56]. These data have led to the initiation of a large randomized trial of aspirin and PPI to test their impact on the development of EAC in BE patients. Retrospective analysis of two cohort studies document the reduction of the development of dysplasia by PPI therapy 4 to 5 fold [57], [58].

With the continuing rise in the incidence of EAC, there is a continuing stimulus to technologic and molecular breakthroughs. These will ultimately provide more effective risk stratification of patients with BE. Emerging information from large chemoprevention trials may offer the necessary breakthroughs to alter the neoplastic progression of BE.

References

[1] Sampliner RE (2002) Practice Parameters Committee ACG. Updated guidelines for the diagnosis, surveillance, and therapy of Barrett's esophagus. Am J Gastroenterol 97: 1888–1895

[2] Blot W, Devesa SS, Kneller RW, Fraumeni JF (1991) Rising incidence of adenocarcinoma of the esophagus and gastric cardia. JAMA 265(10): 1287–1289

[3] Brown LM, Devesa SS (2002) Epidemiologic trends in esophageal and gastric cancer in the United States. Surg Oncol Clin N Am 11: 235–256

[4] Boyce HW (2000) Endoscopic definitions of esophagogastric junction regional anatomy. Gastrintest Endosc 51(5): 586–592

[5] Cameron AJ (2002) Epidemiology of Barrett's esophagus and adenocarcinoma. Dis Esophagus 15: 106–108

[6] Gerson LB, Sheltler K, Triadafilopoloulos G (2002) Prevalence of Barrett's esophagus in asymptomatic individuals. Gastroenterology 123: 461–467

[7] Rex DK, Cummings OW, Shaw M, Cumings MD, Wong RKH, Vasudeva RS et al (2003) Screening for Barrett's esophagus in colonoscopy patients with and without heartburn. Gastroenterology 125: 1670–1677

[8] Drewitz DJ, Sampliner RE, Garewal HS (1997) The incidence of adenocarcinoma in Barrett's esophagus – a prospective study of 170 patients followed 4.8 years. Am J Gastroenterol 92(2): 212–215

[9] Shaheen NJ, Crosby MA, Bozymski EM (2000) Is there publication bias in the reporting of cancer risk of Barrett's esophagus? Gastroenterology 119: 333–338

[10] Anderson LA, Murray LJ, Murphy SJ, Fitzpatrick DA, Johnston BT, Watson RGP et al (2003) Mortality in Barrett's oesophagus: results from a population based study. Gut 52: 1081–1084

[11] Conio M, Blanchi S, Lapertosa G, Ferraris R, Sablich R, Marchi S et al (2003) Long-term endoscopic surveillance of patients with Barrett's esophagus. Incidence of dysplasia and adenocarcinoma: a prospective study. Am J Gastroenterol 98: 1931–1939

[12] Dulai GS, Guha S, Kahn KL, Gornbein J, Weinstein WM (2002) Preoperative prevalence of Barrett's esophagus in esophageal adenocarcinoma: a systematic review. Gastroenterology: 26–33

[13] Lagergren J, Bergstrom R, Lindgren A, Nyren O (1999) Symptomatic gastroesophageal reflux as a risk factor for esophageal adenocarcinoma. N Engl J Med 340(11): 825–831

[14] Lieberman DA, Oehlke M, Helfand M, G.O.R.E. (1997) Risk factors for Barrett's esophagus in community-based practice. Am J Gastroenterol 92(8): 1293–1297

[15] Eisen GM, Sandier IS, Murray S, Gottfried M (1997) The relationship between gastroesophageal reflux disease and its complications with Barrett's esophagus. Am J Gastroenterol 92: 27–31

[16] Breslin NP, Thompson ABR, Bailey RJ, Blustein PK, Meddings J, Lalor E et al (2000) Gastric cancer and other endoscopic diagnoses in patients with benign dyspepsia. Gut 46: 93–97

[17] Cameron AJ, Lomboy CT (1992) Barrett's esophagus: age, prevalence and extent of columnar epithelium. Gastroenterology 103: 1241–1245

[18] Soni A, Sampliner RE, Sonnenberg A (2000) Screening for high grade dysplasia in gastroesophageal reflux disease: is it cost effective? Am J Gastroenterol 95: 2086–2093

[19] Robertson CS, Mayberry JF, Nicholson DA, James P, Atkinson M (1988) Value of endoscopic surveillance in the detection of neoplastic change in Barrett's oesophagus. Br J Surg 75: 760–763

[20] Miros M, Kerlin MM, Walker N (1991) Only patients with dysplasia progress to adenocarcinoma in Barrett's oesophagus. Gut 32: 1441–1446

[21] Reid B, Levine D, Longton G, Blount P, Rabinovitch P (2000) Predictors of progression to cancer in Barrett's esophagus: baseline histology and flow cytometry identify low and high risk patient subsets. Am J Gastroenterol 95: 1669–1676
[22] Weston AP, Badr AS, Hassanein RS (1999) Prospective multivariate analysis of clinical, endoscopic, and histological factors predictive of the development of Barrett's multifocal high grade dysplasia or adenocarcinoma. Am J Gastroenterol 94(12): 3413–3419
[23] Schnell TG, Sontag SJ, Chejfec G, Aranha G, Metz A, O'Connell S et al (2001) Long-term nonsurgical management of Barrett's esophagus with high-grade dysplasia. Gastroenterology 120: 1607–1619
[24] O'Connor JB, Falk GW, Richter JE (1999) The incidence of adenocarcinoma and dysplasia in Barrett's esophagus. Am J Gastroenterol 94(8): 2037–2042
[25] Conio M, Cameron AJ, Romero Y, Branch CD, Schleck CD, Burgart LJ et al (2001) Secular trends in the epidemiology and outcome of Barrett's oesophagus in Olmsted County, Minnesota. Gut 48: 304–309
[26] Streitz JM, Andrews CW, Ellis FH (1993) Endoscopic surveillance of Barrett's esophagus: does it help? J Thorac Cardiovasc Surg 105: 383–388
[27] Peters JH, Clark GWB, Ireland AP, Chandrasoma P, Smyrk TC, DeMeester TR (1994) Outcome of adenocarcinoma arising in Barrett's esophagus in endoscopically surveyed and nonsurveyed patients. J Thorac Cardiovasc Surg 108: 813–822
[28] Corley DA, Levin TR, Habel LA, Weiss NS, Buffler PA (2002) Surveillance and survival in Barrett's adenocarcinomas: a population-based study. Gastroenterology 122: 633–640
[29] Cooper GS, Yuan Z, Chak A, Rimm AA (2002) Association of prediagnosis endoscopy with stage and survival in adenocarcinoma of the esophagus and gastric cardia. Cancer 95: 32–38
[30] Fass R, Sampliner RE, Malagon IB, Hayden CW, Camargo L, Wendel CS et al (2000) Failure of oesophageal acid control in candidates for Barrett's oesophagus reversal on a very high dose of proton pump inhibitor. Aliment Pharmacol 14: 597–602
[31] Sharma P, Weston A, Keeton S, Camargo L, Sampliner RE (2001) Control of esophageal acid exposure in patients with Barrett's esophagus on rabeprazole. Am J Gastroenterol 96: S36(110)
[32] Holscher AH, Bollschweiler E, Schneider PM, Siewert JR (1997) Early adenocarcinoma in Barrett's oesophagus. Br J Surg 84: 1470–1473
[33] Ruol A, Merigliano S, Baldan N, Santi S, Petrin GF, Bonavina L et al (1997) Prevalence, management and outcome of early adenocarcinoma (pT1) of the esophagogastric junction. Comparison between early cancer in Barrett's esophagus (type I) and early cancer of the cardia (type II). Dis Esophagus 10: 190–195
[34] Stein HJ, Feith M, Mueller J, Werner M, Siewert JR (2000) Limited resection of early adenocarcinoma in Barrett's esophagus. Ann Surg 6: 733–742
[35] Begg CB, Cramer LD, Hoskins WJ, Brennan MF (1998) Impact of hospital volume on operative mortality for major cancer surgery. JAMA 280: 1747–1751
[36] Birkmeyer JD, Siewers AE, Finlayson EVA, Stukel TA, Lucas FL, Batista I et al (2002) Hospital volume and surgical mortality in the United States. N Engl J Med 346: 1128–1137
[37] Hofstetter WL, Peters JH, DeMeester T, Hagen JA, DeMeester SR, Crookes PF et al (2001) Long-term outcome of antireflux surgery in patients with Barrett's esophagus. Ann Surg 234: 532–539
[38] Corey KE, Schmitz SM, Shaheen NJ (2003) Does a surgical anti-reflux procedure decrease the incidence of esophageal adenocarcinoma in Barrett's esophagus? A meta-analysis. Am J Gastroenterol 98(11): 2390–2394
[39] Parilla P, Martinez de Haro L, Ortiz A, Munitiz V, Molina JB, Bermejo J et al (2003) Long-term results of a randomized prospective study comparing medical and surgical treatment of Barrett's esophagus. Ann Surg 237(1): 291–298
[40] Csendes A (2004) Surgical treatment of Barrett's esophagus: 1980–2003. World J Surg 28: 225–231
[41] Ell C, May A, Gossner L, Pech O, Gunter E, Mayer G et al (2000) Endoscopic mucosal resection of early cancer and high grade dysplasia in Barrett's esophagus. Gastroenterology 118: 670–677
[42] May A, Gossner L, Pech O, Fritz A, Gunter E, Mayer G et al (2002) Local endoscopic therapy for intraepithelial high-grade neoplasia and early adenocarcinoma in Barrett's oesophagus: acute-phase and intermediate results of a new treatment approach. Eur J Gastroenterol Heptaol 14: 1085–1091
[43] Overholt B, Lightdale C, Wang K, Canto M, Burdick S, Barr H et al (2003) International, multicenter, partially blinded, randomised study of the efficacy of photodynamic therapy (PDT) using porfimer sodium (POR) for the ablation of high-grade dysplasia (HGD) in Barrett's esophagus (BE): results of 24-month follow-up. Gastroenterology 124: A20
[44] Overholt BF, Panjehpour M, Halberg DL (2003) Photodynamic therapy for Barrett's esophagus with dysplasia

and/or early carcinoma: long-term results. Gastrointest Endosc 58: 183–188

[45] Attwood SEA, Lewis CJ, Caplin S, Hemming K, Armstrong GRA (2003) Argon plasma coagulation as therapy for high-grade dysplasia in Barrett's esophagus. Clin Gastroenterol Hepatol 1: 258–263

[46] Gossner L, Stolte M, Sroka R, Rick K, May A, Hahg EG et al (1998) Photodynamic ablation of high-grade dysplasia and early cancer in Barrett's esophagus by means of 5-aminolevulinic acid. Gastroenterology 114: 448–455

[47] Etienne J, Dorme N, Bourg-Heckly G, Raimbert P, Filijou JF (2004) Photodynamic therapy with green light and m-tetrahydroxyphenyl chlorin for intramucosal adenocarcinoma and high-grade dysplasia in Barrett's esophagus. Gastrintest Endosc 59(7): 880–889

[48] Buttar NS, Wang KK, Burgart LJ, Song LMMWK, Lutzke LS, Wandersee SM et al (2003) Endoscopic appearance and extent of high-grade dysplasia in Barrett's esophagus can predict the presence of cancer at esophagectomy. Am J Gastroenterol 98 (9 Suppl): S28 (81)

[49] Nigro JJ, Hagen JA, DeMeester TR, DeMeester SR, Theisen J, Peters JH et al (1999) Occult esophageal adenocarcinoma. Extent of disease and implications for effective therapy. Ann Surg 230: 433–440

[50] Tseng EE, Wu TT, Yeo CF, Heitmiller RF (2003) Barrett's esophagus with high grade dysplasia: surgical results and long-term outcome – an update. J Gastrointest Surg 7: 164–171

[51] Garcia RT, Cello JP, Nguyen MH, Rogers SJ, Rodas A, Trinh HN et al (2003) Unsedated ultrathin EGD is well accepted when compared with conventional sedated EGD: a multicenter randomized trial. Gastroenterology 125: 1606–1612

[52] Inadomi JM, Sampliner RE, Lagergren J, Lieberman D, Fendrick M, Vakil N (2003) Screening and surveillance for Barrett's esophagus in high-risk groups: a cost-utility analysis. Ann Intern Med 138(3): 176–186

[53] Reid B, Prevo L, Galipeau P, Sanchez CA, Longton G, Levine D et al (2001) Predictors of progression in Barrett's esophagus II: baseline 17p (p53) loss of heterozygosity identifies a patient subset at increased risk for neoplastic progression. Am J Gastroenterol 96: 2839–2848

[54] Shirvani VN, Ouatu-Lascar R, Kaur B, Omary B, Triadafilopoloulos G (2000) Cyclooxygenase 2 expression in Barrett's esophagus and adenocarcinoma: ex vivo induction by bile salts and acid exposure. Gastroenterology 118: 487–496

[55] Buttar NS, Wang KK, Leontovich O, Westcott JY, Pacifico RJ, Anderson MA et al (2002) Chemoprevention of esophageal adenocarcinoma by COX-2 inhibitors in an animal model of Barrett's esophagus. Gastroenterology 122: 1101–1112

[56] Corley DA, Kerlikowske K, Verma R, Buffler PA (2003) Protective association of aspirin/NSAIDs and esophageal cancer: a systematic review and meta-analysis. Gastroenterology 124: 47–56

[57] Hillman LC, Chiragakis L, Shadbolt B, Kaye GL, Clarke AC (2004) Proton-pump inhibitor therapy and the development of dysplasia in patients with Barrett's oesophagus. Med J Aust 180(8): 387–391

[58] El-Serag HB, Aguirre TV, Davis S, Kuebeler M, Bhattacharyya A, Sampliner RE (2004) Proton pump inhibitors are associated with reduced incidence of dysplasia. Am J Gastroenterol (in press)

Chapter 6

THE INTRIGUING RELATIONSHIP OF *HELICOBACTER PYLORI* INFECTION AND GASTRO-OESOPHAGEAL REFLUX DISEASE

C. Knippig and P. Malfertheiner

Otto-von-Guericke-Universität Magdeburg, Department of Gastroenterology, Hepatology and Infectiology, Magdeburg, Germany

Introduction

The contrary epidemiological trends of an increase of gastro-oesophageal reflux disease (GORD) and a decrease of *Helicobacter pylori* infection have induced the suggestion that *Helicobacter pylori* is a possible etiologic factor contributing to the increase of GORD prevalence. These have forwarded several hypothesis to explain the phenomenon, but none is convincing. Furthermore eradication of *Helicobacter pylori* leads to an increase of oesophagitis in patients with ulcer disease as reported by some authors, but not confirmed by others. Finally there are several implications of *Helicobacter pylori* infection to gastric physiology that need to be considered in search for a satisfacting explanation.

This article shall give insights into the complex relationship of *Helicobacter pylori* infection with GORD and its implications for the clinical management.

Epidemiology

There is not a gold standard for the definition of GORD [1]. As 24 hour pH-metry studies have shown that only a minority of acid episodes are associated with GORD symptoms and correlate only somewhat with the presence of oesophagitis, definition of GORD has been a point of discussion during the last decade. The Geneval workshop defined GORD pragmatically as "heartburn symptoms sufficient to impair quality of life" knowing that there is an overlap with the definition of dyspepsia and that this definition will cause confusion between the definition of a disease entitiy and a working diagnostic criteria for clinical use.

Heartburn prevalence ranges from 9% in Europe to 38% in Northern Europe and 42% in the US [2]. Frequency of oesophagitis has been described with a prevalence from 4–76.9% [1]. One of the predisposing factors for GORD is the hiatal hernia (*Fig. 1*), which can be found in 2.9–20% of patients if it is smaller than 2 cm and from 4.1–40% if the hiatal hernia is more than 2 cm [1].

In patients with reflux symptoms or oesophagitis a lower prevalence of *Helicobacter pylori* infection was found in some studies, suggesting a possible protective effect of *Helicobacter pylori* infection [3]–[6]. A systematic review evaluating 20 studies found the average prevalence of *Helicobacter pylori* infection in patients with GORD to be 38% from a world perspective [1], [7]. The pooled estimate of the odds ratio for the prevalence of *Helicobacter pylori* in patients with GORD was 0.60 (0.47–0.78 CI, Table 1). However evidence for this protective role was equivocal. Whereas a lower prevalence of *Helicobacter pylori* infection was found among asian GORD patients [8], [9], this effect is less prominent in caucasian populations.

These ethnic differences may be attributed to different patterns of *Helicobacter pylori* gastritis among these populations and therefore may also explain different study results.

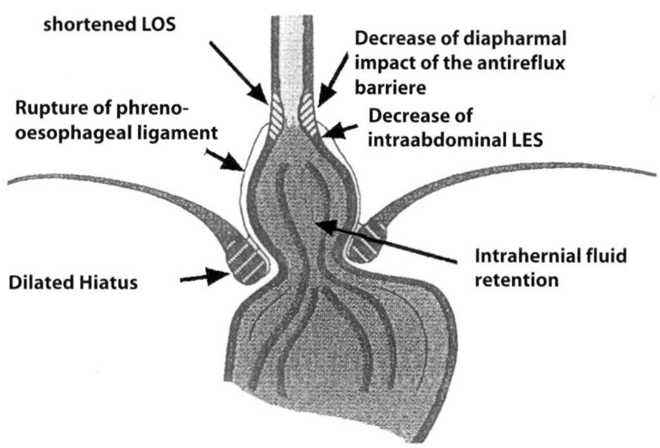

Fig. 1. The impact of hiatal hernia in the pathophysiology of GORD (LOS: lower oesophageal sphincter)

Type of gastritis and impact on gastric physiology

One reason for the variable effect of *Helicobacter pylori* infection and its eradication on acid secretion is the dependence on the type and distribution of gastritis [10]. Non-atrophic predominantly antral gastritis results in hypergastrinaemia and acid hypersecretion. Corpus predominant or atrophic pangastritis lead to decreased acid production and therefor can play a somehow protective role for oesophageal acid exposure ([11]–[13], *Figs. 2* and *3*).

If *Helicobacter pylori* is eradicated, gastritis with low acid output is healed leading to higher acid exposure of the esophagus and possibly resulting in GORD [3] if gastro-oesophageal reflux barrier is impaired [14]. As many *Helicobacter pylori* infected patients without disease have a mixed pattern of gastritis, the elevated gastrin resulting from antral inflammation fails to cause gastric acid secretion because of corpus inflammation.

Table 1. Odds ratio for prevalence of *Helicobacter pylori* in patients with esophagitis [1], [7]

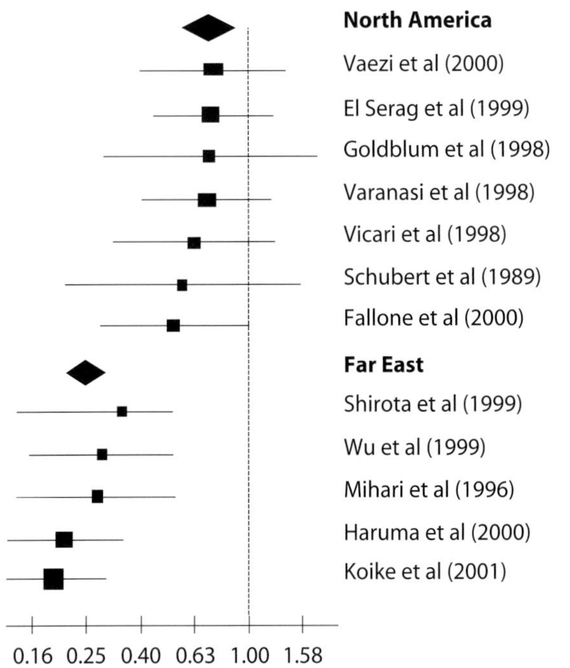

Clinical observations

The clinical effect of the above described relationship has to be analysed under six different aspects:

- The effect of *Helicobacter pylori* eradication on GORD symptoms and severity
- The effect of *Helicobacter pylori* infection and its eradication on proton pump inhibitor (PPI) efficacy
- The effect of *Helicobacter pylori* infection and its eradication on histology if long term PPI therapy is required for GORD maintenance therapy
- *Helicobacter pylori* infection and its role in Barrett's oesophagus
- The role of cagA-positive-strains in patients with Barrett's oesophagus
- The role of cagA-positive-strains in patients with oesophageal adenocarcinoma.

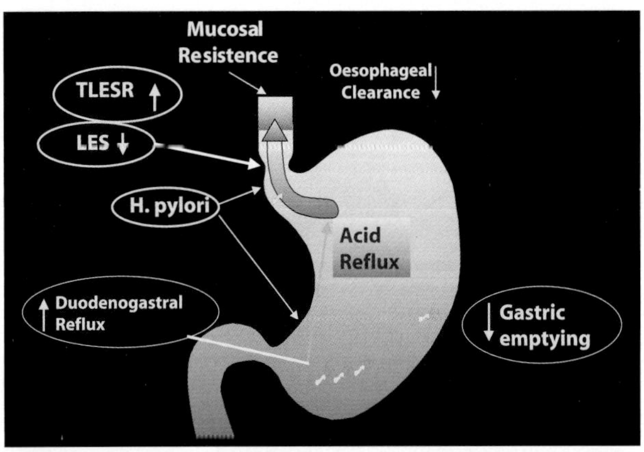

Fig. 2. The pathophysiology of GORD (TLESR: transient lower esophageal sphincter relaxation; LES: lower esophageal sphincter pressure)

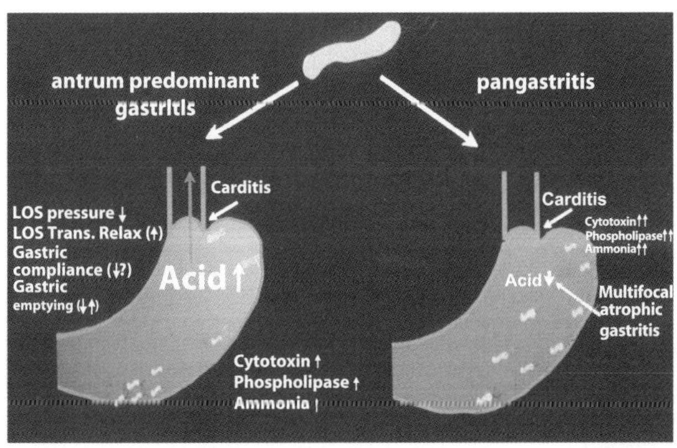

Fig. 3. Impact of the pattern of gastritis: antrum predominant gastritis vs. pangastritis

Effect of *Helicobacter pylori* eradication on GORD symptoms and severity

The actual data range from a more beneficial to an harmful or simply no effect of *Helicobacter pylori* eradication on GORD.

The first report of Labenz et al on an increase of the incidence of oesophagitis in ulcer patients after *Helicobacter pylori* eradication has been confirmed by further studies in patients with corpus predominant gastritis and associated hypochlorhydria. The effect was attributed to the recovery of acid secretion after *Helicobacter pylori* eradication [15], [16]. Further studies confirmed the increase of gastro-oesophageal reflux [17], [18] after eradication. A recent prospective, double blind, placebo controlled, randomised trial including 104 *Helicobacter pylori* infected GORD patients could show that *Helicobacter pylori* eradication was the only predictor of treatment failure of GORD. The authors explained the worsening control of reflux disease after *Helicobacter pylori* eradication with the ammonia production of *Helicobacter pylori* infection which augments the acid suppressing effect of medication. After successful eradication rebound acid secretion on reduced dosage of PPI may have caused relapse of GORD [19]–[21].

Additionaly the resolution of corpus gastritis after successful *Helicobacter pylori* eradication and recovery of gastric acid secretion itself [11], [22], [23] have to be mentioned as the main pathophysiological factors.

However not all studies could confirm these findings. A prospective, controlled trial could demonstrate a GORD relapse rate of 83% within one year of follow up independent of *Helicobacter pylori* status [24]. Additionaly further studies did not find any changes in 24-hour oesophageal acid exposure after successful eradication [24], [25]. A recent prospective randomised study on 231 patients aimed to investigate the influence of *Helicobacter pylori* eradication on gastritis during long term omeprazole therapy for GORD [26] did not find a worsening of reflux disease, nor a need for increased omeprazole maintenance dose.

There are even studies reporting a benefit after *Helicobacter pylori* eradication: Schwizer et al report of a benefit during a six month follow up in which patients with GORD and persistent *Helicobacter pylori* infection relapsed earlier than patients in whom *Helicobacter pylori* had been eradicated [27]. The authors explain their result with the pattern of gastritis which functionaly can be linked to normal or increased acid secretion, which possible can change to lower acid output following eradication [28]. These results have been confirmed by Kupcinskas et al [29].

The discrepancy of the results of the above mentioned studies is probably due to different study designs, such as inclusion criteria, timing of follow up investigations and ethnic differences in the pattern of *Helicobacter pylori* gastritis. There are suggestions that the incidence of patients with predominant corpus gastritis is increased in populations with predominantly cagA+ strains, leading to a worsening of gastro-oesophageal reflux [30], [31]. Although this point is still under discussion, it hints to the importance of respect of ethnicity [32].

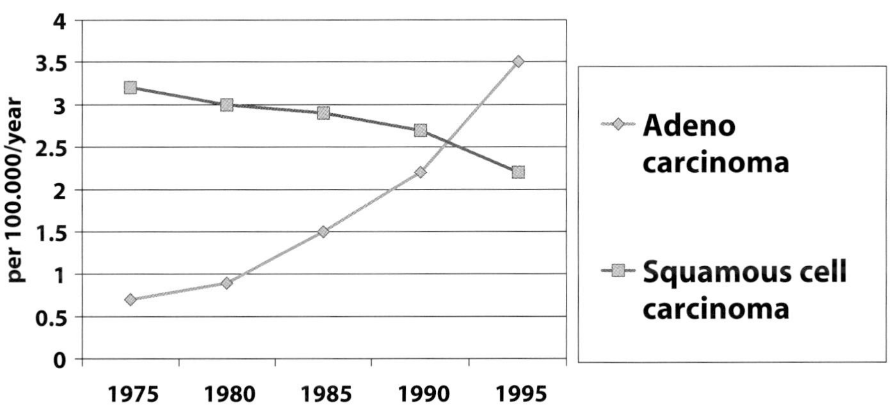

Fig. 4. Epidemiology of oesophageal adenocarcinoma (from [63])

The effect of *Helicobacter pylori* on PPI efficacy

More than 70% of patients suffering from GORD are dependent on long term use of acid suppressants [33].

It is well known that *Helicobacter pylori* infection leads to a higher intragastric pH during PPI treatment [19], [20], [34], [35]. Patients with *Helicobacter pylori* infection treated with pantoprazole have better symptom relief and better healing of severe forms of erosive oesophagitis [36]. These results have been confirmed in a study with 483 patients with uninvestigated heartburn [37].

However in clinical reality most patients have mild to moderate severity of GORD and in most studies a difference in the efficacy of PPI is neither detectable, nor required [38], [39]. Carlsson and colleagues reported from 1350 patients with GORD treated with omeprazole similar symptom relief and healing rates in patients with or without *Helicobacter pylori* infection [40]. These data have been confirmed from other studies [41], [42]. Maintenance dose after healing of erosive oesophagitis was independent of *Helicobacter pylori* status [39].

In summary most treatment trials with PPI do not show an effect of *Helicobacter pylori* on symptom relief, healing of acute oesophagitis or maintenance treatment of erosive oesophagitis.

The effect of *Helicobacter pylori* infection and its eradication on histology if long term PPI therapy is required for GORD maintenance therapy

Considering the effect of persistent *Helicobacter pylori* infection on the type of gastritis under long term PPI therapy Kuipers et al first reported progression of atrophic gastritis in *Helicobacter pylori* infected patients receiving long term PPI [43].

Atrophic gastritis itself is a well recognised risk factor for gastric cancer in *Helicobacter pylori* infected subjects. The paper of Kuipers was criticised for weakness in design [44] and his results have not been confirmed in a subsequent randomised trial by Lundell et al [45]. However anxiety did not relieve as Lundell et al also reported of evidence of accelerated development of moderate and severe atrophy in the *Helicobacter pylori* infected group on PPI therapy.

Subsequently in a new prospective, randomised trial in 231 patients Kuipers himself could not confirm findings of progression of atrophic gastritis, same as other authors [46]–[49]. However he could demonstrate that corpus gastritis progressed on long term omeprazole treatment if *Helicobacter pylori* had not been eradicated [50].

As a consequence there is only little evidence that PPI therapy accelerates corpus atrophy in *Helicobacter pylori* positive patients but PPI therapy moves the predominant type of gastritis from the antrum to the corpus. This may be of importance as Uemura et al recently showed that the strongest risk factor for cancer is the presence of corpus predominant gastritis [51].

As a consequence recommendation for *Helicobacter pylori* eradication before prescribing long term PPI is indicated [52].

Helicobacter pylori infection and Barrett's oesophagus

The definition of Barrett's oesophagus is a subject of controversy over the last years. It is applied to a columnar-lined oesophagus with biopsy specimens that contain specialized intestinal epithelium. This definition applies to patients with long segment and short segment Barrett's oesophagus and those with circumferential disease or tongues. Barrett's oesophagus is the consequence of gastroesophageal reflux.

A prospective evaluation of Barrett's oesophagus in 550 patients found three factors being significantly associated with index diagnosis of Barrett's high-grade dysplasia or adenocarcinoma: larger size hiatal hernia, Barrett's length and absence of *Helicobacter pylori* infection [53].

Another study from Japan underlined the protective role of *Helicobacter pylori* infection in the development of Barrett's oesophagus especially in the development of long segment Barrett's oesophagus in 112 reflux patients [54]. This group additionally included endoscopic gastrin test finding that gastric acid hypersecretion may be concerned with the development of Barrett's oesophagus in addition to the absence of *Helicobacter pylori*. However there is no evidence that *Helicobacter pylori* status itself does affect the presence of Barrett's complications such as stricture or ulcer [55].

The role of cagA-positive-strains in patients with Barrett's oesophagus

An important marker of the virulence of *Helicobacter pylori* strains is cagA encoding the cytotoxin-associated gene protein (cagA) [4]. Almost all *Helicobacter pylori* isolates from patients with peptic ulcers, atrophic gastritis and gastric cancer are cagA+ [56]. As there is an inverse relation between carcinoma in the cardia and lower oesophagus and colonization with cagA+ strains [57] it has been proposed that *Helicobacter pylori* colonization with especially cagA+ strains may protect against the development of GORD and its complications.

These suggestions have been underlined by the results of a cross-sectional study in 736 consecutive patients examining the relation between cagA+ and cagA− *Helicobacter pylori* strains in patients with reflux oesophagitis and Barrett's oesophagus [4]. The authors found a significant lower prevalence of *Helicobacter pylori* (34,9%) in reflux patients than in controls with a prevalence of 59% cagA+ strains in the control group vs. 35% in the reflux group.

In conclusion cagA+ strains may on the one side be most harmful by increasing the risk of ulceration and distal cancer but on the other side be most beneficial by protecting against reflux oesophagitis and its sequelae. Further studies proved this concept [58].

The role of cagA-positive-strains in patients with oesophageal adenocarcinoma

Different studies hint on a protective role of *Helicobacter pylori* infection – especially cagA+-strains – against the development of oesophageal adenocarcinoma.

The incidence of oesophageal adenocarcinoma increased over the last years [59] reaching 4–12 per 100.000. This is in contrast to the decreasing incidence of non-cardia gastric cancer (*Fig. 3*), [63].

Quddus et al did not find any *Helicobacter pylori* infected in 19 patients with Barrett's adenocarcinoma [60]. In a larger study population *Helicobacter pylori* again has been identified in significantly higher proportion of patients with benign Barrett's oesophagus than in those with dysplastic Barrett's oesophagus or Barrett's adenocarcinoma (34% vs. 17%) [61].

A multicenter study did not find a difference in the prevalence of *Helicobacter pylori* infection in patients with oesophageal adenocarcinoma when compared to age- and sex-matched controls. However infection with the cagA+ strain of the bacteria resulted in a reduced odds ratio for developing oesophageal adenocarcinoma [57]. These results have been confirmed in a smaller study by Vicari et al [5] and may be explained by *Helicobacter pylori* induced apoptosis in Barrett derived oesophageal adenocarcinoma cells which is mainly dependent on the presence of the cagA and picB/cagE gene products [62].

Conclusion

The interesting pathophysiological interaction between *Helicobacter pylori* infection, type of gastritis, acid secretion and GORD complicated by weakness of study designs with small numbers of patients should not lead to confusion. The risk of gastric carcinogenesis and peptic ulcer formation against the need for possible higher doses of acid suppressive therapy for symptom control after eradication should be balanced carefully and can only lead us to one conclusion: there are more reasons that favour *Helicobacter pylori* eradication than to leave the bug in the stomach of your patients.

References

[1] Kang JY (2004) Geographical and ethnic differences in gastro-oesophageal reflux disease. Aliment Pharmacol Ther 20: 705–717

[2] Delaney BC (2004) Prevalence and epidemiology of gastro-oesophageal reflux disease. Aliment Pharmacol Ther 20 (Suppl 8): 2–4

[3] Koike T, Ohara S, Sekine H (2001) *Helicobacter pylori* infection prevents erosive reflux oesophagitis by decreasing gastric acid secretion. Gut 1: 330–334

[4] Loffeld FJLF, Werdmuller BFM, Kuster JA (2000) Colonization with cagA positive *Helicobacter pylori*

strains inversely associated with reflux esophagitis and Barrett's esophagus. Digestion 62: 95–99
[5] Vicari JJ, Peek RM, Falk GW (1998) The seroprevalence of cagA positive *Helicobacter pylori* strains in the spectrum of gastroesophageal reflux disease. Gastroenterology 115: 50–57
[6] Fallone CA, Barkun AW, Friedman G (2000) Is *Helicobacter pylori* eradication associated with gastroesophageal reflux disease? Am J Gastroenterol 95: 914–920
[7] Raghunath A, Pali A, Hungin S (2003) Prevalence of *Helicobacter pylori* in patients with gastro-oesophageal reflux disease: systematic review. BMJ 326: 737–739
[8] Wu JCY, Sung Jy, Ng EK (1999) Prevalence and distribution of *Helicobacter pylori* in gastroesophageal reflux disease: a study from the East. Am J Gastroenterol 94: 1790–1794
[9] O'Connor HJ (1999) *Helicobacter pylori* and gastro-oeosphagela reflux disease – clinical implications and management. Aliment Pharmacol Ther 13: 117–127
[10] Labenz J, Malfertheiner P (1997) *Helicobacter pylori* in gastro-oesophageal reflux disease: causal agent, independent or protective factor? Gut 41: 277–280
[11] Koike T, Ohara S, Sekine H (1999) *Helicobacter pylori* infection inhibits reflux oesophagitis by inducing atrophic gastritis. Am J Gastroenterology 94: 3468–3472
[12] Yamaji Y, Mitsushima T, Ikuma H (2001) Inverse background of *Helicobacter pylori* antibody and pepsinogen in reflux oeosphagitis compared with gastric cancer: analysis of 5732 Japanese subjects. Gut 49: 335–340
[13] El Serag Hb, Sonnenberg Am, Jamal MM (1999) Corpus gastritis is protective against reflux oesophagitis. Gut 45: 181–185
[14] Hamada H, Haruma K, Mihara M (2000) High incidence of reflux oesophagitis after eradication therapy for *Helicobacter pylori*: impacts of hiatal hernia and corpus gastritis. Aliment Pharmacol Ther 14: 729–735
[15] Koike T, Ohara S, Sekine H (2001) Increased gastric acid secretion after *Helicobacter pylori* eradication may be a factor for developing reflux oeosphagitis. Aliment Pharmacol Ther 15: 813–820
[16] El-Omar EM, Oien K, El-Nujumi A (1997) *Helicobacter pylori* infection and chronic gastric acid hyposecretion. Gastroenterology 113: 15–24
[17] Feldman M, Cryer B, Sammer D (1999) Influence of *Helicobacter pylori* infection on meal stimulated gastric acid secretion and gastroesophageal reflux. Am J Physiol 277: G1159–G1164
[18] Wu JC, Chan FK, Wang SK (2002) Effect of *Helicobacter pylori* eradication on oesophageal acid exposure in patients with reflux esophagitis. Aliment Pharmacol Ther 16: 545–552
[19] Verdu EF, Armstrong D, Fraser R (1995) Effect of *Helicobacter pylori* status on intergastric pH during treatment with omeprazole. Gut 37: 743–748
[20] Bercik P, Verdu EF, Armstrong D (2000) The effect of ammonia on omeprazole induced reduction of gastric acidity in subjects with *Helicobacter pylori* infection. Am J Gastroenterol 95: 947–955
[21] Gillen D, Wirz AA, Ardill JE (1999) Rebound hypersecretion after omeprazole and its relation to on-treatment acid suppression and *Helicobacter pylori* status. Gastroenterology 116: 239–247
[22] Adamek RJ, Behrendt J, Wenzel C (2001) Relapse and prevention in reflux oeosphagitis with regard to *Helicobacter pylori* status: a double-blinded randomised, multicenter trial to compare the efficacy of pantoprazole versus ranitidine. Eur J Gastroenterol Hepatol 13: 811–817
[23] Labenz J, Blum AL, Bayerdorffer E (1997) Curing *Helicobacter pylori* infection in patients with duodenal ulcer may provoke reflux esophagitis. Gastroenterology 112: 1442–1447
[24] Telfera S, Hatlebakk JG, Berstad A (1999) The effect of *Helicobacter pylori* eradication on gastro-oesophageal reflux. Aliment Pharmacol Ther 13: 915–920
[25] Moayyedi P, Bardhan C, Young L (2001) *Helicobacter pylori* eradication does not exacerbate reflux symptoms in gastroesophageal reflux disease. Gastroenterology 121: 1120–1126
[26] Manifold DK, Anggiansah A, Rowe I (2001) Gastro-oesophageal reflux and duodenogastric reflux before and after eradication in *Helicobacter pylori* gastritis. Eur J Gastroenterol Hepatol 13: 535–539
[27] Kuipers EJ, Nelis GF, Klinkenberg-Knol EC, Snel P, Goldfain D, Kolkman JJ, Festen HPM, Dent J, Zeitoun P, Havu N, Lamm M, Walan A (2004) Cure of *Helicobacter pylori* infection in pateintes with reflux oesophagitis treated with long term omeprazole reverses gastritis without exacerbation of reflux disease: results of a randomised controlled trial. Gut 53: 12–20
[28] Schwizer W, Thurmshirn M, Dent J (2001) *Helicobacter pylori* and symptomatic relapse of gastro-esophageal reflux disease: a randomized controlled trial. Lancet 357: 1738–1742
[29] El Omar E, Perman I, Dorrian CA (1993) *Helicobacter pylori* infection lowers gastrin mediated acid secretion by two thirds in duodenal ulcer patients. Gut 34: 1060–1065
[30] Kupcinskas L, Jonaitis L, Kudelis G (2004) A 1 year follow-up study of the consequences of *Helicobacter pylori* eradication in duodenal ulcer patients: unchanged frequency of erosive oesophagitis and decreased preva-

lence of non-erosive gastro-oesophageal reflux disease. Eur J Gastroenterol Hepatol 16: 369–374

[31] Rokkas T, Ladas S, Triantafyllou K (2001) The association between CagA status and the development of esophagitis after the eradication of *Helicobacter pylori*. Am J Med 110: 703–707

[32] Warburton-Timms VJ, Charlett A, Valori RM (2001) The significance of cagA+ *Helicobacter pylori* in reflux oesophagitis. Gut 49: 341–346

[33] Jakobs R, Riemann JF (2004) CagA-positive *Helicobacter pylori* strains and gastrooesophageal erflux disease: still puzzling. European Jounal of Gastroenterol Hepatol 16: 635–637

[34] Wu JCY, Chan FKL, Ching JYL, Leung W-K, Hui Y, Leong R, Chung SCS, Sung JJY (2004) Effect of *Helicobacter pylori* eradication on treatment of gastro-oesophageal reflux disease: a double blind, placebo controlled, randomised trial. Gut 53: 174–179

[35] Labenz J, Tillenburg B, Peitz U (1996) *Helicobacter pylori* augments the pH-increasing effect of omeprazole in patients with duodenal ulcer. Gastroenterology 110: 725–732

[36] Martinek J, Kuzela I, Spicak J (2000) Review article: the clinical influence of *Helicobacter pylori* in effective acid suppression – implications for the treatment of gastroesophageal reflux disease. Aliment Pharmacol Ther 14: 979–990

[37] Holtmann G, Cain C, Malfertheiner P (1999) Gastric *Helicobacter pylori* infection accelerates healing of reflux esophagitis during treatment with the proton pump inhibitor pantoprazoel. Gastroenterology 117: 11–16

[38] Hatlebakk JG, Hyggen A, Madsen PH (1999) Heartburn treatment in primary care: randomised double-blind study for 8 weeks. BMJ 319: 550–554

[39] Malfertheiner P, Stolte M, Willich SN (submitted 2004) Prognostic influence of Barrett's epithelium and of *Helicobacter pylori* infection on healing of erosive and non-erosive gastro-esophageal reflux disease – Report from the PROGORD Study

[40] Schenk BE, Kuipers EJ, Klinkenberg-Knol EC (1999) *Helicobacter pylori* and the efficacy of omeprazole therapy for gastroesophageal reflux disease. Am J Gastroenterol 94: 884–887

[41] Carlsson R, Bate C, Dent J (1997) Does *Helicobacter pylori* infection influence the response to treatment with acid inhibition in patiens with GORD? Scand J Gastroenterol 32 (Suppl 224): F70

[42] Peter FTM, Kuipers EJ, Ganesh S (1999) The influence of *Helicobacter pylori* on oesophageal acid exposure in GORD during acid supressive therapy. Aliment Pharmacol Ther 13: 921–926

[43] Vakikl N, Kahrilas P, Magner D (2000) Does baseline *Helicobacter pylori* status impact erosive esophagitis healing rates? Am J Gastroenterol 95: 2438A

[44] Kuipers EJ, Lundell L, Klinkenberg-Knol EC (1996) Atrophic gastritis and *Helicobacter pylori* infection in patients with reflux esophagitis treated with omeprazole or fundoplication. N Engl J Med 334: 1018–1022

[45] McColl (2004) *Helicobacter pylori* infection and long term proton pump inhibitor therapy, Gut 53: 5–7

[46] Lundell L, Miettinen P, Myrvold HE (1999) Lack of effect of acid suppression therapy on gastric atrophy. Nodic GORD Study Group. Gastroenterology 117: 319–326

[47] Uemura N, Okamoto S, Ymamoto S (2000) Changes in *Helicobacter pylori*-induced gastritis in the antrum and corpus during long-term acid – suppressive treatment in Japan. Aliment Pharmacol Ther 14: 1345–1352

[48] Geboes K, Dekker W, Mulder Cjj (2001) Longterm lansoprazole treatment for gastroesophageal reflux disease: clinical efficacy and influence on gastric mucosa. Aliment Pharmacol Ther 18: 1819–1826

[49] Stolte M, Meining A, Schmitz JM (1998) Changes in *Helicobacter pylori*-induced gastritis in the antrum and corpus during 12 months of treatment with omeprazole and lansoprazole in patients with gastroesophageal reflux disease. Aliment Pharmacol Ther 12: 247–253

[50] Singh P, Indaram A, Greenberg R (2000) Long term omeprazole therapy for reflux esophagitis: follow-up in serum gastin levels, EC cell hyperplasia and neoplasia. World J Gastroenterol 6: 789–792

[51] Kuipers EJ, Nelis GF, Klinkenberg-Knol EC (2001) Helicobacter eradication for the prevention of atrophic gastritis during omeprazole therapy; a prospective randomised trial. Gastroenterology 120 (Suppl 1): A14

[52] Uemura N, Okamoto S, Yamamoto S (2001) *Helicobacter pylori* infection and the development of gastric cancer. N Engl J Med 345: 784–789

[53] Malfertheiner P, Megraud F, O'Morain C (2002) Current concepts in the management of *Helicobacter pylori* infection – the Maastricht 2-2000 Consensus Report. Aliment Pharmacol Ther 16: 167–180

[54] Weston AP, Sharma P, Mathur S, Banerjee S, Jafri K, Cherian R, McGregor D, Hassanein RS, Hall M (2004) Risk stratification of Barrett's esophagus: updated prospective multivariate analysis. Am J Gastroenterol 99: 1657

[55] Abe Y, Ohara S, Koike T, Sekine H, Lijima K, Kawamura M, Imatani A, Kato K, Shimosegawa T (2004) The prevalence of *Helicobacter pylori* infection and the status of gastric acid secretion in patients with

Barrett's esophagus in Japan. Am J Gastroenterol 99: 1222–1225

[56] Clark GWB (2003) Effect of *Helicobacter pylori* infection in barrett's esophagus and the genesis of esophageal adenocarcinoma. World J Surgery

[57] Pearsonnet J, Friedman GD, Orentrich N, Vogelman H (1997) Risk for gastric cancer in people with cagA-positive or cagA-negative *Helicobacter pylori* infection. Gut 40: 297–301

[58] Chow WA, Blaser MJ, Blot WJ, Gammon MD, Vaughan TL, Risch HA (1998) An inverse relation between cagA+ strains of Helicobcter pylori infection and risk of esophageal and gastric cardia adenocarcinoma. Cancer Res 58: 588–590

[59] Ackermark P, Kuipers EJ, Wolf C, Breuemlhof R, Seldenrijk CA, Timmer R, Segeren KC, Kusters JG, Smout AJ (2003) Colonization with cagA-positive *Helicobacter pylori* strains in intestinal metaplasia of the esophagus and the esophagogastric junction. Am J Gastroenterol 98: 1719–1724

[60] Forman D (2004) Review article: oesophago-gastric adenocarcinoma – an epidemiological perspective. Aliment Pharmacol Ther 20 (Suppl 5): 55–60

[61] Quddus MR, Henley JD, Sulaiman RA (1997) *Helicobacter pylori* infection and adenocarcinoma arising in Barrett's esophagus. Hum Pathol 28: 1007–1009

[62] Wright TA, Myskow M, Kingsnorth AN (1997) *Helicobacter pylori* colonization of Barrett's esophagus and its progression to cancer. Dis Esophagus 10: 196–200

[63] Jones AD, Bacon KD, Jobe BA, Sheppard BC, Deveney CW, Rutten JM (2003) *Helicobacter pylori* induces apoptosis in Barrett's derived esophageal adenocarcinoma cells. J Gastrointest Surg 7: 68–76

[64] Deves SS, Blot WJ, Fraumeni JF Jr (1998) Changing patterns in the incidence of esophageal and gastric carcinoma in the United States. Cancer 83(10): 2049–2053

Chapter 7

EGJ DYSFUNCTION AND GERD

P. J. Kahrilas and J. E. Pandolfino

Department of Medicine, Northwestern University's Feinberg School of Medical School, Chicago, IL, USA

Introduction

The defining abnormality in gastroesophageal reflux disease (GERD) is exposure of esophageal epithelium to gastric juice to an extent sufficient to result in either histopathological injury or bothersome symptoms. Implicit in this definition is that some degree of reflux and esophageal acid exposure is normal or "physiological" and that the esophagogastric junction (EGJ) is normally permissive of some degree of retrograde flow. However, the normal processes of acid clearance and the inherent impermeability of the esophageal epithelium are such that this is easily tolerated. With reflux disease, this tolerance is exceeded because of excessive reflux events, the effect of which may be accentuated by impaired acid clearance. Of the primary defensive factors preventing the clinical manifestations of GERD, EGJ competence is the most fundamental. Given that cardinal importance, this chapter will focus on mechanisms of function and dysfunction of the EGJ as an antireflux barrier.

The integrity of the EGJ as an antireflux barrier is the product of a number of anatomical and physiological properties: the intrinsic lower esophageal sphincter (LES) pressure, extrinsic compression of the LES by the crural diaphragm, the intra-abdominal location of the LES, integrity of the phrenoesophageal ligament, and maintenance of the acute angle of His promoting a "flap valve" function. Physiological investigations have revealed that individual reflux events occur by one of three mechanisms: (1) transient LES relaxation, (2) strain-induced reflux in the setting of a hypotensive LES, or (3) free reflux during periods of low LES pressure or deglutitive relaxation. Each of these reflux mechanisms occurs in the setting of specific anatomical and physiological determinants. The more aberrant those determinants, the worse the antireflux integrity of the EGJ. Thus, each functional component of the EGJ will be discussed individually in terms of its role in preventing gastroesophageal reflux and the mechanisms that lead to abnormal gastroesophageal reflux.

Antireflux function of the EGJ

The distal end of the esophagus is anchored to the diaphragm by the phrenoesophageal membrane that inserts circumferentially into the esophageal musculature around the squamocolumnar junction (SCJ). Viewed as a barrier to reflux, the EGJ is generally conceptualized as the locus of a high-pressure zone within this anatomically complex region (*Fig. 1*). Maintenance of that high-pressure zone assures that the distal esophagus is sealed off from the stomach and protected from contact with caustic gastric juice. However, the EGJ pressure profile is the composite of three key elements: the intrinsic LES, the influence of the surrounding diaphragmatic hiatus and crural diaphragm, and the muscular architecture of the gastric cardia that constitutes the distal aspect of the overall EGJ high-pressure zone. Furthermore, the tubular esophagus joins the stomach in almost a tangential fashion with the shared medial wall functioning as a flap valve under normal circumstances. Consider each of these contributions to the EGJ high-pressure zone.

Lower esophageal sphincter

The LES is a 3–4 cm segment of tonically contracted smooth muscle in the distal esophagus. Among normal individuals basal LES tone varies from 10–30 mmHg relative to intragastric pressure and exhibits substantial temporal variation. Studies utilizing concurrent fluoroscopy and manometry, localize the proximal aspect of the EGJ high-pressure zone 1–1.5 cm proximal to the SCJ and the distal aspect extending about 2 cm distal to it (1) (*Fig. 1*). Anatomical studies suggest that the EGJ component distal to the SCJ is largely attributable to the sling and clasp fibers of the middle layer of gastric musculature in the cardia [2], [3]. In this region, the lateral wall of the esophagus meets the medial aspect of the stomach at an acute angle, defined as the angle of His.

Large fluctuations of LES pressure occur during phase III of the migrating motor complex during which LES pressure may exceed 80 mmHg during this phase. Minor fluctuations occur throughout the day with pressure decreasing in the post-prandial state and increasing during sleep [4]. Basal LES tone is a property of both the smooth muscle itself and of its extrinsic innervation [5]. Consequently, LES pressure may be altered by myogenic factors, intra-abdominal pressure, gastric distention, peptides, hormones, various foods, and many medications. To maintain the delicate balance between antegrade and retrograde flow, the LES has a complex neurological control mechanism involving both the CNS and peripheral enteric nervous system. LES pressure is modulated by reflexes involving both vagal and sympathetic nerves [6]. Efferent function is mediated through neurons of the myenteric plexus that can effect either LES contraction or relaxation. Synapses between the efferent vagal fibers and the myenteric plexus employ a cholinergic system. The post-ganglionic transmitter effecting contraction is acetylcholine while several studies suggest that NO is the dominant inhibitory nonadrenergic-noncholinergic transmitter with VIP serving some type of modifying role [7], [8].

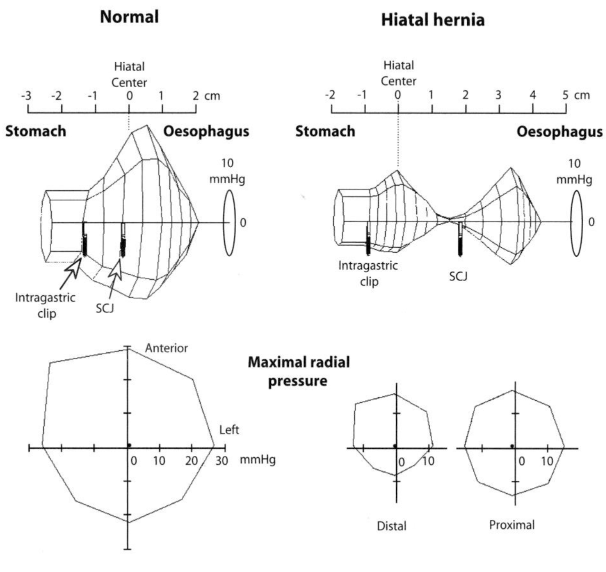

Fig. 1. Pressure topography of the EGJ of normal subjects (left) and hiatus hernia patients (right). Position zero on the axial scale is the midpoint of the diaphragmatic hiatus. The proximal clip indicates the position of the squamocolumnar junction (SCJ) and the distal clip marks the median position of the intragastric aspect to the EGJ as imaged endoscopically. All values of length and pressure are the medians of seven subjects in each subject study group. The bottom tracings represent maximal radial pressure for normals (left) and hiatus hernia subjects (right). Note the two peaks in the hiatus hernia group correlating to the above axial topography figures. (From [1]: Kahrilas PJ, Lin S, Chen J et al (1999) The effect of hiatus hernia on gastro-oesophageal junction pressure. Gut 44: 476–482, with permission)

Crural diaphragm

The hiatal orifice is an teardrop shaped opening through the diaphragm through which the esophagus and vagus nerves gain access to the abdomen. Although minor variants are recognized, the most common anatomy is for the hiatus to be formed by elements of the right diaphragmatic crus with partial contribution from the left crus [9]. The crura arise from tendinous fibers emerging from the anterior longitudinal ligament over the upper lumbar vertebrae (*Fig. 2*). The crura pass upward in close contact with the vertebral bodies for most of their course and only incline anteriorly as they arch around the esophagus [9]. Once muscle fibers emerge from the tendinous origin of the right crus, they form two overlying ribbon-like bundles separated from each other by connective tissue. The dorsal bundle forms the left limb of the right crus and the ventral bundle becomes the right limb of the right crus. As they approach the hiatal canal, the muscle bands diverge and cross each other in a scissor like fashion and merge anterior to the esophagus. The lateral fibers of each hiatal limb insert directly into the central tendon of the diaphragm but the medial fibers, that form the hiatal margins, incline toward the midline and decussate with each other in a trellis-like fashion anterior to the esophagus (*Fig. 3*) [9]. Normally there is about a centimeter of muscle separating the anterior rim of the hiatus from the central tendon of the diaphragm.

Under normal circumstances, the esophagus is anchored to the crural diaphragm by the phrenoesophageal ligaments (membranes) and the stomach cannot be displaced through the hiatal canal into the thoracic cavity [10], [11]. The phrenoesophageal membrane is formed from the fascia transversalis on the under surface of the diaphragm and fused elements of the endothoracic fascia. This membrane inserts circumferentially into the esophageal musculature, close to the squamocolumnar junction, and extends for about a centimeter proximal to the EGJ at which point it merges with the perivisceral fascia of the esophagus [12]. Thus, the axial position of the squamocolumnar junction is normally within or slightly distal to the diaphragmatic hiatus [13].

Independent control of the crural diaphragm can be demonstrated during esophageal distension, belching and vomiting when electrical activity in the crural diaphragm is selectively inhibited [14], [15]. This reflex inhibition of crural activity is eliminated with vagotomy. On the other hand, crural diaphragmatic contraction is amplified during abdominal compression, straining or coughing [16]. Additional evidence of the sphincteric function of the hiatus comes from manometric recordings in patients after distal esophagectomy for esophageal cancer [17]. These patients still exhibited an EGJ high-pressure zone of about 6 mmHg within the hiatal canal despite having had the entire smooth muscle intrinsic sphincter removed.

Hiatus hernia

Hiatal hernia is a perturbation of EGJ anatomy such that elements normally confined within the abdomen traverse the hiatal canal. The most comprehensive classification scheme recognizes 4 types of hiatal hernia and the main distinction is the difference between types-I and II (*Fig. 4*). Type-I or sliding hiatal hernias are associated with a widening of the muscular hiatal tunnel and circumferential laxity of the phrenoesophageal membrane, allowing a portion of the gastric cardia to herniate upward. Due to the inherent subjectivity in defining type-I hiatal hernia, estimates of prevalence vary substantially, from 10% to 80% of the adult population in North America [18]. Most type-I hiatal hernias are asymptomatic and, even with larger type-I hernias, the main clinical implication is the predilection to develop reflux disease, the likelihood of which increases with increasing hernia size. With a well de-

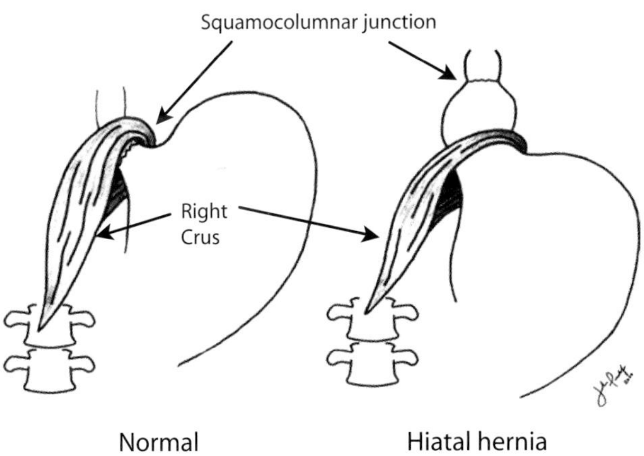

Fig. 2. Anatomy of the diaphragmatic hiatus. The right crus makes up the muscular component of the crural diaphragm. Arising from the anterior longitudinal ligament overlying the lumbar vertebrae. A single muscle band splits into an anterior and posterior muscular band, which cross each other to form the walls of the hiatal canal and then fuse anteriorly. With hiatus hernia the muscle becomes thin and atrophic limiting its ability to function as a sphincter. ([53]: Pandolfino JE, Kahrilas PJ (2001) Esophageal motility abnormalities in Barrett's esophagus. In: Barrett's esophagus and esophageal adenocarcinoma (Sharma P, Sampliner RE, eds). Malden: Blackwell Science, pp 35–44, with permission)

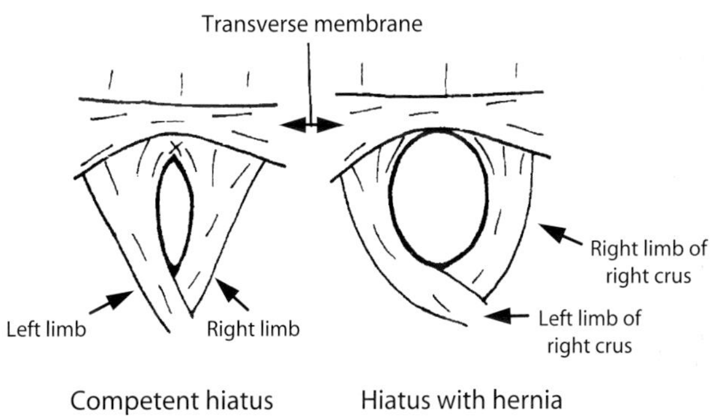

Fig. 3. The most common anatomy of the diaphragmatic hiatus in which the muscular elements of the crural diaphragm derive from the right diaphragmatic crus. The right crus arises from the anterior longitudinal ligament overlying the lumbar vertebrae. Once muscular elements emerge from the tendon, two flat muscular bands form which cross each other in scissor-like fashion, form the walls of the hiatus, and decussate with each other anterior to the esophagus. (Modified from Marchand P (1959) The anatomy of esophageal hiatus of the diaphragm and the pathogenesis of hiatus herniation. Thorac Surg 37: 81–92, with permission)

veloped hernia, the esophageal hiatus abuts directly on the transverse membrane of the central tendon of the diaphragm and the anterior hiatal muscles are absent or reduced to a few atrophic strands [9]. The hiatus itself is no longer a sagittal slit but a rounded opening whose transverse diameter approximates its sagittal diameter in size (*Fig. 3*). This change in caliber of the hiatus is most apparent during distention (*Fig. 5*) [19]. Associated with the widening of the hiatal orifice, the phrenoesophageal membrane also becomes attenuated. However, the phrenoesophageal membrane remains intact and the associated herniated gastric cardia is contained within the posterior mediastinum [18].

Although there are instances in which trauma, congenital malformation, and iatrogeny can be implicated, most evidence suggests that type-I hiatus hernia is usually an acquired condition. Allison observed that the typical age of onset was in the fifth decade of life [20] and pregnancy has long been suspected to be an inciting factor [21]. Marchand theorized that the compounded stresses of age-related degeneration, pregnancy, and obesity take their toll on the supporting structures of the EGJ. The positive peritoneo-pleural pressure gradient acts to push the abdominal contents into the chest and is opposed by the entire surface of the diaphragm. In this respect, only the esophageal hiatus is vulnerable to visceral herniation because it faces directly into the abdominal cavity. Furthermore, since the esophagus does not fill the entire hiatal canal, the integrity of this opening depends upon its intrinsic structures, especially the phrenoesophageal membrane [22]. Add to this susceptibility the repetitive stresses of deep inspiration, Valsalva, vomiting, physiologic herniation with swallowing, and tonic contraction of longitudinal muscle induced by gastroesophageal reflux, and then compound this stress by filling the abdominal cavity with adipose tissue or a gravid uterus and eventually the integrity of the hiatus is gradually compromised.

The type-I, or "sliding", hiatal hernia described above accounts for the vast majority of hiatal hernias, while less common types (II, III and IV) are varieties of "paraesophageal hernias." Together, paraesophageal hernias account for approximately 5–15% of all hiatal hernias [24]–[26]. Although these hernias may also be associated with significant gastroesophageal reflux their more worrisome clinical consequence lies in the poten-

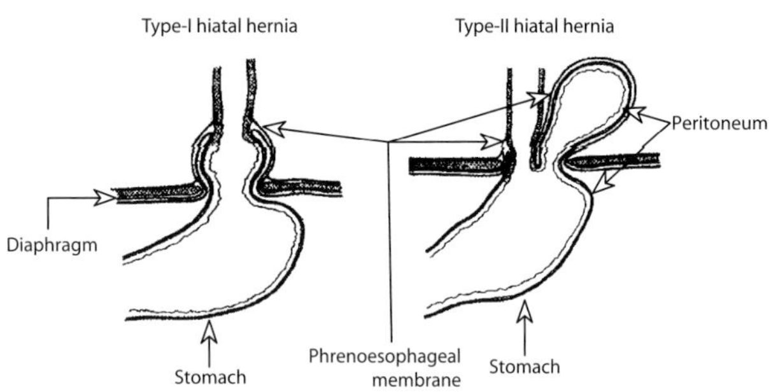

Fig. 4. Alteration of the hiatal anatomy associated with sliding hiatal hernia. Note that the main change is a widening of the hiatal canal. Associated with this there can be substantial atrophy of the abutting muscular elements, thinning and elongation of the phrenoesophageal membrane, and axial displacement of the gastric cardia. Sliding verses paraesophageal hiatal hernia. With sliding or axial hiatal hernia there is thinning and elongation of the phrenoesophageal membrane leading to herniation of the stomach into the posterior mediastinum. As such, there is no potential for incarceration or strangulation. With paraesophageal herniation, visceral elements herniate through a focal weakness in the phrenoesophageal membrane with the potential to lead to the usual array of complications associated with visceral herniation through a constricted aperture [Modified from Skinner DB (1985) Hernias (hiatal, traumatic, and congenital). In: Gastroenterology (Berk JE, ed). Philadelphia: Saunders, p 705, with permission]

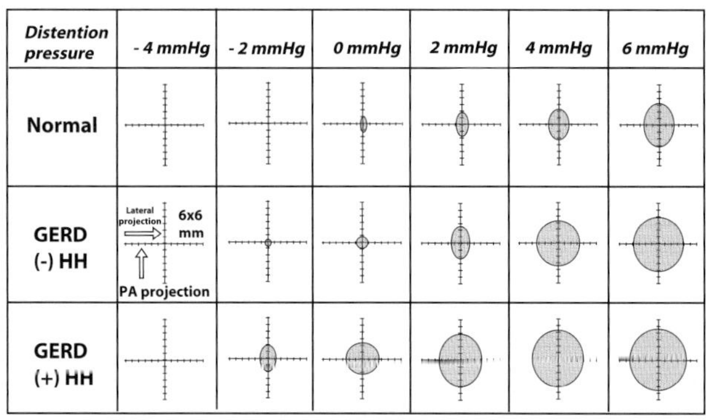

Fig. 5. (A) Dimensions and radial symmetry of the EGJ. Measurements of EGJ opening diameters were made from PA and lateral fluoroscopic projections and are plotted for each intrabag pressures relative to intragastric pressure distention pressure. Some degree of radial asymmetry of the hiatus was seen in all three groups; the lateral diameters were similar among the three groups but the hiatal hernia (HH) and non-hiatal hernia (NHH) GERD patients had increased PA diameters compared to normal subjects (NLS) (From [51]: Pandolfino et al (2003) Gastroenterology 125(4): 1018–1024, with permission)

tial for mechanical and ischemic complications. A type-II paraesophageal hernia results from a localized defect in the phrenoesophageal membrane while the EGJ itself remains fixed to the preaortic fascia and the median arcuate ligament (*Fig. 4*) [18]. The gastric fundus then becomes the leading point of herniation and the natural history of a type-II hernia is progressive enlargement so that the entire stomach eventually herniates into the chest, inverting as it does so with the pylorus juxtaposed to the gastric cardia. Type-III, or mixed, paraesophageal hernias have elements of both types-I and -II hernias with both axial displacement of the EGJ above the diaphragm and a focal defect within the phrenoesophageal membrane adding a paraesophageal element (*Fig. 3*). Type-IV hiatus hernia is associated with a large defect in the phrenoesophageal membrane, through which other abdominal organs, such as colon, spleen, pancreas and small intestine to enter the hernia sac. Type-IV hernias are usually encountered only in individuals with prior surgical procedures involving the left upper quadrant. In general, paraesophageal hernias are associated with abnormal laxity of structures normally preventing displacement of the stomach; the gastrosplenic and gastrocolic ligaments and are a recognized complication of surgical manipulation of the hiatus.

Proximal gastric musculature

In addition to the intrinsic sphincter and crural diaphragm described above, another mechanism of barrier function at the EGJ lies in the positioning of the distal esophagus in the intra-abdominal cavity. A flap valve is formed by a musculo-mucosal fold created by the entry of the esophagus into the stomach along the lesser curvature. Increased intra-abdominal or intragastric pressure can acutely decrease the angle of His thereby compressing and collapsing the subdiaphragmatic portion of the esophagus, preventing reflux during periods of abdominal straining. Viewed intraluminally, this region extends within the gastric lumen, appearing as a large fold that has been referred to as a flap valve because increased intragastric pressure would force the fold against the medial wall of the stomach, sealing off the entry to the esophagus [27], [28] (*Fig. 6*). As evidenced in Fig. 6, this distal aspect of the EGJ is particularly vulnerable to disruption as a consequence of anatomical changes at the hiatus and axial migration of the EGJ.

Mechanisms of EGJ dysfunction in GERD

Reflux occurs with either intermittent or constant compromise of the EGJ high-pressure zone. An added element to EGJ competence is EGJ opening and the degree to which the EGJ opens during periods in which the high-pressure zone is compromised. Just as with the upper esophageal sphincter, it has become apparent that sphincter opening is not synonymous with sphincter relaxation. During swallowing, despite being neurally inhibited, the EGJ must open to facilitate the esophago-gastric flow of a swallowed bolus while at the same time intermittently closing to prevent reflux of gastric contents into esophagus. During rest the EGJ must contain gastric juice but also be able to transiently relax and open enough to selectively permit gas venting without allowing reflux of caustic gastric juice. These functions are accomplished by the delicate interplay of the anatomical components and physiological responses of the EGJ. The dominant mechanism protecting against reflux will vary with physiological circumstance. For example, the intra-abdominal segment of the LES may be important in preventing reflux associated with swallowing, the crural diaphragmatic may be of primary importance during episodes of increased intragastric pressure, and basal LES pressure may be of cardinal importance during sleep. As these protective

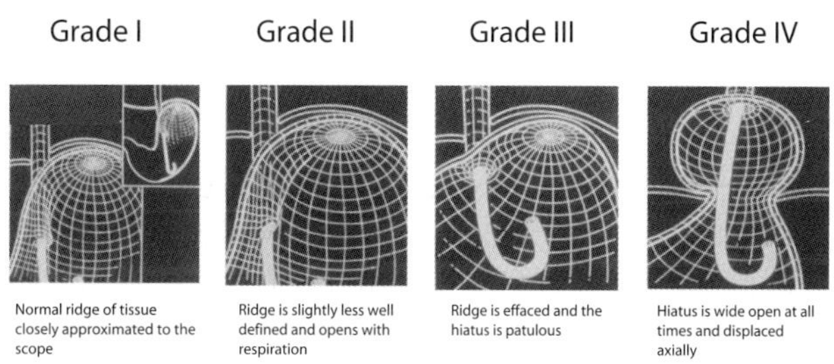

Fig. 6. Three-dimensional representation of the progressive anatomical disruption of the gastroesophageal flap valve along with corresponding endoscopy photos (Grade I). Normal ridge of tissue closely approximated to the shaft of the retroflexed scope (Grade II). The ridge is slightly less well defined and opens with respiration (Grade III). The ridge is barely present and the hiatus is patulous (Grade IV). There is no muscular ridge and the hiatus is wide open at all times (Modified from [28]: Hill LD, Kozarek RA, Kraemer SJ et al (1986) The gastroesophageal flap valve: in vitro and in vivo observations. Gastrointest Endosc 44: 541–547, with permission)

mechanisms are compromised, the deleterious effect is additive resulting in an increasing number of reflux events and consequently an increased amount of esophageal acid exposure.

Investigations have focused on three dominant mechanisms of EGJ incompetence (1) transient LES relaxations, without anatomic abnormality, (2) LES hypotension, again without anatomic abnormality, or (3) anatomical and mechanical distortion of the EGJ inclusive of, but not limited to, hiatus hernia. Which reflux mechanism dominates depends upon a number of factors, the most important being the anatomy of the EGJ.

Transient lower esophageal relaxations

Compelling evidence exists that transient LES relaxations are the most frequent mechanism for reflux during periods of normal LES pressure (> 10 mmHg). Transient LES relaxations occur independently of swallowing, are not accompanied by peristalsis, are accompanied by crural diaphragmatic inhibition, and persist for longer periods than do swallow-induced LES relaxations (> 10 seconds) [29], [30]. The dominant stimulus for transient LES relaxation is distension of the proximal stomach, not surprising given that transient LES relaxation is the physiological mechanism for belching [31]. Transient LES relaxation can be experimentally elicited by either gaseous distension of the stomach or distension of the proximal stomach with a barostat bag. Gastric distension activates vagal afferent mechanoreceptors in the gastric cardia that project to the nucleus tractus solitarii in the brainstem and subsequently to the dorsal motor nuclei of the vagus and finally to the myenteric plexus.

With respect to the role tLESRs play in GERD, it appears that it is not the number but the quality of the refluxate associated with these events. Prolonged manometric recordings have not consistently demonstrated an increased frequency of transient LES relaxations in GERD patients compared to normal controls [32]. However, the frequency of acid reflux (as opposed to gas reflux) during transient LES relaxations has consistently been reported to be greater in GERD patients [32]. The cause for this difference in the frequency of acid reflux during tLESRs is unclear and hypotheses include differences in EGJ morphology and differences in the acid environment of the proximal stomach.

While tLESRs typically account for up to 90% of reflux events in normal subjects or in GERD patients without hiatus hernia, patients with hiatus hernia have a more heterogeneous mechanistic profile with reflux episodes frequently occurring in the context of low LES pressure, straining, and swallowing [33]. These observations support the hypothesis that the functional integrity of the EGJ is dependent on both the intrinsic LES and extrinsic sphincteric function of the diaphragmatic hiatus. In essence, gastroesophageal reflux requires a "two hit phenomenon" to the EGJ. Patients with a normal EGJ require inhibition of both the intrinsic LES and extrinsic crural diaphragm for reflux to occur: physiologically this occurs only in the setting of a tLESR. In contrast, GERD patients, especially those with a hiatal hernia may exhibit pre-existing compromise of the hiatal sphincter. In that setting reflux can occur with only relaxation of the intrinsic LES, as may occur during periods of LES hypotension or even deglutitive relaxation.

Lower esophageal sphincter (intrinsic sphincter) hypotension

Gastroesophageal reflux disease can occur in the context of diminished LES pressure either by strain-induced or free reflux. Strain-induced reflux occurs when a hypotensive LES is overcome and "blown open" in association with an abrupt increase of intra-abdominal pressure [34]. Manometric data suggest that this rarely occurs when the LES pressure is greater than 10 mmHg [34], [35]. It is also a rare occurrence in patients without hiatus hernia [33]. Free reflux is characterized by a fall in intra-esophageal pH without an identifiable change in either intragastric pressure or LES pressure. Episodes of free reflux are observed only when the LES pressure is within 0–4 mmHg of intragastric pressure. A wide open or patulous hiatus will predispose to this free reflux as both the intrinsic and extrinsic sphincter are compromised.

A puzzling clinical observation, and one that supports the importance of transient LES relaxations, is that only a minority of patients with gastroesophageal reflux disease have a fasting LES pressure value of < 10 mmHg [36]. This observation can be partially reconciled when one considers the dynamic nature of LES pressure. The isolated fasting measurement of

LES pressure is probably useful only for identifying patients with a grossly hypotensive sphincter; individuals constantly susceptible to stress and free reflux. However, there is probably a larger population of patients susceptible to strain induced or free reflux when their LES pressure periodically decreases as a result of specific foods, drugs, or habits (Table 1).

The diaphragmatic sphincter and hiatus hernia

Endoscopic and radiographic studies suggest that 50–94% of patients with gastroesophageal reflux disease (GERD) have a type-I hiatal hernia while the corresponding prevalence in control subjects ranges from 13–59% [37]–[40]. Most patients with severe esophagitis have a hiatal hernia [41], [42] and 96% of patients with Barretts esophagus have a ≥ 2 cm hiatus hernia [43]. However, the importance of a type-I hiatal hernia is obscured by the misconception that this is an all or none phenomenon. It is more useful to view type-I hiatal hernia as a continuum of progressive disruption of the gastroesophageal junction, as illustrated in *Fig. 6*. Type-I hiatus hernia impacts on reflux both by affecting the competence of the gastroesophageal junction in preventing reflux and in compromising the process of esophageal acid clearance once reflux has occurred.

Physiological studies by Mittal have clearly demonstrated that the augmentation of EGJ pressure observed during a multitude of activities associated with transient increases in intra-abdominal pressure is attributable to contraction of the crural diaphragm [44]. With hiatus hernia, crural diaphragm function is potentially compromised both by its axial displacement (1) and potentially by atrophy consequent from dilatation of the hiatus [45]. The impact of hiatus hernia on EGJ susceptibility to reflux elicited by straining maneuvers was demonstrated in studies in normal volunteers compared to

Table 1. Factors that influence lower esophageal sphincter pressure and tLESR frequency

	Increase LES pressure	Decrease LES pressure	Increase transient LES relaxations	Decrease transient LES relaxations
Foods	Protein	Fat Chocolate Ethanol Peppermint	Fat	
Medications	Metoclopramide Domperidone Prostaglandin $F_{2\alpha}$ Cisapride	Nitrates Calcium channel blockers Theophylline Morphine Meperidine Diazepam Barbituates	Sumatriptan	Atropine Morphine Loxiglumide
Hormones and neural agents	Gastrin Motilin Substance P α-Adrenergic agonists β-Adrenergic antagonists Cholinergic agonists	Secretin Cholecystokinin Glucagon Gastric inhibitory polypeptide Vasoactive intestinal polypeptide Progesterone α-Adrenergic antagonists β-Adrenergic agonists Cholinergic antagonists Serotonin	Cholecystokinin L-arginine	Baclofen L-NAME Serotonin

GERD patients with and without hiatus hernia [34]. Of several physiological and anatomical variables tested, the size of hiatus hernia was shown to have the highest correlation with the susceptibility to strain-induced reflux (*Fig. 7*). The implication of this observation is that patients with hiatus hernia exhibit progressive impairment of the diaphragmatic component of EGJ function proportional to the extent of axial herniation [1].

Another effect that hiatus hernia exerts on the anti-reflux barrier is to diminish the intraluminal pressure within the EGJ. Relevant animal experiments revealed that simulating the effect of hiatus hernia by severing the phrenoesophageal ligament reduced the LES pressure and that the subsequent repair of the ligament restored the LES pressure to levels similar to baseline [46]. Similarly, manometric studies in humans using a topographic representation of the EGJ high pressure zone of hiatus hernia patients revealed distinct intrinsic sphincter and hiatal canal pressure components, each of which was of lower magnitude

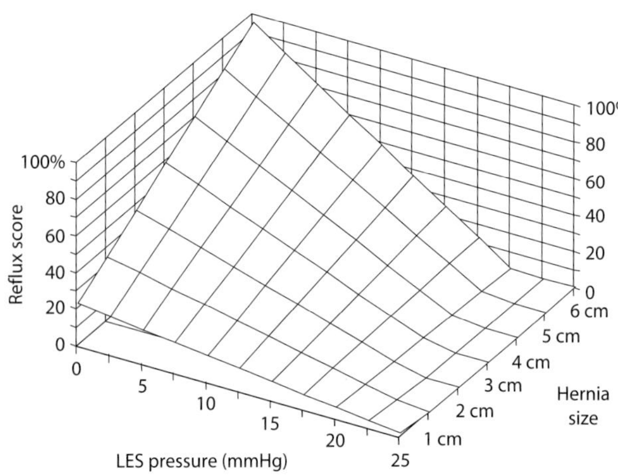

Fig. 7. Model of the relationship between the lower esophageal sphincter (LES) pressure, size of hernia, and the susceptibility to gastroesophageal reflux induced by provocative maneuvers as reflected by the reflux score on the Z-axis. The overall equation of the model is: reflux score- = 22.64 + 12.05 (hernia size) − 0.83 (LES pressure) − 0.65 (LES pressure × hernia size). The hernia size is in cm, and the LES pressure is in mmHg. The multiple correlation coefficient of this equation for the 50 subject data set was 0.86 ($R^2 = .75$). Thus, the susceptibility to stress reflux is dependent upon the interaction of the instantaneous value of LES pressure and the size of the hiatus hernia (From [34]: Sloan S, Rademaker AW, Kahrilas PJ (1992) Determinants of gastroesophageal junction incompetence: hiatal hernia, lower esophageal sphincter, or both? Ann Intern Med 117: 977–982, with permission)

than the EGJ pressure of a comparator group of normal controls [47] (*Fig. 1*). However, simulating reduction of the hernia by arithmetically repositioning the intrinsic sphincter back within the hiatal canal resulted in calculated EGJ pressures that were practically indistinguishable from those of the control subjects. Along with previous investigations these data also demonstrated that hiatus hernia reduced the length of the EGJ high pressure zone [1]. This is likely due to disruption of the EGJ segment distal to the SCJ attributable to the opposing sling and clasp fibers of the gastric cardia [2].

Gastroesophageal flap valve

Although the clinical relevance of the gastroesophageal flap valve (GEFV) concept has been controversial, several studies have helped bolster its validity. Hill et al demonstrated the presence of a gastroesophageal pressure gradient in cadavers without a hiatal hernia [28]. They also showed that ability of the cadaveric EGJ to prevent reflux in the setting of increased intra-abdominal pressure could be increased by surgically accentuating the length of the flap valve. Hill and colleagues then went on to define a GEFV classification grading scheme based on endoscopic inspection (*Fig. 6*). Two endoscopic studies have reported that this grading scheme correlated with the severity of reflux disease [28], [48]. In addition, a recent study assessing exercise induced gastroesophageal reflux using a radiotelemetry pH probe in 20 subjects revealed a strong correlation between exercise-induced acid exposure and GEFV grade [49]. This relationship remained strong even when subjects with overt hiatus hernia (grade IV) were excluded. In contrast, the relationship between esophageal acid exposure during exercise and basal LES pressure was not statistically significant.

The exact mechanism by which disruption of the GEFV leads to increasing reflux severity is unclear, however, most theories focus on the effect it has on the subdiaphragmatic segment of the esophagus. Grade-3 and -4 flap valves are associated with decreased prominence of the musculo-mucosal fold that abuts the esophageal inlet [28]. Consequently, the angle of His is also increased and there is no longer a subdiaphragmatic segment of the esophagus to be compressed when intra-abdominal pressure rises.

Mechanical properties of the relaxed EGJ

In contemplating the occurrence of reflux in the setting of a relaxed or hypotensive sphincter it is also necessary to consider other mechanical attributes of the system that may account for a relaxed sphincter remaining closed in one case and physically open in another; one such attribute is compliance, or distensibility of the sphincter. Acquired anatomic changes inclusive of, but not restricted to, hiatus hernia may alter the compliance at the relaxed EGJ thereby decreasing the resistance to gastroesophageal flow.

Recent physiologic studies exploring the role of compliance in GERD reported that GERD patients with and without hiatus hernia had increased compliance at the EGJ compared to normal subjects [50], [51]. These experiments utilized a combination of barostat-controlled distention, manometry, and fluoroscopy to directly measure the compliance of the relaxed EGJ. Several parameters of EGJ compliance were shown to be increased in hiatus hernia patients with GERD: (1) the EGJ opened at lower distention pressure, (2) the relaxed EGJ opened at distention pressures that were at or near resting intra-gastric pressure, and (3) for a given distention pressure the EGJ opened about 0.5 cm wider (*Fig. 8*). These alterations of EGJ mechanics are likely secondary to a disrupted, distensible crural aperture and may contribute to the physiological aberrations associated with hiatus hernia and GERD.

Increased EGJ compliance may help explain why patients with hiatus hernia have a distinct mechanistic reflux profile compared to patients without hiatus hernia [52]. Anatomical alterations, such as hiatal hernia, dilatation of the diaphragmatic hiatus, and disruption of the gastroesophageal flap valve may alter the elastic characteristics of the hiatus such that this factor is no longer protective in preventing gastroesophageal reflux. In that setting, reflux no longer requires "two hits" because the extrinsic sphincteric mechanism is already disrupted. Thus, the only prerequisite for reflux becomes LES relaxation, be that in the setting of swallow-induced relaxation, tLESR, or a period of prolonged LES relaxation.

Increased compliance may also help explain why GERD patients may be more likely to sustain acid reflux in association with tLESRs compared to asymptomatic subjects. In an experiment that sought to quantify this difference, normal subjects exhibited acid reflux with 40–50% of tLESRs compared to 60–70% in patients with GERD [32]. This difference may be the result of increased EGJ compliance and its effect on trans-EGJ flow.

$$\textit{Trans-EGJflow} = \Delta P \times R^4/C \times L \times \eta$$

In the flow equation, flow is directly proportional to EGJ diameter to the 4th power and inversely proportional to the length of the narrowed segment and the viscosity of the gas or liquid traversing the segment. Should tLESRs occur in the context of an EGJ with increased compliance, wider opening diameters will occur under a given set of circumstances and trans-EGJ flow will increase. Patients without obvious hiatus hernia may still have increased compliance secondary to more subtle defects at the EGJ not readily evident using current radiographic or endoscopic methods of evaluation. These defects may be more akin to minor anatomical variants of the EGJ such as a grade-2 gastroesophageal flap valve or defects in the LES musculature.

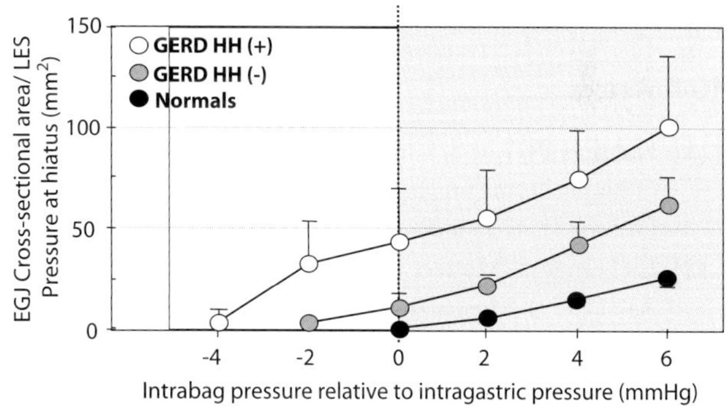

Fig. 8. EGJ cross sectional area as a function of distention pressure. Cross-sectional area at intrabag pressures > 0 mmHg was significantly increased in the NHH GERD patients compared to normal subjects ($p < 0.0001$) and in the HH patients compared top the NHH patients ($p < 0.005$). At pressures ≤ 0 mmHg the EGJ cross-sectional area of HH GERD patients was significantly greater than both the NHH GERD patients and NLs ($p < 0.05$). At pressures below 0 mmHg there was no significant difference between NHH GERD patients and NLs (From [51]: Pandolfino et al (2003) Gastroenterology 125(4): 1018–1024, with permission)

Conclusion

Theories of the mechanism of gastroesophageal junction competence have seesawed between strictly anatomic explanations, focusing on type-I hiatus hernia, and physiologic explanations focusing on the vigor of LES contraction while ignoring the significance of anatomic factors. As detailed above, current thinking recognizes contributions from both sphincteric components. Furthermore, there is an increasing understanding of mechanical elements of the antireflux barrier, inclusive of, but nor restricted to hiatus hernia and the intrinsic LES. Thus, our view of GERD pathogenesis as it pertains to EGJ competence is now focusing on quantifying the mechanical properties of this complex anatomical zone. Future research will likely focus on methods to measure EGJ compliance and elasticity, as these are the mechanical parameters that influence gastroesophageal reflux.

Acknowledgement

This work was supported by grant nos. RO1 DC00646 (PJK) and K23 DK062170-01 (JEP) from the Public Health Service.

References

[1] Kahrilas PJ, Lin S, Chen J, Manka M (1999) The effect of hiatus hernia on gastro-oesophageal junction pressure. Gut 44(4): 476–482
[2] Liebermann-Meffert D, Allgower M, Schmid P, Blum AL (1979) Muscular equivalent of the lower esophageal sphincter. Gastroenterology 76(1): 31–38
[3] Kahrilas PJ (1997) Anatomy and physiology of the gastroesophageal junction. Gastroenterol Clin North Am 26(3): 467–486
[4] Dent J, Dodds WJ, Friedman RH et al (1980) Mechanism of gastroesophageal reflux in recumbent asymptomatic human subjects. J Clin Invest 65(2): 256–267
[5] Goyal RK, Rattan S (1976) Genesis of basal sphincter pressure: effect of tetrodotoxin on lower esophageal sphincter pressure in opossum in vivo. Gastroenterology 71(1): 62–67
[6] Goyal RK, Rattan S (1975) Nature of the vagal inhibitory innervation to the lower esophageal sphincter. J Clin Invest 55(5): 1119–1126
[7] Yamato S, Saha JK, Goyal RK (1992) Role of nitric oxide in lower esophageal sphincter relaxation to swallowing. Life Sci 50(17): 1263–1272
[8] Richards WG, Sugarbaker DJ (1995) Neuronal control of esophageal function. Chest Surg Clin N Am 5(1): 157–171
[9] Marchand P (1959) The anatomy of the esophageal hiatus of the diaphragm and the pathogenesis of hiatus herniation. Thorac Surg 37: 81–92
[10] Barrett NR (1932) Discussion on hiatus hernia. Proc R Soc Med 122: 736–796
[11] Schatzki R (1932) Die Hernien des Hiatus oesophageus. Deutsches Arch F Klin Med 173: 85–103
[12] Low A (1907) A note on the crura of the diaphragm nd the muscle of treitsz. J Anatomy Lond 42: 93–96
[13] Kahrilas PJ, Wu S, Lin S, Pouderoux P (1995) Attenuation of esophageal shortening during peristalsis with hiatus hernia. Gastroenterology 109(6): 1818–1825
[14] De Troyer A, Sampson M, Sigrist S, Macklem PT (1982) Action of costal and crural parts of the diaphragm on the rib cage in dog. J Appl Physiol 53(1): 30–39
[15] Altschuler SM, Boyle JT, Nixon TE, Pack AI, Cohen S (1985) Simultaneous reflex inhibition of lower esophageal sphincter and crural diaphragm in cats. Am J Physiol 249(5 Pt 1): G586–G591
[16] Mittal RK, Fisher M, McCallum RW, Rochester DF, Dent J, Sluss J (1990) Human lower esophageal sphincter pressure response to increased intra-abdominal pressure. Am J Physiol 258(4 Pt 1): G624–G630
[17] Klein WA, Parkman HP, Dempsey DT, Fisher RS (1993) Sphincterlike thoracoabdominal high-pressure zone after esophagogastrectomy. Gastroenterology 105(5): 1362–1369
[18] Skinner DB (1985) Hernias (hiatal, traumatic and congnital). In: Gastroenterology (Berk JE, ed), 4th ed. Philadelphia: W. B. Saunders, pp 705–716
[19] Pandolfino JE, Shi G, Cisler J, Joehl RJ, Brasseur JG, Kahrilas PJ (2002) Opening characteristics of the relaxed EGJ during low-pressure distention in normal subjects and hiatus hernia patients. Gastroenterology 122(4): 430–450
[20] Allison PR (1951) Reflux esophagitis, sliding hiatal hernai and the anatomy of repair. Surg Gynecol Obstet 92: 419–431
[21] Rigler LG, Eneboe JB (1935) Incidence of hiatus hernia in pregnant women and its significance. J Thorac Surg 4: 262–268
[22] Marchand P (1957) A study of the forces productive of gastroesophageal regurgitation through the diaphragmatic hiatus. Thorax 12: 189–202
[23] Paterson WG, Kolyn DM (1994) Esophageal shortening induced by short-term intraluminal acid perfusion in

opossum: a cause for hiatus hernia? Gastroenterology 107(6): 1736–1740

[24] Kahrilas PJ (1993) Hiatus hernia: fact or fiction? Gullet 3 (Suppl): 21

[25] Perdikis G, Hinder RA (1995) Paraesophageal hernia. In: Hernia (Nyhus LM, Condon RE, eds). Philadelphia: J. B. Lippincott, p 544

[26] Postlethwait RW (1979) Surgery of the esophagus. Norwalk: Appleton Century-Crofts

[27] Thor KB, Hill LD, Mercer DD, Kozarek RD (1987) Reappraisal of the flap valve mechanism in the gastroesophageal junction. A study of a new valvuloplasty procedure in cadavers. Acta Chir Scand 153(1): 25–28

[28] Hill LD, Kozarek RA, Kraemer SJ et al (1996) The gastroesophageal flap valve: in vitro and in vivo observations. Gastrointest Endosc 44(5): 541–547

[29] Mittal RK, Holloway RH, Penagini R, Blackshaw LA, Dent J (1995) Transient lower esophageal sphincter relaxation. Gastroenterology 109(2): 601–610

[30] Holloway RH, Penagini R, Ireland AC (1995) Criteria for objective definition of transient lower esophageal sphincter relaxation. Am J Physiol 268(Pt 1): G128–G133

[31] Wyman JB, Dent J, Heddle R, Dodds WJ, Toouli J, Downton J (1990) Control of belching by the lower oesophageal sphincter. Gut 31(6): 639–646

[32] Sifrim D, Tack J, Lerut T, Janssens J (2000) Transient lower esophageal sphincter relaxations and esophageal body muscular contractile response in reflux esophagitis. Dig Dis Sci 45(7): 1293–1300

[33] van Herwaarden MA, Samsom M, Smout AJ (2000) Excess gastroesophageal reflux in patients with hiatus hernia is caused by mechanisms other than transient LES relaxations. Gastroenterology 119(6): 1439–1446

[34] Sloan S, Rademaker AW, Kahrilas PJ (1992) Determinants of gastroesophageal junction incompetence: hiatal hernia, lower esophageal sphincter, or both? Ann Intern Med 117(12): 977–982

[35] Dent J, Holloway RH, Toouli J, Dodds WJ (1988) Mechanisms of lower oesophageal sphincter incompetence in patients with symptomatic gastrooesophageal reflux. Gut 29(8): 1020–1028

[36] Kahrilas PJ, Dodds WJ, Hogan WJ, Kern M, Arndorfer RC, Reece A (1986) Esophageal peristaltic dysfunction in peptic esophagitis. Gastroenterology 91(4): 897–904

[37] Ott DJ, Gelfand DW, Wu WC et al (1984) Esophagogastric region and its rings. Amer J Roentgenol 142: 281–287

[38] Berstad A, Weberg R, Froyshov Larsen I, Hoel B, Hauer-Jensen M (1986) Relationship of hiatus hernia to reflux oesophagitis. A prospective study of coincidence, using endoscopy. Scand J Gastroenterol 21(1): 55–58

[39] Wright RA (1979) Relationship of hiatal hernia in endoscopically proved reflux esophagitis. Dig Dis Sci 24: 311–313

[40] Petersen H, Johannessen T, Sandvik AK et al (1991) Relationship between endoscopic hiatus hernia and gastroesophageal reflux symptoms. Scand J Gastroenterol 26(9): 921–926

[41] Sontag SJ, Schnell TG, Miller TQ et al (1991) The importance of hiatal hernia in reflux esophagitis compared with lower esophageal sphincter pressure or smoking. J Clin Gastroenterol 13(6): 628–643

[42] Jones MP, Sloan SS, Rabine JC, Ebert CC, Huang CF, Kahrilas PJ (2001) Hiatal hernia size is the dominant determinant of esophagitis presence and severity in gastroesophageal reflux disease. Am J Gastroenterol 96(6): 1711–1777

[43] Cameron AJ (1999) Barrett's esophagus: prevalence and size of hiatal hernia. Am J Gastroenterol 94(8): 2054–2059

[44] Mittal RK, Rochester DF, McCallum RW (1987) Effect of the diaphragmatic contraction on lower oesophageal sphincter pressure in man. Gut 28(12): 1564–1568

[45] Marchand P (1970) The surgery for hiatus hernia: is vagotomy rational? S Afr Med J 44(2): 35–39

[46] Michelson E, Siegel C (1964) The role of the phrenicoesophageal ligament in the lower esophageal sphincter. Surg Gynecol Obstet 118: 1291–1294

[47] Kahrilas PJ, Lin S, Manka M, Shi G, Joehl RJ (2000) Esophagogastric junction pressure topography after fundoplication. Surgery 127(2): 200–208

[48] Contractor QQ, Akhtar SS, Contractor TQ (1999) Endoscopic esophagitis and gastroesophageal flap valve. J Clin Gastroenterol 28(3): 233–237

[49] Pandolfino JE, Bianchi L, Lee TJ, Hirano I, Kahrilas PJ (2004) Esophagogastric junction morphology predicts susceptibility to exercise-induced reflux. Am J Gastroenterol (accepted)

[50] Pandolfino JE, Shi G, Manka M, Joehl RJ, Brasseur JG, Kahrilas PJ (2000) EGJ opening with hiatal hernia: lower-pressure threshold, wider diameter. Gastroenterology 118: A860

[51] Pandolfino JE, Shi G, Trueworthy B, Kahrilas PJ (2003) Esophagogastric junction opening during relaxation distinguishes nonhernia reflux patients, hernia patients, and normal subjects. Gastroenterology 125(4): 1018–1024

[52] van Herwaarden MA, Samsom M, Smout AJ (2001) Prolonged manometric recordings of oesophagus and lower oesophageal sphincter in achalasia patients. Gut 49(6): 813–821

[53] Pandolfino JE, Kahrilas PJ (2001) Esophagel motility abnormalities in Barrett's esophagus. In: Barrett's esophagus and esophageal adenocarcinoma (Sharma P, Sampliner RE, eds). Malden: Blackwell Science, pp 35–44

[54] Kahrilas PJ (1992) Cigarette smoking and gastroesophageal reflux disease. Dig Dis 10(2): 61–71

Chapter 8

NON-EROSIVE REFLUX DISEASE (NERD) AND FUNCTIONAL HEARTBURN

E. M. M. Quigley

Head of the Medical School, National University of Ireland, Cork, Ireland

Introduction

Most individuals with symptoms compatible with gastroesophageal reflux disease (GERD) who undergo endoscopy will not show evidence of erosive esophagitis. Indeed, it is now clear that non-erosive or negative-endoscopy reflux disease (NERD) [also referred to as endoscopy-negative reflux disease (ENRD)], may account for up to 70% of patients with GERD in the community [1]–[3]. This contrasts with the spectrum of patients seen in a gastroenterological practice or tertiary referral center, where esophagitis and complicated GERD may predominate. However, until recently, most studies of diagnostic or therapeutic interventions in GERD were performed in the latter setting and may well, therefore, not be representative of the true spectrum of GERD. It is appropriate, therefore, to review our understanding of the clinical features, natural history, pathophysiology, evaluation and management of GERD, recognizing that the majority of patients have NERD and not erosive reflux disease (ERD) or one of its complications.

Definitions

1. NERD

Patients with NERD do not, by definition, have esophagitis and appear to be at low risk to develop esophagitis; NERD is best defined, therefore, on the basis of symptoms and/or their impact on an individual's health-related quality of life (QOL) [4]. Indeed, it is apparent that NERD patients can, and do, suffer from symptoms as severe as those with ERD, and the impact on quality of life can be at least as disabling in NERD as in other manifestations of GERD [5], [6]. It is appropriate, therefore, that recent definitions of GERD incorporate the issue of quality of life [4]. In defining NERD, one must be cognizant of prior therapy; an esophagus rendered free of esophagitis by acid-suppressive therapy does not constitute NERD. Attempts to define GERD on the basis of histological findings, in those in whom the mucosa is endoscopically normal, have also proven disappointing [7], [8].

Fass and colleagues have suggested that NERD may be further defined and sub-classified based on the results of 24-hour pH recordings in to three distinct groups [9] (*Fig. 1*):

(i) Those with an abnormal acid exposure time (AET); these individuals appear to behave, in terms of therapeutic response, in a manner analogous to those with obvious esophagitis,

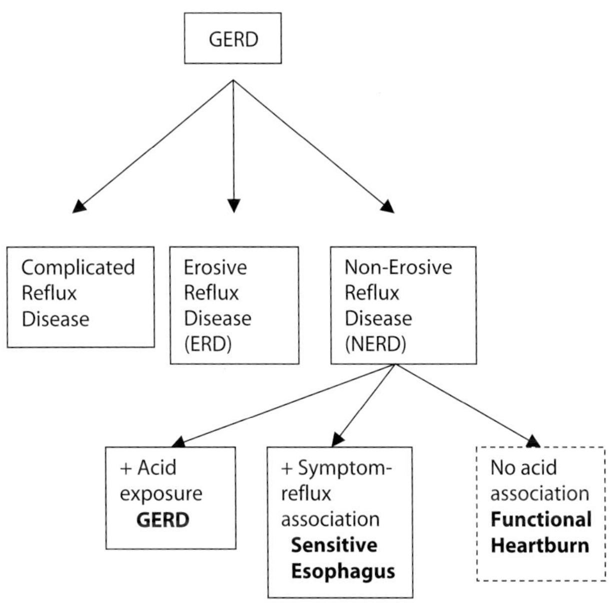

Fig. 1. GERD subgroups

(ii) Those who demonstrate a normal AET but in whom symptoms and reflux events are significantly correlated (as estimated by some form of symptom index or other measure of symptom-reflux event association); these individuals have been referred to as "the sensitive esophagus" [10],

(iii) Those with typical reflux symptoms (i.e., heartburn and acid regurgitation), yet in whom all parameters of the pH study are normal. These individuals appear highly resistant to acid-suppressive therapy [10] and are more likely to demonstrate psychopathology [11].

The definition of functional heartburn is especially problematic and confusing. For example, the second iteration of the "Rome" criteria [12] and other experts [13]–[15] incorporate groups (ii) and (iii), above, in the definition of functional heartburn. Given that classification should advise diagnostic and therapeutic decisions and predict pathophysiology, most clinicians would reserve this term for group (iii) alone. This is also the opinion of this author; it is, to my mind, counterproductive and well as counterintuitive to include two quite distinct groups of patients (i.e., those who do and do not demonstrate an association with acid exposure and a response to acid suppression) in the same category.

This reliance on pH data could be construed to imply that this test plays a pivotal and essential role in the evaluation of NERD. If one accepts that the true NERD patient (as distinct from the individual with therapeutically-resolved esophagitis) is at low risk for progression to such worrisome complications as Barrett's esophagus, then a therapeutic trial (also referred to as the PPI test) emerges as a valid diagnostic alternative [16]. This approach has the additional benefit of rapidly identifying those who are likely to benefit from long-term PPI therapy.

2. Functional heartburn

Among the various manifestations of GERD described so far in this review, functional heartburn may represent the greatest challenge to the clinician. Affected patients present with typical reflux symptoms, yet, as described above, all diagnostic modalities fail to reveal either evidence of pathological acid reflux or an association between symptoms and acid exposure; needless to say, there is no macroscopic or microscopic evidence of acid-related mucosal injury. The precise prevalence of this disorder is unknown; estimates suggest that approximately 40% of NERD patients (or 20% of all GERD) will fall into this category [3], [17]–[19] and its pathophysiology remains virtually unexplored [20]. Clinical impressions suggest that there is considerable overlap with other functional disorders such as irritable bowel syndrome and non-cardiac chest pain; one can assume, therefore, that such phenomena as visceral hypersensitivity and abnormal cerebral perception of visceral events may be involved. Anecdotal evidence, derived largely from referral centres, suggests a significant role for psychological factors; given the context of this observation and of prior experience with the perils of extrapolating from a referral sample to the community in other functional disorders, one needs to exert extreme caution in the interpretation of this association, however.

Pathophysiology

While gender and age are by no means absolute discriminators for any group of GERD, it is noteworthy that, in contrast to GERD, in general, females do predominate in NERD, a group who, on the whole, tend to be younger, by a factor of about a decade, than their erosive GERD counterparts. Existing data on the pathophysiology of NERD suggest that while, as in ERD, acid and pepsin play a central role in the induction of symptoms, abnormal esophageal acid exposure cannot be the sole mechanism. Thus, on ambulatory esophageal pH testing, the acid exposure time (AET), expressed as the total percentage of time that the pH is less than 4, is abnormal in only one-half to two-thirds of NERD patients [9], [21]. In the remainder, GERD may be defined on the basis of a positive correlation between symptom onset and reflux events [22]. As a result, it has been suggested that these individuals are hypersensitive to physiological degrees of esophageal acid exposure. Experimental evidence to support this concept comes from studies which have demonstrated that these patients are hypersensitive to intra-esophageal balloon inflation, in comparison to both control subjects and to GERD patients with abnormal AET [22], [23]. Fass and colleagues failed, however, to demonstrate an effect of acid exposure on mechano-sensitivity, in their study; they did, however, describe an accentuation of the chemo-sensitive response to acid following prolonged acid exposure [24]. Visceral hypersensitivity has, of course, been invoked as an important factor in the etiology of such functional gastrointestinal disorders as non-cardiac chest pain, functional dyspepsia and the irritable bowel syndrome. It should come as no surprise, therefore, that there is accumulating evidence to indicate an overlap between NERD and functional dyspepsia [25], [26]; in our own experience, up to 50% of NERD patients have dysmotility/dyspeptic symptoms [27].

Is NERD truly non-erosive? Ultrastructural studies on human tissues, as well as experimental animal models, have demonstrated dilatation of the intercellular spaces in the esophageal epithelium in esophagi that look macroscopically normal [28]–[30]. Such changes could increase permeability and facilitate access for acid to submucosal neurons, thereby, inducing either spasm and/or visceral hypersensitivity [9]. Given the very low rate of progression, among NERD patients, to more obvious mucosal disease [31]–[39], it seems most unlikely that these subtle changes are the harbingers of esophagitis to come. Recent studies employing magnification and other techniques have revealed subtle abnormalities at the gastro-esophageal junction in NERD [40], [41]; how these findings relate to symptoms and to possible disease progression remain to be defined.

What is the etiology of functional heartburn? Given that acid exposure is, by definition, normal in affected patients and episodes of acid exposure do not predict symptoms, one must look elsewhere to explain the precipitation of heartburn in this population. Pending definitive study and based on our experience with other functional gastrointestinal disorders, it seems reasonable to propose likely roles for visceral hypersensitivity, abnormal central perception and psychopathology, among others [20]. It is also clear that stimuli other than acid can evoke typical heartburn [24] and that the pathophysiology of heartburn even in "classical" GERD is complex [42], [43]. Utilising miniaturised intraluminal ultrasound probes, Mittal and colleagues have, for example, revealed acid-induced episodes of shortening of the longitudinal muscle layer in relation to the occurrence of heartburn, thereby, revealing another mechanism whereby acid may induce symptoms [42]–[44]. Whether this and other methodologies, such as intra-luminal impedance measurements [45]–[47], to detect reflux of gas and non-acid liquid components of the refluxate, and brain mapping studies [48], to identify the cortical representation of esophageal symptoms, will reveal as yet unrecognised associations between luminal acid, bile or other agents in the refluxate and symptoms in functional heartburn, remains to be defined. Even in functional heartburn, where acid exposure is normal and temporal associations between acid reflux and symptoms are not readily identified, acid cannot be discounted. Prior, or even remote, episodes of physiological reflux may sensitise the esophagus, in predisposed individuals, to the subsequent development of symptoms in relation to non-acid stimuli [43], [49]. Hyperensitivity to acid may, indeed, reflect sensitization of afferent neurons leading from the esophagus to the central nervous system [20].

Available evidence does indicate that the more one strays into the realm of those with normal pH studies in a heartburn population, the lower the response to acid suppression and the greater the overlap with other functional disorders. To date, however, most studies of NERD pathophysiology have failed to differentiate between the various subgroups of NERD and, in particular, to separate out those with functional heartburn. Those that have indicate, as one would predict, that NERD patients with abnormal acid exposure and acid hypersensitivity resemble patients with erosive and complicated esophagitis whereas parameters of esophageal physiology are more closely akin to normal subjects among those with functional heartburn [50]. Fass and Tougas suggest that symptom induction in the functional heartburn patient represents a complex interaction between the intraluminal stimulus, esophageal receptors, visceral afferent neurons and central perception [20]. In keeping with other functional disorders, it is to be expected that a hypervigilant brain, sensitized, perhaps, by environmental or intrinsic stressors may play a significant role.

For all of these reasons, this author proposes that future definitions of this subpopulation will remove functional heartburn patients from the spectrum of GERD and place them where they belong, among the functional gastrointestinal disorders.

NERD and dyspepsia

As overlap between these functional syndromes comes to be accepted as a clinical reality, it has posed a dilemma for those who seek to develop precise clinical definitions for the individual functional disorders. For example, where does NERD end and functional dyspepsia begin? [51] This is far more than an issue of semantics; the inclusion of patients with predominant heartburn in a dyspepsia study population which examines the response to an acid-suppressing agent will significantly bias the study in a positive direction [52], [53]; as a corollary, the exclusion of heartburn, as advocated by some [54], will lessen the impact of the same agents. The approach to definition will similarly have a significant impact on studies of the epidemiology, pathophysiology and natural history of the respective disorders. The need to delineate succinct patient categories notwithstanding, the clinical reality is that many NERD patients complain of heartburn and dyspepsia; attempts to separate patients on the basis of the relative "predominance" of one or other symptom complex seems unrealistic, if not impossible. Other data supports the overlap between the disorders.

Firstly, the intimacy of physiological relationships between the lower esophagus and the upper stomach continues to be revealed. Thus, fundic distension is a primary mechanism of induction of transient lower esophageal relaxations (TLESR's) [55]; which are, in turn, responsible for most episodes of reflux in both health and in GERD [26]. Secondly, similar disturbances in upper gut motility, including gastric emptying delay, have been described in NERD and functional dyspepsia [26]. In functional dyspepsia, impaired fundic accommodation appears to be a prominent feature [56]. Very recent data suggest that dysfunction of the upper stomach may occur in NERD also [57], [58]. Just as the overlap with functional dyspepsia, and the potential role of motility and or sensory dysfunction in symptom generation, have been implicated to explain the relatively inferior response to proton pump inhibitors in NERD, these same factors have encouraged investigation of a potential role for prokinetic agents. To date there have been few studies of prokinetic agents in NERD; those that have been performed have not proven encouraging [27], [59], [60].

Assessment

Can one predict NERD on the basis of clinical evaluation? While the NERD patient is, on average, younger and more likely to be female that the individual with complicated GERD, these demographic features are not sufficiently discriminating to be of diagnostic value. In terms of typical GERD symptoms, neither severity nor duration can discriminate between NERD and GERD, or predict complications or manometric or pH study results. Some atypical or extraesophageal symptoms, in contrast, tend to be associated with NERD and may in of themselves predicate a different therapeutic strategy. It has been suggested, for example, that both laryngitis and asthma related to GERD require more intensive and more prolonged acid-suppressive therapy in order to optimise symptomatic response. It is also abundantly clear that this area continues to suffer from a striking paucity of data derived from randomised controlled clinical trials.

Many approaches may be taken to the evaluation of the individual presenting, for the first time, with symptoms indicative or suggestive of GERD. Decisions regarding the extent of assessment are based on individual patient factors and on some generic issues. With regard to the former, patient age and nature of symptomatology are fundamental; few would dispute the appropriateness of endoscopy in a 63-year old patient with heartburn and dysphagia referred to the lower esophagus. More controversial are the generic issues and one, in particular, Barrett's esophagus. One's assessment of the role of Barrett's in the pathogenesis of esophageal adenocarcinoma and one's attitude to the efficacy and appropriateness of screening and surveillance policies for this manifestation of GERD will determine enthusiasm for such approaches to GERD as "once in a life-time endoscopy for every GERD patient" or "endoscopy for all over 50". In the absence of conclusive data, approaches are largely empiric and extend from one of recommending endoscopy in all GERD patients to a position which, unimpressed by the efficacy of either screening or surveillance, would not factor Barrett's into the equation when making decisions on evaluation. Endoscopy may have other roles in assessment. These include the obvious value of defining GERD, on the basis of endoscopic findings, in a patient with atypical or non-responsive symptoms and also the less well-defined role of endoscopic features in predicting long-term prognosis and therapeutic response. If, as some evidence suggests, GERD phenotypes remain stable, over time, this has fundamental implications from a management perspective. In choosing a therapeutic strategy for a NERD patient, for example, one can do so confident that progression to esophagitis or Barrett's esophagus is so unlikely that the effect of a particular treatment modality on natural history is not an issue. Several studies from Lagergren and colleagues, in Sweden, have raised a note of caution in this regard. Their suggestion that the risk for adenocarcinoma of the esophagus, in the patient with GERD, relates to heartburn frequency, severity and duration and not to such mucosal pathologies as Barrett's epithelium [61], certainly requires confirmation but cannot be ignored.

Management

Of interest, several studies as well as recent reviews and meta-analyses, while confirming a significant response, in terms of symptom relief, to proton pump inhibitors in NERD, have demonstrated, with some consistency, that these agents are somewhat less effective in NERD [3], [9], [59], [62]–[68] than in ERD [69]. Several factors might explain this somewhat unexpected finding and include the relatively greater importance of abnormal acid exposure in ERD and the significant overlap with functional dyspepsia and other functional disorders [64], in NERD; a disorder where acid suppressing agents have a far smaller impact than in GERD [51], [52]. This is not to say that NERD patients with dyspepsia do not respond to proton pump inhibitors; indeed, functional dyspepsia patients with heartburn are perhaps those most likely to respond to acid suppression [51]–[53]. At the present time there is relatively little information on the use of non-acid suppressing approaches in NERD [62]. In terms of other forms of acid suppression, studies of histamine H2-receptor antagonists in NERD [62], [65], [70] suggested a response rate similar to, and as disappointing as, that seen in ERD [71], [72]. For the moment, at least, potent acid suppressing agents, such as proton pump inhibitors, remain the first-line option for these patients. The response is not optimal and other approaches to restore normal motor function and modulate sensation may be of value to those with normal esophageal acid exposure or who demonstrate significant dyspeptic symptoms.

While the natural history of NERD remains poorly documented, available evidence suggests a benign course. Symptom control and restoration of quality of life become the primary therapeutic goals, therefore [73]. These concepts, together with the expense of sustained proton pump inhibitor therapy, have prompted an evaluation of on-demand therapy for NERD patients [74]–[77]. This approach proved effective using omeprazole 20 mg per day; only 50% of patients required the proton pump inhibitor, in addition to antacids, to maintain quality of life. On-demand therapy may represent a more cost effective approach to management for this large group of GERD patients. The adoption of this strategy necessitates an acceptance of the benign nature of NERD; it must be stated that available data, though consistent in this regard [31]–[39], are far from adequate to permit a definitive statement on the natural history of this disorder. The recent suggestion that adenocarcinoma risk relates to heartburn frequency, severity and duration and not mucosal pathology [61], must also be taken into account.

The introduction of the laparoscopic approach has revolutionized the surgical approach to GERD and has led to a virtual epidemic of fundoplication procedures. Not surprisingly, many patients with NERD are being considered for, and subjected to, laparoscopic fundoplication. The precise proportion of NERD patients in surgical series is often difficult to discern as the effects of prior acid-suppressive medication is usually not accounted for in describing preoperative endoscopic findings. Several recent pieces of evidence indicate that the clinician needs to exert cautious and careful judgement in considering the surgical option in the NERD patient. Firstly, it has become clear that the best results from surgery are obtained in those with typical GERD symptoms, an abnormal esophageal pH study and a good symptomatic response to acid suppression [78], [79]; features not common to all NERD patients. Secondly, it is evident that the NERD patient with prominent dyspeptic features may fare especially poorly and become crippled by gas-bloat and other symptoms post-fundoplication. There is, indeed, a potential pathophysiological explanation for these unfortunate occurrences. As mentioned, functional dyspepsia is associated with impaired gastric accommodation; a phenomenon which is further restricted by fundoplication [58], [80]. Delayed gastric emptying, present in some GERD patients at baseline (review) and, perhaps, more prevalent among those with NERD, may also be further impaired by fundoplication, if vagal injury occurs.

If one accepts the definition of functional heartburn proposed in this review, one is faced with a patient with disabling heartburn which is totally unresponsive to proton pump inhibitor therapy. There are few, if any, studies to guide therapeutic choices in this population, apart from the critical observation that one cannot expect a favourable response to fundoplication among these patients. Indeed, I would go so far as to state that one should be guided by the principle that fundoplication is contraindicated in functional heartburn. For this reason, I appeal to my surgical colleagues to remove "failure to respond to medical therapy" from their list of indications for fundoplication in GERD. Indeed, the removal of functional heartburn from within the spectrum of GERD, as advocated above, would similarly prevent the consideration of a surgical option for these unfortunate patients. Pending definitive study in functional heartburn, per se, one must look elsewhere for guidance in the management of these disorders. The overlap with dyspepsia may attract one to therapies that have been advocated in these disorders, be they prokinetics, fundic relaxants or visceral analgesics. Unfortunately, there is as yet little evidence of real therapeutic efficacy for any of the agents in functional dyspepsia, not to mind functional heartburn, where they have been scarcely evaluated. One is left then with agents that have been evaluated, albeit to a limited and often unsatisfactory extent, in functional disorders, in general. I am referring here to such pharmacological approaches as tricyclic antidepressants and serotonin re-uptake inhibitors and such alternative therapies as hypnosis and psychotherapy. While it is my personal practice to treat these patients empirically with tricylics, such as amitriptyline, and I remain impressed by the results of hypnosis in irritable bowel syndrome, I cannot call on a single, randomized, controlled study to support either approach for a patient with functional heartburn. This is clearly an area deserving of study.

Conclusion

NERD is a real entity and its importance in the spectrum of GERD must be appreciated. Functional heartburn needs to be further differentiated as that subgroup of patients in which there appears to be no relationship between symptoms, albeit "typical" of GERD, and acid exposure. Several aspects of NERD need to be appreciated including the overlap with functional dyspepsia and potential differences in response to such therapeutic interventions as acid suppressive therapy and fundoplication. While definitive studies on this issue are yet to be completed, it remains quite possible that our failure to separate functional heartburn from NERD, in general, has contributed in large measure to diagnostic difficulties and therapeutic disappointment in GERD. This author contends that functional heartburn should be removed from the spectrum of GERD and relocated to the functional gastrointestinal disorders; only then will effective approaches to the assessment and therapy of this challenging disorder emerge.

References

[1] Spechler SJ (1992) Epidemiology and natural history of gastroesophageal reflux disease. Digestion 51 (Suppl 1): 24–29

[2] Smout AJPM (1997) Endoscopy-negative acid reflux disease. Aliment Pharmacol Ther 11 (Suppl 2): 81–85

[3] Lind T, Havelund T, Carlsson R et al (1997) Heartburn without esophagitis: efficacy of omeprazole therapy and features determining therapeutic response. Scand J Gastroenterol 32: 974–979

[4] Dent J, Brun J, Fendrick AM, Fennerty MB, Janssens J, Kahrilas PJ, Lauritsen K, Reynolds JC, Shaw M, Talley NJ (1999) An evidence-based appraisal of reflux disease management: the Genval Workshop Report. Gut 44 (Suppl 2): S1–S16

[5] Lind T, Havelund T, Lundell L, Glise H, Lauritsen K, Pedersen SA, Anker-Hansen O, Stubberod G, Carlsson R, Junghard O (1999) On-demand therapy with omeprazole for the long-term management of patients with heartburn without oesophagitis – a placebo-controlled randomized trial. Aliment Pharmacol Ther 13: 907–914

[6] Tew S, Jamieson GG, Pilowsky I et al (1997) The illness behavior of patients with gastroesophageal reflux

disease with and without endoscopic esophagitis. Dis Esophagus 10: 9–15

[7] Tummala V, Barwick KW, Sontag SJ, Vlahcevic RZ, McCallum RW (1987) The significance of intraepithelial eosinophils in the histologic diagnosis of gastroesophageal reflux. Am J Clin Path 87: 43–48

[8] Schindlbeck NE, Wiebecke B, Klauser AG, Voderholzer WA, Muller-Lissner SA (1996) Diagnostic value of histology in non-erosive gastroesophageal reflux disease. Gut 39: 151–154

[9] Fass R, Fennerty MB, Vakil N (2001) Non-erosive reflux disease (NERD) – current concepts and dilemmas. Am J Gastroenterol 96: 303–314

[10] Watson RGP, Tham TCK, Johnston BT, McDougall NI (1997) Double blind cross-over placebo controlled study of omeprazole in the treatment of patients with reflux symptoms and physiological levels of acid reflux – the "sensitive oesophagus". Gut 40: 587–590

[11] Johnston BT, Lewis SA, Collins JSA et al (1997) Acid perception in gastro-oesophageal reflux disease is dependent on psychological factors. Scand J Gastroenterol 32: 974–979

[12] Clouse RE, Richter JE, Heading RC, Janssens J, Wilson JA (1999) Functional esophageal disorders. Gut 45 (Suppl II): II31–II36

[13] Smout AJPM (1997) Endoscopy-negative acid reflux disease. Aliment Pharmacol Ther 11 (Suppl 2): 81–85

[14] Kahrilas PJ (2004) Review article: gastro-oesophageal reflux disease as a functional gastrointestinal disorder. Aliment Pharmacol Ther 20 (Suppl 7): 50–55

[15] Tack J, Janssens J (2002) Functional heartburn. Curr Treat Options Gastroenterol 5: 251–258

[16] Fass R (2000) Empirical trials in treatment of gastroesophageal reflux disease. Dig Dis 18: 20–26

[17] Schenk BE, Kuipers EJ, Klinkenberg-Knol EC et al (1997) Omeprazole as a diagnostic tool in gastroesophageal reflux disease. Am J Gastroenterol 92: 1997–2000

[18] Johnsson F, Weywadt L, Solhaug J-H et al (1997) One-week omeprazole treatment in the diagnosis of gastro-oesophageal reflux disease. Scand J Gastroenterol 33: 15–20

[19] Fass R, Ofman JJ, Gralnek IM et al (1999) Clinical and economic assessment of the omeprazole test in patients with symptoms suggestive of gastroesophageal reflux disease. Arch Intern Med 159: 2161–2168

[20] Fass R, Tougas G (2002) Functional heartburn: the stimulus, the pain, and the brain. Gut 51: 885–892

[21] Dent J (1998) Gastro-oesophageal reflux disease. Digestion 59: 433–445

[22] Trimble KC, Pryde A, Heading RC (1995) Lowered oesophageal sensory thresholds in patients with symptomatic but not excess gastro-oesophageal reflux: evidence for a spectrum of visceral sensitivity in GORD. Gut 37: 7–12

[23] Shi G, des Varannes SB, Scarpignato C, Le Rhun M, Galmiche JP (1995) Reflux related symptoms in patients with normal esophageal exposure to acid. Gut 37: 457–464

[24] Fass R, Naliboff B, Higa L et al (1998) Differential effect of long-term esophageal acid exposure on mechano-sensitivity and chemo-sensitivity in humans. Gastroenterology 115: 1363–1373

[25] Talley NJ, Zinsmeister AR, Schleck CK, Melton III LJ (1992) Dyspepsia and dyspepsia subgroups: a population-based study. Gastroenterology 102: 1259–1268

[26] Quigley EMM (1997) Motility, heartburn and dyspepsia. Aliment Pharmacol Ther 11 (Suppl 2): 41–50

[27] DiBaise JK, Lof J, Akromis I, Quigley EMM (1999) An open-label comparison of omeprazole and cisapride in endoscopy-negative reflux disease. Am J Gastroenterol 94: A2583

[28] Hopwood D, Milne G, Logan KR (1979) Electron microscopic changes in human oesophageal epithelium in oesophagitis. J Pathol 129: 161–167

[29] Carney CN, Orlando RC, Powell DW, Dotson MM (1981) Morphologic alterations in early acid-induced epithelial injury of the rabbit esophagus. Lab Invest 45: 198–208

[30] Tobey NA, Carson JL, Alkiek RA, Orlando RC (1996) Dilated intracellular spaces: a morphological feature of acid reflux-damaged human esophageal epithelium. Gastroenterology 111: 1200–1205

[31] Pace F, Santalucia F, Bianchi Porro G (1991) Natural history of gastro-oesophageal reflux disease without oesophagitis. Gut 32: 845–848

[32] Schindlbeck NE, Klauser AG, Berghammer G, Londong W, Muller-Lissner SA (1992) Three-year follow-up of patients with gastro-esophageal reflux disease. Gut 33: 1016–1019

[33] Ollyo JB, Monnier P, Fontolliet C et al (1993) The natural history, prevalence and incidence of reflux oesophagitis. Gullet 3 (Suppl): 3–10

[34] Kuster E, Ros E, Toledo-Pimentel V et al (1994) Predictive factors of the long-term outcome in gastro-oesophageal reflux disease: six-year follow-up of 107 patients. Gut 35: 8–14

[35] Trimble KC, Douglas S, Pryde A, Heading RC (1995) Clinical characteristics and natural history of symptomatic but not excess gastroesophageal reflux. Dig Dis Sci 40: 1098–1104

[36] McDougall NI, Johnston BT, Kee F et al (1996) Natural history of reflux esophagitis: a 10-year follow-up of patient symptomatology and quality of life. Gut 38: 491–486
[37] Isolauri J, Luostarinen M, Isolauri E et al (1997) Natural course of gastro-oesophageal reflux disease: 17–22 year follow-up of 60 patients. Am J Gastroenterol 92: 37–41
[38] McDougall NI, Johnston BT, Collins JS et al (1997) Disease progression in gastro-oesophageal reflux disease as determined by repeat oesophageal pH monitoring and endoscopy 3 to 4.5 years after diagnosis. Eur J Gastroenterol Hepatol 9: 1161–1167
[39] McDougall NI, Johnston BT, Collins JS et al (1998) Three to 4.5 year prospective study of prognostic indicators in gastro-oesophageal reflux disease. Scand J Gastroenterol 33: 1016–1022
[40] Fockens P (2002) Future developments in endoscopic imaging. Best Pract Res Clin Gastroenterol 16: 999–1012
[41] Klesslich R, Kanzler S, Vieth M, Moehler M, Neidig J, Thanka Nadar BJ, Schilling D, Burg J, Nafe B, Neurath MF, Galle PR (2004) Minimal change esophagitis: prospective comparison of endoscopic and histological markers between patients with non-erosive reflux disease and normal controls using magnifying endoscopy. Dig Dis 22: 221–227
[42] Pehlivanov N, Liu J, Mittal RK (2001) Sustained esophageal contraction: a motor correlate of heartburn. Am J Physiol 281: G743–G751
[43] Bhalla V, Liu J, Puckett JL, Mittal RK (2004) Symptom hypersensitivity to acid infusion is associated with hypersensitivity of esophageal contractility. Am J Physiol 287: G65–G71
[44] Rhee PL, Liu J, Puckett JL, Mittal RK (2002) Measuring esophageal distension by high-frequency intraluminal ultrasound probe. Am J Physiol 283: G886–G892
[45] Sifrim D, Castell D, Dent J, Kahrilas PJ (2004) Gastro-oesophageal reflux monitoring: review and consensus report on detection and definitions of acid, non-acid, and gas reflux. Gut 53: 1024–1031
[46] Shay S, Tutuian R, Sifrim D, Vela M, Wise J, Balaji N, Zhang X, Adhami T, Murray J, Castell D (2004) Twenty-four ambulatory simultaneous impedance and pH monitoring; a multicenter report of normal values from 60 healthy volunteers. Am J Gastroenterol 99: 1037–1043
[47] Vela MF, Camacho-Lobato L, Srinivasan R, Tutuian R, Katz PO, Castell DO (2001) Simultaneous intraseophageal impedance and pH measurement of acid and non-acid gastroesophageal reflux: effect of omeprazole. Gastroenterology 120: 1862–1864
[48] Kern M, Hofmann C, Hyde J, Shaker R (2004) Characterization of the cerebral cortical representation of heartburn in GERD patients. Am J Physiol 286: G174–G181
[49] Rodriguez-Stanley S, Ciociola AA, Zubaidi S, Proskin HM, Miner PB Jr (2004) A single dose of ranitidine 150 mg modulates oesophageal acid sensitivity in patients with functional heartburn. Aliment Pharmacol Ther 20: 975–982
[50] Frazzoni M, De Micheli E, Zentilin P, Savarino V (2004) Pathophysiological characteristics of patients with non-erosive reflux disease differ from those of patients with functional heartburn. Aliment Pharmacol Ther 20: 81–88
[51] Quigley EMM (2001) Non-Erosive Reflux Disease (NERD); part of the spectrum of gastro-oesophageal reflux, a component of functional dyspepsia, or both? Eur J Gastroenterol Hepatol 13 (Suppl 13): S13–S18
[52] Talley NJ, Meineche-Schmidt V, Pare P, Raisanen P, Pap A, Kordecki H et al (1998) Efficacy of omeprazole in functional dyspepsia: double-blind, randomized, placebo-controlled trials (the Bond and Opera studies). Aliment Pharmacol Ther 12: 1055–1065
[53] Carlsson R, Dent J, Bolling-Sternevald E, Johnsson F, Junghard O, Lauritsen K et al (1998) The usefulness of a structured questionnaire in the assessment of symptomatic gastroesophageal disease. Scand J Gastroenterol 33: 1023–1029
[54] Talley NJ, Stanghellini V, Heading RC, Koch KL, Malagelada JR, Tytgat GNJ (1999) Functional gastroduodenal disorders. Gut 45 (Suppl II): II37–II42
[55] Mittal R, Holloway R, Penagini R, Plackshaw LA, Dent J (1995) Transient lower esophageal sphincter relaxation. Gastroenterology 109: 601–610
[56] Tack J, Piessevaux H, Coulie B et al (1998) Role of impaired gastric accommodation to a meal in functional dyspepsia. Gastroenterology 115: 1346–1352
[57] Penagini R, Hebbard G, Horowitz M et al (1998) Motor functions of the proximal stomach and visceral perception in gastro-oesophageal reflux disease. Gut 42: 251–257
[58] Vu MK, Straathof JWA, van der Schaar PJ, Arndt JW, Ringers J, Lamers CBHW, Masclee AAM (1999) Motor and sensory function of the stomach in reflux disease and after laparoscopic Nissen fundoplication. Am J Gastroenterol 94: 1481–1490
[59] Galmiche JP, Barthelmy P, Hamelin B (1997) Treating the symptoms of gastroesophageal reflux disease: a double-blind comparison of omeprazole and cisapride. Aliment Pharmacol Therap 11: 765–773

[60] Castell DO, Sigmund C Jr, Patterson D, Lambert R, Hasner D, Clyde C, Zeldis JB (1998) and the CIS-USA-52 Investigator Group. Cisapride 20 mg b.i.d. provides symptomatic relief of heartburn and related symptoms of chronic mild to moderate gastroesophageal reflux disease. Am J Gastroenterol 93: 547–552

[61] Lagergren J, Bergstrom R, Lindgren A, Nyren O (1999) Symptomatic gastroesophageal reflux as a risk factor for esophageal adenocarcinoma. N Engl J Med 340: 825–831

[62] van Pinxteren B, Numans ME, Bonis PA, Lau J (2000) Short-term treatment with proton pump inhibitors, H2-receptor antagonists and prokinetics for gastro-oesophageal reflux disease-like symptoms and endoscopy-negative reflux disease (Cochrane Review). In: The Cochrane Library, vol. 4. Oxford: Update Software

[63] Richter JE, Peura D, Benjamin SB, Joelsson B, Whipple J (2000) Efficacy of Omeprazole for the treatment of symptomatic acid reflux disease without esophagitis. Arch Intern Med 160: 1810–1816

[64] Bate CM, Keeling PWN, Axon ATR, Dronfield MW, Chapman RWG, O'Donoghue D, Calam J, Crowe J, Mountford RA, Watts DA, Taylor MD, Richardson PDI (1996) Reflux symptom relief with omeprazole inpatients without unequivocal oesophagitis. Aliment Pharmacol Ther 10: 547–555

[65] Bate CM, Green JRB, Axon ATR, Murray FE, Tidesley G, Emmas CE, Taylor MD (1997) Omeprazole is more effective than cimetidine for the relief of all grades of gastro-oesophageal reflux disease-associated heartburn, irrespective of the presence or absence of endoscopic oesophagitis. Aliment Pharmacol Ther 11: 755–763

[66] Carlsson R, Dent J, Watts et al (1998) Gastro-oesophageal reflux disease in primary care: an international study of different treatment strategies with omeprazole. Eur J Gastroenterol Hepatol 10: 119–124

[67] Venables TL, Newland RD, Patel AC, Hole J, Wilcock C, Turbitt ML (1997) Omeprazole 10 milligrams once daily, omeprazole 20 milligrams once daily, or ranitidine 150 milligrams twice daily, evaluated as initial therapy for the relief of symptoms of gastro-oesophageal reflux disease in general practice. Scand J Gastroenterol 32: 965–973

[68] Dean BB, Gano AD Jr, Knight K, Ofman JJ, Fass R (2004) Effectiveness of proton pump inhibitors in nonerosive reflux disease. Clin Gastroenterol Hepatol 2: 656–664

[69] Sontag SJ, Hirschowitz BI, Holt S, Robinson MG, Behar J, Berenson MM, McCullogh A, Ippoliti AF, Richter JE, Ahtaridis G et al (1992) Two doses of omeprazole versus placebo in symptomatic erosive esophagitis: the U.S. multicenter study. Gastroenterology 102: 109–118

[70] Hungin APS, Gunn SD, Bate CM, Turbitt ML, Wilcock C, Richardson PDI (1993) A comparison of the efficacy of omeprazole 20 mg once daily with ranitidine 150 mg bd in the relief of symptomatic gastro-oesophageal reflux in general practice. Br J Clin Res 4: 73–88

[71] Spechler SJ and the Department of Veterans Affairs Gastroesophageal Reflux Disease Study Group (1992) Comparison of medical and surgical therapy for complicated gastroesophageal reflux disease in veterans. N Engl J Med 326: 786–792

[72] Vigneri S, Termini R, Leandro G et al (1995) A comparison of five maintenance therapies for reflux esophagitis. N Engl J Med 333: 1106–1110

[73] Glise H (1995) Quality of life and cost of therapy in reflux disease. Scand J Gastroenterol 30 (Suppl 210): 38–42

[74] Bardhan KD, Muller-Lissner S, Bigard MA, Porro GB, Ponce J, Hosie J, Scott M, Weir DG, Gillon KRW, Peacock RA, Fulton C (1999) Symptomatic gastro-oesophageal reflux disease: double blind controlled study of intermittent treatment with omeprazole or ranitidine. The European Study. Br Med J 318: 502–507

[75] Lind T, Havelund T, Lundell L, Glise H, Lauritsen K, Pedersen SA, Anker-Hansen O, Stubberod A, Eriksson G, Carlsson R, Junghard O (1999) On demand therapy with omeprazole for the long-term management of patients with heartburn without oesophagitis – a placebo-controlled randomized trial. Aliment Pharmacol Therap 13: 907–914

[76] Havelund T, Lind T, Wiklund I, Glise H, Hernqvist H, Lauritsen K, Lundell L, Pedersen SA, Carlsson R, Junghard O, Stubberod A, Anker-Hansen O (1999) Quality of life in patients with heartburn but without esophagitis: effects of treatment with omeprazole. Am J Gastroenterol 94: 1782–1789

[77] Bytzer P (2001) On-demand therapy for gastro-oesophageal reflux disease. Eur J Gastroenterol Hepatol 13 (Suppl 1): S19–S22

[78] Campos GM, Peters JH, DeMeester TR, Oberg S, Crookes PF, Tan S, DeMeester SR, Hagen JA, Bremner CG (1999) Multivariate analysis of factors predicting outcome after laparoscopic fundoplication. J Gastrointest Surg 3: 292–300

[79] Eubanks TR, Omelanczuk P, Richards C, Pohl D, Pellegrini CA (2000) Outcomes of laparoscopic antireflux procedures. Am J Surg 179: 391–395

[80] Vu MK, Ringers J, Arndt JW, Lamers CB, Masclee AA (2000) Prospective study of the effect of laparoscopic hemifundoplication on motor and sensory function of the proximal stomach. Br J Surg 87: 338–343

Chapter 9

MEDICAL THERAPY OF GASTRO-OESOPHAGEAL REFLUX DISEASE

H. Koop

II. Innere Klinik, HELIOS Klinikum Berlin-Buch, Berlin, Germany

Treatment of gastro-oesophageal reflux disease (GERD) has to take into account that GERD shows a considerable variation in the way of manifestations: the spectrum ranges from intermittent heartburn of minor severity to severe daily symptoms; additionally, dysphagia and bleeding may be due to complications such as strictures and oesophageal ulcers. Furthermore, gastro-oesophageal reflux has also been linked to a number of symptoms of the respiratory tract (e.g., chronic cough, posterior laryngitis). Thus, the questions arises whether a tailored treatment strategy is necessary for each individual aspect in this broad spectrum. The therapeutic strategy may also be influenced by results from diagnostic procedures, primarily from upper gastrointestinal endoscopy. More than half of the patients undergoing endoscopic evaluation do not reveal any changes of the mucosa (non-erosive reflux disease = NERD). These questions will be answered and a practical guideline based upon published literature as well as personal experience will be given.

Medical treatment primarily relies on drug-induced acid suppression whereas prokinetic agents do not play any role any more (if they ever played a role). A controversy exists as to what lifestyle modification have a role in the management of GERD.

Drugs

Proton pump inhibitors

Today, proton pump inhibitors (PPI) are the drug of choice for the vast majority of patients with GERD. This class of drugs consists of substituted benzimidazoles which are prodrugs activated at low pH in the parietal cell. After entering the acid space of the parietal cell, PPI are transformed to a sulfenamide, a tetracyclic compound which covalently binds to the H^+/K^+-ATPase (proton pump). The ability of the individual parietal cell to regain its function of acid production is restored by newly synthesised H^+/K^+-ATPase. Since only a fraction of parietal cells is simultaneously active and thus possesses an acidic compartment, acid inhibition usually reaches its maximal extent within a couple of days with ongoing therapy.

Since PPI bind irreversibly to the proton pump, its duration of action covers 24 hours; therefore, in most instances a once daily administration is sufficient. However, the degree of acid suppression shows profound interindividual variability. One major reason is the speed of metabolism via the cytochrome P 450 isoenzyme 2C19: it has been shown that slow metabolizers exert more profound inhibition of acid secretion than rapid metabolizers; this effect on acid inhibition is paralleled by differences in healing rates of oesophagitis [1], [34]. Another factor influencing the intragastric pH is the *Helicobacter pylori* (H. p.) status [5]: acid inhibition leads to higher pH levels in individuals infected with H.p. irrespective of drugs employed for acid suppression but most pronounced in patients with PPI of therapy. Whether other factors (e.g., differences in the rate degradation and new synthesis of the proton pump) also influences the pH levels achieved under PPI therapy remains unclear so far.

Largely, standard doses of the racemic PPI omeprazole (20 mg), lansoprazole (30 mg), pantoprazole (40 mg) and rabeprazole (20 mg) are comparable in efficacy. It has been claimed that the more recently developed isomeric PPI esomeprazole at its standard dose (40 mg) may be more effective than the former but this has been shown convincingly only in comparison to omeprazole [17] whereas its superiority over the other racemic PPI remains to confirmed. In this context one common observation is always puzzling: in comparative double-blind (!) trials of (oeconomically highly) competitive drugs the superiority of a particular compounds tested often correlates to the sponsor of the study who simultaneously is the manufacturer of the respective drug; if a similar trial is repeated by the competitor studying the same drugs, the results are often vice versa. Even taking into consideration that some of the differences are without any clinical relevance although they may be statistically significant (and thus supporting the oeconomical expectations of the respective company), those discrepancies remain obscure.

H_2-receptor antagonists

H_2-receptor antagonists competitively inhibit binding of histamine at the respective receptor located at the basolateral membrane of the parietal cell. The stimulatory effects of both gastrin and acetylcholine which are largely mediated via histamine release from the enterochromaffin-like (ECL) cells are also partially blocked by these compounds. However, the class of H_2-receptor blockers are less profound inhibitors of acid secretion than PPI. Particularly, H_2-blockers are inferior in the inhibition of food stimulated acid secretion – a significant disadvantage since the majority of reflux patients suffers predominantly from postprandial reflux symptoms. A further problem arises from a phenomena called tolerance [23]: during prolonged therapy with H_2-receptor antagonists the degree of acid suppression decreases. This further limits its use in the treatment of reflux disease in which more effective acid suppression is necessary compared to gastroduodenal ulcer healing. On the other hand, H_2-blockers are meanwhile cheap compounds which make them attractive from the oeconomical point of view.

Antacids

Antacids act by neutralising acid thus leading to prompt disappearance of symptoms. Therefore, antacids regularly serve as rescue medication in studies on the effect of acid inhibitory compounds and are also preferred by patients with sporadic heartburn. However, antacid consumption several times a day (which indicates the presence of reflux oesophagitis) should not be encouraged: intake of high doses of antacids inherits a lot of problems (diarrhoea due to magnesium, aluminium-induced constipation, interference with other drugs taken etc). Therefore, antacids can only be recommended in patients with infrequent heartburn (which according to the definition of GERD that includes impaired quality of life cannot be regarded as sufferers from reflux *disease* but from sporadic reflux symptoms).

GABA antagonists

The neurotransmitter γ-butyric acid (GABA) has been shown to be involved in the initiation of transient sphincter relaxations of the lower oesophageal sphincter (LES) which are thought to play the major role in the pathophysiology of reflux disease. Attempts have been made to suppress these relaxations not associated with swollowing, e.g. by the prototype of $GABA_B$ receptor agonist, baclofen. In fact, GABAergic stimulation increases the pressure in the lower oesophageal sphincter [7]. So far, clinical trials with $GABA_B$ agonists in patients with GERD show limited clinical efficacy [9], [18], [30], but it seems too early to make a firm judgement about this interesting and maybe promising pharmacological principle.

Clinical efficacy

Lifestyle modifications

Several modifications of habits are recommended for patients with GERD. These include rising of the head of the bed, early evening meals with sufficient time to elapse before going to bed, weight reduction, stopping smoking and avoidance of alcoholic beverages etc (for overview, see [22]). None of these measures have been studied with sufficient quality so far. Therefore, its merits – if there are any – cannot be evaluated based employing the methods of evidence-based medicine. Certainly, some suggestions may have some limited value in an individual patient. It seems, however, questionable to recommend these lifestyle modifications as a prerequisite for starting effective drug therapy. It is completely unknown whether life style modifications have any effect as an adjunct to effective drug therapy.

Drug therapy

Several controlled trials have been performed comparing the effect of different acid inhibitory drugs in the treatment of reflux oesophagitis (erosive reflux disease; ERD). Data on the effect of acid suppression in non-erosive reflux disease (NERD) are less frequent; in particular, studies comparing the effect of PPI and H_2-blockers are scare.

In patients with ERD (Table 1), PPI have been shown to be much more effective than H_2-receptor antagonists in terms of healing of erosions, resolution of heartburn, prevention of relapsing heartburn and endoscopic recurrence of erosions [6], [10], [14]. The differences are even more pronounced with increasing severity of ERD. According to evidence-based medicine [29], the superiority can be regarded as proven at the highest possible level I a (confirmed by multiple randomised, double-blind controlled studies and meta-analyses). In a comparative study, omeprazole was even more effective than a combination of the H_2-blocker ranitidine at a dose of 150 mg three times daily and the prokinetic agent cisapride 10 mg three times daily [33].

A recent updated Cochrane review also showed that empirical treatment of GERD with PPI was significantly more effective than with H_2-blockers [29]. The same applies for a comparison of PPI with prokinetics. Maintenance therapy with PPI was the most effective strategy; whereas H_2-blockers had some symptomatic effect, its ability to prevent relapse was regarded as marginal.

As far as NERD is concerned, it is much more difficult to evaluate the comparative efficacy of H_2-blockers and PPI. Inclusion criteria vary considerably, and in most instances PPI were compared only to placebo (and found to be superior [13]). In an earlier study, the differences between H_2-blockers and 2 doses of omeprazole were small in patients without erosive oesophagitis, but patients with heartburn at least twice a week were allowed to enter the study according to the inclusion criteria [32]. Whether this is a reliable criterion for NERD appears questionable but is seems likely that patients with functional complaints not related to acid reflux may have been included in the study to a significant extent. Within the group of PPI, a dose-depending effect of PPI could not be observed [3]. In all these studies the problem of lacking reliable criteria for the definition of NERD remains.

Other drugs such as sucralfate are difficult to evaluate since they have not been studied to a sufficient degree; therefore, they are not even mentioned in some guidelines or judged as compounds without confirmed evidence of efficacy [2], [12], [20].

Table 1. Efficacy of drug treatment in acute reflux oesophagitis. The therapeutic gain over placebo after 8–12 weeks of therapy are displayed (data from Kahrilas, 2000)

Drug class	Therapeutic gain over placebo
Proton pump inhibitors	40–80%
H_2-receptor antagonists	10–25%

Practical considerations

Treatment of acute reflux symptoms

For practical reasons it seems important to review the optimal strategy in a given patients depending upon presence or absence of information about the results of endoscopy. Thus, empirical therapy and treatment of ERD and NERD are discussed separately.

Another questions also has also to be considered particularly in respect to empirical treatment: should we increase the efficacy of medical therapy in relation to its symptomatic effect ("step-up") or should we initially employ the most effective drugs in order to achieve most efficient and immediate resolution of symptoms and/or most rapid healing of lesions then followed by gradually reducing the intensity of therapy as long as the patient remains symptom-free ("step-down"). So far, this controversy about the most appropriate strategy is present also in the scientific literature: some groups of authors support the escalation scheme [28] whereas others favour the concept of starting with a kind of treatment which brings prompt relief to the greatest possible population [11]. The author of the present chapter discourages the step-up strategy for several reasons: first, most patients have used antacids before they show up in the doctor's office but found antacids to be insufficient (that's why they seek medical attention); therefore, it seems inappropriate to recommend a treatment which the patient has already found to be unsatisfactory. Second, the next step up the ladder would be the administration of H_2-blockers, a class of drugs which have not convincingly shown to be potent enough in patients with GERD; consequently, a significant number of patient will remain symptomatic [4], [16]. Probably after many weeks of inadequate symptomatic responses these patients will finally end up in the therapy they deserve: PPI which will effectively suppress the reflux symptoms. Using the alternative strategy with the step-down approach, the goal of resolution of heartburn can be achieved within several days using PPI in 50–80% of patients. During follow-up, the optimal choice of drug and dosing scheme can be established by reducing the dose according to the patient's individual severity and frequency of symptoms. It is not excluded that some of the patients may eventually be treated with (cheap) H_2-receptor antagonists if these are capable of controlling symptoms.

Empirical therapy

In patients with symptoms suggestive of GERD, in many instances it will be impossible to gain access to immediate endoscopy or prompt endoscopy appears not necessary at an early stage but rather an exaggerated diagnostic procedure. This seems, according to recent data of the CADET-PE study [27], appropriate since reflux disease is by far the dominating endoscopic diagnosis whereas other benign diagnoses (e.g., peptic gastro-duodenal ulcers) were much less frequent and malignancies were rare and occurring only in patients aged over 50 years. Therefore, approaching a given patient with symptoms suggestive of reflux disease but without any alarm symptoms (e.g., dysphagia, weight loss, anaemia etc), the first option will often be empirical therapy; a prescription of a PPI is recommended due to its superiority over alternative drugs.

Therapy of reflux oesophagitis

Treatment of choice is the administration of PPI. Within 6–8 weeks, oesophagitis has healed in up to 90%, and more than half of the patients are free of heartburn after the first week. Though disappearance of symptoms is a valuable predictor of effective healing [8], discrepant results can be detected in up to 20%; however, in such cases residual lesions are predominantly minor in asymptomatic patients or heartburn of little intensity in healed cases.

Healing rates are influenced by the initial degree of severity with slower disappearance of peptic lesions in severe reflux oesophagitis. The EXPO study [21] including more than 3000 patients may serve as an example: after 8 weeks of pantoprazole (40 mg) therapy healing rates were 97% in mild forms (grade A according to the Los Angeles (LA) classification) gradually declining to only 74% in more severe forms (LA grade D). Nevertheless, in patients with lesions of high severity healing rates similar to those in less severe forms can be observed after more extended periods of PPI administration and/or dose escalation. Even patients with peptic strictures can be managed conservatively if PPI therapy (with even more often higher doses necessary) is combined with dilatation.

A small proportion of reflux patients will not adequately respond to standard doses of PPI, though the proportion is small in patients with uncomplicated reflux oesophagitis. In such cases, doubling the dose will lead to healing of lesions in the vast majoritiy. Failure to higher doses are rare and should question the concept that symptoms are related to oesophagitis.

Therapy of non-erosive reflux disease

Since PPI are also the most effective therapy in NERD, it is advisable to start treatment with these compounds. However, results from treatment in patients with NERD are much more complex. This has to be ascribed to the heterogenous population: solely based upon a careful history of symptoms it is not always possible to exclude patients with predominant non-acid reflux or aerophagia who often also report to suffer from heartburn, but who will eventually not respond to acid inhibitory drug. Thus, the outcome from an effective treatment will also generate valuable diagnostic information. Taken these facts into consideration, prompt response to PPI therapy supports the assumption that pathological reflux is the underlying pathophysiological mechanism though placebo effects cannot be excluded. On the other hand, complete failure of PPI therapy casts doubt on the suspected diagnosis of NERD.

Since acid inhibitory effects vary considerably interindividually, PPI dose should be doubled if responses to PPI therapy are unsatisfactory. The optimal intervals after which the dose escalation should be initiated is unclear so far, but should be carried out not later than 6–8 weeks after starting therapy. If doubled or tripled PPI doses (preferentially administered in divided doses which will produce profound and prolonged acid inhibition close to achlorhydria with the exception of only few patients) will not lead to disappearance of reflux symptoms, it can be concluded with almost certainty that acid reflux does not play a significant role for the symptoms. Only in rare cases, pH-metry will be necessary to confirm absence of pathological reflux (for further discussion see chapter on therapeutic failure).

Treatment of therapeutic failure

Several reasons may be responsible for the failure of drugs as antireflux therapy (Table 2). Probably the by far most important factor is inadequate inhibition of acid secretion. This may be due to administration of H_2-recptor antagonists which do not produce sufficient acid suppression to control reflux symptoms and achieve healing of peptic lesion. Furthermore, also standard doses of PPI are not effective either in about 10–20% of subjects. Thus as a logical consequence PPI should be administered as first line treatment, and in case of insufficient responses at standard doses, PPI doses should be doubled (given b.i.d.). In symptomatic reflux reflux disease, lack of compliance is a relatively rare phenomena since interruption of therapy leads to reoccurrence of symptoms. Some patient still will not show adequate responses even to doubled or tripled doses, a scenario more frequently observed in NERD than in ERD patients.

Table 2. Factors which may play a role for therapeutic failure of medical therapy in gastro-oesophageal reflux disease

- insufficient acid inhibition
  - ineffective drug (e.g., H_2-blockers instead of PPI)
  - inadequate dosing (PPI dose to low)
- compliance
- wrong diagnosis (e.g., functional disease instead of reflux disease)
- predominant biliary reflux (after gastric surgery)

PPI = proton pump inhibitors

In *oesophagitis* patients one always assumes that lesions found at endoscopy will also be responsible for a symptom profile which suggests reflux disease; however, detection of minor lesions is not an infrequent observation in patients undergoing endoscopy for other reasons (e.g., work-up for diarrhoea). Thus, there is a population with asymptomatic reflux oesophagitis which has not been characterized well enough until now. It can be speculated that such patients may have upper abdominal or retrosternal symptoms for other reasons, but thought to be related to ERD; under these circumstances PPI therapy even at higher doses might fail. Another reason for PPI failure may occur in patients after gastric surgery which by itself resulted in profound reduction of acid secretion; in such patients a predominant biliary but only little acid reflux may be the underlying mechanism for generating oesophageal lesions and/ or symptoms but which will not well respond to acid inhibitory therapy. In general however, unresponsiveness to individually tailored PPI therapy is a minor problem in ERD [15].

Failure to PPI in *NERD* is a much greater problem. It is well established that demonstration of pathological reflux by pH-metry is associated with much better results of acid suppression thus demonstrating that proven exaggerated acid reflux will be also – analogous to ERD – a predictor for treatment success. In patients with symptoms suggestive of GERD but a reflux

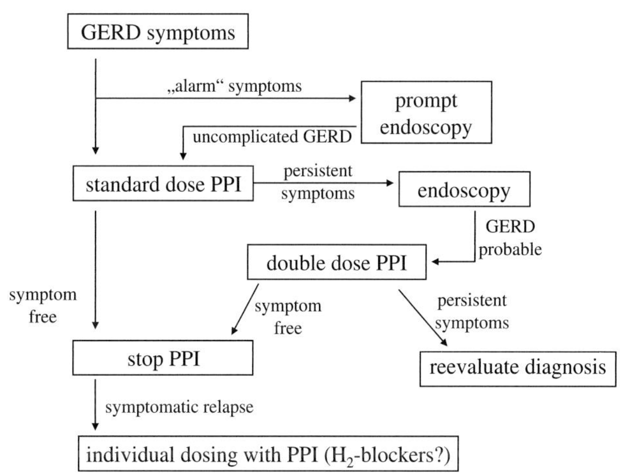

Fig. 1. Management algorhythm for the unendoscoped patient with symptoms suggestive of reflux disease. PPI = proton pump inhibitors

pattern quantitatively within the normal range, the suggested diagnosis is functional heartburn [15]. It is unclear so far whether episodes with heartburn are induced by minute episodes of acid reflux or whether other mechanisms apply (e.g., motor events). Therefore, it is also unproven that acid suppression will benefit those patients. In studies with combined intra-oesophageal impedance and pH monitoring (which allows separate analysis of acid, non-acid, and air regurgitation) it has been shown that in patients with GERD the number of acid reflux episodes can be well reduced by PPI treatment but non-acid reflux persists to the same extent. This observation may explain why some patients report no change in symptoms under the conditions of acid suppression although they well respond to therapy in terms of acidic reflux because they link non-acid reflux to treatment failure. These patients will subsequently not benefit from dose escalation either. Furthermore, many patients with aerophagia and air eructation will often be referred to specialists under the diagnosis of refractory reflux disease after they had (expectedly) not responded to PPI treatment; these patients will not gain any benefit from acid suppressants and have otherwise to be regarded as a demanding population in general. One important rule should be obeyed: transfer of NERD patients refractory to high PPI doses to antireflux surgery should be avoided since functional diseases do not respond to operative procedures but this will lead to an even more complex symptomatology (surgeons should only be involved if a pathophysiological condition can be unequivocally identified which can be corrected by surgery).

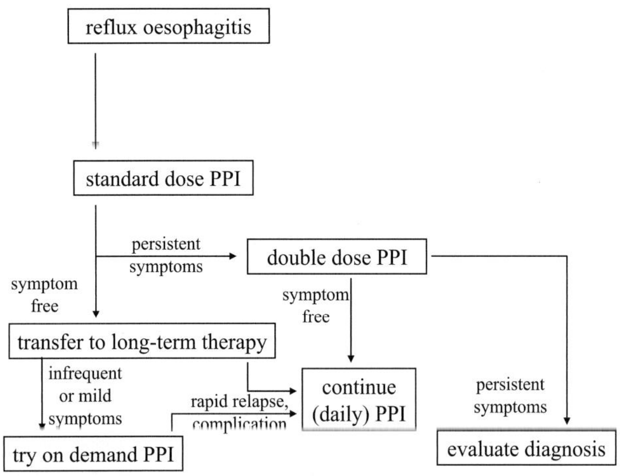

Fig. 2. Management algorhythm for the endoscoped patient with reflux oesophagitis. PPI = proton pump inhibitor

Finally, there is some overlap in patients with GERD and those who otherwise would be assumed to have non-cardiac chest pain (NCCP). A subgroup will also improve when given PPI (which suggests that acid reflux may play a central role) but a significant portion will not (e.g., with motor disorders of the oesophagus) but may subsequently respond to tricyclic antidepressants. Since symptoms are sometimes indistinguishable between reflux disease and NCCP, some patients with refractory retrosternal symptoms may belong to the group of NCCP patients.

Long-term strategy

Once a patient has been shown to improve with acid suppression therapy, the question of long-term management becomes evident. Since GERD is in most instances a chronic (relapsing) disease, a concept for the further treatment is needed in the vast majority. The speed of recurrence of symptoms after cessation of treatment represents a reliable predictor for the necessity of ongoing therapy: those who will become symptomatic within a few days after stopping treatment will probably require (almost) daily doses to achieve prolonged remission whereas those remaining asymptomatic for a considerable period can most likely treated by on demand therapy. Particularly in NERD, cessation of therapy after treatment of an acute episode of reflux symptoms is advisable since about half of the patients will remain in symptomatic remission within a 6-month interval. In symptomatic patients, tailoring of long-term treatment can be well orientated at the presence of symptoms whereas endoscopic guidance is predominantly required only in patients without or with minor reflux symptoms. Reflux oesophagitis initially with high degree of severity as well as complicated reflux disease will most probably require daily administration of PPI.

The strategy with on demand therapy has been developed primarily for patients with NERD since freedom of heartburn and other reflux symptoms is the only therapeutic goal in this group of patients. However, many patients overwhelmingly with mild reflux oesophagitis will also switch voluntarily to an on demand concept as long as they remain symptom free. Since there is no evidence that such a strategy will bear the risk for the development of Barrett's oesophagus or other complications of reflux disease, symptom-orientated drug administration can be well accepted also in patients with low-grade oesophagitis since absence of heartburn is associated with healing of lesions in the vast majority [8] despite the fact that endoscopic investigations may reveal some minor peptic lesions during follow-up.

Whereas PPI are the acute treatment of choice for all forms of reflux disease, the question remains whether other compounds, in particular H_2-blockers which are attractive due to low costs, can be regarded as an alternative in long-term management in accordance with the step-down concept. So far, there are very little reliable data which demonstrate unequivocally the benefits from such an H_2-receptor antagonist treatment e.g. compared to PPI. It seems, however, justified to try such an approach in patients with mild symptoms requiring only minute doses of PPI to remain free of heartburn. Patients should be advised to return to the office if symptom control is unsatisfactory after switching to H_2-blockers.

Treatment in selected conditions

Pregnancy. Though H_2-receptor antagonists have been regarded as the first line therapy during pregnancy, administration of omeprazole to control reflux symptoms can be regarded as a safe treatment option today – at least in those women who will not respond sufficiently to H_2-blockers. Whether this applies for the other PPI compound available remains unclear so far though there has been no evidence for an increased risk from clinical practice as well as from the mode of action regarding this class of acid suppressants.

Peptic strictures. In the era of potent antisecretory drugs the incidence of peptic strictures seems to decrease though reliable data are missing. The combination of PPI with dilatation offers an effective kind of treatment which substitutes formerly necessary surgery in such cases [25], [26]. Obviously, more pronounced acid suppression than in mild form of ERD is required to maintain the success of dilatation, and higher doses than those defined as standard dosing by the manufacturers are needed in up to 20% which have to be administered also in the long-term management of such strictures [19].

Safety of medical therapy

Adverse events. Since the introduction of acid inhibitory drugs, many potential risks have been attributed to the use of these substances, particularly if taken on the long run: bacterial growth in gastric juice and formation of N-nitroso compounds increasing the risk for gastric cancer, hypergastrinaemia with subsequent risk of developing gastric carcinoids arising from ECL cells, development of gastric atrophy in the fundus of the stomach etc. As we know today, most of these hypotheses have been refuted, and only some controversy remains whether gastritis may be accelerated in the presence of *Helicobacter pylori* (H. p.) during prolonged acid inhibition. Data from the ongoing Scandinavian trial in which omeprazole therapy is compared to antireflux surgery, but also from randomised H.p. eradication trials show that progression of atrophy is a rare phenomena which by the way can easily be overcome by eradication therapy if long term acid suppression is likely to be necessary in the future.

Interactions with concomitant medication. In respect to drug interactions, PPI can be regarded as safe drugs with little interaction: all compounds alter pH-dependent absorption of other pharmaceuticals (e.g. konazoles), and some PPI (e.g., omeprazole, esomeprazole) show interaction with drugs which plasma concentration (phenytoin) or clinical effect (warfarine) is under strict control under any circumstances.

In summary, PPI as well as H_2-receptor antagonists (except cimetidine) exert an excellent safety profile which has already led to the availability of both H_2-blockers and the first PPI omeprazole as over-the-counter (OTC) drugs in some countries. It is likely that other PPI will follow in this line.

References

[1] Adachi K, Katsube T, Kawamura A et al (2000) CYP 2C19 genotype status and intragastric pH during dosing with lasoprazole and rabeprazole. Aliment Pharmacol Ther 14: 1259–1266

[2] Armstrong D, Marshall JK, Chiba N et al (2004) Canadian consensus conference on the management of gastroesophageal reflux disease in adults – update 2004. Can J Gastroenterol 19: 15–35

[3] Armstrong D, Talley NJ, Lauritsen K et al (2004) The role of acid suppression in patients with endoscopy-negative reflux disease: the effect of treatment with esomperazole and omeprazole. Aliment Pharmacol Ther 20: 413–436
[4] Armstrong D, Veldhuizenvan Zanten SJO, Barkun AN et al (2005) Heartburn-dominant, univestigated dyspepsia: a comparison of "PPI-start" and "H2-RA-start" management strategy in primary care – the CADET-HR study. Aliment Pharmacol Ther 21: 1189–1202
[5] Blum AL, Martinek J (1999) Interactions of proton pump inhibitors and *Helicobacter pylori* in vivo. In: Proton pump inhibitors (Olbe L, ed). Basel Boston London: Birkhäuser, pp 130–141
[6] Caro JJ, Salas M, Ward A (2001) Healing and relapse rates in gastroesophageal reflux disease treated with newer proton pump inhibitors lansoprazole, rabeprazole, and pantoprazole compared with omeprazole, ranitidine, and placebo: evidence from randomized clinical trials. Clin Ther 23: 998–1017
[7] Cantu P, Carmagnola S, Savojardo D, Aloca M, Penagini R (2003) Effect of non-selective gamma-aminobutyric acid receptor stimulation on motor function of the lower oesophageal sphincter and gastro-oesophageal reflux in healthy human subjects. Aliment Pharmacol Ther 18: 699–704
[8] Carlsson R, Galmiche JP, Dent J, Lundell L, Frison L (1997) Prognostic factors influencing relapse of oesophagitis during maintenance therapy with antisecretory drugs: a meta-analysis of long-term omeprazole trials. Aliment Pharmacol Ther 11: 473–482
[9] Ciccaglione AF, Marzio L (2003) Effect of acute and chronic administration of the $GABA_B$ agonist baclofen on 24 hour pH metry and symptoms in control subjects and in patients with gastro-oesophageal reflux disease. Gut 52: 464–470
[10] Chiba N, de Gara CJ, Wilkinson JM, Hunt RH (1997) Speed of healing and symptom relief in grade-II to -IV gastroesophageal reflux disease: a meta-analysis. Gastroenetrology 112: 1798–1810
[11] Dent J, Brun J, Fendrick AM et al (1999) An evidence-based appraisal of reflux disease management – the Genval Workshop Report. Gut 44 (Suppl. 2): 1–16
[12] DeVault KR, Castell DO (1999) Updated guidelines for the diagnosis and treatment of gastroesophageal reflux disease. The practice parameters committee of the American College of Gastroenterology. Am J Gastroenetrol 94: 1434–1442
[13] Donnellan C, Sharma N, Preston C, Moayyedi P (2005) Medical treatments for maintenance therapy of reflux oesophagitis and endoscopic negative reflux disease. Cochrane Database Syst Rev 2: CD 003245
[14] Eriksson S, Langström G, Rikner L, Carlsson R, Naesdal J (1995) Omeprazole and H_2-receptor antagonists in the acute treatment of duodenal ulcer, gastric ulcer and reflux oesophagitis: a meta-analysis. Eur J Gastroenetrol Hepatol 7: 467–475
[15] Fass, R, Shapiro M, Dekel R, Sewell J (2005) Systematic review: proton pump inhibitor failure in gastro-oesophageal reflux disease – where next? Aliment Pharmacol Ther 22: 79–94
[16] Howden CW, Henning JM, Huang B, Lukasik N, Freston JW (2001) Management of heartburn in a large, randomized, community-based study: comparison of four therapeutic strategies. Am J Gastroenterol 96: 1704–1710
[17] Klok RM, Postma MJ, van Hout BA, Brouwers JR (2003) Meta-analysis: comparing the efficacy of proton pump inhibitors in short-term use. Aliment Pharmacol Ther 17: 1237–1245
[18] Koeck GH, Sifrim D, Lerut T, Janssens J, Tack J (2003) Effect of the GABA(B) agonist baclofen in patients with symptoms and duodeno-gastro-oesophageal reflux refractory to proton pump inhibitors. Gut 52: 1397–1402
[19] Koop H, Katschinski M, Arnold R (1991) Konservative Behandlung der floriden peptischen Ösophagusstenose. Vollständige Beseitigung durch Bougeirung und Omeprazol bei H_2-Blocker-refraktären Fällen. Med Klin 86: 566–568
[20] Koop H, Schepp W, Müller-Lissner S et al (2005) Gastroösophageale Refluxkrankheit – Ergebnisse einer evidenzbasierten Konsensuskonferenz der Deutschen Gesellschaft für Verdauungs- und Stoffwechselkrankheiten. Z Gastroenterol 43: 163–194
[21] Labenz J, Armstrong D, Lauritsen K et al (2005) A randomised comparative study of esomeprazole 40 mg versus pantoprazole 40 mg for healing erosive oesophagtis: the EXPO study. Aliment Pharmacol Ther 21: 739–746
[22] Meining A, Classen M (2000) The role of diet an lifestyle measures in the pathogenesis and treatment of gastroesophageal reflux disease. Am J Gastroenterol 95: 2692–2697
[23] Sandvik AK, Brenna E, Waldum HL (1997) Review article: the pharmacological inhibition of acid secretion – tolerance and rebound. Aliment Pharmacol Ther 11: 1013–1018
[24] Sifrim D, Holloway RH, Silny J, Tack J, Lerut T, Janssens J (2001) Composition of the postprandial

refluxate in patients with gastro-esophageal reflux disease. Amer J Gastroenterol 96: 647–655

[25] Silvis SE, Farahmand M, Johnson JA, Ansel HJ, Ho SB (1996) A randomized blinded comparison of omeprazole and ranitidine in the treatment of chronic esophageal stricture secondary to acid peptic reflux. Gastrointest Endoc 43: 216–221

[26] Smith PM, Kerr GD, Cockel R et al (1994) A comparison of omeprazole and ranitidine in the prevention of recurrance of benign esophageal stricture. Restore Investigator Group. Gastroenterology 107: 1545–1548

[27] Thomson AB, Barkun AN, Armstrong D et al (2003) The prevalence of clinically significant endoscopic findings in primary care patients with uninvestigated dyspepsia: the Canadian Adult Dyspepsia Emperiric Therapy – Prompt Endoscopy (CADET-PE) study. Aliment Pharmacol Ther 17: 1481–1491

[28] Tytgat GN, Heading RC, Müller-Lissner S et al (2003) Contemporary understanding and management of reflux and constipation in the general population and pregnancy: a consensus meeting. Aliment Pharmacol Ther 18: 291–301

[29] van Pinxteren B, Numans ME, Bonis PA, Lau J (2004) Short-term treatment with proton pump inhibitors, H2-receptor antagonists and prokinetics for gastro-oesophageal reflux-like symptoms and endoscopy negative reflux disease. Cochrane Database Sys Rev 4: CD 002095

[30] Vela MF, Tutuian R, Katz PO, Castell DO (2003) Baclofen decreases acid and non-acid post-prandial gastroesophageal reflux measured by combined multichannel intraluminal impedance and pH. Aliment Pharmacol Ther 17: 243–251

[31] Vela MF, Camacho-Lubato L, Srinivasan R, Tutuian R, Katz PO, Castel DO (2001) Simultaneous intraesophageal impedance and pH measurement of acid and nonacid gastroesophageal reflux: effect of omeprazole. Gastroenetrology 120: 1599–1806

[32] Venables TL, Newland RD, Patel AC, Hole J, Wicock C, Turbitt ML (1997) Omeprazole 10 milligrams once daily, omeprazole 20 mg once daily, or ranitidine 150 twice daily, evaluated as initial therapy for the relief of symptoms of gastro-oesophageal reflux disease in general pratice. Scand J Gastroenterol 32: 965–973

[33] Vigneri S, Termini R, Leandro G et al (1995) A comparison of five maintenance therapies for reflux esophagitis. N Engl J Med 333: 1106–1110

[34] Wilkinson GR (2005) Drug metabolism and variability among patients in drug response. N Engl J Med 352: 2211–2221

Chapter 10

DIAGNOSIS OF GASTROESOPHAGEAL REFLUX DISEASE: ROLE OF ENDOSCOPY

A. Bansal and P. Sharma

University of Kansas, School of Medicine and Veteran Affairs Medical Center, Kansas City, MO, USA

Introduction

The diagnosis of gastroesophageal reflux disease (GERD) can be made by a number of methods including endoscopy, patient's symptoms, Bernstein test, 24 hr ambulatory pH and by using a short course of acid suppressive therapy (proton pump inhibitors). Newer techniques including magnetoencephalography, postiron emission tomography and functional magnetic resonance imaging (fMRI) are currently being evaluated for the diagnosis of GERD [1]. None of these tests can be considered as the gold standard for the diagnosis of GERD. The role of endoscopy in GERD is to evaluate changes in the mucosa of the distal esophagus and offers the potential to obtain biopsies, treat reflux induced strictures and rule out other structural lesions in the upper gastrointestinal tract. However, endoscopy is relatively insensitive for making a diagnosis of GERD since only 40–50% of patients with typical reflux symptoms undergoing endoscopy may have GERD induced changes. Utilization of newer techniques like chromoendoscopy, high resolution and magnification endoscopy may play an important role in the endoscopic evaluation of GERD in the near future.

Endoscopic findings suggestive of GERD

The findings at endoscopy that suggest a diagnosis of GERD include the presence of erosive esophagitis, Barrett's esophagus and peptic stricture. In combination with reflux symptoms, these findings are highly suggestive for a diagnosis of GERD. In this chapter, we will discuss the findings of erosive esophagitis, Barrett's esophagus, role of esophageal biopsies and the impact of a negative endoscopy in patients with GERD.

Erosive esophagitis

Multiple studies have shown that only 30–40% of patients with typical reflux symptoms (i.e., heartburn, regurgitation) have evidence of erosive esophagitis (*Fig. 1*) on upper endoscopy whereas the other 60–70% of patients even with troublesome reflux symptoms have no clear-cut esophageal mucosal abnormalities [2]–[7]. Thus, overall endoscopy is an insensitive test for diagnosing reflux disease. However, if detected, erosive esophagitis has a good positive predictive value for the diagnosis of GERD as discussed below.

Role in diagnosis
A number of different classification systems for grading erosive esophagitis have been described including the Savary-Miller, Los Angeles (LA) (Table 1), Hetzel-Dent etc. [8]–[11]. The LA classification is a well validated, widely used system and is listed in Table 1. In general, as the grade of erosive esophagitis worsens, the degree of esophageal acid exposure increases. Lundell et al showed that the severity of esophageal acid exposure was significantly ($p < 0.001$)

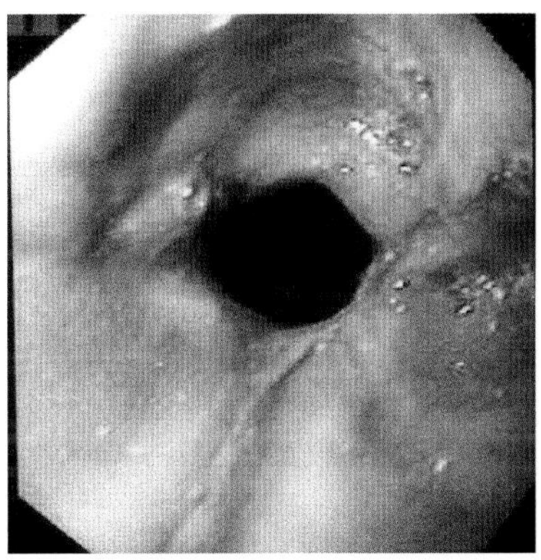

Fig. 1. Endoscopic appearance of erosive esophagitis

related to the grade of esophagitis as judged by the LA classification for erosive esophagitis [10]. Another study of 150 patients demonstrated a significantly higher duration of esophageal acid exposure in patients with grade-III/-IV esophagitis compared to grade-II esophagitis (percent time pH < 4.0 17.5% vs. 10.4%; $p < 0.001$). Both groups (i.e., patients with esophagitis) had significantly higher pH scores compared to control subjects (percent time pH < 4.0 1.8%; $p < 0.0001$) [12].

The presence of erosive esophagitis has a good correlation with results of 24 h pH monitoring showing increased esophageal acid exposure. In a study by DeMeester et al [13], the combination of typical reflux symptoms (i.e., grade-II or -III heartburn and/or regurgitation, scale of severity 0–3) and the presence of erosive esophagitis or Barrett's esophagus on endoscopy had a 64% sensitivity and 97% specificity for accurately diagnosing GERD as defined by a positive 24-hr ambulatory pH result. A study of 24 controls and 64 patients with reflux symptoms (all of whom underwent 24-hr pH monitoring), showed that the distinction in degree of esophageal acid exposure was excellent between asymptomatic controls and patients with severe erosive esophagitis (sensitivity and specificity both 100% by logistic regression) but discrimination was relatively poor when asymptomatic controls were compared to symptomatic patients without esophagitis (71% and 79% by logistic regression) [14].

On the other hand, a study from Spain showed that 34% of patients with grade-I and -II esophagitis showed variable patterns of reflux whereas most patients (76.2%) with grade-III and -IV esophagitis showed a clearly defined pattern of gastroesophageal reflux in both the supine and the upright positions ($p < 0.05$) [15]. In another study of 100 patients with reflux symptoms, 51% and 48% of patients respectively with grades 1 and 2 esophagitis had a normal DeMeester's score (< 14.7) [16]. This raises questions whether milder grades of esophagitis on endoscopy may overdiagnose GERD, if other causes of esophagitis may have been present and last but not the least, if results of 24-hr pH monitoring may have been falsely negative. Furthermore, some patients may be susceptible to esophageal damage at relatively low levels of acid exposure.

Table 1. The Los Angeles Classification System for the endoscopic assessment of grade of esophagitis [10]

(A)	One or more mucosal breaks no longer than 5 mm, none of which extends between the tops of the mucosal folds
(B)	One or more mucosal breaks more than 5 mm long, none of which extends between the tops of two mucosal folds
(c)	Mucosal breaks that extend between the tops of two or more mucosal folds, but which involve less than 75% of the oesophageal circumference
(D)	Mucosal breaks which involve at least 75% of the oesophageal circumference

All these studies have compared endoscopic findings to 24-h ambulatory pH – using it as the gold standard, which is less than a perfect test for the diagnosis of GERD. Studies have shown that 37–60% of patients with non erosive reflux disease (NERD), as defined either by symptom response to PPI or significant symptom correlation with reflux episodes, will have normal ambulatory 24-H esophageal pH results [4], [6], [17], [18]. Moreover, when the reproducibility of prolonged esophageal pH testing is measured on two separate days in patients with reflux symptoms or with esophagitis, the results change the diagnosis (normal or abnormal based on the percentage time pH < 4.0) in 11% of the cases [19]. Thus, comparison with 24-h pH monitoring may lower the sensitivity of milder forms of erosive esophagitis in the diagnosis of GERD. It is possible that these shortcomings may be overcome by using the new Bravo wireless pH device and correlating these pH results to the presence of erosive esophagitis. Results of such studies are as yet awaited.

Overall, in the presence of typical reflux symptoms (i.e. heartburn), detection of macroscopic endoscopic injury is strongly predictive of the diagnosis of GERD.

Role in prognosis

Given the lack of efficacy of non-drug measures and antacids and the relatively low efficacy of H2 receptor antagonists, the majority of patients with erosive esophagitis require acid suppression therapy using PPI's (proton pump inhibitors) [2]. Also, patients with erosive esophagitis, especially those with higher grades are less likely to be effectively managed with less than standard dose of PPI therapy, and step-down attempts in this group are less successful [20]. Castell et al [21] noted in a large study ($n = 5{,}241$) declining efficacy of PPI's in patients with more severe grades of esophagitis (healing at 8 weeks- 92–94% in grades A/B compared to 70–72% in grades C/D).

Multiple studies have also shown that the presence of erosive esophagitis at baseline is predictive of the need for chronic acid suppression [22], [23]. A long term follow up study (> 3 years) in elderly patients (> 65 years) with documented esophagitis as a inclusion criterion suggested that the presence of severe grades of esophagitis at baseline ($p = 0.009$) was a risk factor for relapse of esophagitis, suggesting need for maintenance therapy in this group of patients [24].

Thus, it is clear that more severe grades of esophagitis require more complete acid suppression for intial healing as well as for maintenance of healing [10]. However, GERD is a symptom driven disorder and this information may not be necessary to guide therapy in all patients [25].

Barrett's esophagus

The definition of Barrett's esophagus (BE), as discussed at a recent evidence based workshop, is based on a combination of endoscopic and histologic criteria consisting of an abnormal appearing distal esophageal lining (endoscopic BE) with histologic evidence of intestinal metaplasia (confirmed BE). Barrett's esophagus has been arbitrarily divided into long (≥ 3 cm) and short segment (< 3 cm), although there is no evidence that a risk gradient for complications (i.e., dysplasia/cancer risk) may be demarcated at a particular segment length [26]. The role of gastroesophageal reflux in the development of BE has been consistently shown in animal and human studies. In a rat model, BE could be induced in 80% of the animals following a jejunoesophageal loop. In a recent prospective study of 40 patients who underwent esophagogastrostomy and sub-total esophagectomy (done for adenocarcinoma or squamous cell carcinoma), 10 developed BE above the anastomosis [27].

Role in diagnosis

Longer lengths of BE have been found to be highly predictive of gastro esophageal reflux. In some studies, the sensitivity of pH testing in BE patients is reported to be as high as 90% [28]. Some studies have also found a significant correlation between the percent total time pH < 4 and the length of BE ($r = 0.6234$, $p = 0.0005$) [29], [30]. Other investigators have performed studies correlating esophageal acid exposure in long segment BE and erosive esophagitis patients compared to controls. Most studies have demonstrated that BE patients have more pronounced acid reflux than patients with mild-moderate esophagitis (grades-I and -II Savary-Miller) and controls [31]–[34]. In a study of 150 patients, no significant difference was observed in esophageal acid exposure between patients with grades-III/IV esophagitis and long segment BE, although both groups had significantly higher values compared to controls (17.5% vs. 21.5% vs. 1.8%, respectively) [12]. Similarly, other studies have also shown the duration of reflux in BE patients to be significantly higher compared to controls, but not different than patients with grades-III/-IV erosive esophagitis [35]–[37].

The shorter lengths of BE have attracted considerable attention in recent years. The issues around this are more complex than traditional or long segment BE [2], [3], [38]–[41]. A study comparing 21 patients with short segment BE and 18 with long segment BE showed that the percent time pH < 4.0 was significantly lower in short segment (8.6%) compared to long segment BE (24.4%) patients. These numbers were significantly higher compared to controls (1.8%) arguing that short segment BE may be a true pathological finding albeit reflecting a lower severity of esophageal acid exposure [42]. In a recent interesting study, a group of predominantly male, Caucasian patients undergoing colorectal cancer screening were offered an upper endoscopy. Long segment BE was detected in 0.36% and short segment BE in 5.24% of subjects without any history of heartburn compared to 2.6% and 5.7% respectively in those with a history of heartburn [43]. These results raise many questions, the most relevant to this discussion is whether the finding of BE in asymptomatic individuals is equivalent to pathological reflux.

In conclusion, the presence of longer lengths of BE may be reliable for the diagnosis of GERD but shorter lengths as a diagnostic criterion for GERD by itself may have poor specificity.

Newer endoscopic techniques to increase yield of Barrett's esophagus (BE)

Chromoendoscopy, i.e., endoscopy with dye spraying has been utilized to increase the detection of intestinal metaplasia in the columnar lined segment. Different stains that have been used include methylene blue, indigo carmine and Lugol's iodine. In an intial report of 14 patients with known BE and 12 controls, Canto et al reported a sensitivity of 95%, specificity of 97% and positive predictive value of 98% with methylene blue staining for detecting intestinal metaplasia [44]. Sharma et al showed that methylene blue increased the yield of intestinal metaplasia in shorter segments of BE compared to controls that had undergone random biopsies (61% vs. 42%; $p < 0.02$) [45]. A recent study from Greece also showed that chromoendoscopy done immediately following conventional endoscopy increased the yield of intestinal metaplasia from 1.6% to 3.5% ($p < 0.001$) [46]. On the other hand, in a crossover study by Wo et al [47], the sensitivity and specificity of methylene blue staining to detect intestinal metaplasia were poor at 53% and 51% and for dysplasia 51% and 48%, respectively.

The addition of magnification endoscopy to methylene blue staining may further increase the yield of metaplastic and dysplastic tissue by identifying specific mucosal patterns. Yagi et al [48] found this combination to have a sensitivity of 84.8% and specificity of 91.7% for detecting intestinal metaplasia. The pattern suggestive of intestinal metaplasia on magnification chromoendoscopy was a tubular, cavernous or elliptical appearance of the mucosa. Using a combination of indigo carmine with magnification endoscopy in 80 patients, Sharma et al showed that the presence of a ridge/villous pattern had a sensitivity of 97%, specificity of 76% and PPV of 92% for the detection of intestinal metaplasia [49]. Six patients with an irregular/distorted pattern proved to have high grade dysplasia on biopsies.

Thus, chromo and magnification endoscopy offers great promise in the diagnosis and follow up of patients with BE and further large multicenter trial are awaited in this field.

Endoscopically normal mucosa

The absence of changes in the distal esophagus on conventional endoscopy does not rule out the diagnosis of GERD. It is estimated that upto 70% of patients with typical symptoms of GERD have normal esophageal mucosa on upper endoscopy (NERD) [4], [6], [7]. At least, two different approaches have been attempted in these patients: biopsies of the normal appearing squamous mucosa and evaluation of the distal esophagus with newer techniques such as high resolution and magnification endoscopy.

Role of biopsy
Histologically, acute reflux damage consists of superficial epithelial swelling and/or necrosis accompanied by intraepithelial neutrophilic infiltrates. Chronic reflux induces eosinophilic infiltrates, basal cell hyperplasia, epithelial thickening, and elongation of the vascular papillae (Ismail-Beigi Criteria) [50], [51]. Basal hyperplasia in excess of 15% and papillary elongation in excess of 2/3 of the epithelial thickness have been proposed as criterion to diagnose reflux esophagitis (*Fig. 2*). The number of eosinophils in reflux esophagitis is usually 1–20/high power field. More than 20 eosinophils/HPF should alert the clinician to the possibility of an alternative diagnosis such as eosinophilic esophagitis [52]. However, the lack of eosinophils does not rule out reflux esophagitis [53].

Although, initial reports in 1970s suggested that histologic features of basal cell hyperplasia and location of the papillae close to the epithelial surface correlated well with the presence of GERD [50], [51], other studies directly comparing esophageal 24-hr pH results to histology have attested to the lack of discriminatory value of these histological criteria. In a report of 100 patients, (69 with positive pH studies), Johnson et al [54] found a significant correlation between esophageal acid exposure and the length of both the papillary and basal cell zones, although the correlation coefficients were low (none exceeding 0.33). In

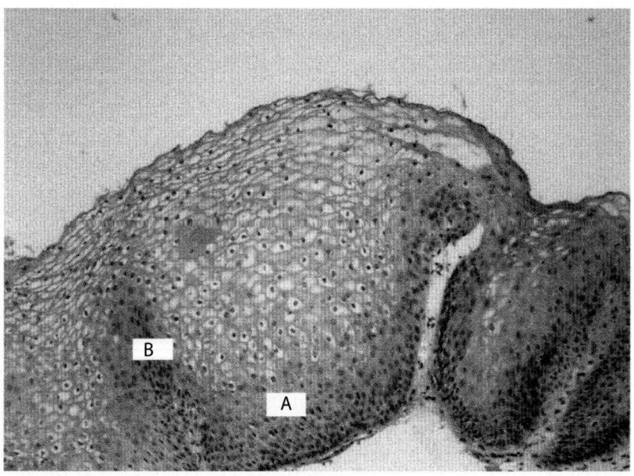

Fig. 2. Biopsy of the squamous mucosa in a patient with reflux symptoms showing histological signs of reflux esophagitis. (**A**) represents Basal cell hyperplasia; (**B**) represents papillary elongation

another study, Schindlbeck and colleagues found only minor differences in the prevalence of histological features between 13 NERD patients, 11 patient controls, and 7 healthy controls [55].

In a recent study, the correlation between the histological criteria and 24 hour pH testing was predominantly negative, with the exception of neutrophil inflammation [56]. However, another recent study, which analyzed data from a large prospective GERD trial (the ProGERD study; n = 1475), found that elongation of papillae and basal cell hyperplasia were seen in 40.7% and 12.7% of NERD patients and 46.1% and 15.7% of patients with erosive esophagitis, respectively, at 2 cm above the z-line. The presence of intraepithelial inflammatory cells showed a high specificity but very low sensitivity [57]. However, the lack of a clearly defined control group makes it hard to make conclusive recommendations as some of these histological findings may be observed in biopsies from asymptomatic individuals.

Some other groups have evaluated the presence of dilated intercellular spaces (DIS) as a marker for GERD. Calabrese et al used transmission electron microscopy to study DIS in patients with GERD and duodenal gastro-esophageal reflux disease (DGER). Patients with GERD and DGER had intercellular spaces dilated to at least two times greater than controls and there was no significant difference in DIS between patients with erosive esophagitis and NERD [58].

At this time, unless histological criteria are updated or better correlated to either symptoms, 24 h pH results or response to acid suppressive therapy, biopsies of the distal normal appearing distal esophageal mucosa cannot be routinely recommended for the diagnosis of GERD.

Role of newer techniques

High resolution and magnification endoscopy has recently been used to develop endoscopic criteria for non-erosive esophageal injury from gastroesophageal reflux [59]. Lugol's Iodine was used in 13 patients with heartburn and pathologic 24-hour esophageal acid exposure but with no erosions on standard endoscopy and in 10 asymptomatic volunteers with normal esophageal acid exposure. A few subtle endoscopic findings, such as pin-point vessels and triangular indentation of the squamocolumnar junction upward into the squamous mucosa, were found in NERD patients using high-resolution magnification chromoendoscopy with Lugol's staining [60]. These preliminary findings demonstrate that NERD patients may show minimal mucosal changes on high-resolution endoscopy.

A recent elegant study correlated histologic and endoscopic findings in patients with NERD with the help of magnification endoscopy before and after PPI treatment [61]. Patients with NERD, more often than controls, showed endoscopic changes of minimal change esophagitis with punctate erythema as the most important finding, which resolved after PPI therapy. A sensitivity of 64%, specificity of 85% and a positive predictive value of 80% were determined for these findings on magnifying endoscopy. In the same study, an increased length of papillae (14/39 with NERD vs. 2/39 in controls; $p < 0.005$) and basal cell hyperplasia (17/39 vs. 4/39; $p < 0.009$) were seen in the NERD group which resolved in the majority of patients after PPI therapy. These new techniques appear very promising for the future but are not yet ready for routine clinical practice.

Utility of endoscopy in addition to confirmation of diagnosis

In patients with atypical symptoms or symptoms over and above those of typical reflux, endoscopy may also have utility in ruling out alternative diseases, such as peptic ulcer disease, eosinophilic esophagitis and complications like adenocarcinoma. Eosinophilic esophagitis, also known as primary eosinophilic esophagitis or idiopathic eosinophilic esophagitis, occurs in adults and in children and represents a subset of eosinophilic gastroenteritis with an isolated severe esophageal eosinophilia. Patients with eosinophilic esophagitis present with symptoms similar to those of gastroesophageal reflux but may be less responsive to antireflux medication. The importance of recognizing this entity, especially in children is underscored by the need for different treatment approaches, e.g., dietary restriction or corticosteroids and in preventing unnecessary fundoplication [62]. Dyspepsia and GERD may overlap and sometimes they may be difficult to distinguish by symptoms alone. Many patients with upper gastrointestinal symptoms have significant anxiety about their diagnosis, including fear of cancer, and that some of that anxiety and anxiety-related impairment of quality of life could be improved with the knowledge of a normal upper endoscopy [63].

An additional benefit of endoscopy in GERD patients is that it provides the opportunity for therapeutic stricture dilation, as well as biopsy confirmation of any tumors or Barrett esophagus. It can also identify the subset of patients who may need future surveillance, although this is controversial. An index endoscopy for GERD may also obviate need for future screening procedures as BE is almost always diagnosed at its full extent at the first endoscopy [64] and rarely, if ever, develops after a normal endoscopy. Therefore, those who respond to a treatment trial and have no erosive esophagitis or BE on the initial endoscopy would be able to enter a maintenance treatment program with no further fears of significant pathology.

However, any new onset of gastrointestinal symptoms including reflux symptoms, in patients older than 60–65 years also requires further investigation (i.e., endoscopy) as do patients with dysphagia, weight loss, anemia, and atypical symptoms [2], [3], [65].

Conclusions

Endoscopy is relatively insensitive for making the diagnosis of gastro esophageal reflux disease. However, the presence of erosive esophagitis and/or BE is highly suggestive of GERD. The presence of normal mucosa at endoscopy does not rule out the diagnosis of GERD. At present, the role of biopsies in these situations is unsettled and more data are needed. Newer endoscopic techniques such as chromoendoscopy, magnification and high resolution may demonstrate minimal changes in the distal squamous mucosa such as punctate erythema, pinpoint vessels etc. not seen by standard endoscopy. Some of these changes may respond to therapy with proton pump inhibitor. Endoscopy remains the best test to rule out complications of GERD and allows histological confirmation of esophageal pathology such as intestinal metaplasia, dysplasia and adenocarcinoma. Identifying the patient group with severe erosive esophagitis, BE and peptic strictures may help focus aggressive management that may potentially prevent future complications in these patient groups. Finally, endoscopy may be useful to rule out other diseases in the upper gastrointestinal tract.

References

[1] Kahrilas PJ (2003) Diagnosis of symptomatic gastroesophageal reflux disease. Am J Gastroenterol 98: S15–S23

[2] Dent J, Brun J, Fendrick AM et al (1999) An evidence-based appraisal of reflux disease management – the genval workshop report. Gut 44 (Suppl 2): 1–16

[3] Jian R, Galmiche JP, Bretagne JF (1999) Gastroesophageal reflux in adults: will a consensus be possible?. Gastroenterol Clin Biol 23: 1–2

[4] Jones R (1995) Gastro-oesophageal reflux disease in general practice. Scand J Gastroenterol (Suppl 211): 35–38

[5] Kahrilas PJ, Quigley EM (1996) Clinical esophageal pH recording: a technical review for practice guideline development. Gastroenterology 110: 1982–1996

[6] Lind T, Havelund T, Carlsson R et al (1997) Heartburn without oesophagitis: efficacy of omeprazole therapy and features determining therapeutic response. Scand J Gastroenterol 32: 974–979

[7] Spechler SJ (1992) Epidemiology and natural history of gastro-oesophageal reflux disease. Digestion 51 (Suppl 1): 24–29

[8] Hatlebakk JG, Berstad A, Carling L et al (1993) Lansoprazole versus omeprazole in short-term treatment of reflux oesophagitis. Results of a Scandinavian multicentre trial. Scand J Gastroenterol 28: 224–228

[9] Hetzel DJ, Dent J, Reed WD et al (1988) Healing and relapse of severe peptic esophagitis after treatment with omeprazole. Gastroenterology 95: 903–912

[10] Lundell LR, Dent J, Bennett JR et al (1999) Endoscopic assessment of oesophagitis: clinical and functional correlates and further validation of the Los Angeles classification. Gut 45: 172–180

[11] Ozzello L, Savary M, Roethlisberger B (1977) Columnar mucosa of the distal esophagus in patients with gastroesophageal reflux. Pathol Annu 12 (Pt 1): 41–86

[12] Coenraad M, Masclee AA, Straathof JW et al (1998) Is Barrett's esophagus characterized by more pronounced acid reflux than severe esophagitis? Am J Gastroenterol 93: 1068–1072

[13] Tefera L, Fein M, Ritter MP et al (1997) Can the combination of symptoms and endoscopy confirm the presence of gastroesophageal reflux disease? Am J Surg 63. 933–936

[14] Ghillebert G, Demeyere AM, Janssens J et al (1995) How well can quantitative 24-hour intraesophageal pH

monitoring distinguish various degrees of reflux disease? Dig Dis Sci 40: 1317–1324
[15] Sanchez-Gey Venegas S, Yerro Paez VM, Pellicer Bautista FJ et al (1999) Relationship between endoscopic esophagitis and patterns of gastroesophageal reflux in ambulatory pHmetry. Rev Esp Enferm Dig 91: 125–132
[16] Arango L, Angel A, Molina RI et al (2000) Comparison between digestive endoscopy and 24-hour esophageal pH monitoring for the diagnosis of gastroesophageal reflux esophagitis: "presentation of 100 cases". Hepatogastroenterology 47: 174–180
[17] Bate CM, Griffin SM, Keeling PW et al (1996) Reflux symptom relief with omeprazole in patients without unequivocal oesophagitis. Aliment Pharmacol Ther 10: 547–555
[18] Shi G, Bruley des Varannes S, Scarpignato C et al (1995) Reflux related symptoms in patients with normal oesophageal exposure to acid. Gut 37: 457–464
[19] Wiener GJ, Morgan TM, Copper JB et al (1988) Ambulatory 24-hour esophageal pH monitoring. Reproducibility and variability of pH parameters. Dig Dis Sci 33: 1127–1133
[20] Vigneri S, Termini R, Leandro G et al (1995) A comparison of five maintenance therapies for reflux esophagitis. N Engl J Med 333: 1106–1110
[21] Castell DO, Kahrilas PJ, Richter JE et al (2002) Esomeprazole (40 mg) compared with lansoprazole (30 mg) in the treatment of erosive esophagitis. Am J Gastroenterol 97: 575–583
[22] Kuster E, Ros E, Toledo-Pimentel V et al (1994) Predictive factors of the long term outcome in gastro-oesophageal reflux disease: six year follow up of 107 patients. Gut 35: 8–14
[23] McDougall NI, Johnston BT, Collins JS et al (1998) Three- to 4.5-year prospective study of prognostic indicators in gastro-oesophageal reflux disease. Scand J Gastroenterol 33: 1016–1022
[24] Pilotto A, Franceschi M, Leandro G et al (2002) Long-term clinical outcome of elderly patients with reflux esophagitis: a six-month to three-year follow-up study. Am J Ther 9: 295–300
[25] Fass R, Ofman JJ (2002) Gastroesophageal reflux disease – should we adopt a new conceptual framework? Am J Gastroenterol 97: 1901–1909
[26] Sharma P, McQuaid K, Dent J et al (2004) A critical review of the diagnosis and management of Barrett's esophagus: the AGA Chicago Workshop. Gastroenterology 127: 310–330
[27] Dresner SM, Griffin SM, Wayman J et al (2003) Human model of duodenogastro-oesophageal reflux in the development of Barrett's metaplasia. Br J Surg 90: 1120–1128
[28] Martinez SDMI, Fass R (2001) Non-erosive reflux disease (NERD)-is it really just a mild form of gastroesophageal disease (GERD). Gastroenterology 120 (Suppl 1)
[29] Fass R, Hell RW, Garewal HS et al (2001) Correlation of oesophageal acid exposure with Barrett's oesophagus length. Gut 48: 310–313
[30] Tharalson EF, Martinez SD, Garewal HS et al (2002) Relationship between rate of change in acid exposure along the esophagus and length of Barrett's epithelium. Am J Gastroenterol 97: 851–856
[31] Iascone C, DeMeester TR, Little AG et al (1983) Barrett's esophagus. Functional assessment, proposed pathogenesis, and surgical therapy. Arch Surg 118: 543–549
[32] Attwood SE, DeMeester TR, Bremner CG et al (1989) Alkaline gastroesophageal reflux: implications in the development of complications in Barrett's columnar-lined lower esophagus. Surgery 106: 764–770
[33] Fiorucci S, Santucci L, Farroni F et al (1989) Effect of omeprazole on gastroesophageal reflux in Barrett's esophagus. Am J Gastroenterol 84: 1263–1267
[34] Champion G, Richter JE, Vaezi MF et al (1994) Duodenogastroesophageal reflux: relationship to pH and importance in Barrett's esophagus. Gastroenterology 107: 747–754
[35] Robertson D, Aldersley M, Shepherd H et al (1987) Patterns of acid reflux in complicated oesophagitis. Gut 28: 1484–1488
[36] Gillen P, Keeling P, Byrne PJ et al (1987) Barrett's oesophagus: pH profile. Br J Surg 74: 774–776
[37] Stein HJ, Barlow AP, DeMeester TR et al (1992) Complications of gastroesophageal reflux disease. Role of the lower esophageal sphincter, esophageal acid and acid/alkaline exposure, and duodenogastric reflux. Ann Surg 216: 35–43
[38] Nandurkar S, Talley NJ (1999) Barrett's esophagus: the long and the short of it. Am J Gastroenterol 94: 30–40
[39] Sharma P, Morales TG, Sampliner RE (1998) Short segment Barrett's esophagus – the need for standardization of the definition and of endoscopic criteria. Am J Gastroenterol 93: 1033–1036
[40] Sharma P, Sampliner RE (1998) Short segment Barrett's esophagus and intestinal metaplasia of the cardia – it's not all symantics! Am J Gastroenterol 93: 2303–2304
[41] Spechler SJ (1997) Short and ultrashort Barrett's esophagus – what does it mean? Semin Gastrointest Dis 8: 59–67
[42] Loughney T, Maydonovitch CL, Wong RK (1998) Esophageal manometry and ambulatory 24-hour pH

monitoring in patients with short and long segment Barrett's esophagus. Am J Gastroenterol 93: 916–919

[43] Gerson LB, Shetler K, Triadafilopoulos G (2002) Prevalence of Barrett's esophagus in asymptomatic individuals. Gastroenterology 123: 461–467

[44] Canto MI, Setrakian S, Petras RE et al (1996) Methylene blue selectively stains intestinal metaplasia in Barrett's esophagus. Gastrointest Endosc 44: 1–7

[45] Sharma P, Topalovski M, Mayo MS et al (2001) Methylene blue chromoendoscopy for detection of short-segment Barrett's esophagus. Gastrointest Endosc 54: 289–293

[46] Kouklakis GS, Kountouras J, Dokas SM et al (2003) Methylene blue chromoendoscopy for the detection of Barrett's esophagus in a Greek cohort. Endoscopy 35: 383–387

[47] Wo JM, Ray MB, Mayfield-Stokes S et al (2001) Comparison of methylene blue-directed biopsies and conventional biopsies in the detection of intestinal metaplasia and dysplasia in Barrett's esophagus: a preliminary study. Gastrointest Endosc 54: 294–301

[48] Yagi K, Nakamura A, Sekine A (2003) Accuracy of magnifying endoscopy with methylene blue in the diagnosis of specialized intestinal metaplasia and short-segment Barrett's esophagus in Japanese patients without *Helicobacter pylori* infection. Gastrointest Endosc 58: 189–195

[49] Sharma P, Weston AP, Topalovski M et al (2003) Magnification chromoendoscopy for the detection of intestinal metaplasia and dysplasia in Barrett's oesophagus. Gut 52: 24–27

[50] Ismail-Beigi F, Horton PF, Pope CE, 2nd (1970) Histological consequences of gastroesophageal reflux in man. Gastroenterology 58: 163–174

[51] Ismail-Beigi F, Pope CE, 2nd (1974) Distribution of the histological changes of gastroesophageal reflux in the distal esophagus of man. Gastroenterology 66: 1109–1113

[52] Belafsky PC, Postma GN, Koufman JA et al (2002) Stevens-Johnson syndrome with diffuse esophageal involvement. Ear Nose Throat J 81: 220

[53] Steiner SJ, Gupta SK, Croffie JM et al (2004) Correlation between number of eosinophils and reflux index on same day esophageal biopsy and 24-hour esophageal pH-monitoring. Am J Gastroenterol 99: 801–805

[54] Johnson LF, Demeester TR, Haggitt RC (1978) Esophageal epithelial response to gastroesophageal reflux. A quantitative study. Am J Dig Dis 23: 498–509

[55] Schindlbeck NE, Wiebecke B, Klauser AG et al (1996) Diagnostic value of histology in non-erosive gastro-oesophageal reflux disease. Gut 39: 151–154

[56] Bowrey DJ, Williams GT, Clark GW (2003) Histological changes in the oesophageal squamous mucosa: correlation with ambulatory 24-hour pH-monitoring. J Clin Pathol 56: 205–208

[57] M.Veith UP, Labenz J (2004) What parameters are relevant for the histological diagnosis of Gastroesophageal reflux disease without Barrett's mucosa? Dig Dis 22: 196–201

[58] Carlo Calabrese AF, Mauro Bortolotti (2003) Comparative results of esophageal damage in GERD and DGER: dilation of intercellular spaces as a marker of esophageal injury [abstract]. Gastro

[59] Tam WCE DJ, Conroy-Hiller TA (2001) Proposed new Endoscopic criteria for minimal change reflux esophagitis based on magnification endoscopy [abstract]. Gastrointes Endosc 53: AB119

[60] Tam WEA, Bruno M (2002) Endoscopy-negative reflux disease: high-resolution endoscopic and histological signs [abstract]. Gastro 122: A74

[61] Kiesslich R, Kanzler S, Vieth M et al (2004) Minimal change esophagitis: prospective comparison of endoscopic and histological markers between patients with non-erosive reflux disease and normal controls using magnifying endoscopy. Dig Dis 22: 221–227

[62] Liacouras CA, Markowitz JE (1999) Eosinophilic esophagitis: a subset of eosinophilic gastroenteritis. Curr Gastroenterol Rep 1: 253–258

[63] Wiklund I, Glise H, Jerndal P et al (1998) Does endoscopy have a positive impact on quality of life in dyspepsia? Gastrointest Endosc 47: 449–454

[64] Sampliner RE, Garewal HS, Fennerty MB et al (1990) Lack of impact of therapy on extent of Barrett's esophagus in 67 patients. Dig Dis Sci 35: 93–96

[65] Szarka LA, DeVault KR, Murray JA (2001) Diagnosing gastroesophageal reflux disease. Mayo Clin Proc 76: 97–101

DIAGNOSTIC PROCEDURES IN GERD: PRINCIPLES AND VALUES OF ESOPHAGEAL MANOMETRY AND pH-MONITORING

R. Tutuian and D. O. Castell

Division of Gastroenterology – Hepatology, Medical University of South Carolina, Charleston, SC, USA

Introduction

Gastroesophageal reflux disease (GERD) is a highly prevalent disease in industrialized countries. In the US alone, 40% of the adult population frequently complains of heartburn, one of the cardinal symptoms of GERD [1]. In a recent study by Sandler et al [2] gastroesophageal reflux disease (GERD) has been reported to be the 4th most prevalent GI disease in the US (19 million cases/year), being surpassed only by non-food-borne gastroenteritis and other gastrointestinal infections (135 million cases/year), food-borne illness (76 million cases/year) and cholelithiasis (20 million cases/year). In the same study, GERD was found to be the most costly gastrointestinal disease with direct and indirect costs estimated at $ 9.8 billion 1998 US Dollars, surpassing the costs of treatment for cholelithiasis ($5.8 billions), colorectal cancer ($4.9 billions) and peptic ulcer disease ($3.1 billions).

Reflux esophagitis, a term first introduced by Allison [3] in 1946, was considered for many years to provide the evidence of gastroesophageal disease. As clinicians became more familiar with the spectrum of GERD it became clear that esophageal symptoms (heartburn, regurgitation, dysphagia, chest pain, etc.) might be caused by gastroesophageal reflux in the absence of endoscopic evidence of esophageal lesions. With this understanding it became clear that other tests for the diagnosis of GERD were needed. Over time esophageal manometry, pH monitoring and more recently multichannel intraluminal impedance (MII) combined with pH (MII-pH) were added to the clinical armamentarium to diagnose GERD.

Esophageal manometry

Esophageal manometry has been used as a diagnostic test for esophageal disease for over 40 years [4] and is currently considered the gold standard to diagnose esophageal motility abnormalities. Esophageal manometry provides information on amplitude and coordination of esophageal contractions and the relaxation and coordination of the upper and lower esophageal sphincter. Simultaneous video-fluoroscopy and manometry studies have been used to document bolus transit dependence on esophageal peristalsis (*Fig. 1*) [5]. Even though it is not used to primarily diagnosed GERD, esophageal manometry is frequently used in patients with GERD in order to support the diagnosis in a complex patient, to evaluate patients with atypical symptoms, to detect defective peristalsis prior to fundoplication, to exclude scleroderma or achalasia as cause of the patient's symptoms and to assist placing of pH-probes.

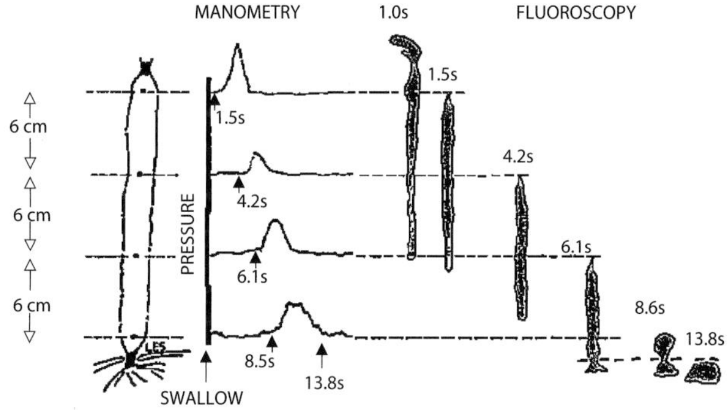

Fig. 1. Manometric/videofluoroscopic comparison during normal swallows. Schematic representation of esophageal peristalsis as measured by manometry corresponding to the time when the barium column is advancing through the esophagus. The timings (in sec) indicate that effective peristaltic contractions are responsible for bolus transit through the esophagus

Esophageal manometry equipment

The main components of a manometry system are (1) the esophageal manometry catheter, (2) pressure transducers, (3) signal acquisition, and (4) information storage devices. The majority of esophageal laboratories use either water-perfused catheters with external transducers or catheters with solid-state transducers. Water perfused systems include a thin, flexible catheter with small capillary orifices connected to an external water supply and pump and external pressure transducers. The pressure measured by external, water-column, transducers reflects the pressure that the water pump has to generate in order to overcome the pressure with which the esophageal wall occludes the capillary orifice. These systems have the advantage of relatively low-cost catheters but have the disadvantage of requiring additional equipment (water supply, pump) and are more difficult to operate and maintain. Another disadvantage of water-perfused systems is that the external, water-column transducers require the patient's body to be aligned with the pressure sensors, often limiting esophageal motility testing to the recumbent position.

Solid-state transducer systems include equally thin, flexible catheters with pressure transducers mounted directly on the catheter. The solid-state transducers use small, oil-filled chambers with extremely high compliance to transmit esophageal pressure to miniature sensors incorporated in the catheter. The increased cost of solid-state transducer catheters is compensated by easier, more convenient operability of the system without additional equipment (pumps and supplies). Solid-state transducer systems can also be used for ambulatory monitoring and motility testing in upright positions.

Signal acquisition devices consist of sets of amplifiers and converters while, these days, computer systems have long replaced polygraphs as data storage devices.

In addition to this primary equipment certain smaller equipment (calibration chamber) and secondary consumable supplies (disinfection and sterilization materials, tape, lubricating gel, viscous lidocaine, emesis basins, syringes, testing substances, etc.) are needed to perform esophageal manometry.

Performing esophageal manometry

Esophageal manometry is usually performed as an outpatient procedure and patients are requested to fast for at least 4–6 hours prior to testing. After calibrating the esophageal manometry catheter outside the patient, the tube is typically inserted transnasally after applying viscous lidocaine to decrease the discomfort as the catheter passes the nasal cavity. The esophageal catheter is advanced into the stomach where gastric baseline pressures are measured as reference and then slowly pulled back (stationary pull-through) to identify the lower esophageal sphincter. Depending on the configuration of the catheter LES dynamics and esophageal body activity can be measured during the same or during separate swallows. In our laboratory we use a solid-state transducer catheter that allows evaluation of esophageal peristalsis and LES relaxation during the same swallow (*Fig. 2*). Once the catheter is placed in the right position ten 5 ml swallows are administered at 20–30 second intervals and the subject is asked to swallow once. The 20–30 second interval is necessary to avoid falsely low contraction amplitudes determined by deglutitive inhibition. Double swallow and/or

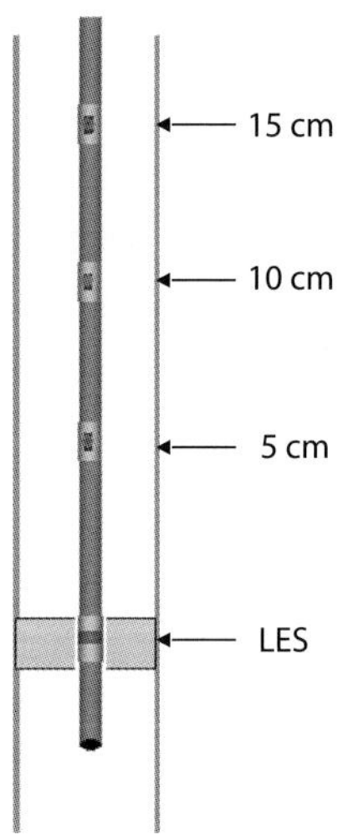

Fig. 2. Solid-state sensor esophageal manometry catheter. The distal pressure transducer has a circumferential sensor collecting 360 degrees data from the lower esophageal sphincter. Unidirectional sensors placed in the esophagus 5, 10 and 15 cm above the LES allow measurement of esophageal peristalsis. This system allows measuring esophageal body peristalsis and LES relaxation during the same swallow

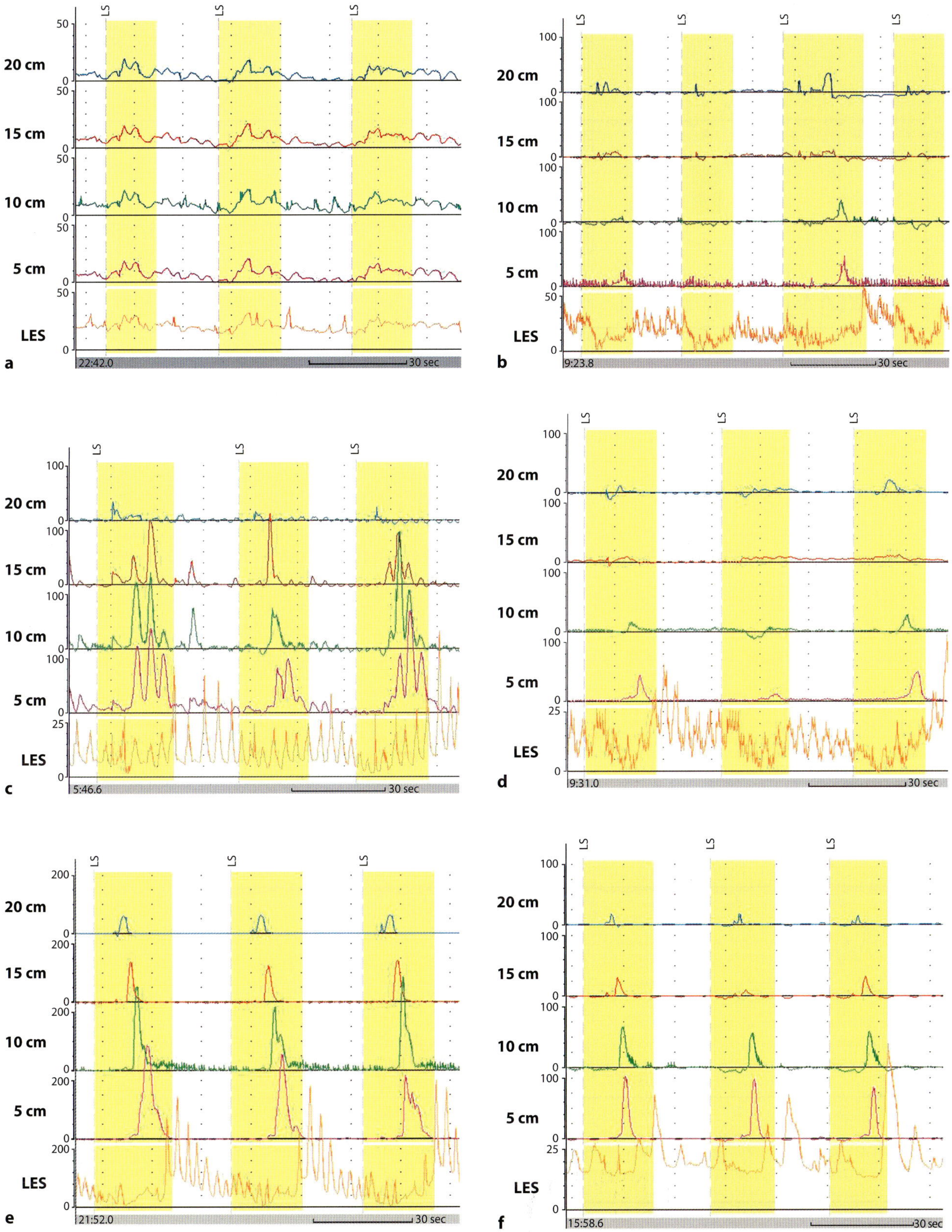

Fig. 3 *(continued)*

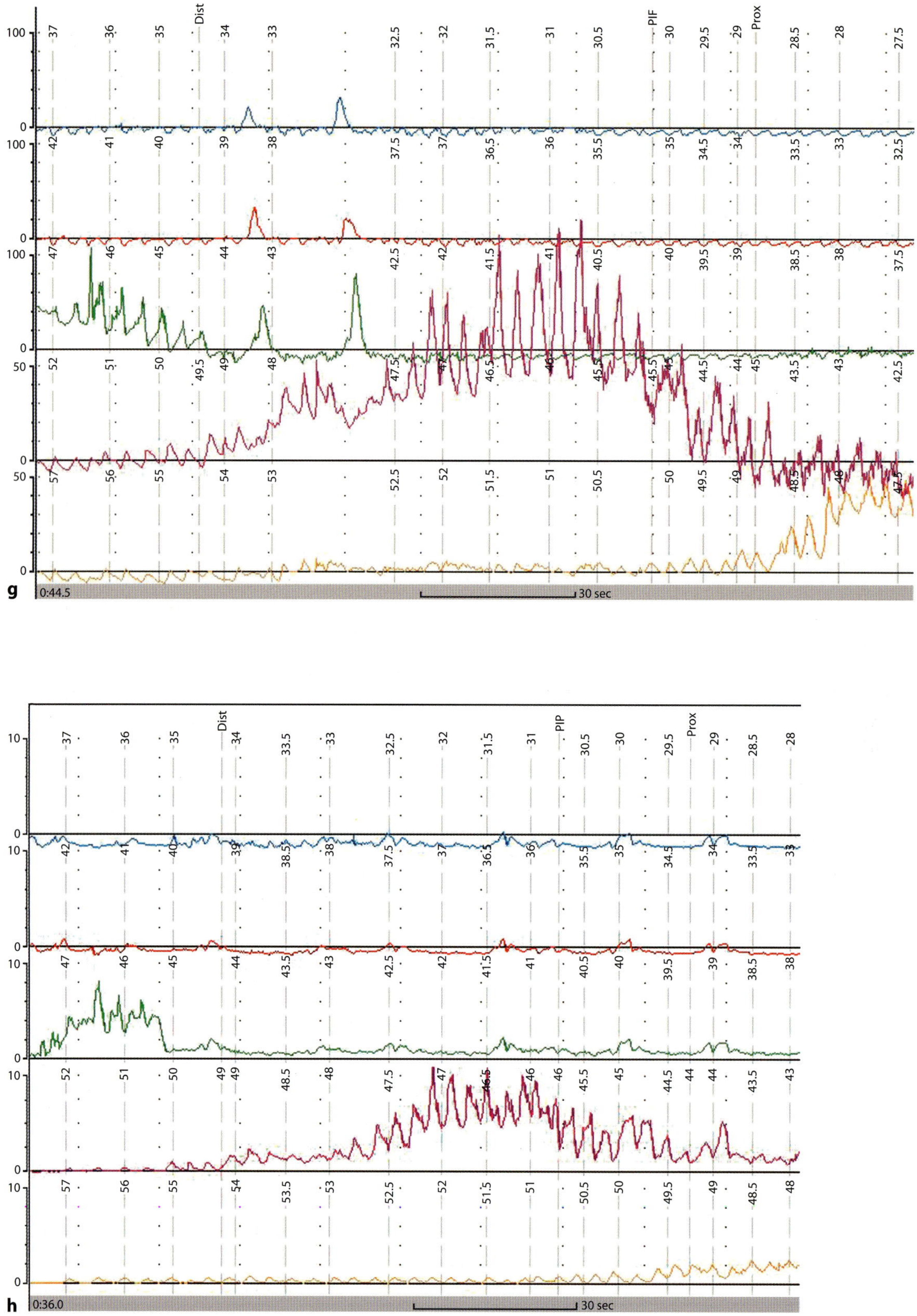

Fig. 3 (*continued*)

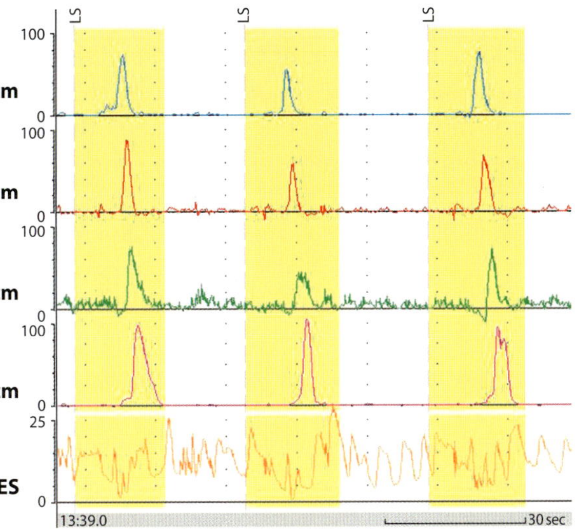

i

Fig. 3. Manometric diagnoses: (**a**) Achalasia is defined by absent esophageal body peristalsis and, if present, poorly relaxing LES. (**b**) Scleroderma is defined based on an appropriate clinical diagnosis and confirmed by low amplitude or absent contractions in the distal esophagus with or without a low LES pressure. (**c**) Distal esophageal spasm is defined as 20% or more simultaneous contractions. (**d**) Ineffective esophageal motility is defined as 30% or more swallows with contraction amplitude less than 30 mmHg in either of the two distal sites located at 5 and 10 cm above the LES. (**e**) Nutcracker esophagus is defined as normal peristalsis of the esophageal body with average distal esophageal amplitude (DEA) exceeding 180 mmHg. (**f**) Poorly relaxing LES is defined as average LES residual pressure exceeding 8 mmHg associated with normal esophageal body contractions. (**g**) Hypertensive LES is defined as LES resting pressure exceeding 45 mmHg with normal esophageal body contractions. (**h**) Hypotensive LES is defined as LES resting pressure below 10 mmHg with normal esophageal body contractions. (**i**) Normal esophageal manometry is defined as not more than 20% ineffective and not more than 10% simultaneous swallows with DEA $<$ 180 mmHg and with normal LES resting and residual pressures

closely spaced swallows are discarded and repeated. Liquid swallows of a fixed volume (i.e., 5 ml) are preferred over dry swallows since the pressure generates is more reproducible. The administration of 10 liquid swallows allows a more convenient determination of the percentage of normal peristaltic, ineffective and simultaneous swallows.

Interpreting esophageal manometry

The interpretation of esophageal manometry data is based on comparing information about swallows against data collected in normal volunteers [6]. It is important to recognize that different laboratories may use slightly different manometric criteria based on their individual experience. In our laboratory, individual swallows are classified as normal peristaltic if their contraction amplitude exceeds 30 mmHg in the distal esophagus and the velocity of the contraction onset does not exceed 8 cm/sec. Swallows are declared ineffective if the contraction amplitude is less than 30 mmHg in the distal esophagus. This definition allows including in the manometric ineffective category swallows classified by other authors as “failed peristalsis” or “non-transmitted”. Swallows are classified as manometric simultaneous if their amplitude exceeds 30 mmHg in the distal esophagus and have a simultaneous or retrograde onset of contraction or the velocity of the contraction onset in the distal esophagus exceeds 8 cm/sec.

For the overall interpretation of manometric findings we recommend using criteria published by Spechler and Castell [7] (*Fig. 3*). Achalasia is defined by absent esophageal body peristalsis and, if present, poorly relaxing and hypertensive LES. Patients with GERD may have a variety of esophageal manometric abnormalities, low amplitude contractions (i.e., ineffective esophageal motility; IEM) being particularly frequent. Abnormal esophageal acid exposure has also been associated with incoordinated esophageal peristalsis (distal esophageal spasm), high amplitude contractions (nutcracker esophagus) but also with normal esophageal body peristalsis. Decreased resting LES pressure (i.e., hypotensive LES) has been associated and is a pathophysiologically plausible cause of abnormal gastroesophageal reflux, but is a rather infrequent finding.

Some of the currently used definitions are challenged by functional information obtained from combined multichannel intraluminal impedance and manometry [8]. Data from our laboratory suggest that the manometric definition of IEM may be too sensitive as approximate half of the patients with 3 or more manometric ineffective swallows have normal bolus transit for liquid. Stricter criteria for IEM, i.e., requiring 5 or more low-amplitude contractions before classifying a study as manometric ineffective should increase the specificity of these findings.

Clinical implications of esophageal manometry findings in GERD patients

Esophageal manometry can detect esophageal body or LES abnormalities associated with GERD. Hiatal hernias and low LES resting pressure (i.e., hypotensive LES) can be detected during stationary pull-through and abnormal esophageal peristalsis during standardized swallows.

Gastroesophageal reflux episodes are very difficult to identify during esophageal manometry. It has been proposed that a rapid rise of 4–10 mmHg at multiple levels in the esophagus a phenomenon known as "common cavity", could be used to detect the presence of gastroesophageal refluxate in the esophagus [9] (*Fig. 4*). This finding is difficult to identify and has recently been shown to be not very sensitive in identifying reflux episodes [10].

On the other hand, manometry can be adapted to identify transient lower esophageal relaxations, currently thought to be the most important pathophysiologic mechanism of GERD [11]. During conventional manometry the detection of tLESR's can be very difficult since the position of the LES is moving with respiration. Therefore, for prolonged measurements of the LES pressure either pressure sleeves [12] or closely spaced pressure measuring sites [13] should be used. While these measurements are very important in understanding the pathophysiology of GERD, their clinical applicability during routine clinical practice is limited.

For many clinicians esophageal manometry is an important tool in evaluating GERD patients who are considering surgical antireflux procedures. A complete, 360 degree wrap of the gastric fundus around the distal esophagus (Nissen fundoplication) creates a higher resistance to flow compared to a partial, 270 degree wrap (Toupet fundoplication) [14]. Since patients with esophageal peristaltic dysfunction may have poor bolus clearance [15] tailoring the surgical approach towards a

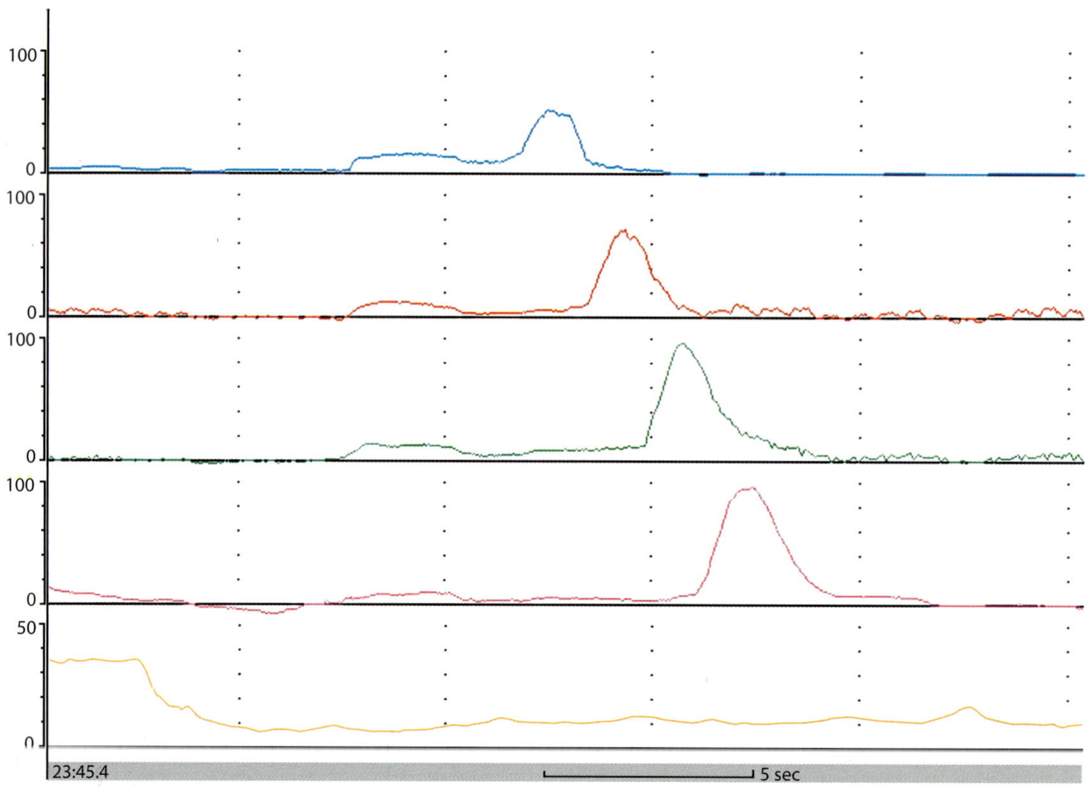

Fig. 4. Gastroesophageal reflux episode identified on manometry as a rapid rise of 4–10 mmHg at multiple levels in the esophagus ("common cavity") while the lower esophageal sphincter is relaxed. The refluxate is subsequently cleared by an esophageal peristalsis

partial wrap in patients with abnormal esophageal peristalsis is a rational approach [16]. This concept was challenged by the recently published publication by Fibbe et al [17]. In a prospective study they stratified 200 patients with longstanding GERD into those with and without esophageal dysmotility and then randomized them to undergo either Nissen or Toupet fundoplication. While finding similar proportion of patients with dysmotility complaining of post-operative dysphagia after either full or partial fundoplication they concluded that pre-operative identification of esophageal dysmotility does not affect the outcome and that tailoring of the surgical approach is not needed.

Esophageal pH monitoring

It was in the late 1960ies when Spencer first reported on prolonged intraesophageal pH monitoring to study gastroesophageal reflux disease [18] and not until the mid 1970ies when Johnson and DeMeester established the first normal values for this technique [19]. Intraesophageal pH monitoring allows study of the role of gastroesophageal reflux in patients with esophageal symptoms in the absence of endoscopic visible lesions (i.e., endoscopy negative reflux disease). Over the years many experts have accepted this as the gold standard in diagnosing GERD.

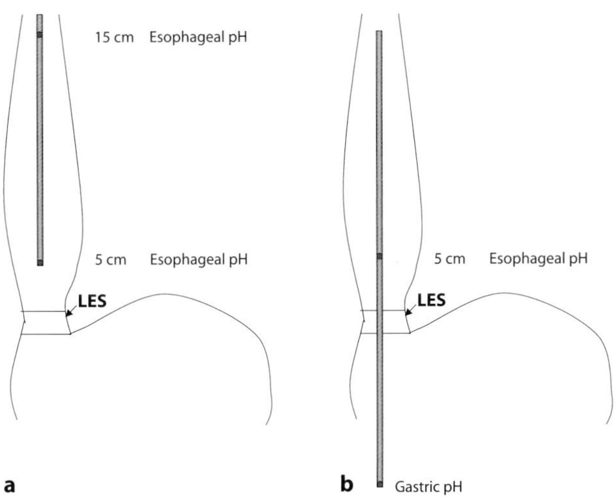

Fig. 5. Ambulatory pH catheter placement. (**a**) Dual channel proximal and distal esophageal pH monitoring is used to monitor patients with reflux symptoms off therapy. (**b**) Dual channel distal esophageal and gastric pH monitoring is used to monitor patients with reflux symptoms on acid suppressive therapy

Conventional, catheter-based pH-monitoring

The main components of catheter based pH monitoring systems are (1) flexible catheter with pH-sensors, and (2) data logger. Esophageal pH catheters distinguish themselves based on the type of pH sensor (i.e., glass vs. antimony) and the location of the reference electrode (i.e., external reference or built-in reference). Systems using external reference electrodes typically use a cutaneous reference and are therefore influenced by the contact between the skin and the external reference. Occasionally loosening of the skin contact or perspiration-induced changes in the ionic composition surrounding the reference electrode can lead to artifacts. In vitro studies suggest that the more expensive, glass-electrodes are superior to monocrystaline antimony electrodes as they respond much quicker to changes in pH, have less drift and a better linear response [20]. However, in clinical studies the less expensive antimony electrodes provide similar results and better insertion comfort compared to the larger (up to 4.5 mm) glass-electrodes [21].

Prior to ambulatory pH monitoring the pH electrodes are calibrated using buffer solutions with distinct pH values. The catheter is then passed transnasally into the esophagus and one sensor is positioned 5 cm above the previously determined proximal border of the lower esophageal sphincter. This position was reached by global consensus and is considered at an optimal depth in order to monitor distal esophageal acid exposure while preventing accidental slipping into the stomach. While virtually all laboratories use this location (*Fig. 5*), individual groups prefer using also a second proximal esophageal site (15 or 20 cm above the LES) to better characterize reflux episodes. In other circumstances (i.e., on acid suppressive therapy) the second pH sensor is placed in the stomach, 10 cm below the LES in order to monitor intragastric acidity. After positioning of the pH sensors and taping the catheter in place the patient is instructed to reproduce as much as possible daily scenarios during which she or he experiences symptoms. Patients are provided with diaries and asked to record the timing and contents of ingested meals, periods of upright and recumbent position and the time of symptoms. They are then discharged from the clinic and asked to return the data logger the following day. Typically ambulatory pH data is recorded over 24 hours although recent data suggest that 16-hour studies provide accurate information and improve patient tolerance [22].

Catheter-free pH-monitoring (Bravo® system)

The clinical acceptability of ambulatory pH-monitoring is limited by the discomfort of the pH catheter reported by the patient and perception of clinicians. While telemetric intragastric pH recordings (the Heidelberg capsule) were first reported in mid 1960ies [23], [24] it was not until recently that catheter-free pH monitoring was approved for clinical use by the US Food and Drug administration [25]. The Bravo system (Medtronic Inc. USA) includes a 26 mm × 5.5 mm × 6.5 mm capsule containing an antimony pH electrode with internal reference, miniaturized electronics with radiofrequency transmitter and battery, a capsule delivery system and an external receiver to monitor intraesophageal pH (*Fig. 6*). The capsule delivery system is passes trans-

Bravo capsule and delivery system

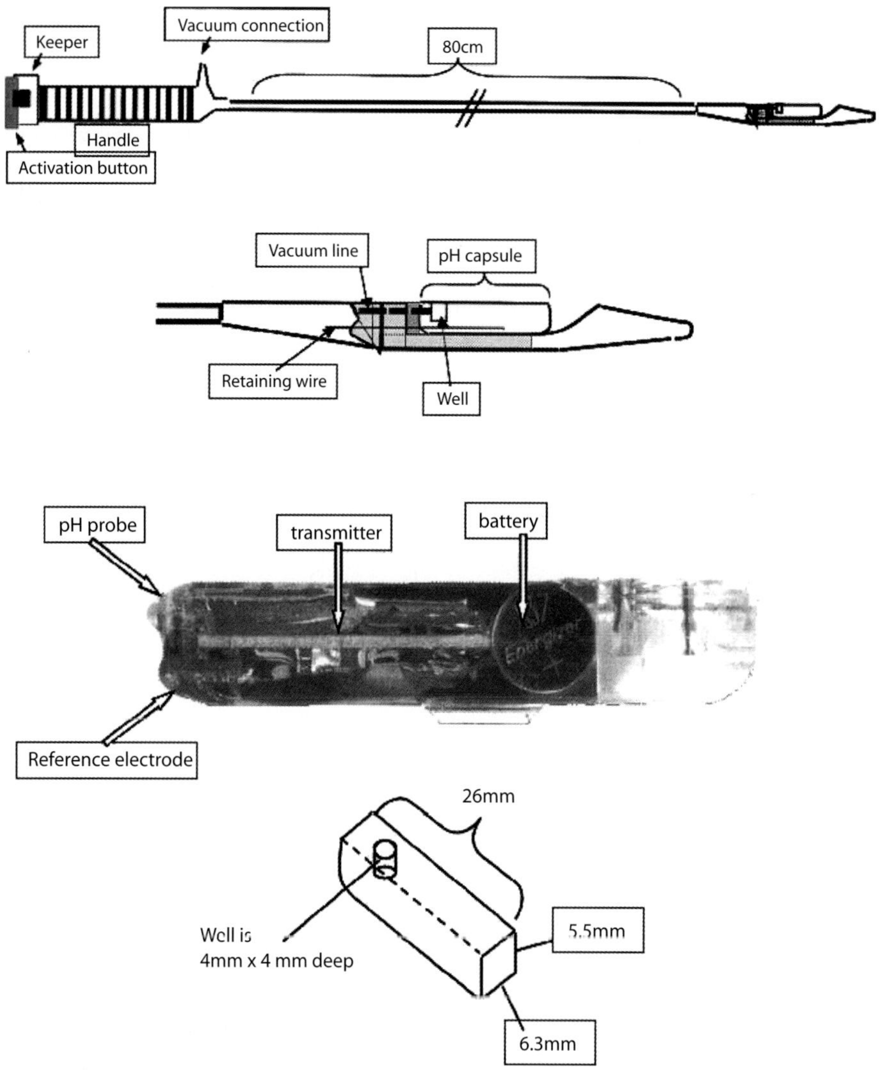

Fig. 6. Catheter free pH-monitoring system (Bravo System)

orally and the capsule is positioned 6 cm above the endoscopic determined gastro-esophageal mucosal separation ("Z-line"). Once the capsule is "pierced" to the esophageal mucosa the delivery system is removed and pH data is recorded from the distal esophageal site. In addition to improved patient comfort this system has the advantage of a fixed placement of the pH electrode, eliminating the risk of "slipping" into the stomach and also prolonged (48–72 hour) recording. These advantages are unfortunately offset by the high cost of the pH capsule, need of endoscopy for accurate placement and impracticality of multiple recording sites.

Esophageal pH-data interpretation

Both, catheter based and catheter free pH monitoring provide prolonged intraesophageal pH data. The interpretation of pH monitoring should attempt to answer 2 questions: (1) Does the amount of gastroesophageal reflux exceed normal values, and (2) are the symptoms reported by the patient during pH monitoring associated with gastroesophageal reflux?

By consensus, gastroesophageal reflux during pH monitoring is detected by a sudden decrease in intraesophageal pH to below 4.0 (*Fig. 7*). The rational for choosing this cutoff value are observations that the proteolytic enzyme pepsin is inactive above this value [26] and because patients with reflux symptoms are more likely to report heartburn at an intraesophageal pH below 4.0 [27]. This cutoff value has been challenged over the years by studies suggesting that a pH value of 5 may provide better discrimination between healthy volunteers and patients with reflux symptoms [28], by studies suggesting that the best discrimination between patients with reflux symptoms and healthy volunteers occurs within the full range between pH 3 and 6 rather than a single pH value [29] or by studies proposing different pH threshold values for different electrode positions based on pH distribution curves [30]. Still, the widespread acceptance of the cutoff pH value of 4.0 to identify gastroesophageal reflux prevails.

Based on the cutoff value of pH 4 several parameters can be defined to quantify the amount of gastroesophageal reflux: number of episodes of drop in pH below 4, number of episodes of certain duration (i.e., > 5 minutes) of drop in pH below 4, duration intraesophageal pH below 4. Currently, the most widely used parameter to quantify gastroesophageal reflux is the proportion of time that the pH is below 4, also known as acid exposure time. Recognizing that body position and the degree of activity including state of consciousness (i.e., awake vs. asleep) can affect intragastric pressure, LES resting pressure, bolus clearance and salivary acid neutralization, acid exposure time is reported separately depending on the body position (upright vs. recumbent). Further, observing that times spent upright and recumbent by individual patients vary, reporting a "normalized" percent time (i.e. duration of intraesophageal pH

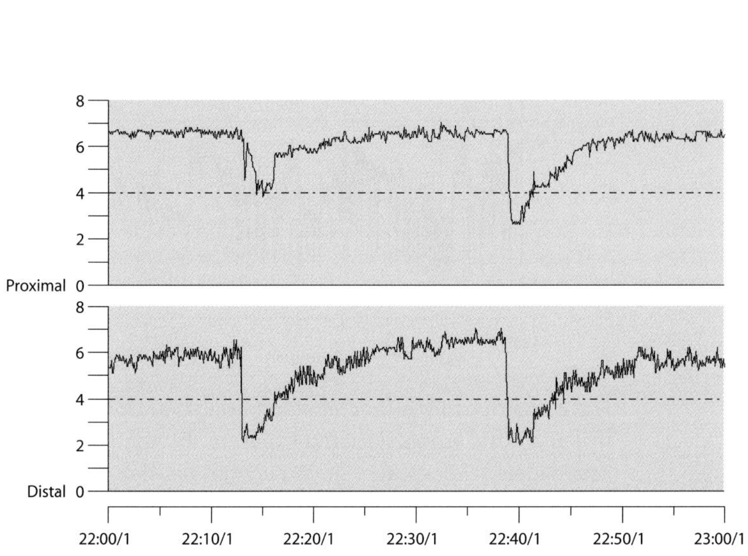

Fig. 7. Reflux episode identified by pH monitoring as a rapid drop in pH from above to below 4.0 distally longer than proximal

less than 4 divided by the total recording time in one position) is preferred. A final detail in reporting acid exposure time (percent time pH less than 4) relates to excluding meal periods from the recording time. The rationale for this is the understanding that some foods, especially drinks (carbonated beverages, wine, juices), have pH values below 4 and, if not excluded, will artifactually increase the esophageal acid exposure time. Excluding meals is preferred over limiting the ingested food since one of the goals of the patient during pH monitoring is inducing situations (including ingesting meals) that may generate symptoms.

Normal values for percent time pH less than 4 have been established for both catheter-based and catheter-free system based on studies in healthy volunteers (Table 1). Intraesophageal pH data from individual patients are compared against these values and esophageal acid exposure times are reported as normal or abnormal (*Fig. 8*).

Table 1. Normal values for ambulatory pH-monitoring. *Catheter* based dual probe (distal and proximal) esophageal pH monitoring [19]

Variable	**Normal**	
	Proximal	Distal
Time pH < 4 (%)		
Total period	< 0.9%	< 4.2%
Upright period	< 1.2%	< 6.3%
Recumbent period	< 0.0%	< 1.2%

Distal = 5 cm above manometric defined proximal border of the LES
Proximal = 20 cm above manometric defined proximal border of the LES

Catheter free distal esophageal pH-monitoring [25]

Variable	**Normal** Distal
Time pH < 4 (%)	
Total period	< 5.3%
Upright period	< 6.9%
Recumbent period	< 6.7%

Distal = 6 cm above endoscopic defined gastroesophageal junction

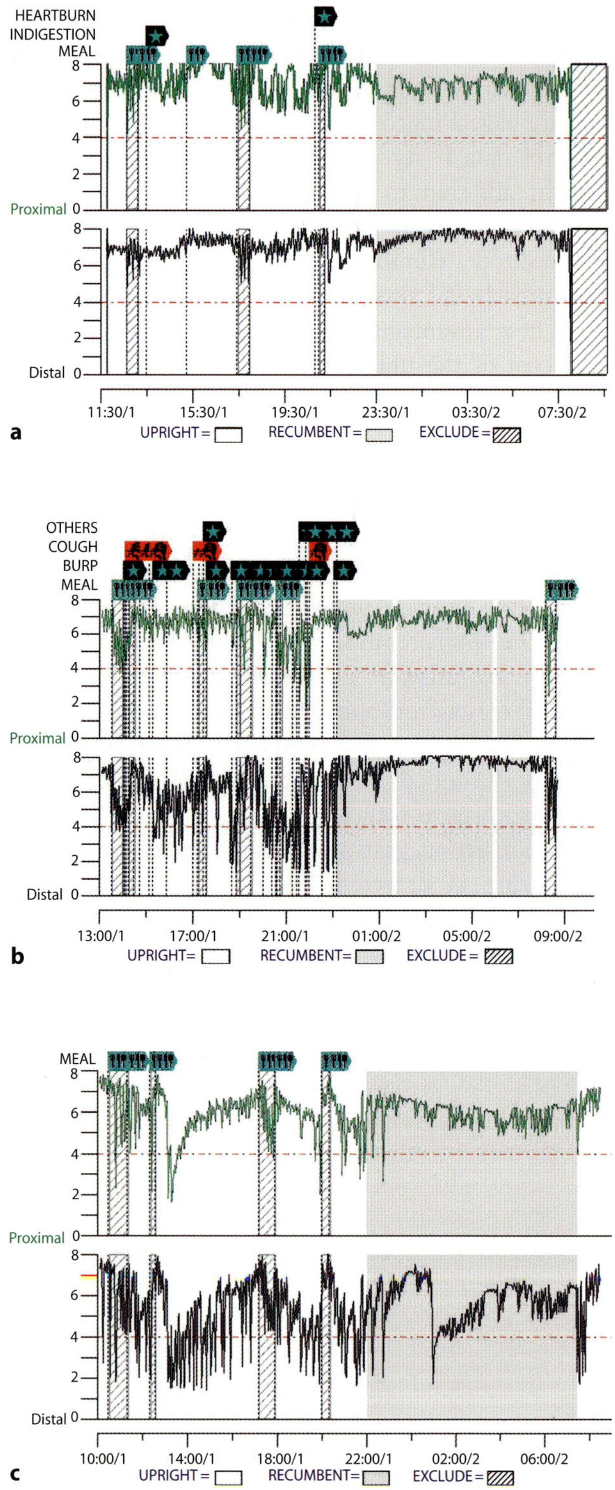

Fig. 8. Ambulatory pH-monitoring tracings. (**a**) Normal proximal and distal esophageal acid exposure. (**b**) Abnormal distal esophageal acid exposure during upright position. (**c**) Abnormal distal esophageal acid exposure during upright and recumbent position

Another method in reporting esophageal acid exposure, particularly popular in the surgical literature is a cumulative score originally established by Johnson and DeMeester (JD score). The JD score take into account and weighs 6 different parameters: (1) total percent time pH less than 4, (2) percent time pH less than 4 in the upright period, (3) percent time pH less than 4 in the recumbent period, (4) the total number of reflux episodes, (5) the total number of reflux episodes longer than 5 minutes and (6) the duration of the longest reflux episode. To date, commercially available pH software programs report this score along with individual exposure times. Studies comparing the composite score against time pH less than 4 have indicated that the later discriminates at least as well as the score between healthy volunteers and GERD patients [31], [32]. Regardless whether one uses the composite score or individual acid exposure times a detailed evaluation of the pH tracing is of pivotal importance to recognize and exclude artifacts (*Fig. 9*) and to assess symptom association.

Equally important information from intraesophageal pH monitoring is evaluating the relationship between symptoms and acid reflux. Like the pH threshold and reflux parameters to quantify GER, there are different ways to assess the association between symptoms and reflux episodes. The simplest way to evaluate this association is by reporting the symptom index. First described by Wiener et al [33] the symptom index is the percentage of symptoms preceded by a drop in esophageal pH below 4 within a 5-minute time window divided by the total number of symptoms. The symptom index should be determined separately for each different

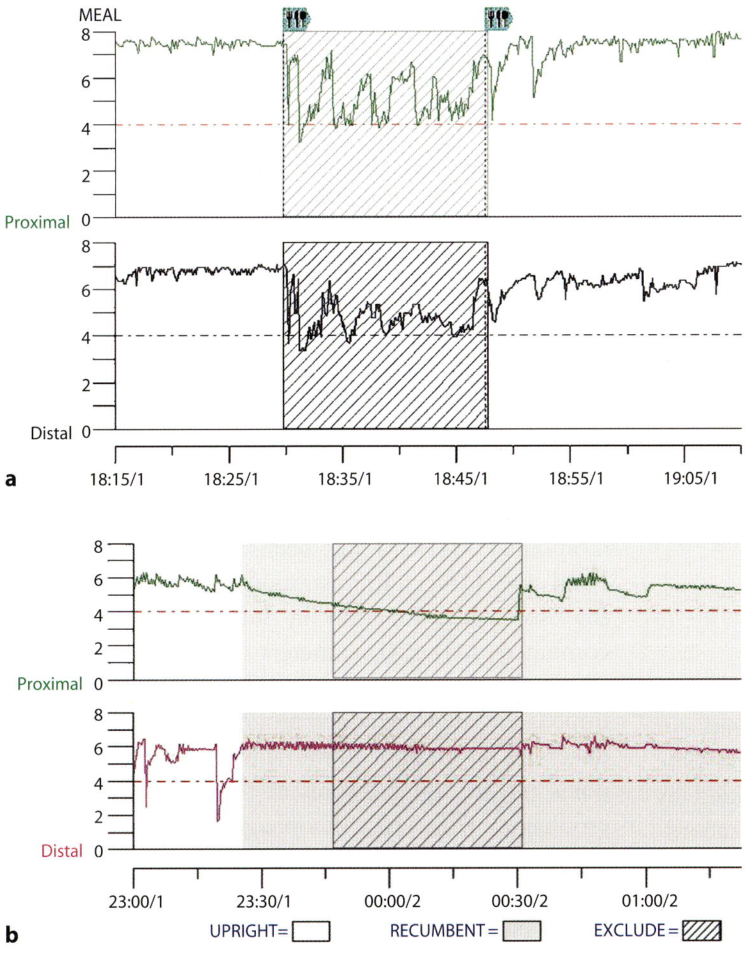

Fig. 9. Artifacts during pH monitoring: (**a**) meal artifact, and (**b**) pseudoreflux (slow drift in proximal pH channel only)

symptom and a positive symptom association is declared if the symptom index is greater or equal to 50% (i.e., at least half of the reported symptoms are preceded within a 5-minute time window by an intraesophageal pH below 4). Over the years the definition and use of the symptom index have been challenged. Based on a sensitivity analysis in patients with chest pain Lam et al [34] have proposed using a shorter, 2-min time window after the onset of a reflux episode in which a symptom has to occur in order for it to be consider associated with reflux.

Recognizing that in patients with multiple reflux episodes and few symptoms the association may occur by chance other authors have advocated using, in addition to the symptom index, a symptom sensitivity index. The symptom sensitivity index is defined as the percentage of reflux episodes associated with symptoms out of the total number of reflux episodes. A symptom sensitivity index greater than 10% would further strengthen the symptom association with reflux.

In a more complex approach, Weusten et al [35] have proposed using the symptom association probability (SAP). The SAP tries to evaluate if, from a statistical approach, the pattern of reflux and symptoms during the monitoring period may have occurred by chance or if the association of symptoms and reflux episodes is not by chance. Commercially available software programs have the ability to report the SAP in percentage based on the methodology used by Weusten et al. When interpreting the SAP it is important to remember that this parameter indicates the statistical probability with which symptoms and reflux episodes are associated. Therefore only an SAP greater than 95% (i.e., the probability of this association having occurred by chance is less than 5%) is considered positive.

Multichannel intraluminal impedance

Esophageal manometry and catheter-based or catheter-free esophageal pH monitoring have some inherent limitations. The information provided by esophageal manometry is limited to pressure recordings within the esophagus with only indirect information about the functional aspect of esophageal contractions, i.e., bolus transit. Esophageal pH monitoring can detect reflux episodes during which the pH drops below 4 but provides limited information about the refluxate bolus and reflux episodes during which the pH does not drop below 4.

The ability to detect intraluminal bolus movement using multichannel intraluminal impedance (MII) was first described by Silny in 1991 [36]. Recognizing that the presence of boluses in the esophagus changes the electrical conductivity of the intraluminal content measured between two rings separated by an isolator, Silny described this method that allows detection of intraesophageal bolus movement without the use of radiation. The appearance of liquid bolus is detected by a drop in the impedance from baseline to a nadir value that is recorded as long as the bolus is present in the impedance-measuring segment. The intraluminal impedance will then rise back to baseline once the bolus leaves the impedance-measuring segment [37]. Using multiple impedance measuring segments on a catheter the direction of bolus movement can be determined: a rapid decline in impedance progressing from proximal to distal suggests aboral (antegrade) bolus movement as seen during swallowing while a rapid decline in impedance progressing from distally to proximally is indicative of oral (retrograde) bolus movement as seen during reflux episodes (*Fig. 11*). Multichannel intraluminal impedance can be added to esophageal manometry (combined MII-EM) in order to evaluate bolus transit during swallowing or added to pH catheters (combined MII-pH) in order to obtain information about refluxate boluses and to detect reflux episodes during which the pH is not below 4.

Combined MII-EM

Combined MII-EM has been approved by the US Food and Drug administration as a diagnostic test for esophageal function in July 2002. Solid state combined MII-EM catheters are very similar to conventional solid-state manometry catheters where impedance rings are added around the pressure transducers. This design allows simultaneous measuring bolus transit and pressures at the same level in the esophagus (*Fig. 10*). Esophageal function testing using combined MII-EM helps clarify the functional defect in patients with esophageal motility abnormalities. Normal values have been established by a multicenter study in 43 healthy volunteers [38]. Normal liquid esophageal bolus transit is declared if at least 80% of liquid swallows have a defined entry in the proximal esophagus and exit the region between 5 and 15 cm above the LES. During viscous swallows 70% of swallows have to fulfill these criteria in order to declare normal bolus transit.

Studying a group of patients with various manometric abnormalities [8] we identified abnormal bolus transit in all patients with achalasia and scleroderma esophagus, and normal bolus transit for liquid in virtually all patients with normal manometry, nutcracker esophagus and isolated LES abnormalities (i.e., poorly relaxing LES, hypertensive or hypotensive LES). In this study, approximately half of patients with ineffective esophageal motility

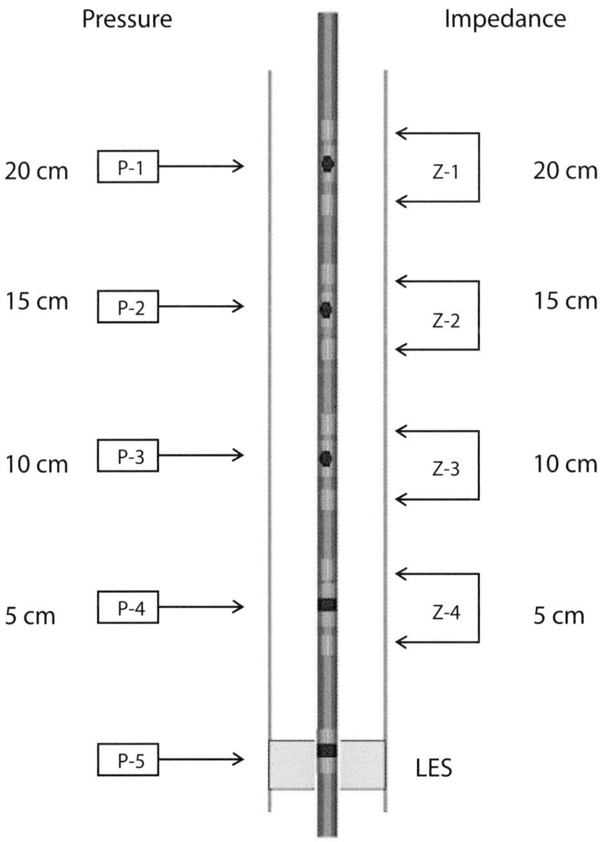

Fig. 10. Esophageal function catheter. Circumferential solid-state pressure sensors located in LES high-pressure zone (P5) and 5 cm above it (P4), unidirectional solid-state pressure sensors located 10 cm (P3), 15 cm (P2) and 20 cm (P1) above LES. Impedance measuring segments centered at 5 cm (Z4), 10 cm (Z3), 15 cm (Z2) and 20 cm (Z1) above LES

(IEM) and distal esophageal spasm (DES) had normal bolus transit. Studying in more detail patients with IEM we identified that there is no perfect (i.e., highly sensitive and highly specific) manometric pressure cutoff that would predict complete bolus transit, that the current manometric criteria for diagnosing IEM (i.e., 30% or more manometric ineffective swallows) may be too sensitive and lacks the specificity of identifying patients with abnormal bolus transit. In addition approximately one third of patients with IEM have normal bolus transit for liquid and viscous (suggesting a mild functional defect), approximately one third have abnormal bolus transit for either liquid or viscous (i.e., moderate functional defect) and the remaining third of IEM patients have abnormal bolus transit for both liquid and viscous (i.e., severe functional defect) [39].

Combined MII-EM provides information about bolus transit in patients with post-fundoplication dysphagia [40]. Combined impedance-manometry and videofluoroscopy studies in patients with post-fundoplication dysphagia indicate the ability of MII-EM to identify bolus pooling above the wrap and retrograde escape of the bolus into the proximal esophagus after the completion of an otherwise normal-peristaltic contraction.

While prospective studies evaluating the role of combined MII-EM in assisting in the selection of patients for anti-reflux surgery and evaluating post-operative dysphagia are underway the above mentioned data suggest that combined MII-EM, through its capability of assessing bolus transit without the use of radiation during esophageal manometry, has great potential.

Combined MII-pH

While the majority of clinicians and investigators consider esophageal pH monitoring to be the "gold standard" in diagnosing GERD they also acknowledge its limitation in detecting only gastroesophageal reflux when the pH of the intraluminal content produces a rapid decline in pH from above to below 4.0. Gastroesophageal reflux with pH above 4.0 is difficult to detect by conventional pH-monitoring and different approaches (i.e., bilirubin monitoring, scintigraphy, manometry, etc.) have been proposed to overcome this limitation. Recently multichannel intraluminal impedance has been described

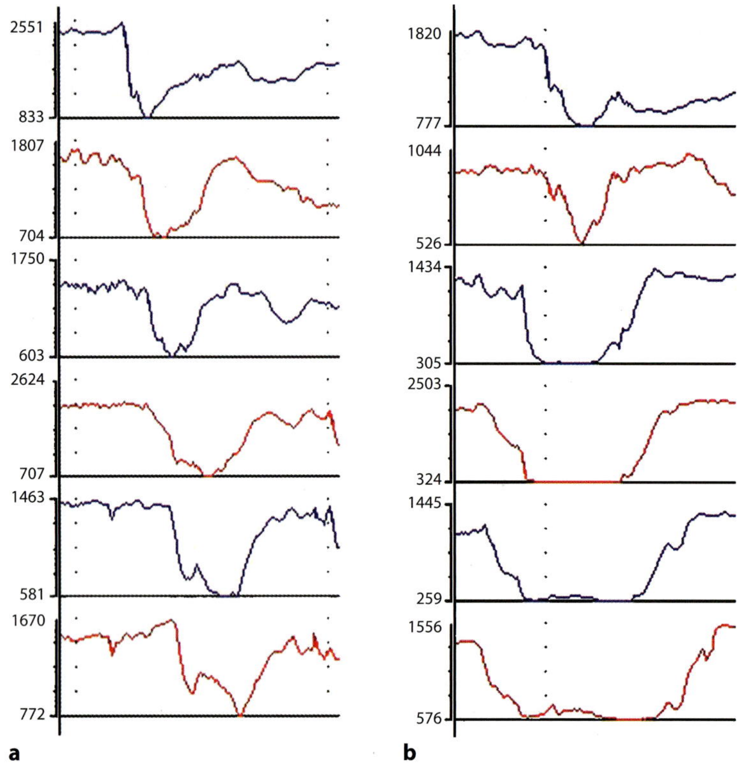

Fig. 11. Direction of intraluminal bolus movement as detected by multichannel intraluminal impedance. Drops in impedance starting proximally and moving distally are indicative of antegrade bolus movement as seen during swallowing (**a**). Drops in impedance starting distally and moving proximally are indicative of retrograde bolus movement as seen during reflux (**b**)

as a new method in monitoring gastroesophageal reflux.

Similar to combined MII-EM, multiple impedance measuring segments can be mounted on a regular 2.1 mm pH catheter (*Fig. 12*) and gastroesophageal reflux monitored by combined multichannel intraluminal impedance and pH (MII-pH). Combined MII-pH represents a shift in the GERD testing paradigm. Gastroesophageal reflux episodes are detected by retrograde (i.e., distal to proximal) progressing declines in intraluminal impedance determined by the increased conductivity of the liquid GER while the pH sensor is simply used to categorize the reflux into acid or non-acid. Traditionally, gastroesophageal reflux with a pH above 4.0 is considered non-acid in order to underscore the difference to the acid reflux episodes detectable by conventional pH monitoring (*Fig. 13*). In an attempt to comply to the chemical definition of acid and non-acid a group of leading esophageal experts have proposed separating gastroesophageal reflux detected by MII into acid, if the pH drops from above to below 4.0, weakly acidic if the pH is between 4.0 and 7.0 and non-acid if the intraesophageal pH during an MII-detected reflux episode remains above 7.0.

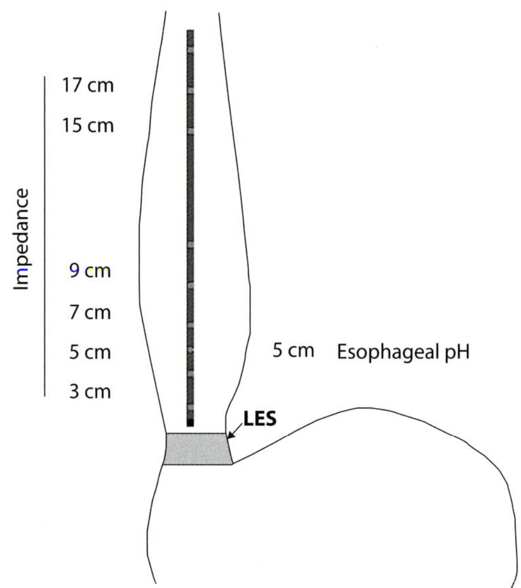

Fig. 12. Combined multichannel intraluminal impedance and pH catheter

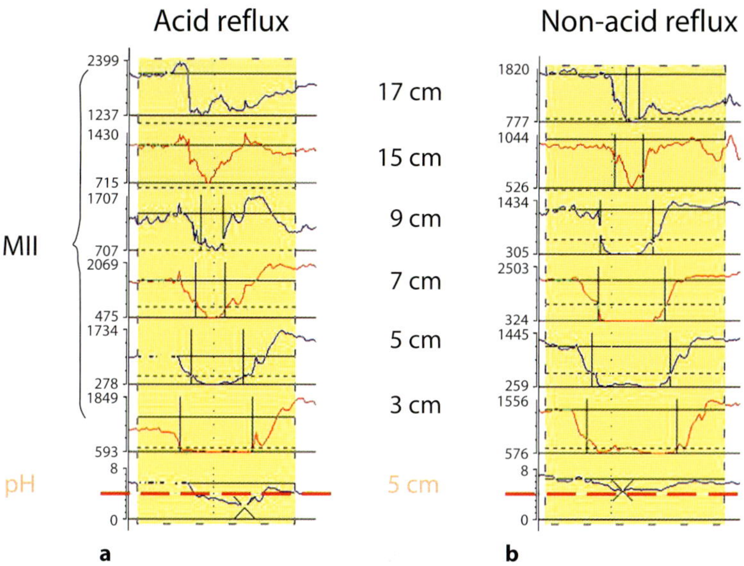

Fig. 13. Gastroesophageal reflux detected by combined MII-pH monitoring. Impedance-detected reflux episodes during which the intraesophageal pH drops from above to below 4.0 are considered acid (**a**) while impedance-detected reflux episodes during which the intraesophageal pH remains above 4.0 are considered non-acid (**b**)

Non-acid reflux is relatively infrequent in subjects not taking acid suppressive therapy. In individuals off acid suppressive therapy it occurs primarily in the post prandial periods [41] and rarely at night. On the other hand in individuals taking acid suppressive therapy the medications primarily change the composition of the gastroesophageal refluxate without affecting the total number of GER episodes [42]. Since esophageal mucosal healing occurs in up to 90% of patients taking potent acid suppressive therapy the question of the clinical relevance of non-acid reflux is appropriate. While non-acid reflux may have a limited contribution to esophageal structural lesions, it has a role in causing persistent symptoms in patients on acid suppressive therapy. In a large trial including over 5000 GERD patients once daily acid suppressive therapy controlled the symptoms in only 60–65% of patients [43] and non-acid reflux has been documented to be associated with esophageal symptoms [40].

Current clinical practice guidelines favor empiric trials of PPI over pH testing to diagnose GERD. Esophageal pH testing is then recommended primarily in patients with persistent symptoms despite acid suppressive therapy. In these circumstances the decision to test the patient on or off therapy becomes difficult since, on one hand esophageal pH testing is more accurate when performed off therapy, but on the other hand esophageal pH testing cannot exclude non-acid reflux in patients. In our opinion combined MII-pH has the potential of overcoming this impasse and we propose the algorithm depicted in *Fig. 14* in evaluating patients with GERD symptoms.

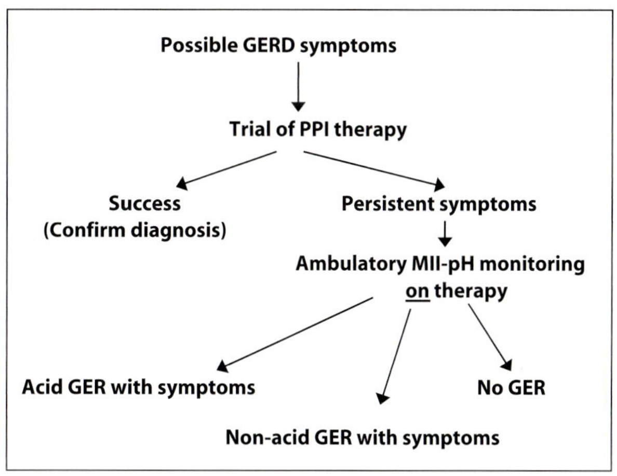

MII-pH = combined multichannel intraluminal impedance and pH
GER = gastroesophageal reflux
PPI = proton pump inhibitor

Fig. 14. Suggested diagnostic GERD algorithm

Table 2. Diagnostic modalities for GERD

	Endoscopy	Manometry	pH monitoring	MII-pH-monitoring
Erosive esophagitis	Yes	No	No	Suggestive but not diagnostic
Barrett's esophagus	Yes (with biopsy)	No	No	Suggestive but not diagnostic
GERD symptoms due to acid reflux in the absence of esophagitis	No	Not feasible	Yes	Yes
GERD symptoms due to non-acid reflux	No	Not feasible	No	Yes

MII-pH = combined multichannel intraluminal impedance and pH-monitoring

Conclusions

Gastroesophageal reflux disease is a common condition encountered in clinical practice. Upper GI endoscopy remains the best modality to diagnose erosive esophagitis and Barrett's esophagus but recognizing that GERD can be present in the absence of esophageal lesions other techniques are employed in documenting an abnormal amount of gastroesophageal reflux and the relation between reflux and symptoms (Table 2). Esophageal manometry is an important test in supporting the diagnosis in complex GERD patients and can be used to clarify the pathophysiologic mechanisms of GERD. The role of manometry in evaluating patients prior to undergoing antireflux surgery has been recently challenged although combined multichannel intraluminal impedance and manometry (MII-EM) may help refine the diagnostic abilities to identify patients at risk of developing post-fundoplication dysphagia.

Gastroesophageal reflux monitoring using pH electrodes is an important tool in evaluating patients with GERD symptoms not taking acid suppressive therapy. Combined multichannel intraluminal impedance and pH (MII-pH) may be the preferred method to evaluate patients with persistent symptoms on acid suppressive therapy.

References

[1] Locke GR, Talley NJ, Fett SL et al (1997) Prevalence and clinical spectrum of gastroesophageal reflux: a population based study in Olmsted County, Minnesota. Gastroenterology 112: 1448–1456

[2] Sandler RS, Everhart JE, Donowitz M et al (2002) The burden of selected digestive diseases in the United States. Gastroenterology 122: 1500–1511

[3] Allison PR (1946) Peptic ulcer of the esophagus. J Thorac Cardiovasc Surg 15: 308–317

[4] Nagler R, Spiro HM (1961) Serial esophageal motility studies in asymptomatic young subjects. Gastroenterology 41: 371–379

[5] Kahrilas PJ, Dodds WJ, Hogan WJ (1988) Effect of peristaltic dysfunction on esophageal volume clearance. Gastroenterology 94: 73–80

[6] Richter JE, Wu WC, Johns DN, Blackwell JN, Nelson JL 3rd, Castell JA, Castell DO (1987) Esophageal manometry in 95 healthy adult volunteers. Dig Dis Sci 32: 583–592

[7] Spechler SJ, Castell DO (2001) Classification of esophageal motility abnormalities. Gut 49: 145–151

[8] Tutuian R, Castell DO (2004) Combined multichannel intraluminal impedance and manometry clarifies esophageal function abnormalities. Study in 350 patients. Am J Gastroenterol 99: 1011–1019

[9] Butterfield DG, Struthers JE Jr, Showalter JP (1972) A test of gastroesophageal sphincter competence. The common cavity test. Am J Dig Dis 17: 415–421

[10] Shay SS, Richer JE (2003) Direct comparison of impedance, common cavity and pH probe in detecting daytime GER's and their characteristics. Gastroenterology 124 S1: A534 (Abstract)

[11] Dodds WJ, Dent J, Hogan WJ, Helm JF, Hauser R, Patel GK, Egide MS (1982) Mechanisms of gastroesophageal reflux in patients with reflux esophagitis. N Engl J Med 307: 1547–1552

[12] Dent J, Dodds WJ, Friedman RH, Sekiguchi T, Hogan WJ, Arndorfer RC, Petrie DJ (1980) Mechanism of gastroesophageal reflux in recumbent asymptomatic human subjects. J Clin Invest 65: 256–267

[13] Pandolfion JE, Shi G, Zhang Q, Ghosh S, Brasseur JG, Kahrilas PJ (2004) Measuring EGJ opening patterns using high-resolution intraluminal impedance. Neurogastroenterol Motil; DOI: 10.1111/j.1365-2982.2004.00589.x
[14] Wetscher GJ, Glaser K, Wieschemeyer T, Gadenstaetter M, Prommegger R, Profanter C (1997) Tailored antireflux surgery for gastroesophageal reflux disease: effectiveness and risk of postoperative dysphagia. World J Surg 21: 605–610
[15] Kahrilas PJ, Doods WJ, Hogan WJ (1988) Effect of peristaltic dysfunction on esophageal volume clearance. Gastroenterology 94: 73–80
[16] Incarbone R, Bonavina L, Reitano M, Peracchia A (1999) Esophageal function studies in the management of gastroesophageal reflux disease. Int J Surg Investig 1: 351–356
[17] Fibbe C, Layer P, Keller J, Strate U, Emmermann A, Zornig C (2001) Esophageal motility in reflux disease before and after fundoplication: a prospective, randomized, clinical, and manometric study. Gastroenterology 121: 5–14
[18] Spencer J (1969) Prolonged pH recording in the study of gastro-oesophageal reflux. Br J Surg 56: 912–914
[19] Johnson LF, DeMeester TR (1974) Twenty-four-hour pH monitoring of the distal esophagus. A quantitative measure of gastroesophageal reflux. Am J Gastroenterol 62: 325–332
[20] McLauchlan G, Rawlings JM, Lucas ML, McCloy RF, Crean GP, McColl KE (1987) Electrodes for 24 hours pH monitoring – a comparative study. Gut 28: 935–939
[21] Ward BW, Wu WC, Richter JE, Lui KW, Castell DO (1986) Ambulatory 24-hour esophageal pH monitoring. Technology searching for a clinical application. J Clin Gastroenterol 8 (Suppl) 1: 59–67
[22] Dobhan R, Castell DO (1992) Prolonged intraesophageal pH monitoring with 16-hr overnight recording. Comparison with "24-hr" analysis. Dig Dis Sci 37: 857–864
[23] Gureneis P, Orleanski A (1964) On determination of the pH value of gastric juice by means of the internal radio sound, according to the H. G. Noeller (Heidelberg capsule). Wien Z Inn Med 45: 368–372
[24] Connell AM, Waters TE (1964) Assessment of gastric function by pH-telemetring capsule. Lancet 189: 227–230
[25] Pandolfino JE, Richter JE, Ours T, Guardino JM, Chapman J, Kahrilas PJ (2003) Ambulatory esophageal pH monitoring using a wireless system. Am J Gastroenterol 98: 740–749
[26] Piper DW, Fenton BH (1965) pH stability and activity curves of pepsin with special reference to their clinical importance. Gut 6: 506–508
[27] Tuttle SG, Rufin F, Bettarello A (1961) The physiology of heartburn. Ann Intern Med 55: 292–300
[28] Stanciu C, Hoare RC, Bennett JR (1977) Correlation between manometric and pH tests for gastro-oesophageal reflux. Gut 18: 536–540
[29] Vitale GC, Sadek S, Tulley FM, Rimmer AR, Hunter BE, Phelan J, Cuschieri A (1985) Computerized 24-hour esophageal pH monitoring: a new ambulatory technique using radiotelemetry. J Lab Clin Med 105: 686–693
[30] Weusten BL, Roelofs JM, Akkermans LM, Vanberge-Henegouwen GP, Smout AJ (1996) Objective determination of pH thresholds in the analysis of 24-h ambulatory esophageal pH monitoring. Eur J Clin Invest 26: 151–158
[31] Johnsson F, Joelsson B, Isberg PE (1987) Ambulatory 24-hour intraesophageal pH-monitoring in the diagnosis of gastroesophageal reflux disease. Gut 28: 1145–1150
[32] Schindlbeck NE, Heinrich C, Konig A, Dendorfer A, Pace F, Muller-Lissner SA (1987) Optimal thresholds, sensitivity, and specificity of long-term pH-metry for the detection of gastroesophageal reflux disease. Gastroenterology 93: 85–90
[33] Wiener GJ, Richter JE, Copper JB, Wu WC, Castell DO (1988) The symptom index: a clinically important parameter of ambulatory 24-hour esophageal pH monitoring. Am J Gastroenterol 83: 358–361
[34] Lam HG, Breumelhof R, Roelofs JM, Van Berge Henegouwen GP, Smout AJ (1994) What is the optimal time window in symptom analysis of 24-hour esophageal pressure and pH data? Dig Dis Sci 39: 402–409
[35] Weusten BL, Roelofs JM, Akkermans LM, Van Berge-Henegouwen GP, Smout AJ (1994) The symptom-association probability: an improved method for symptom analysis of 24-hour esophageal pH data. Gastroenterology 107: 1741–1745
[36] Silny J (1991) Intraluminal multiple electric impedance procedure for measurement of gastrointestinal motility. J Gastrointest Motil 3: 151–162
[37] Srinivasan R, Vela MF, Katz PO, Tutuian R, Castell JA, Castell DO (2001) Esophageal function testing using multichannel intraluminal impedance. Am J Physiol 280: G457–G462
[38] Tutuian R, Vela MF, Balaji N, Wise JL, Murray JA, Peters JH, Shay SS, Castell DO (2003) Esophageal function testing using combined multichannel intraluminal impedance and manometry. Multicenter study of healthy volunteers. Clin Gastroenterol Hepatol 1: 174–182

[39] Tutuian R, Castell DO (2004) Clarification of the esophageal function defect in patients with manometric ineffective esophageal motility: studies using combined impedance-manometry. Clin Gastroenterol Hepatol 2: 230–236

[40] Imam H, Baker M, Shay S (2004) Simultaneous barium esophagogram (Ba), impedance monitoring (Imp) and manometry (Ba-Imp-Manometry) in patients with dysphagia due to tight fundoplication. Gastroenterology 126 (Suppl) 2: A-639 (Abstract)

[41] Wildi SM, Tutuian R, Castell DO (2004) The influence of rapid food intake on postprandial reflux: studies in healthy volunteers. Am J Gastroenterol 99: 1645–1651

[42] Vela MF, Camacho-Lobato L, Srinivasan R, Tutuian R, Katz PO, Castell DO (2001) Simultaneous intraesophageal impedance and pH measurement of acid and nonacid gastroesophageal reflux: effect of omeprazole. Gastroenterology 120: 1599–1606

[43] Castell DO, Kahrilas PJ, Richter JE, Vakil NB, Johnson DA, Zuckerman S, Skammer W, Levine JG (2002) Esomeprazole (40 mg) compared with lansoprazole (30 mg) in the treatment of erosive esophagitis. Am J Gastroenterol 97: 575–583

Chapter 12

ENDOSCOPIC ANTI-REFLUX THERAPY

E. Günter and Ch. Ell

Klinik Innere Medizin II, HSK Wiesbaden, Germany

Introduction

Gastro-esophageal reflux disease (GERD) has increased substantially in the developed world over the past 30 years [1]. Epidemiological data show a prevalence of heartburn at least once weekly of about 20% [2]. GERD seriously affects quality of life. Variables such as daily fitness, vitality, emotional control, and quality of sleep are notably diminished compared with the healthy population [3], [4].

The severity and frequency of symptoms correlates not only with the presence and extent of organic lesions. Some 50–60% of patients do not have visible tissue changes on endoscopy [5], [6], which means that they have endoscopically negative reflux disease (NERD, stage 0, according to Savary and Miller). The role of endoscopy is to help in staging the disease and, quintessentially, in the early recognition of complications such as Barrett's esophagus or adenocarcinoma, which have become increasingly common in tandem with the increase in reflux disease [7], [8].

The treatment of choice is acid suppression with a medical drug, preferably with a proton pump inhibitor. Some 90% of patients are completely complaint free on such a regimen [9]. General measures such as weight reduction, sleeping with a raised upper body, and dietary changes have shown only marginal or no effects in studies [10]–[13]. Even with long-term use, the side effects of drug treatment are negligible relative to their usefulness [14].

For selected patients, an alternative to medical drugs is surgical treatment, i.e., laparoscopic fundoplication after Nissen or Toupet. The indications for surgical anti-reflux treatment according to the European Study Group for Antireflux-Surgery are the following:

- Persistent or recurring symptoms in spite of optimal drug treatment
- Persistent or recurring complications of the disease in spite of treatment
- Negative effects on quality of life because of dependence on medical drug treatment or adverse effects from the drugs
- Restricted quality of life and presence of a large, symptomatic hiatus hernia (regurgitation, feeling of pressure after meals).

The reported primary success rate of laparoscopic fundoplication is 85–95% [16]. Thirty day mortality is 0.0–0.6%. Typical complications, such as postoperative dysphagia, gas-bloating syndrome, and meteorismu have been reported in 25–30% of patients. In the long term, up to 38% of patients will require drug treatment with proton pump inhibitors because of typical reflux symptoms [16]–[19].

The different methods of reflux therapy have to be assessed against this background. Some procedures have been approved by the regulators, and some have already disappeared from the market. The following overview presents the currently available therapies and their published results.

Principles of endoscopic treatment methods

All endoscopic anti-reflux therapies aim at strengthening the lower esophageal sphincter. The three different fundamental principles used to achieve this objective are:

(1) Suture techniques
Endoscopic gastroplasty (EndoCinch, BARD®, USA)
Full-thickness plication (Plicator®, NDO-Surgical, USA)

(2) Injection and implantation techniques
Injection of biopolymers (Enteryx®, Boston Scientific, USA)
Implantation treatment (Gatekeeper®, Medtronic, USA)

(3) Radiofrequency application (Stretta®, Curon Medical, USA)

Endoscopic gastroplasty (EndoCinch®)

During endoscopic gastroplasty (ELGP), the esophageal junction is being narrowed through the creation of mucous pleats immediately below the lower esophageal sphincter. The folds are being created with a special suturing device that is attached to a standard endoscope. The technique is derived from the endoscopic suturing method developed by Paul Swain [20]. A metal capsule with a side opening is attached to the tip of the endoscope and applies suction to the esophageal wall, which is then sutures with a hollow needle, which is handled via a manual grip attached to the endoscope. The endoscope will have to be pulled out and reinserted several times for this, which is done via a tube that has been put into position first, whose outer diameter is 19.7 mm. To achieve sufficient gathering and narrowing of the esophageal junction, two or three mucous folds will normally have to be created. The pleats are either applied at the same level or at different levels immediately on top of each other. The procedure is reversible, and the sutures can be removed at any time. More than 5000 patients have so far been treated with this procedure worldwide.

Studies

The first multicentre study from the United States included 64 patients and was published in 2001. The study included patients with at least three episodes of heartburn per week that required drug treatment and with pathological reflux as proved by pH measurement. Exclusion criteria were severe reflux esophagitis (grade 3 or 4), extreme obesity (BMI > 40, or a hiatus hernia with a diameter of > 2 cm. After six months, 62% of patients required no or only occasional (three times or less per month) drug treatment. The reflux and heartburn severity scores had improved significantly (1.81 ± 0.8 *v* 0.61 ± 0.6, $P < 0.0001$ and 62.7 ± 18.6 *v* 17.0 ± 20.2, $P < 0.0001$). The objective variables, however, had improved much less markedly. Pressure measurement in the lower esophagus showed no significant improvement. The endoscopically determined stage of reflux esophagitis was also unchanged; pH measurements showed a significant but small reduction in reflux time ($9.6\% \pm 6.8\%$ *v* $8.5\% \pm 8.3$, $P < 0.011$). Complications included a perforated stitch in one patient, which could be managed conservatively. Reported complaints after the treatment included pharyngitis in 31% patients, stomach pains in 14%, chest pain in 16%, and vomiting in 14%. The procedure had to be repeated in 11 patients as one or several stitches had loosened (the authors gave no details). The patients had been randomised into two groups according to suture technique: in one group the sutures followed a circular arrangement, in the other, a linear one. Results between the two treatment arms did not differ [21].

Because of the positive effect of the reflux symptoms the procedure gained FDA approval in the United States after this study had been published.

Another study from 2001 is worth mentioning, although it was reported only as an abstract on the occasion of the DDW and was never published. The study is a European multicentre study, which included 142 patients. Inclusion and exclusion criteria are not given but presumably do not differ much from those of the US study. The mean observation time after the procedure was only 12 weeks. A significant reduction in the use of proton pump inhibitors was observed, the DeMeester score dropped from a median of 5 to 1 ($P < 0.05$), and the pressure measured in the lower esophageal sphincter rose from 5 mm Hg to 8 mm Hg ($P < 0.05$). pH measurements showed a reduction of acid exposure in the lower esophagus from 8.5% to 3.7% ($P < 0.05$). Complications included light bleeds in two cases, transient dysphagia in three cases, sedation that had been too deep in one case, and two perforations that necessitated surgical fundoplication [22].

A study from 2003 reported 26 patients undergoing treatment, of whom 22 had a follow-up examination after one year. Inclusion and exclusion criteria were similar to the studies mentioned earlier. The results after a year showed significant improvement of the subjective variables such as heartburn severity score (19.22 *v* 7.5, $P < 0.0001$) and regurgitation score (2.27 *v* 0.86, $P < 0.001$). The DeMeester score was measured after three months and showed a significant but slight improvement (44.1 ± 4.3 *v* 33.32 ± 4.73, $P < 0.028$). Use of proton pump inhibitors had fallen by only 64% after 12 months. Complications after the treatment included pharyngitis in 27% of patients, thoracic pain in 19%, abdominal pain in 12%, and dysphagia, nausea, and meteorism in 8% of patients each. Severe complications included a tear to the mucosa (without further consequences) and two bleeds, one of which necessitated blood transfusion [23].

Data about the long-term development after treatment are available only in abstract form. A Canadian study with a follow-up period of two years reports treatment failure in 11 of 25 patients [24]. A US study reached similar conclusions at two year follow-up. Of 33 patients, only 25% were without acid suppressing drugs, 28% were able to reduce the dose by half. The remaining 47% had to start taking their original medication again because the treatment had been ineffective [25].

An interesting study comparing endoscopic gastroplasty and laparoscopic fundoplication was published in early 2004. Eighty seven patients with typical reflux disease were divided into two non-randomized groups: one (n = 47) was treated by intraluminal gastroplication and the other (n = 40) by laparoscopic fundoplication. Measurements before the procedure (duration and severity of symptoms, DeMeester score) were the same in both groups. In 10 patients of the groups treated by endoscopy the procedure had to be stopped for various reasons (hypoxia, bleeding, vomiting, delayed emptying of the stomach). Five of these patients then underwent laparoscopic fundoplication. At the follow-up examination after seven or eight months, 32% of patients who had had endoscopy treatment were taking acid suppressing drugs, compared with 13% in the group treated by laparoscopy. In the endoscopy group, 66% of patients expressed satisfaction with their treatment, compared with 93% in the laparoscopy group. The authors conclude that laparoscopic fundoplication is superior to endoscopic gastroplasty [26].

Endoscopic reflux therapy is now also used in children and adolescents. A study from December 2004 reports results in 17 patients aged between 6 and 16 years. Inclusion criteria were dependency on proton pump inhibitors for at least 12 months or treatment failure of drugs. Three plicatures each were positioned with the EndoCinch procedure immediately below the lower esophageal sphincter. The treatment had to be repeated in three patients because the effects were not strong enough. Complications included a self limiting bleed. After a median follow-up period of 23 month, 14 of 17 patients were free of medication. pH measurements in 14 of 16 patients were normal immediately after treatment and in six out of nine patients after one year. The authors conclude that the method is safe and effective to use in children and adolescents [27].

Full-thickness plication (Plicator®)

Endoscopic full-thickness plication is the most recent treatment procedure. In contrast to ELGP, the entire gastric wall from the cardia to the serosa is gripped with an endoscopic tissue retractor and a double, transmural stitch is placed. The suturing device is inserted into the stomach with the endoscope, which is used to supervise the procedure, in a 60F tube. In inversion, the gastric wall is being gripped 1–2 cm below the esophageal junction, and retracted into the suturing device with a special corkscrew shaped retractor. A transmural plicature is then applied.

Studies

In a first feasibility study that was published in 2002, the system was tested on an animal model and used without complications. The expected effect on the gastro-esophageal reflux dependent in the pressure in the stomach could be demonstrated. All plicatures were unchanged and in place after 12 weeks, without any complication such as ischaemia or ulceration [28]. The same study group reported first experiences with seven patients in 2003. Six of these had been treated successfully, but the procedure had to be stopped in one patient because of problems with sedation. Inclusion criteria were reflux symptoms for at least six months, pathological pH values, and an at least partial response to treatment with proton pump inhibitors. Exclusion criteria were more severe esophagitis and a hiatus hernia > 2 cm. After 2 months, five patients were re-examined, the sixth patient underwent laparoscopic fundoplication after six months because his symptoms had deteriorated. After 12 months, the clinical scores were significantly improved (HRQL and SF-36). Three of five patients did not need any more antisecretory medication. The others were able to reduce their drug dosage notably. The study protocol did not include systematic pH measurements, but according to the authors this had not improved markedly after treatment. Endocopic controls after three and six months confirmed that the plicatures were intact in all patients [29].

The first multicentre Plicator study was published in 2004. The exclusion and inclusion criteria were the same as above. Sixty four patients had treatment; the mean duration of treatment was 17.2 minutes. Complications included pharyngitis in 41% of patients, thoracic pain in 17%, other abdominal pain in 17%, hiccups in 14%, dysphagia in 11%, and vomiting in 6%. Six serious complications were reported: in two patients, acute dyspnoea occurred after the tube had been inserted so that the treatment had to be stopped and later performed under full intubation anaesthesia. One patient developed pneumothorax and one pneumoperitoneum. Perforation could be excluded in both cases; the plicature was removed in one of the patients. Both recovered without the need for further interventions. Perforation of the stomach occurred in one patients, but this was managed successfully with endo-clips. Six months after treatment, 74% of patients were without acid suppressing treatment, the clinical score (GERD-HRQL, $P < 0.001$) had improved significantly, pH measurements had also improved ($P < 0.008$), and in 30% of patients, pH measurements had normalised [30].

Injection of biopolymers (Enteryx®)

The principle underlying this procedure is that of strengthening the lower esophageal sphincter by injecting an inert biopolymer into the musculature of the esophageo-cardial junction. The substance used for this purpose (Enteryx®) is well known in medicine. It is used in neurosurgery and conventional radiology to embolise blood vessels. A bio-polymer (ethylene-vinyl-alcohol), the substance is chemically inert and biologically non-degradable and has no antigenic properties. After being injected into the tissue the liquid substance assumes a sponge-like, elastic consistency. It has to be used in a special solution (dimethyl sulphide) and can then be injected through the endoscope with a needle into the wall of the esophageo-cardial junction. The injection is monitored on X ray. In the ideal scenario the polymer will form a ring around the injection site. As the polymer enters in the esophageal wall it cannot be removed; the procedure is thus not reversible. Fundoplication at a later stage is not affected, however.

A first animal experiment about the injection of a polymer into the cardia to increase sphincter pressure was published in 2002. In 12 minipigs, 1–1.5 ml polymer was injected into three or four sites circumferentially into the cardial area. The stomach pressure needed for esophageal reflux increased significantly six weeks after the injection. At necropsy, the implant was found unchanged in the cardia only when the injection had been strictly intramuscular. After submucosal injection, the polymer could not be located in most cases [31]. In 2002, a pilot study was published that reported the results in 15 patients. These patients had been treated in two centres, in Brussels and Rom. The injection succeeded in 10 of 15 cases and the polymer dispersed under radiological control in a ring shape in the cardial muscles. In the remaining five patients the polymer was not optimally distributed. At a median follow-up of six months, reflux symptoms had fallen significantly (heartburn score 4.3 ± 0.13 *v* $1.9 \pm .26$, $P < 0.01$). Eleven patients were not treated with drugs at this point in time. More than 50% of the injected polymer was detectable in only nine of 15 patients. Among the 10 patients with optimum distribution of the polymer at injection, more than 50% was visible in eight [32].

The six month and 12 month results of an international multicentre study with 85 patients were published in 2003. Treatment was given on an outpatient basis and patients were discharged two-four hours after the procedure. The mean treatment time was 33.8 ± 10 minutes. Side effects in 84% of patients included slight to medium grade retrosternal pain for up to a week. Twelve per cent had a slight fever for one to three days. Treatment had to be repeated after one to three months in 22% of patients because it was insufficiently effective. After six and 12 months, 81 patients were re-examined. After six months, 74% of patients were not taking proton pump inhibitors and after 12 months, 70.4%. The proportion of patients who could reduce their proton pump inhibitor dosage by more than 50% was 9.8% after six and 12 months. Radiological identification of the implant showed a loss in volume to about 75% of the original quantity after three months, after which the polymer did not incur further losses. The authors explain this with quantities of polymer that were injected submucosally and had dispersed. The polymer in the muscle layer seems to be stable [33], [34].

Exact injection of Enteryx® into the cardial muscle is not always possible, as two case studies from

2004 show. One reports a para-esophageal abscess after injection [25], and the other describes the anatomical situation in four patients after unsuccessful injection of Enteryx® and subsequent laparoscopic fundoplication. In three patients, the polymer was found intraoperatively, in a para-esophageal position and had fibrosed [36].

Hydrogel implantation (Gatekeeper®)

Implantation therapy is similar to injection in that is aims at narrowing the esophageo-cardial junction. By strengthening the wall around the lower esophageal sphincter. The Gatekeeper® reflux repair system uses several prostheses, 20 mm in length and 1.5 mm in thickness, made from dehydrated hydrogel based on polyacrylonitril, which are inserted into the submucosal layer. They absorb moisture and expand within 24 hours to reach a thickness of 5–6 mm. Up to eight prostheses can be implanted in one session. This is done through a tube that has a chamber at its distal end and is sucked into the esophageal mucosa. A needle is inserted along the inner wall of the tube and used to inject 3–6 ml salt solution into the submucosa fixated in the chamber. The implant is then inserted via the same canal. The procedure is performed under endoscopic supervision. For this purpose, a normal gastroscope is pushed through to the tube's distal end.

A first pilot study included 10 patients and was published merely in abstract form in 2002. This study reports significant improvements in reflux symptoms; seven patients were able to reduce or even cease acid suppressing drugs [37]. In the meantime, the initial results from a European multicentre study were published in 2004. This included 68 patients with typical reflux symptoms who responded to treatment with proton pump inhibitors. Pathological pH measurements had to be available over 24 hours. Patients with a hiatus hernia larger than 3 cm or high higher-grade esophagitis were excluded. In one patient, insertion of the tube resulted in perforation of the pharynx, which was managed conservatively; 67 patients were treated and followed up. Altogether, 77 procedures were performed and the implants were placed correctly in 93.1%. One patient had recurrent vomiting and the implants had to be removed three weeks after the procedure. Sixty six patients were followed up, 12 of whom were lost to follow-up. After six months, only 54 patients were available for reexamination. Clinical scores had improved significantly (GERD-HRQL 24.0 *v* 5.0, SF-36 43.4 *v* 52.4; $P < 0.05$). Fifty three per cent of patients did not need proton pump inhibitors after six months, and 16% took these only as needed. pH measurements had improved significantly (pH < 4 from 9.1% to 6.1%, $P < 0.05$). Of the implanted polymer prostheses, in 35.2% of patients all implants were in situ, in 22.2% of patients 75–99%, in 29.6% of patients 50–75%, and in 11.1% of patients fewer than 50%.

Radio frequency application (Stretta®)

Radio frequency application/ablation in the esophageo-cardial junction heats the muscle layer in a circumscribed area and results in tissue restructuring and remodelling, with the aim of strengthening the lower esophageal sphincter. Simultaneously, vagal nerve fibres are ablated locally, which reduces transient sphincter relaxation, a crucial pathogenetic factor in lighter reflux disease [39].

The procedure is performed via a special catheter system, consisting of a balloon with four steel needle electrodes that are placed radially at 90% angles above the balloon. The needles are inserted into protective sheaths, which additionally include a water cooling facility for each position of a needle. The temperature is measured at the tip of the pin and also at its base, and the treatment is monitored continually. The catheter has a diameter of only 20F. After the level of the Z-line (mucosal junction) has been endoscopically determined and a guiding wire has been placed, the system is inserted via the wire. The needle electrodes are then deployed in several locations according to a set algorithm. Typically, 12 positions above and below the Z line and in the cardial area are being treated for about 90 seconds, and 56 lesions are applied. The mucosa is being irrigated with water at the basis of the needle during the entire procedure, and the water is suctioned off through an opening at the tip of the catheter. The whole procedure takes 45–60 minutes. Some 3500 patients worldwide have been treated with this method, most of those in the United States.

Studies
The developers of the Stretta® system convincingly showed the feasibility and effectiveness of the procedure in a first animal experimental study in 2000, as measured in the increased pressure in the lower esophageal sphincter nine weeks after treatment [40]. In 2001, the initial results of a US multicentre study were published. The study included 47 patients with typical reflux symptoms, who responded at least partially to acid suppressing treatment and had a pathological pH measurement over 24 hours. Ninety per cent of patients had no hiatus hernia and the remaining 10% an axial hernia with a diameter of less than 2 cm. Forty seven per cent of patients had no esophagitis at endoscopy, only 23% and 21% had reflux esophagitis of grade I or II, respectively. After six months, clinical scores showed highly significant improvement (median heartburn score 4 *v* 1, $P < 0.0001$, HERD score 26 *v* 7, $P < 0.0001$; physical SF-36 41.1 *v* 51.9, $P < 0.0001$). pH measurements were also significantly improved ($P < 0.0001$). Manometry did not find a significant increase of pressure in the lower esophageal sphincter. Light to medium grade esophagitis was found at endoscopy in only eight patients (17%; $P < 0.005$). Eighty seven of the patients were able to stop taking proton pump inhibitors. Only three self limiting complications occurred (slight fever, odynophagia, and injury to the mucosa) [41]. Because of these favourable data, the procedure gained FDA approval in the United States in 2000.

The 12 month results of a US multicentre study of 118 patients were published in 2002. The results in essence confirmed those already described from the 20021 publication. In addition to a highly significant improvement in the clinical scores, pH measurement had also improved significantly. Only 30% of patients had to continue taking a proton pump inhibitor, compared with 88.1% before treatment. 75% of patients had no hiatus hernia, and 70% had no esophagitis at endoscopy. Ten slight and self limiting complications were reported (slight fever, thoracic pain, dysphagia, hypotension, and a localised allergic reaction to local anaesthesia) [42].

A retrospective analysis of patients treated with Stretta®, which was published in 2002, follows 558 patients who had been treated in 33 institutions. Median follow-up was eight months. A standardised questionnaire was administered by the treating doctor to the patient. Improved reflux symptoms within the first two months were reported by 68.7% of patients; 14.6% reported an improvement after two to six months, and 8.1% after six months. Before treatment, 50% complained of symptoms in spite of taking acid suppressing drugs; this fell to 10% after treatment. The patients categorised the severity of their reflux symptoms as medium to severe in 73.7%; this fell to 23.0% after treatment. Patients were able to reduce their use of proton pump inhibitors significantly or step down to less strong drugs, such as H_2 receptor blockers or antacid drugs [43].

An interesting study was published in 2003. This study compared the effectiveness of the Stretta treatment with a sham treatment. During the sham treatment, the Stretta catheter was inserted and the balloon blown up, but the radiofrequency needles were not deployed. Results were compared after six months. Patients whom had initially received the sham treatment only were then able to choose active treatment. Initially, 35 patients had received active treatment and 29 the sham treatment. After six months the scores in the groups receiving active treatment were significantly better than those in the sham treatment group (reflux: $P < 0.05$; quality of life: 0.03%). The need for medication was the same in both groups; as was the median acid exposure of the distal esophagus as determined by pH measurement. Only subgroup analysis of patients with clinical improvement after active therapy showed a significant fall in acid exposure compared with the baseline value ($P < 0.01$) [44].

Conclusion and evaluation

Although gastro-esophageal reflux disease present a multifactorial and complex pathology, treatment with drugs has become simple, effective, and successful since the proton pump inhibitors were introduced. Only a minority of patients taking a high-dose regimen still complains about symptoms or has to switch to other, less effective drugs because of adverse effects associated with the proton pump inhibitors. The recommendation for these patients is usually surgical therapy, namely laparoscopic fundoplication. In addition, a particular group of patients may seek an alternative to a permanent drug regimen if they tolerate the proton pump inhibitors well.

Endoscopic reflux procedures offer an attractive alternative. Their advantages are obvious: they can be performed an outpatient basis and under sedation. Some of the procedures are reversible. In case of treatment failure, laparoscopic fundoplication is possible without presenting problems, despite previous treatment. Even multiple procedures are possible. However, in spite of this, endoscopic treatment should be recommended cautiously and under several provisos. Only patients who have typical reflux symptoms that respond to proton pump inhibitors and no (or only a small) hiatus hernia should have endoscopic treatment. The sparse data assessing the success rates of the individual procedures were collected on such patients. Whether patients with larger hiatus hernias and/or volume reflux might benefit from endoscopic treatment remains unknown. It is also unknown whether complications of reflux disease, such as Barrett's esophagus or adenocarcinoma, are influenced by endoscopy treatment.

Sufficient data are available only for two endoscopic procedures-gastroplasty (EndoCinch®) and radiofrequency ablation (Stretta®). Both therapies have been approved in the United States in 2000, and several thousand patients per treatment have been treated. About two-thirds of patients can expect a successful outcome, although this applies only to reflux symptoms. An improvement of the objective variables, such as acid load of the distal esophagus or esophagitis cannot be expected. Long-term data are not available. Initial observations imply that the effect of these treatments wear off over the years – similar to laparoscopic fundoplication – and that drug treatment will become necessary, albeit possible at reduced dosages [19], [25].

References

[1] El-Serag HB, Sonnenberg A (1999) Opposing time trends of peptic ulcer and reflux disease. Gut 43: 327–333

[2] Locke G, Talley N, Fett S et al (1997) Prevalence and clinical spectrum of gastroesophageal reflux: a population-based study in Olmsted County, Minnesota. Gastroenterology 112: 1448–1452

[3] Madisch A, Kulich KR, Malfertheiner P, Ziegler K, Bayerdörffer E, Miehlke S, Labenz J, Carlsson J, Wiklund IK (2003) Impact of reflux disease on general and disease-related quality of life-evidence from a recent comparative methodological study in Germany. Z Gastroenterol 41: 1137–1143

[4] Revicki DA, Wood M, Maton PN, Sorensen S (1998) The impact of gastroesophageal reflux disease on health related quality of life. Am J Med 104: 252–258

[5] Dent J, Brun J, Fendrick F, Fennerty MB et al (1995) On behalf of the Genval workshop group: an evidence-based appraisal of reflux disease management–the Geneval workshop report. Gut 44 (Suppl 2)

[6] Dent J (1998) Gastro-oesophageal reflux disease. Digestion 59: 433–445

[7] Lagergren J, Bergstrom R, Lindgren A et al (1999) Symptomatic gastroesophageal reflux as a risk factor for esophageal adenocarcinoma. New Engl J Med 340: 825–831

[8] Bytzer P, Christensen PB, Damkier P, Vinding K, Seersholm N (1999) Adenocarcinoma of the esophagus and Barrett's esophagus: a population-based study. Am J Gastroenterol 94: 86–91

[9] Schilling D, Riemann JF (2003) Evidenzbasierte konservative Therapie der gastroösophagealen Refluxkrankheit. Internist 44: 21–27

[10] Lagergren J, Bergström R, Nyren Q (2000) No relation between body mass and gastro-oesophageal reflux symptoms in a swedish population based study. Gut 47: 26–29

[11] Harvey RF, Gordon PC, Hadley N et al (1987) Effects of sleeping with be head raised and ranitidine in patients with severe peptic esophagitis. Lancet 2: 1200–1203

[12] Pehl C, Pfeiffer A, Wendl B, Kaess H (1997) Effect of decaffeination of coffee on gastroesophageal reflux in patients with reflux disease. Aliment Pharmacol Ther 11: 483–486

[13] Pehl C, Waizenhofer A, Wendl B, Schmidt T, Schepp W, Pfeiffer A (1999) Effect of low and high fat meals on lower esophageal sphincter motility and gastroesophageal reflux in healthy subjects. Am J Gastroenterol 94: 1192–1196

[14] Klinkenberg-Knol EC, Nelis F, Dent J et al (2000) Long-term omeprazole treatment in resistant gastroesophageal reflux disease: efficacy, safety, and influence on gastric mucosa. Gastroenterology 118: 661–669

[15] E.A.E.S. (1997) Laparoscopic antireflux surgery for gastroesophageal reflux disease (GERD). Results of a consensus development conference. Surg Endosc 11: 413–426

[16] Fuchs KH, Feussner H (2003) Laparoskopische Fundoplikatio. Internist 44: 36–42

[17] Terry M, Smith CD, Branum GD, Galloway K, Waring JP, Hunter JG (2001) Outcomes of laparoscopic fund-

oplication for gastroesophageal reflux disease and paraesophageal hernia. Surg Endosc 15: 691–699

[18] Sullivan EM, Pelletier EM, Richter JE (2002) Use of acid reduction therapy and medical costs among medically vs. surgically managed GERD patients. Am J Gastroenterol 97: S239

[19] Spechler SJ, Lee E, Ahnen D, Goyal RK, Hiano I, Ramirez F, Raufman JP, Sampliner R, Schnell T, Sontag S, Vlahcevic ZR, Young R, Williford W (2001) Long-term outcome of medical and surgical therapies for gastroesophageal reflux disease: follow-up of a randomized controlled trial. JAMA 285: 2331–2338

[20] Swain C (1999) Endoscopic suturing. Ballière's Clinical Gastroenterology 13: 97–108

[21] Filipi C, Lehman G, Rothstein R et al (2001) Transoral, flexible endoscopic suturing for treatment of GERD: a multicenter trial. Gastrointest Endosc 51: 416–422

[22] Park P, Kjellin T, Kadirkamanthan S, Appleyard MN, Swain P (2001) Results of endoscopic gastroplasty for gastroesophageal reflux disease. Gastrointest Endosc 53: AB 115

[23] Mahmood Z, McMahon BP, Arfin Q, Byrne PJ, Reynolds JV, Murphy EM, Weir DG (2003) Endocinch therapy for gastro-oesophageal reflux disease: a one year prospective follow up. Gut 52(1): 34–39

[24] Haber GB, Marcon NE, Kortan P, Kandel G, Cirocco M, Basset N (2001) A 2 year follow-up of 25 patients undergoing endoluminal gastric plication (ELPG) for gastroesophageal reflux disease (GERD). Gastrointest Endosc 53: AB116

[25] Rothstein R, Pohl H, Growe M et al (2001) Endoscopic gastric plication for the treatment of GERD: Two year follow-up results. Am J Gastroenterol 96: S35

[26] Chadalavada R, Lin E, Swafford V, Sedghi S, Smith CD (2004) Comparative results of endoluminal gastroplassty and laparoscopic antireflux surgery for the treatment of GERD. Surg Endosc 18: 261–265

[27] Thomson M, Fritscher-Ravens A, Hall S, Afzal N, Ashwood P, Swain CP (2004) Endoluminal gastroplication in children with significant gastro-oesophageal reflux disease. Gut 53: 1745–1750

[28] Chuttani R, Kozarek R, Critchlow J, Lo S, Pleskow D, Brandwein S, Lembo T (2002) A novel endoscopic full-thickness plicator for treatment of GERD: an animal model study. Gastrointest Endosc 56: 116–122

[29] Chuttani R, Sud R, Sachdev G, Puri R, Kozarek R, Haber G, Pleskow D, Zaman M, Lembo A (2003) A novel endoscopic full-thickness plicator for the treatment of GERD: a pilot study. Gastrointest Endosc 58 (5): 770–776

[30] Pleskow D, Rothstein R, Lo S, Hawes R, Kozarek R, Haber G, Gostout C, Lembo A (2004) Endoscopic full-thickness plication for the treatment of GERD: a multicenter trial. Gastrointest Endosc 59: 163–171

[31] Mason RJ, Hughes M, Lehman GA, Chiao G, Deviere J, Silverman DE, DeMeester TR, Peters JH (2002) Endoscopic augmentation of the cardia with a biocompatible injectable polymer (Enteryx) in a porcine model. Surg Endosc 16: 386–391

[32] Deviere J, Pastorelli A, Louis H, de Maertelaer V, Lehman G, Cicala M, Le Moine O, Silverman D, Costamagna G (2002) Endoscopic implantation of a biopolymer in the lower esophageal sphincter for gastroesophageal reflux: a pilot study. Gastrointest Endosc 55: 335–341

[33] Johnson DA, Ganz R, Aisenberg J, Cohen LB, Deviere J, Foley TR, Haber GB, Petrs JH, Lehman GA (2003) Endoscopic, deep mural implantation of Enteryx for the treatment of GERD: 6-month follow-up of a multicenter trial. Am J Gastroenterol 98: 250–258

[34] Johnson DA, Ganz R, Aisenberg J, Cohen LB, Deviere J, Foley TR, Haber GB, Petrs JH, Lehman GA (2003) Endoscopic implantation of enteryx for treatment of GERD: 12-month results of a prospective, multicenter tral. Am J Gastroenterol 98: 1921–1930

[35] Tintillier M, Chaput A, Kirch L, Martinet JP, Pochet JM, Cuvelier C (2004) Esophageal abscess complicating endoscopic treatment of refractory gastroesophageal reflux disease by Enteryx injection: a first case report. Am J Gastroenterol 99: 1856–1858

[36] El Nakadi I, Closset J, De Moor V, Coppens E, Zalcman M, Deviere J, Gelin M (2004) Laparoscopic Nissen fundoplication after failure of Enteryx injection into the lower esophageal sphincter. Surg Endosc 18: 818–820

[37] Fockens P, Bruno M, Kirsch D et al (2002) Endoscopic augmentation of the lower esophageal sphincter. Pilot study with the gatekeeper reflux repair system in patients with GERD. Gastrointest Endosc 55:AB257

[38] Fockens P, Bruno MJ, Gabbrielli A, Odegaard S, Hatlebakk J, Allescher HD, Rosch T, Rhodes M, Bastid C, Rey J, Boyer J, Muehldorffer S, van den Hombergh U, Costamagna G (2004) Endoscopic augmentation of the lower esophageal sphincter for the treatment of gastroesophageal reflux disease: multicenter study of the gatekeeper reflux repair system. Endoscopy 36: 682–689

[39] Hirsch DP, Tytgat GNJ, Boeckxstaens GEE (2002) Review article: transient lower oesophageal sphincter relaxations – a pharmacological target for gastro-oesophageal reflux disease. Aliment Pharmacol Ther 16: 17–26

[40] Utley DS, Kim M, Mark A, Vierra A, Triadafilopoulos G (2000) Augmentation of lower esophageal sphincter pressure and gastric yield pressure after radiofrequency energy delivery to the gastroesophageal junction: a porcine model. Gastrointest Endosc 52: 81–86

[41] Triadafilopoulos G, Dibaise JK, Nostrant TT, Stollman NH, Anderson PK, Edmundowicz SA, Castell DO, Kim MS, Rabine JC, Utley DS (2001) Radiofrequency energy delivery to the gastroesophageal junction for the treatment of GERD. Gastrointest Endosc 53: 407–415

[42] Triadafilopoulos G, DiBaise JK, Nostrant TT, Stollman NH, Anderson PK, Wolfe MM, Rothstein RI, Wo JM, Corley DA, Patti MG, Antignano LV, Goff JS, Edmundowicz SA, Castell DO, Rabine JC, Kim MS, Utley DS (2002) The Stretta procedure for the treatment of GERD: 6 and 12 month follow-up of the U.S. open label trial. Gastrointest Endosc 55: 149–156

[43] Wolfsen HC, Richards WO (2002) The stretta procedure for the treatment of GERD: a registry of 558 patients. J Laparoendosc Adv Surg Tech 12: 395–402

[44] Corley DA, Kath P, Wo JM, Stefan A, Patti M, Rothstein R, Edmundowicz S, Kline M, Mason R, Wolfe MM (2003) Improvement of gastroesophageal reflux symptoms after radiofrequency energy: a randomized, Sham-controlled trial. Gastroenterology 125: 668–676

[45] Islam S, Geiger JD, Coran AG, Teitelbaum DH (2004) Use of radiofrequency ablation of the lower esophageal sphincter to treat recurrent gastroesophageal reflux disease. J Pediatr Surg 39: 282–286

Chapter 13

INDICATION FOR ANTIREFLUX SURGERY

K.-H. Fuchs[1] • M. Fein[2] • J. Maroske[2] • W. Breithaupt[1] • I. Hammer[1]

1 Department of Surgery, Markus-Krankenhaus, Frankfurter Diakonie-Kliniken, Frankfurt am Main, Germany
2 Department of Surgery, University of Würzburg, Würzburg, Germany

Introduction

It is an understandable request of gastroenterologists and surgeons in clinical practice to have a precise list of indications for antireflux surgery. This is rather difficult because it is in contrast to the multifactorial aspects that should be summarized in such a list of indications in order to respond to the different needs in a differentiated therapeutic spectrum to individualize antireflux therapy. Currently there is a remarkable number of randomized trials available focusing on technical aspects of antireflux surgery [1]–[5]. However, there is very little evidence based information to justify certain factors for the indication of antireflux surgery. This chapter reflects all the different aspects which are part of the management of gastroesophageal reflux disease and play a role in the indication for surgery.

The following factors are major issues in the discussion about the indication for laparoscopic antireflux surgery:

(1) a precise definition of the disease,
(2) the therapeutic aim of medical and surgical therapy,
(3) the analysis of results of different therapeutic strategies in order to identify patient subgroups which would benefit more from one or the other therapeutic regiment,
(4) a risk analysis and
(5) cost-benefit-considerations.

With the advent of minimal access technique antireflux surgery has boomed in the past ten years. In most western countries, where the disease is more prevalent, the number of antireflux operations have more than tripled compared to the time before the introduction of minimal access techniques [6]–[9]. This has happened in a time, when the most potent antisecretory drugs were on the market, which stimulates the controversal discussion between gastroenterologists and surgeons regarding the indication for surgery [10], [11]. In several consensus projects in the past ten years indication for surgery has been more or less addressed but no widely accepted rules exist [12]–[14]. Therefore it is necessary to address this issue with a thorough analysis.

Definition of the disease

If an indication for surgery is established, one needs to base this on validated criteria. Most important are criteria for the presence of the disease. However, a general validated definition of GERD does not exist. The disease can be defined by different components and it all depends on the evaluation methods that are used to detect disease. In general, gastroesphageal reflux disease could be defined as the process, in which an abnormal amount of gastric contents or an abnormal composition of a normal amount of gastric fluid is moving back into the esophageal lumen [15], [16]. This contact can cause symptoms and/or erosions of the esophageal mucosa. The disease is clinically present, when there is a risk for complications by excessive reflux and/or a significant impact on health-related well-being because of the patients reflux-related symptoms [14]. The process of reflux and its damage is more complex and multifactorial determined and even a complicated monitoring system such as 24-hour-pH-monitoring, bilirubin-monitoring and/or aspiration-analysis would still have its limitations in determining the precise borderline between normal and abnormal [17]–[19]. In addition little is known about the ability of the esophageal mucosa to resist this abnormal exposure to toxic agents and little is known if a given patient has a low or a high threshold of sensitivity to develop symptoms. As a consequence, it is impossible especially with limited economic resources to diagnose and classify every patient in detail regarding all the above mentioned criteria. Instead, diagnostic work-up must be minimized to a few most useful and reasonable investigations in order to establish the decision for surgery.

In order to obtain more information about the definition of gastroesophageal reflux disease used in clinical practice, the definitions of the disease used in randomized trials for antireflux therapy were analysed. It is surprising what a variety of definitions for the disease have been used by several authors performing randomized trials in the past decades. Table 1 demonstrates the difference in these definitions [20]–[44]. In 25 randomized trials, focusing on surgical therapy of the disease, in the majority of the studies the presence of symptoms and esophagitis were used. Only in about one third of the studies, positive pH-monitoring as a more specific tool to verify pathologic esophageal acid exposure was applicated for the definition. Only a few studies have relied on symptoms only, since symptoms can be an unreliable guide for the presence of gastroesophageal reflux disease [45].

On the other hand it must be emphasized that the presence of typical symptoms such as heartburn and acid or fluid regurgitation has been shown to be a very specific symptom with a positive predictive value for therapeutic success [46]. The authors of this study have shown that a good result of laparoscopic antireflux surgery is more probable in patients with preoperative presence of typical symptoms of reflux such as

Table 1. Application of different criteria for definition of GERD in randomized trials

Author year	Comparison	Criteria for presence of GERD
DeMeester (1974)	Nissen vs Belsey vs Hill	symptoms, pH, endoscopy
Behar (1975)	Angelchick vs surgery	symptoms
Stuart (1989)	Nissen vs Angelchick	pH, symptoms, endo, mano
Thor (1989)	Nissen vs Toupet	symptoms, endo, mano
Kmiot (1991)	Nissen vs Angelchick	symptoms, pH, mano, endo + x-ray
Lundell (1991)	Toupet vs Nissen	symptoms, endoscopy, pH
Spechler (1992)	H2 blocker vs Nissen	symptoms, pH, mano, endo + x-ray
Eyre-Brook (1993)	Nissen vs Angelchick	symptoms, endoscopy, x-ray
Janssen (1993)	Nissen vs ... cardio ...	symptoms, endoscopy, pH
Hill (1994)	Nissen vs Angelchick	symptoms
Ortiz (1996)	H2 blocker vs Nissen (Barrett)	Barrett, pH
Lundell (1996)	Nissen vs Toupet	symptoms
Rydberg (1997)	Nissen vs Toupet	symptoms, mano, endo, pH
Watson (1997)	lap. Nissen vs lap. Nissen ... short gastrics	manometry, endoscopy (selective pH)
Laws (1997)	lap. Nissen vs lap. Toupet	endo, mano, pH, x-ray
Anderson (1998)	lap. nissen vs lap. anterior fundoplication	endoscopy, pH, manometry
Lundell (1998)	Omeprazol vs surgery	symptoms, endoscopy
Rydberg (1999)	Nissen vs Toupet (tailored)	symptoms, endo, mano
Watson (1999)	lap. Nissen vs lap. anterior	symptoms, endoscopy, manometry (pat. selective)
Luostarinen (1999)	Nissen vs Nissen ...	symptoms, endoscopy, pH
Csendes (2000)	Nissen vs Hill	symptoms, mano, pH, endo
Nilsson (2000)	lap. Nissen vs open Nissen	endoscopy, pH
Bais (2000)	lap. Nissen vs open Nissen	symptoms, endoscopy, pH
Lundell (2001, continued)	Omeprazol vs surgery	symptoms, endoscopy
Luostarinen (2001)	lap. AF vs open AF	endoscopy, pH
Spechler (2001, continued)	H2 blocker vs Nissen	symptoms, pH, mano, endo, x-ray

heartburn and regurgitation, a preoperative positive test in 24-hour-esophageal-pH-monitoring showing a pathologic acid exposure in the esophagus and a positive response to proton-pump-inhibitors, indicating that medical acid reduction will also reduce at least to some of the heartburn of the patient.

Regarding the diagnostic requirements, pH-monitoring and endoscopy are necessary for the objective documentation of the disease [12], [13], [45]. With manometry other esophageal functional disorders can be excluded, which potentially cause a postoperative failure, especially spastic disorders [12], [13], [47]. Since a weak lower esophageal sphincter has been shown to be a prognostic bad sign regarding the future prognosis of GERD, one could use this criterium for the indication [48]. In addition, selection of patients with preoperative normal lower esophageal sphincter parameters can be indicative for worse postoperative results [49]. However, several studies have shown, that its predictive value for the postoperative results remains controversial and is therefore not recommended by gastroenterologists [50], [51].

Currently gastroesophageal reflux diease has been redefined in three subgroups [14], [48]. These subgroups are nonerosive reflux disease, erosive reflux disease and Barrett's esophagus. This is a reasonable separation. However, it must be kept in mind that there is some overlapping especially between patients with Barrett's esophagus and erosive gastroesophageal reflux disease, since it has been shown that this overlapping is present in at least 30% of the Barrett's patients in several series [16], [19].

This classification of reflux patients is very important because it reflects an increasing severity of the disease and this should be especially kept in mind by surgeons when discussing indication for a patient [13], [47]. There should be a general trend to operate severe cases of gastroesophageal reflux disease with a reduced quality of life because for most patients with a mild or moderate expression of the disease, proton-pump-inhibitors are well sufficient for symptom control.

For several years Barrett's esophagus has been one of the main focuses within the complex of gastroesophageal reflux disease due to its association with the adenocarcinoma of the cardia and the esophagus [19], [52]–[55]. Some authors have proposed Barrett's esophagus as a clear indication for surgery independent from reflux disease in order to prevent the development of adenocarcinoma [56]. From publications of recent years, it can be deducted that neither proton-pump-inhibitor therapy nor antireflux surgery can guarantee the prevention of the progression towards cancer [57]. In a recent meta-analysis it has been shown that the probability of developing cancer after antireflux surgery is not significant different from proton-pump-inhibitor therapy. Therefore, it must be stated that Barrett's esophagus alone is not an indication for antireflux surgery. However, many patients with severe reflux disease also suffer from Barrett's esophagus [16], [19], [58]. The severity of the underlying reflux disease is a leading criteria for the establishment of an indication for antireflux surgery. Gastroenterologists have used the arguement against fundoplication since it would be less favorable to perform endoscopic controlls in Barrett's patients after a fundoplication. This argument is not valid, since experienced endoscopists have no problem to visualize the distal esophageal area and the gastroesophageal junction after a fundoplication.

Therapeutic aims

Currently there is even a controversal discussion between gastroenterologists and surgeons regarding the therapeutic aims in controling gastroesophageal reflux. Two decades ago the undoubtable aim of the therapy for the management was the healing of esophagitis, the removal of symptoms ant the removal and/or prevention of complications of the disease [15]. The presence of severe esophagitis was for many surgeons an indication for surgery. Today many gastroenterologists are convinced that the only criteria for therapeutic success is the removal of symptoms, may it occur with healing of esophagitis or not [14]. In surgical literature, both removal of symptoms and healing of esophagitis is necessary to determine a successful surgical therapy [12], [13]. In some papers even the documentation of a negative 24-hour-esophageal-pH-monitoring is used as definitive criteria for success.

This discussion is important in the controversy about the indication for laparoscopic antireflux surgery, since many gastroenterologists have the opinion that there is hardly any indication for antireflux surgery because after antireflux surgery patients still need in a high percentage proton-pump-inhibitor therapy [44]. This question will be addressed in detail further below.

In summary, for the establishment of the indication of a surgical procedure, gastroenterologists and surgeons should use more than one criteria for the definition and the verification of gastroesophageal reflux disease. In several consensus projects, it was documented that endoscopic signs of esophagitis should have been documented at present or in the past at least once. In addition, a positive 24-hour-pH-monitoring together with typical symptoms of the disease such as heartburn and/or regurgitation are important criteria for the presence of disease, which are needed for indication.

Analysis of results of laparoscopic antireflux surgery, identification of subgroups with therapeutic benefit

Failure to medical therapy was used as indication for some time. Today, this approach regarding the relation between therapeutic success and indication needs more differentiation. There has always been an attempt to identify certain subgroups of patients with gastroesophageal reflux disease, who especially benefit from surgery compared to prolonged conservative therapy.

There are only two relevant randomized trials comparing operative versus medical therapy [25], [42], [44]. Both trials compared the open technique in antireflux surgery to medical therapy. The first trial was performed in the late 1980ies comparing Nissen open fundoplication versus medical therapy with antacids in H2-blocker [25]. The results of this trial have shown an advantage for the Nissen fundoplication evaluating a clinical score as well as reduction in the presence of esophagitis after one year and the mean of the percentage of esophageal acid exposure after one year. Ten years later, in which many patients had switched towards a proton-pump-inhibitor treatment, these patients were re-evaluated and did not show any significant difference when comparing surgical patients without drugs and the medical group patients under proton-pump-inhibitor treatment [44]. However approximately 30% of the patients in the surgical group were taking proton-pump-inhibitors. The authors concluded that the indication for surgery to exclude the necessity of long-term medication would be no longer valid. The results of this study were discussed very controversally since the spectrum of the patients treated in this trial was not representative for the average reflux patients in western countries.

In a Scandinavian randomized trial, comparing medical versus surgical therapy, the measurement of success was time interval until a failure occured, in which the failure was defined as severe heartburn and regurgitation and/or esophagitis grade 2 as well as severe dysphagia and odynophagia [42]. The results of this trial showed, that if dosage of proton-pump-inhibitor Omeprazol is not restricted, there was no significant difference in failure rate between the antireflux surgery and Omeprazol. Recently the authors have presented seven year follow-up data, indicating that after seven years the slight advantage of the operative versus Omeprazol treatment has reached the level of significance.

So far, there is no randomized trial available comparing laparoscopic antireflux surgery with proton-pump-inhibitors. From the randomized trials, where laparoscopic antireflux surgery is involved, the results show much more favorable results regarding reflux recurrence than the above mentioned study with a recurrence rate of 30%. Table 2 demonstrates these results [59]–[61]. It can be summarized, that the failure rate is at approximately around 15% after three to five years if the operation is performed in centers that are able to do studies. It must be also emphasized that in none of these series regarding randomized studies patients died from laparoscopic antireflux surgery while in greater prospective or retrospective series the mortality was approximately 0,2 to 0,6%.

Considering the prognosis of the disease, it has been shown that the severity of the disease is accompanied with a higher incidence of complications [62]. It has also been proven that the presence of mechanical incompetence of the sphincter is associated with a worse prognosis of the reflux disease over the years [48]. Severity of the disease, mechanical incompetence of the lower esophageal sphincter as well as the presence of a hiatal hernia are factors which can aggravate the disease and therefore are considered to be criteria which encourage the indication for surgery [12], [13], [47], [63], [64].

Risk analysis

It must be emphasized that antireflux surgery is usually a choice for elective surgery after well prepared diagnostic work-up in order to verify the criteria for indication of surgery. A risk analysis of the general condition of the patient should be added especially in patients with concomitant disease or in the elderly. There is recent evidence that patients with concomitant disease and patients older than 70 years face a higher risk of probability of fatal outcome. Therefore, the decision for surgery should be well adjusted according to a previous risk analysis based on the evaluation of the associated factors [65].

Cost benefit considerations

If one of the possible therapies would have a substantial better cost-benefit-ratio, this would have an influence on indication for surgery. In the past ten years several cost benefit analyses have been published, comparing medical and surgical therapy [66]–[68]. These analyses are usually based on the economic systems of the different countries where the studies were performed. The results vary dramatically with a break even point, where costs of conservative therapy match with surgical therapy between two years and ten years. Only one study was based on a randomized trial in Scandinavia [68]. In this analysis, there were even differencies between the four different Scandinavian countries in costs for surgical and medical therapy. In three of these countries surgical therapy was remarkably more expensive over three year follow-up basis compared to medical therapy. In one country these data were comparable. As a consequence with decreasing expenses for medical therapy because of the use of generic proton-pump-inhibitors and possible increasing cost for disposable instruments in laparoscopic surgery it seems to be difficult to use cost benefit analyses as an argument for the indication of laparoscopic surgery.

In countries where the economic advantage of short reconvalescence resulting in a short hospital stay and early return to work pays off regarding health insurance, laparoscopic surgery indeed could be advantageous. But this waits to be proven in large series.

Synapsis of factors for the indication of surgery

From all data available it must be concluded that gastroesophageal reflux disease can be treated sufficiently both by proton-pump-inhibitors and by anti-

Table 2. Randomized trials comparing open versus laparoscopic antireflux surgery

Author recruitment	Random-group		Morbidity N (%)	Patient follow-up	Reflux recurrence N (%)	Dysphagia N (%)
Laine	Open	55	7 (13)	30 (12mo)	3 (10)	4 (13)
(1992–95)	Lap	55	3 (8)	18 (12mo)	0	0
Heikkinen	Open	20	5 (25)	19 (24mo)	2 (11)	11 (58)
(1995–96)	Lap	22	3 (14)	19 (24mo)	0	9 (48)
Bais	Open	46	8 (17)	46 (3mo)	1 (2)	0
(1997–98)	Lap	57	5 (9)	57 (3mo)	2 (4)	7 (12)
Luostarinen	Open	15	0	13 (17mo)	0	6 (46)
(1994–95)	Lap	13	1 (8)	13 (17mo)	0	4 (31)
Chrysos	Open	50	38 (76)	50 (12mo)	1 (2)	2 (4)
(1993–98)	Lap	56	12 (21)	56 (12mo)	2 (4)	2 (4)
Nilsson	Open	30	0	23 (60mo)	4 (17)	5 (22)
(1995–97)	Lap	30	0	17 (60mo)	2 (12)	7 (41)

reflux surgery preferably in a minimal access technique. However, surgical therapy can have severe complications and even fatalities and therefore the indication for surgery must be well adjusted. It should be a general rule, independent of subgroups (non-erosive reflux disease, erosive reflux disease, Barrett's esophagus), that prior to any surgical considerations, the patient should be treated by adequate dosage of proton-pump-inhibitors. Following this treatment line most of the patients will be satisfied and should be followed by the rules of medical therapy as published by many gastroenterologic societies. The more severe reflux symptoms and the disease clinically is, the more precise diagnostic work-up should be preformed in order to evaluate the condition of the patient. It can not be overemphasized, that preoperative diagnostic work-up should include endoscopy and pH-monitoring to document the disease and in addition manometry to exclude any other esophageal motility disorder. If medical therapy provides only limited symptom control and limited prevention of complications, the more the surgical alternative should be prefered.

Following these ideas an indication for surgery in patients with a none erosive reflux disease is an exception. However, there have been reports that laparoscopic antireflux surgery is successful in cases with nonerosive reflux disease in controlling symptoms. Therefore, the decision for antireflux surgery in a NERD-patient with refractory treatment can be establish only after an adequate long segment of medical therapy with no success and the willingness of the patient to undergo a possible risk of operative morbidity. The majority of the indications are established in patients with erosive reflux disease with or without Barrett esophagus. The overlap between these two groups is large and reaches up to 30% in some series. Several gastroenterologic and surgical societies or initiatives have discussed and published lists of indication for antireflux surgery. Common criteria among these publications are:

(1) patients with persistent or recurrent symptoms usually non-acid related such as volume reflux, food and fluid regurgitation, respiratory symptoms as hoarseness, chronic cough under adequate sufficient proton-pump-inhibitor therapy.
(2) Persistent or recurrent complications despite adequate proton-pump-inhibitor therapy such as persistent esophagitis, chronic ulceration and strictures.
(3) Side effects of medication despite changing medication with adequate dosage resulting in reduced quality of life due to symptoms.
(4) Anatomical changes such as large hiatal hernias, completely incompetent lower esophageal sphincter, massive combined acid and duodenogastroesophageal reflux.

A questionable indication is a patient with unwillingness to accept a long-term medication despite the fact that the adequate proton-pump-inhibitor therapy is successfull and reduces symptoms.

In summary, indication for antireflux surgery should be based on several facts such as the objectified presence of the disease by sufficient diagnostic testing, the presence of symptoms to satisfy the patients after surgery with the relief of symptoms, the sufficient and adequate medical treatment prior to surgery in order to ensure that all conservative attempts have been fulfilled, which usually increases the patient`s motivation for surgery. Prior to surgery, a risk analysis should be performed especially in patients with concomitant disease and those patients above 70 years of age. In addition, it must be emphasized that psychologic influences are possible on the patient's clinical presentations of symptoms on esophagus and stomach and could overlap the clinical picture. If there is any doubt concerning this matter, psychologic evaluation is important.

References

[1] Patterson EJ, Herron DM, Hansen PD, Ramzi N, Standage BA, Swanstrom LL (2000) Effect of an esophageal bougie on the incidence of dysphagia following nissen fundoplication; a prospective, blinded, randomized clinical trial. Arch Surg 135(9): 1055–1061; Discussion 1061–1062
[2] Peillon C, Manouvrier JL, Labreche J, Kaeffer N, Testart DP (1994) Should be vagus nerves be isolated from the fundoplication wrap? A prospective study. Arch Surg 129(8): 814–818
[3] Watson DI, Pike GK, Baigrie RJ, Mathew G, Devitt PG, Britten-Jones R, Jamieson GG (1997) Prospective

double-blind randomized trial of laparoscopic Nissen fundoplication with division and without division of short gastric vessels. Ann Surg 226(5): 642–652

[4] Patterson EJ, Herron DM, Hansen PD, Ramzi N, Standage BA, Swanstrom LL (2000) Effect of an esophageal bougie on the incidence of dysphagia following nissen fundoplication; a prospective, blinded, randomized clinical trial. Arch Surg 135(9): 1055–1061; Discussion 1061–1062

[5] Zornig C, Strate U, Fibbe C, Emmermann A, Layer P (2002) Nissen vs Toupet laparoscopic fundoplication. Surg Endosc 16(5): 758–766

[6] Jamieson GG, Watson DI, Britten-Jones R, Mitchell PC, Anvari M (1994) Laparoscopic Nissen fundoplication. Ann Surg 220: 137–145

[7] Dallemagne B, Weerts JM, Jehaes C, Markiewicz S (1996) Causes of failures of laparoscopic antireflux operations. Surg Endosc 10: 305–310

[8] Perdikis G, Hinder RA, Lund RJ, Raiser F, Katada N (1997) Laparoscopic Nissen fundoplication: Where do we stand? Surg Laparoscopy Endoscopy 7: 117–121

[9] Hüttl TP, Hohle M, Meyer G, Schildberg FW (2002) Antirefluxchirurgie in Deutschland. Chirurg 73(5): 451–461

[10] Vigneri S, Termini R, Leandro G, Badalamenti S, Pantalena M, Savarino V, Di Mario F, Battaglia G, Mela GS, Pilotto A (1995) A comparison of five maintenance therapies for reflux esophagitis. N Engl J Med 326: 1106–1110

[11] Klinkenberg-Knol EC, Nelis F, Dent J et al (2000) Long-term Omeprazole treatment in resistant gastroesophageal reflux disease: efficacy, safety, and influence on gastric mucosa. Gastroenterology 118: 661–669

[12] Eypasch E, Neugebauer E, Fischer F, Troidl H (1997) Laparoscopic antireflux surgery for gastroesophageal reflux disease (GERD). Results of a consensus development conference. Surg Endoscopy 11: 413–426

[13] Fuchs KH, Feussner H, Bonavina L, Collard JM, Coosemans W for the European Study Group for Antireflux Surgery (1997) Current status and trends in laparoscopic antireflux surgery: results of a consensus meeting. Endoscopy 29: 298–308

[14] Dent J, Brun J, Fendrick AM, Fennerry MB, Janssens J et al (1999) Genval Workshop Group: An evidence-based appraisal of reflux disease management. Gut 44: S1–S16

[15] DeMeester TR, Johnson LF, Kent AH (1974) Evaluation of current operations for the prevention of gastroesophageal reflux. Ann Surg 180: 511–525

[16] Fuchs KH, Freys SM, Heimbucher J, Fein M, Thiede A (1995) Pathophysiologic spectrum in patients with gastroesophageal reflux disease in a surgical GI function laboratory. Diseases of the Esophagus 8: 211–217

[17] DeMeester TR, Johnson LS, Joseph GJ, Toscano MS, Hall AW, Skinner DB (1976) Patterns of gastroesophageal reflux in health and disease. Ann Surg 184: 459–470

[18] Vaezi MF, Richter JE (1995) Synergism of acid and duodeno-gastro-esophageal reflux in complicated Barrett's esophagus. Surgery 117: 699–704

[19] Fein M, Ireland AP, Ritter MP, Peters JH, Hagen JA, Bremner CG, DeMeester TR (1997) Duodenogastric reflux potentiates the injurious effects of gastroesophageal reflux. J Gastrointest Surg 1: 27–33

[20] Behar J, Sheahan DG, Biancani P, Spiro HM, Storer EH (1975) Medical and surgical management of reflux esophagitis. New Engl J Med: 263–268

[21] Stuart RC, Dawson K, Keeling P, Byrne PJ, Hennessy TP (1989) A prospective randomized trial of Angelchik prosthesis versus Nissen fundoplication. Br J Surg 76: 86–89

[22] Thor KBA, Silander T (1989) A long-term randomized prospective trial of the Nissen procedure versus a modified Toupet technique. Ann Surg 210: 719–724

[23] Kmiot WA, Kirby RM, Akinola D, Temple JG (1991) Prospective randomized trial of Nissen fundoplication and Angelchik prosthesis in the surgical treatment of medically refractory gastro-oesophageal reflux disease. Br J Surg 78: 1181–1184

[24] Lundell L, Abrahamsson H, Ruth M, Sandberg L, Olbe L (1991) Lower esophageal sphincter characteristics and esophageal acid exposure following partial or 360° fundoplication: Results of a prospective, randomized, clinical study. World J Surg 15: 115–121

[25] Spechler SJ and the department of veterans affairs gastroesophageal reflux disease study group (1992) Comparison of medical and surgical therapy for complicated gastroesophageal reflux disease in veterans. N Engl J Med 326,12: 786–792

[26] Eyre-Brook IA, Codling BW, Gear MWL (1993) Results of a prospective randomized trial of the Angelchik prosthesis and of a consecutive series of 119 patients. Br J Surg 80: 602–604

[27] Janssen IMC, Gouma DJ, Klementschitsch P, van der Heyde MN, Obertop H (1993) Prospective randomized comparison of teres cardiopexy and Nissen fundoplication in the surgical therapy of gastro-oesophageal reflux disease. Br J Surg 80: 875–878

[28] Hill ADK, Walsh TN, Bolger CM, Byrne PJ, Hennessy TPJ (1994) Randomized controlled trial comparing Nissen fundoplication and the Angelchik prosthesis. Br J Surg 81: 72–74

[29] Ortiz EA, Martinez de Haro LF, Parrilla P, Morales G, Molina J, Bermejo J, Liron R, Aguilar J (1996) Conservative treatment versus antireflux surgery in Barrett's oesophagus: long-term results of a prospective study. Br J Surg 83(2): 274–278
[30] Lundell L, Abrahamsson H, Ruth M, Rydberg L, Lonroth H, Olbe L (1996) Long-term results of a prospective randomized comparison of total fundic wrap (Nissen-Rossetti) or semifundoplication (Toupet) for gastro-oesophageal reflux. Br J Surg 83(6): 830–835
[31] Rydberg L, Ruth M, Lundell L (1997) Does oesophageal motor function improve with time after successful antireflux surgery? Results of a prospective, randomized clinical study. Gut 41: 82–86
[32] Watson DI, Pike GK, Baigrie RJ, Mathew G, Devitt PG, Britten-Jones R, Jamieson GG (1997) Prospective double-blind randomized trial of laparoscopic Nissen fundoplication with division and without division of short gastric vessels. Ann Surg 226(5): 642–652
[33] Laws HL, Clements RH, Swillie CM (1997) A randomized, prospective comparison of the Nissen fundoplication versus the Toupet fundoplication for gastroesophageal reflux disease. Ann Surg 225(6): 647–653; Discussion 654
[34] Anderson JA, Myers JC, Watson DI, Gabb M, Mathew G, Jamieson GG (1998) Concurrent fluoroscopy and manometry reveal differences in laparoscopic Nissen and anterior fundoplication. Dig Dis Sci 43(4): 847–853
[35] Lundell L, Dalenbäck J, Hattlebakk J et al (1998) Outcome of open antireflux surgery as assessed in a nordic multicentre, prospective clinical trial. Eur J Surg 164: 751–757
[36] Rydberg L, Ruth M, Abrahamsson H, Lundell L (1999) Tailoring antireflux surgery: a randomized clinical trial. World J Surg 23: 612–618
[37] Watson DI, Jamieson GG, Pike GK, Davies N, Richardson M, Devitt PG (1999) Prospective randomized double-blind trial between laparoscopic Nissen fundoplication and anterior partial fundoplication. Br J Surg 86: 123–130
[38] Luostarinen MES, Isolauri JO (1999) Randomized trial to study the effect of fundic mobilization on long-term results of Nissen fundoplication. Br J Surg 86: 614–618
[39] Csendes A, Burdiles P, Korn O, Braghetto I, Huertas C, Rojas J (2000) Late results of a randomized clinical trial comparing total fundoplication versus calibration of the cardia with posterior gastropexy. Br J Surg 87. 289–297
[40] Bais JE, Bartelsman JF, Bonjer HJ, Cuesta MA, Go PM, Klinkenberg-Knol EC, van Lanschot JJB, Nadorp JH, Smout AJ, van der Graaf Y (The Netherlands Antireflux Surgery Study Group) (2000) Laparoscopic or conventional Nissen fundoplication for gastroesophageal reflux disease: randomized clinical trial. Lancet 355: 170–174
[41] Nilsson G, Larsson S, Johnsson F (2000) Randomized clinical trial of laparoscopic versus open fundoplication: blind evaluation of recovery and discharge period. Br J Surg 87: 873–878
[42] Lundell L, Miettinen P, Myrvold HE, Pedersen SA, Liedman B, Hatlebakk JG, Julkonen R, Levander K, Carlsson J, Lamm M, Wiklund I (2001) Continued (5-year) followup of a randomized clinical study comparing antireflux surgery and omeprazole in gastroesophageal reflux disease. J Am Coll Surg 192(2): 172–179; Discussion 179–181
[43] Luostarinen M, Virtanen J, Koskinen M, Matikainen M, Isolauri J (2001) Dysphagia and oesophageal clearance after laparoscopic versus open Nissen fundoplication. A randomized, prospective trial. Scand J Gastroenterol 6: 565–571
[44] Spechler SJ, Lee E, Ahnen D, Goyal RK, Hirano I, Williford WO (2001) Long-term outcome of medical and surgical therapies for gastroesophageal reflux disease. JAMA 285: 2331–2338
[45] Costantini M, Crookes PF, Bremner RM, Hoeft SF, Ehsan A, Peters JH, Bremner CG, DeMeester TR (1993) Value of physiologic assessment of foregut symptoms in a surgical practice. Surgery 114(4): 780–786
[46] Campos GM, Peters JH, DeMeester TR, Oberg S, Crookes PF, Tan S, DeMeester SR, Hagen JA, Bremner CG (1999) Multivariate analysis of factors predicting outcome after laparoscopic Nissen fundoplication. J Gastrointest Surg 3(3): 292–300
[47] Peters JH, DeMeester TR, Crookes P, Oberg S, de Vos Shoop M, Hagen JA, Bremner CG (1998) The treatment of gastroesophageal reflux disease with laparoscopic Nissen Fundoplication. Ann Surg 228(1): 40–50
[48] Kuster E, Ros E, Toledo-Pimentel V, Pujol A, Bordas JM, Grande IC (1994) Predictive factors of the long term outcome in gastro-oesophageal reflux disease: six year follow up of 107 patients. Gut 35(1): 8–14
[49] Blom D, Peters JH, DeMeester TR, Crookes P, Hagen JA, DeMeester SR, Bremner CG (2002) Physiologic mechanism and preoperative prediction of new-onset dysphagia after laparoscopic Nissen fundoplication. J Gastrointest Surg 6(1): 22–27
[50] Fang J, Bjorkman D (2002) Prefundoplication testing: is manometry needed? Am J Gastroenterol 97(4): 1056–1058

[51] Fibbe C, Layer P, Keller J et al (2001) Esophageal motility in reflux disease before and after fundoplication: a prospective, randomized, clinical and manometric study. Gastroenterology 121: 5–14
[52] Haggit RC, Tryzelaar J, Ellis FH, Colcher H (1978) Adenocarcinoma complicating columnar-epithelium-lined (Barrett's) esophagus. Am J Clin Pathol 70: 1
[53] Hameeteman W, Tytgat GNJ, Houthoff HJ, Van Den Tweel JG (1989) Barrett's esophagus: development of dysplasia and adenocarcinoma. Gastroenterology 96: 1249–1256
[54] Pera M, Cameron AJ, Trastek VF, Carpenter HA, Zinsmeister AR (1993) Increasing incidence of adenocarcinoma of the esophagus and esophagogastric junction. Gastroenterology 104: 510–513
[55] Lagergren J, Bergström R, Lindgren A, Nyrén O (1999) Symptomatic gastroesophageal reflux as a risk factor for esophageal adenocarcinoma. The New England J of Medicine 340: 825–831
[56] DeMeester SR, DeMeester TR (2000) Columnar mucosa and intestinal metaplasia of the esophagus: fifty year controversy. Ann Surg 231(2): 303–321
[57] Corey KE, Schmitz SM, Shaheen NJ (2003) Does a surgical antireflux procedure decrease the incidence of esophageal adenocarcinoma in Barrett's esophagus? A meta-analysis. Am J Gastroenterol 98(11): 2390–2394
[58] Tigges H, Fuchs KH, Maroske J, Fein M, Freys SM, Muller J, Theide A (2001) Combination of endoscopic argon plasma coagulation and antireflux surgery for treatment of Barrett's esophagus. J Gastrointest Surg 5(4): 251–259
[59] Laine S, Rantala A, Gullichsen R, Ovaska J (1997) Laparoscopic vs conventional Nissen fundoplication. A prospective randomized study. Surg Endosc 11: 441–444
[60] Heikkinen TJ, Hakipuro K, Bringman S (2000) Comparison of laparoscopic and open Nissen fundoplication 2 years after operation. A prospective randomized trial. Surg Endosc 355: 170–174
[61] Chrysos E, Tsiaoussis J, Athanasakis E, Vassilakis J, Xynos E (2002) Laparoscopic versus open approach for Nissen fundoplication. Surg Endosc 16: 1679–1684
[62] Stein HJ, Barlow AP, DeMeester TR, Hinder RA (1992) Complications of gastroesophageal reflux disease. Role of the lower esophageal sphincter, esophageal acid and acid/alkaline exposure, and duodenogastric reflux. Ann Surg 216(1): 35–43
[63] Fein M, Ritter MP, DeMeester TR, Oberg S, Peters JH, Hagen JA, Bremner CG (1999) Role of the lower esophageal sphincter and hiatal hernia in the pathogenesis of gastroesophageal reflux disease. J Gastrointest Surg 3(4): 405–410
[64] Jones MS, Sloan SS, Rabine JC, Ebert CC, Huang CF, Kahrilas PJ (2001) Hiatal hernia size is the dominant determinant of esophagitis presence and severity in gastroesophageal reflux disease. Am J Gastroenterol 96(6): 1711–1717
[65] Flum DR, Koepsell T, Heagerty P, Pellegrini CA (2002) The nationwide frequency of major adverse outcomes in antireflux surgery and the role of surgeon experience, 1992–1997. J Am Coll Surg 195(5): 611–618
[66] Heudebert GR, Marks R, Wilcox CM et al (1997) Choice of long-term strategy for the management of patients with severe esophagitis: a cost-utility analysis. Gastroenterology 112: 1078–1086
[67] Fuchs KH, Tigges H, Heimbucher J et al (1997) Laparoskopische Eingriffe bei gastroösophagealer Refluxkrankheit – eine Nutzen-Kosten-Analyse. Zentralbl Chir 122: 1072–1077
[68] Myrvold HE, Lundell L Nordic GERD Study Group (2001) The cost of long-term therapy for gastroesophageal reflux disease: a randomized trial comparing omeprazole and open antireflux surgery. Gut 49(4): 462–463

Chapter 14

THE HISTORY OF SURGERY FOR HIATAL HERNIA AND GASTROESOPHAGEAL REFLUX

R. P. Turk and Alex G. Little

Department of Surgery, Wright State University School of Medicine, Dayton, OH, USA

The surgical treatment of GERD is based on the concept of the bathing of the esophageal epithelium with gastric acid. This understanding is the culmination of both studies of anatomy, physiology, and pathology and radiography of the esophagus, and the clinical experience of treating patients. Each of these disciplines was an incomplete chapter awaiting the development of new technologies. A retrospective review of this progress is helpful in understanding the present state of the surgical treatment of GERD.

The understanding of the function of the esophagus from ancient times is evident from the construction of the word from the Greek as "*oisophagos*" (from "*oisein*" = carry and "*phagema*" = food). In Old English and Old French the Latin *gula* for throat became gullet and that word has been used interchangeably in the old medical literature [1]. The Oxford English Dictionary records the earliest English usage of Ysophagus as 1398 and in a 1541 surgical treatise by Guydon, he states "the Meri called Ysophagus is ye way of the mete and this Meri commeth out of the throte and thyrtem the mydryfe unto ye bely or stomacke." The English continue to use oesophagus, probably to acknowledge the Greek origin of the word.

The oldest medical treatise to mention the gullet is the Edwin Smith Papyrus. This papyrus, one of the four principal medical papyri, deals almost exclusively with wounds or surgical conditions. Edwin Smith, an American Egyptologist, discovered this papyrus at Thebes in 1862. It was translated by Henry Breasted in 1930 and contains 48 surgical case histories classified by the organs affected and is organized from cephalad to caudad [2]. The papyrus ends abruptly at case 48 at the level of the chest. All the cases follow a formula where the "Title" names the condition, "The Examination" describes the findings, followed by the "Diagnosis". All the cases are classified as an "illness which I will treat, contend or not contend", i.e., curable, possibly curable or incurable.

Case 28 has the title "Instructions concerning a wound in his throat". The examination states "If thou examinest a man having a gaping wound of the throat, piercing through his gullet; if he drinks water he chokes and it comes out of the mouth of the wound; it is greatly inflamed, so that he develops fever from it; thou should draw together that wound with stitching." Under diagnosis, "Thou should say concerning him 'One having a wound in his throat, piercing throu to his gullet. An ailment with which I will contend.'" This last statement indicated that it was a possibly curable condition.

Although the physicians of antiquity such as Galen and Aulus Cornelius Celsus must have known something of the anatomy and the pathology of the esophagus, nothing is reported until the publication of the dissections of Andreus Vesalius. Vesalius of Brussels studied at Paris but was unsatisfied with his education and immigrated to Padua. A year after his arrival he was appointed Professor of Anatomy at Padua in 1542 at age 28. Woodblocks of his anatomical dissections were made by Jan Stephen Calcar, a countryman of Vesalius and a pupil of Titian. Although the blocks were carved in Italy, they were sent to Basel to be printed in 1543 by Johannes Oporinus [3]. The book was entitled *De Humani Corporis Fabrica* (*Libri Septum*) or the "structure of the human body in seven books." In the fifth book (*Tabulae Libri Quinti: Organis Nutrioni Quae Cibo Potugu Fit . . .*) "Concerning the Organs Which Minister to Nutrition by Food and Drink," both the anterior aspect of the entire stomach and esophagus together with the veins arteries and nerves inserted into the stomach, and the posterior aspect of the stomach and esophagus are illustrated [4].

Another 150 years passed before Anton Maria Valsalva published his treatise *De Aure Humana*

Tractatus, "Treatise on the Human Ear" in 1704 to describe the upper esophageal sphincter. In this book he described a new description of the soft palate and musculature of the pharynx. He was the first to delineate the cricopharyngeus muscle as a discrete muscle separated by the constrictors of the pharynx and lacking a median raphe [5].

The lower esophageal sphincter has been described as a ring of muscular fibers which act as a valve. This has been called the cardiac sphincter because of its proximity to the heart which lies just across the thickness of the diaphragm. A fold in the lining of the esophagus over the cardiac sphincter is sometimes called Braune's valvule, after Christian Braune, a professor of surgery and anatomy at Leipzig who described it in 1875 [6].

In the age of GERD, the anatomical controversies have mostly involved the distal esophagus. Some questions are the presence or absence of a sphincter, the exact location of the esophago-gastric junction, and the structure of the phreno- esophageal membrane. Friedland, a radiologist, has researched these areas by reviewing the original sources [7]. Thomas Willis in the late 1600's described the sling fibers of the stomach which cause a notch between the left lower esophagus and the stomach and in 1903 Wilhelm His, embryologist and professor of anatomy at Leipzig, called it the incisura cardiaca. In 1906, DJ Cunningham began calling it the angle of His. (The "bundle of His" in the heart was discovered by Wilhelm His Junior while a medical student.) [8]. The phrenoesophageal membrane attaches the esophagus to the diaphragm and was originally described by Galen. The British surgeon Allison emphasized the role of this membrane in preventing the formation of a hiatus hernia. In 1973, Eliska described four types of phreno- esophageal membrane classified by age into the fetal type, the juvenile type, the old age type and the transitional type. These different types are produced by the loss of elastic tissue and fatty infiltration of the membranes which allows for the development of a hiatus hernia [9].

Although, Ambroise Pare' has been attributed as the first to describe a diaphragmatic hernia, his description was not of a hiatus hernia, but of two traumatic hernias of the diagram both discovered at autopsy [10]. The first case was that of a mason "who was wounded in the middle of the diaphragm in its nervous part, of which he died on the third day. I opened the belly and could not find the stomach. This made me marvel greatly, thinking it a monstrous thing to be without a stomach. Then I considered diligently and realized that it must have entered the thorax even though the wound in the diaphragm was no larger than enough to admit the thumb. On opening the thorax I found the stomach filled with air and containing little fluid."

The second case described an artillery captain who was shot through the chest, the wound healed externally but he continued to have a stomach disorder, "like a sort of colic so he could eat only sparingly. Eight months later he developed a severe colic like pain in the epigastrium . . . and died." At autopsy "in the thorax was found a large part of the colon, filled with air; it had entered through a hole only large enough to admit the tip of the little finger, made through the diaphragm by the wound."

When Giovanni Battista Morgagni was almost eighty years old he published a book "*De sedibus, et causis morborum per anatomen indagatis*" (The Origins and Causes of Disease Anatomically Investigated) in which he recorded the findings of 700 autopsies and linked them to the complaints of the patients and the symptoms of their diseases [11]. This marked the advent of anatomic pathology as a separate medical discipline. Morgagni described Pare's case of the mason with the diaphragmatic hernia as well as other's dissections. In Letter LIV Article 13, he first described a paraesophageal hernia. "But in the case of Schoberus we are not wanting in these particulars, as, without any wound, a very vehement cardialgia came on in the morning, at the break of day; attended by very frequent vomiting of an incredible amount of blackish matter, and straining to vomit, so that the young man died on the following night: and within his thorax was found, together with the omentum, and *intestine duodenum* . . . the stomach so distended with that matter, and with flatus, as to compress into a very narrow compass the heart and lungs; having been admitted into that cavity by the same foramen through which the gula is brought down, this foramen being greatly dilated and deprived of its tone." These were considered pathologic curiosities observed at autopsy and no connection was made between the presence of a hernia and the possibility of acid reflux and/or esophageal disease.

Esophageal hiatus hernia was uncommonly described before the advent of radiographic techniques.

One reason was that the classic autopsy technique was to divide the esophagus just above the diaphragm and remove it along with the heart and lungs, thus losing its connections to the abdominal segment and with the stomach. Another was that at autopsy the muscles were relaxed and intra-abdominal pressure diminished and therefore the condition would be overlooked. It required the development of contrast radiography in the first decade of the twentieth century to identify hiatus hernia. This required examination in the recumbent and sometimes in the Trendelenburg position to demonstrate the condition. Once the study was standardized the relative frequent occurrence of hiatus hernia was recognized.

Although neither curiosity about or understanding of GERD were in evidence during the 1800's, there was in 1853 by Bowditch perhaps the first identification of what we now call hiatal hernia [12]. Bowditch reviewed the extant literature on both hiatal hernia and other types of diaphragmatic hernias and as well reported his observations and descriptions of his anatomic findings with these entities as encountered during performance of autopsies. Again, however, there was no attempt to connect these anatomic findings with the presence of either anatomic disease such as esophagitis or with premortem symptoms of esophageal disease.

There is no evidence that there was any connection made in the medical community between any type of post prandial symptoms to either the phenomenon of gastroesophageal reflux disease (GERD) or to hiatal hernia prior to the 19th century. In fact, in retrospect it is hard to imagine any physician having the acuity to connect gastric acid to esophageal disease or symptomatology prior to Beaumont's demonstration of the digestive and corrosive capability of gastric contents in 1833 [13]. Although, there is no evidence directly linking Beaumont's observations to subsequent understanding of acid reflux and its sequelae it seems likely that this evidence of the injurious efficacy of gastric contents would have informed subsequent speculations about the pathophysiology of esophageal injury and/or related symptoms.

In 1925, Friedenwald and Feldman did describe the typical symptoms of GERD, especially heartburn. They edged closer than their predecessors to recognizing the entity of GERD when they related these symptoms to the presence of an anatomic hiatal hernia. However, they stopped short of definitively associating the symptoms with the possibility of gastric acid reflux [14]. A year later, in 1926, Robbins and Jankelson actually demonstrated gastroesophageal reflux by radiographic techniques and observed that this produced epigastric and/or substernal discomfort in 90% of patients in which reflux occurred [14]. The stage was now set as the occurrence of reflux of gastric contents into the esophagus was documented and its association with symptoms demonstrated. This understanding could be linked to earlier observations as regards esophagitis and hiatal hernia.

In February 1929, Chevalier Jackson reported on "Peptic Ulcer of the Esophagus" and gave the incidence as eighty-eight out of more than 4000 cases of esophageal disease in 42 years of his experience and in speculating on the etiology included "retrograde flow of gastric juice" as a possible cause [15].

At the 85th Annual Session of the American Medical Association in Cleveland in June of 1934 Asher Winkelstein (1893–1972) presented a paper entitled "Peptic esophagitis: A new clinical entity." Dr. Winkelstein was the chief of Gastroenterology at Mount Sinai Hospital in New York and subsequently his paper was published in the Journal of the American Medical Association in March of 1935. Dr. Winkelstein's report consisted of five cases with biopsy proven esophagitis. Dr. Chevalier Jackson in discussing the paper remarked that "the chief reason, I think, why so little has been heard of peptic esophagitis is that so few esophagoscopies are done in patients with gastric symptoms" [16].

The ease of studying the distal esophagus and upper gastrointestinal tract was markedly advanced by the invention by Basil Hirschowitz of the fiberoptic endoscope. At the 1957 meeting of the American Gastroenterointestinal Endoscopy Society, the president of that society relinquished his presidential address so that Dr. Hirschowitz could present his first studies [9].

In 1906, perhaps the first true identification of GERD occurred. Tileston in 1906 collected and reported on 44 patients found to have pathologic esophagitis at the time of autopsy [17]. He went so far as to speculate that insufficiency of the cardia or the gastroesophageal junction would be a prerequisite to development of esophagitis. He did not however, use the expression reflux or clearly attempt to connect this pathologic finding to premortem symptoms.

Although progress was made during the latter half of the 20th century in first identifying and subsequently elucidating the pathophysiology and pathogenesis of GERD, as recently as 1913 a review of one of the leading medical texts of the day, Garrison's *An Introduction to the History of Medicine* [18] failed to reveal any mention in either the text or index of any of the following terms: heartburn, gastroesophageal reflux, reflux, or hiatal hernia. This suggests that well into the 20th century there was no understanding of or even speculation about the possibility of acid reflux into the esophagus as a disease entity.

At about this same time, surgeons began to become at least indirectly involved in this area through interest in and repair of hiatal hernia. For example, though apparently not reported until Soutter in 1947 when he published the first review of the Massachusetts General Hospital cumulative surgical experience with hiatal hernia, the first elective repair of a hiatal hernia was performed at Massachusetts General Hospital in 1920 [13]. These operations were hernia repairs; justification for them was, as for any hernia, the perceived risks of incarceration and strangulation. GERD was not a consideration. In other words, operations for the repair of diaphragmatic hernia were based on anatomic rather than physiologic principles. Similarly, in 1928 Harrington reported 51 cases of diaphragmatic hernia seen at the Mayo Clinic since 1908, 27 of which were repaired surgically [19]. These two reports initiated and incited surgical interest in diaphragmatic hernias.

In the 1940's and 1950's, the contributions of Philip Allison in Great Britain were of major importance in furthering the understanding of the pathophysiology of GERD and hiatal hernia as well as the pursuit of their surgical treatment. His seminal report in 1951 was entitled "Reflux Esophagitis, Sliding Hiatal Hernia and the Anatomy of Repair" [20]. This article begins with a classic description of a 59 year old woman with heartburn and regurgitation. The second paragraph begins with the statement, "The symptoms are those of esophagitis from the reflux of gastric contents into the esophagus, due to incompetence of the gastroesophageal junction." With the minor cavil that we now are well aware that symptoms can occur with reflux without anatomic esophagitis, this is a clear and unequivocal description of the pathophysiology of GERD. However, without the ability to distinguish hiatal hernia from intrinsic gastroesophageal incompetence as the important surgical consideration, Allison understandably focused on the hiatal hernia and the anatomy of hernia repair. The operation he performed was to reunite the two halves of the crus of the right diaphragm and to reattach the phreno- esophageal membrane to the undersurface of the diaphragm. Although this operation successfully repaired the esophageal sliding hernia, it did not prevent acid reflux. Consequently, while he made major contributions to the understanding of pathophysiology and began to address the challenge of surgical repair, his operation was not a successful one as patients retained their reflux symptoms despite surgical elimination of their hiatal hernia.

The next stage in the evolution of surgical correction of reflux esophagitis took two separate paths- one of serendipity and the other of trial and error and scientific study over a long period of time. Ronald Belsey began his series of observations at the Frenchay Hospital in Bristol. His examination of the seated, sedated patient with a rigid esophagoscope led him to observe a gaping cardia with gastric contents rising into the esophagus with deep inspiration. This observation of the gaping cardia suggested the operative goal of fixing the gastroesophageal junction 2–3 cm below the diaphragm. His Mark-I operation was essentially the same as the Allison approach. The Mark-II and Mark-III procedures were various degrees of fundoplication. These first 3 types of operations took place between 1949 and 1955 and about a third of the patients had poor results. He modified his operation based on long term outcomes and this experience culminated with the Mark-IV. This operation was based on his intuitive concepts derived from his personal experience. The operation was based on his belief in the importance of establishing an intra-abdominal segment of esophagus and creating a flap valve anti-reflux mechanism at the restored gastroesophageal junction and was performed through the left chest with a 270 degree fundoplication fixed to the undersurface of the diaphragm. Belsey's long term cumulative results were published after 20 years with over 1000 patients being treated and showed a better than 85% success rate [21]. It is remarkable to note that these results were obtained on astute observations long before the availability of manometry, pH studies and flexible endoscopy. This landmark publication made several important contributions. Based upon the reported experience with 1,030 patients, the pathophysiology of GERD was discussed and analyzed. This report is important for emphasizing the conversion of surgical thinking from a focus on anatomy to an appreciation of physiology. Grades of esophagitis were defined and correlated with clinical outcomes, showing for the first time that the more diseased the esophagus the worse the surgical results and the more likely the need for reoperation. The evolution of the indications for operation was discussed and criticized, identifying the need to properly select patients to obtain satisfactory outcomes. Finally, the results of what Belsey termed his Mark-IV procedure were provided. This discussion emphasized the evolution of the operative technique based on careful follow-up of patients undergoing earlier modifications of the operation and of the delay in reporting on this operation until genuine long term follow-up, allowing certainty about long term results, had been obtained.

The serendipity path fell to Rudolph Nissen (1896–1981). Nissen was born in Niesse, Prussia, served and was wounded in WWI and was trained in medicine in a number of German universities. He was trained in Surgery by Ferdinand Sauerbruch in Munich and in Berlin. Sauerbruch was a protégé of Mickulcz who encouraged his work in chest surgery by the use of a pressure chamber until endotracheal anesthesia was developed. As a result Nissen was a competent thoracic surgeon who performed the first pneumonectomy. He resigned his position at the Charite in 1933 under pressure from the National Socialist Party. At about this time Ataturk was engineering a cultural revolution in Turkey and Sauerbruch arranged his appointment as Chief and Professor of Surgery at the University of Istanbul. In 1936 he was presented with a 28 year old male who had a distal esophageal ulcer penetrating into the pericardium. Nissen resected this area and reanastamosed the esophagus to the stomach using a Witzel tunneling technique. Fearing an anastomotic leak, he folded the anterior wall of the stomach over the gastroesophagel anastomosis as a fundoplication. He had the opportunity to follow up this patient and specifically noted the absence of esophagitis. During WW II Nissen was in Boston as a research fellow under Churchill and in Brooklyn Jewish Hospital as chief of surgery and after the war was offered the position of Professor and Chair of Surgery in Basle, Switzerland. It was in December 1955 that he encountered a 49 year old female patient with a 3 year history of reflux esophagitis *without* a hiatal hernia. Based on his previous experience, using a transabdominal approach he mobilized the distal esophagus and wrapped the distal 6 cm of it with the gastric fundus (he called it a gastroplication) [22].

Although the operation proved to be effective, there were a number of complications including postoperative dysphagia, disruption of the wrap, inability to belch ("gas bloat syndrome") and gastric motility problems. As a result a number of modifications have been proposed. The Rosetti-Nissen fundoplication uses the anterior wall for the total wrap. In 1977, Donahue and Bombeck emphasized the "short floppy cuff" [23]. This modification proposed complete mobilization of the fundus and GE junction, a wrap of short length and preservation of the vagus nerves. This reduced the incidence of dysphagia and gas bloat symptoms. Partial fundoplication wraps placed either anterior or posterior to the gastroesophageal junction, have been described such as the crurally fixed partial fundoplication of Toupet. There is also an anterior 180 degree fundoplication developed by Dor. A fundoplication described by Watson consists of full mobilization of the lower esophagus and gastroesophageal junction, crural repair, fixation of the esophagus to the crura and an anterior 180 degree Dor-type fundoplication. While retaining the eponym, both Nissen and other surgeons have modified his original operation to its present form. The hiatus is closed. A relatively short, no more than a three cm. wrap, of posterior to anterior fundus around the distal esophagus is constructed by passing the posterior fundus behind the esophagus and the suturing it to the anterior fundus.

The technique and application of both these operations have evolved over time. While the Belsey procedure is quite effective it is only occasionally performed at present because of the need for a painful thoracotomy. The Nissen procedure has achieved widespread utilization because it can be performed from either the abdomen or the chest, with good results, and can be accomplished laparoscopically, thus sparing the patient even a laparotomy.

Throughout the 1970's and 1980's both the gastroenterology and surgical communities exhibited increased interest in GERD. Multiple publications have advanced the understanding of pathophysiology and of treatment, both medical and surgical. Some operative techniques were established by the end of the 1980's as essential parts of a successful antireflux operation, most frequently a Nissen fundoplication, and some were more controversial. Securely established are the need: (1) to perform a sufficient mediastinal dissection to release the esophagus from tissue creating cephalad distraction, (2) to close the esophageal hiatus to prevent postoperative herniation, (3) to construct a relatively short (one to three cm) gastric wrap to balance control of reflux with the likelihood of dysphagia, and (4) to ensure a correct preoperative diagnosis with utilization of esophageal function tests when the clinical picture is ambiguous. Continuing to be debated are the need to divide the short gastric vessels, the benefits of performing the wrap with an esophageal dilator in place, the questions of identifying and treating the so-called short esophagus, and the need to modify the operation in the presence of impaired esophageal peristalsis.

The burgeoning field of laparoscopic surgery has transformed the field of antireflux surgery. Short and medium term followup of operated patients shows comparable surgical outcomes to those achieved with the open operation [24]. Because of the well documented benefits of the laparoscopic approach over an open operation, including but not limited to diminished postoperative pain, a shorter hospitalization and an attenuated inflammatory response, patient interest in laparoscopic antireflux surgery has been considerable. This increase in the number of patients seeking and actually undergoing antireflux surgery has likewise widened and stimulated the pool of both thoracic and general surgeons interested in this disease.

Increasingly sophisticated techniques of endo-esophageal study are being utilized to analyze the function and dysfunction of the lower esophageal sphincter and the esophageal body. These investigations serve the need to appreciate, understand and have physiologic as well as anatomic information when planning and executing functional surgery. The modern battery of esophageal functional investigations are the descendants of earlier studies such as the Bernstein test, Skinner's Standard Acid Reflux Test, esophageal manometry and esophageal pH monitoring [25]. The current ability to detect and quantitate not only acid reflux, but also bile reflux, non specific liquid reflux and gas reflux have opened new doors into the understanding of esophageal function and dysfunction and will be effecting medical and surgical therapy in profound ways in subsequent years.

References

[1] Sebastian A (1999) A dictionary of the history of medicine. Pearl River, NY: Parthenon Publishing Group, p 294

[2] Breasted JH (1984) The Edwin Smith Papyrus. Birmingham, AL: Gryphon Editions, pp 312–316

[3] Walton JN, Beeson PB, Scott RB (1986) The Oxford companion to medicine. Oxford University Press, p 1436

[4] Rosenberg JC (1959) A Vesalian woodcut of the esophagus and stomach. Surgery 46: 469–474

[5] Marchese-Ragona R (2002) Valsalva and the upper esophageal airway. Dysphagia 17: 250–251

[6] Knight B (1980) Discovering the human body. London. Imprint Books

[7] Friedland GW (1978) A historical review of the changing concepts of lower esophageal anatomy 430 BC–1977. Am J Roentgenol 131: 373–388

[8] Firkin BG (1996) Dictionary of medical eponyms. London: Parthenon Publishing Group, p 181

[9] Modlin IM (2003) Historical perspectives on the treatment of gastroesophageal reflux disease. Gastrointest Endoscopy Clin N Am 13: 19–55

[10] Hamby WB (1960) The case reports and autopsy records of Ambroise Pare'. Translated from JP Malgaigne's "Oeuvres complete d'Ambroise Pare'" Paris 1840. Springfield: Thomas, pp 50–51

[11] Morgagni GB (1983) The seats and causes of diseases. Translated by Benjamin Alexander (1749). Birmingham, AL: Gryphon Editions, Book IV, p 210

[12] Bowditch HL (1853) A treatise on diaphragmatic hernia. Buffalo, NY: Jewett, Thomas and Co

[13] Beaumont W (1833) Experiments and observations on the gastric juice and physiology of digestion. Plattsburgh, NY: FP Allen

[14] Postlethwait RW (1986) Surgery of the esophagus, 2nd ed. Norwalk, Conn.: Appleton-Century-Crofts, pp 211–276

[15] Jackson C (1929) Peptic ulcer of the esophagus. JAMA 92: 369–372
[16] Winkelstein A (1935) Peptic esophagitis, a new clinical entity. JAMA 104: 906–909
[17] Tiletson W (1906) Peptic ulcer of the esophagus. J Am Med Sci 132: 240–265
[18] Garrison JF (1913) An introduction to the history of medicine. Philadelphia: W.B. Saunders
[19] Harrington SW (1928) Diaphragmatic hernia. Arch Surg 16: 386–392
[20] Allison PR (1948) Peptic ulcer of the esophagus. Thorax 3: 20–42
[21] Skinner DB, Belsey RHR (1967) Surgical management of esophageal reflux and hiatus hernia: long term results with 1030 patients. J Thorac Cardiovasc Surg 53: 33–54
[22] Nissen R (1956) Eine einfache Operation zur Beeinflussung der Reflux Oesophagitis. Schweiz Med Wochenschr 86: 590–592
[23] Donahue PE et al (1977) "Floppy" Nisssen fundoplication. Rev Surg 34: 223–224
[24] Peters JH, DeMeester TR, Crookes P, Oberg S, VosShoop M, Hagen JA, Bremmer CG (1990) Ann Surg 228: 40–50
[25] Skinner DB, DeMeester TR (1976) Gastroesophageal reflux in current problems in surgery, Vol XIII, No 1

Chapter 15

COMPARISON OF LAPAROSCOPIC AND OPEN ANTIREFLUX PROCEDURES

V. Velanovich

Division of General Surgery, Henry Ford Hospital, Detroit, MI, USA

Introduction

Antireflux surgery was originally developed as an open operation. With the advent of laparoscopic cholestectomy, fundoplications have been modified to the laparoscopic approach. There have been at least 11 non-randomized comparisons and 6 randomized clinical trials comparing laparoscopic and open antireflux surgery. Overall, these studies have shown that symptomatic relief is similar between these approaches. Short-term quality of life appears superior for the laparoscopic approach. However, the laparoscopic approach may also have a slightly higher complication and side effect rate. Nevertheless, patient satisfaction appears dependent of symptomatic relief, not the type of approach. Therefore, type of approach should be determined by patient and surgeon factors, not dogmatically applied to all patients.

Rudolph Nissen published in 1956 the landmark article pertaining to the fundoplication which now bears his name [1]. Since that time the Nissen fundoplication has become the standard by which all other anti-reflux operations are compared. Most variations of anti-reflux operations have some component of either a partial or complete fundoplication. Up until recently, the two main approaches have been the trans-abdominal approach, through some type of laparotomy, or a trans-thoracic approach, through a left posterior lateral thoracotomy. 1991 ushered in a new era of anti-reflux surgery with the first Nissen fundoplication performed through a laparoscopic approach [2]. Although the laparoscopic fundoplication has rightfully taken its place as a standard of care for gastroesophageal reflux disease, the open approach is still a valuable alternative to the minimally invasive approach. The purpose of this chapter will be to review the comparative data pertaining to laparoscopic and open anti-reflux surgery, and to make recommendations with respect to these approaches.

Indications for antireflux surgery

Although other chapters in this book will deal with the evaluation and treatment planning of patients with gastroesophageal reflux disease, review of acceptable indications for anti-reflex surgery is still warranted. Patients with both typical and atypical symptoms of gastroesophageal reflux disease are amendable to both the laparoscopic and open approach. The minimum requirements to determine the suitably of patients for surgery include a complete history and physical examination to rule out other potential causes for symptoms (e.g., cardiac or respiratory causes), upper endoscopy primarily to rule out other sources of pathology (e.g., esophageal cancer), esophageal manometry primarily to rule out other esophageal motility disorders, and 24 hour pH-monitoring to establish the presence of pathologic reflux and symptoms index. On a selective basis, upper gastrointestinal contrast radiography and gastric emptying scintography can be used to evaluate for potential structural abnormalities, like paraesophageal hernia, or gastroparesis, especially if symptoms of bloating exist. Once the decision has been made to proceed with anti-reflux surgery, the surgeon must choose the approach best suited for the patient.

The majority of patients are good candidates for a laparoscopic fundoplication, and this would be the first choice of most surgeons experienced in this technique. The only areas where an open approach would be considered preferable by some authorities to the laparoscopic approach include patient preference, prior abdominal surgeries where extensive intra-abdominal adhesions would be expected, large paraesophageal hernias, extensive esophageal foreshortening mandating a thoracic approach although the Belsey fundoplication can be done thoracoscepically, or redo fundoplication. This being said, there are many surgeons who would feel perfectly comfortable proceeding with a laparoscopic approach despite the limitations listed above. However, it is imperative that the first choice for the patient be based on the safety and effectiveness of the technique in the surgeon's hands.

I will not go into detail as to the operative techniques as these are reviewed in other chapters.

Comparison of laparoscopic and open fundoplication

As with other laparoscopic operations, it has generally been assumed that patients undergoing laparoscopic fundoplication will have less pain and a faster return to normal activities. Initially there has been some question about whether a laparoscopic fundoplication would be as effective as the open fundoplication in the treatment of gastroesophageal reflux disease. Therefore studies comparing the two have focused on several points. These include symptomatic relief, complications, post-operative side effects, costs, durability of symptom relief, short and long-term quality of life.

Table 1 [3]–[13] lists studies comparing the laparoscopic to the open approach in a non-randomized fashion. Some of these studies are retrospective, others are prospective. Table 2 [14]–[22] lists the six studies in which report randomized prospective comparisons of the laparoscopic to the open approach. In addition, Catarci et al [23], have done a very interesting evidenced based appraisal of anti-reflux operations reviewing in a strict manner the available data pertaining to anti-reflux surgery.

Peters et al [3], in 1995 compared 34 patients who underwent laparoscopic fundoplication compared to 47 who underwent open fundoplication. There was a similar outcome with respect to symptomatic improvement. They found that 84% of patients in both groups were "cured" or improved. However, 87% of the laparoscopic group was satisfied with surgery, compared to 95% of open patients. Lower esophageal sphincter pressure was higher in the laparoscopic group (20.9 mm Hg vs. 12.1 in the open group). In addition lower esophageal sphincter length and prevalence of incomplete relaxation were also higher in the laparoscopic group. Hospital stay was less in the laparoscopic group. Nevertheless these physiologic differences did

Table 1. Non-randomized comparisons

Study/ reference	Year	Open operations (n)	LAP operations (n)	Follow-up
Peters [3]	1995	47	34	7 months (lap) 52 months (open)
Low [4]	1995	25	5	Not specified
Rattner [5]	1995	12	74	12 months
Blomquist [6]	1996	25	25	
Blomquist [8]	1996	28	28	N/A
Eshraghi [7]	1998	114	157	23 months
Velanovich [9]	1999	20	60	1.5 months
Rantanen [10]	1999[a]	27	30	
Rantanen [11]	1999[b]	1162	3993	N/A
Streets [12]	2002	33	72	25 months (lap) 31 months (open)
Stewart [13]	2004			

Table 2. Randomized comparisons

Study/ reference	Year	Open operations	LAP operations	Follow up
Laine [12]	1997	55	55	12 months
Heikkinen [15], [16]	1999 2000	20	22	24 months
Bias [1], [17]	2000	46	57	3 months
Nilsson [18]–[20]	2000 2001 2002	30	30	6 months
Luostarinen [21]	2001	15	13	17 months
Chrysos [22]	2002	50	56	12 months

not seem to translate into higher postoperative side effects. Rattner and Brooks [5] in 1995 also reported similar levels of patient satisfaction, with equal occurrences of the post-operative symptoms of bloating, dysphasia and recurrent heartburn. However, these authors report that patients undergoing laparoscopic fundoplication returned to work sooner than open patients, and overall monetary charges were less for the laparoscopic group. Interestingly, correction of preoperative symptoms and lack of postoperative side effects were more accurate predictors of satisfaction then surgical approach. Eshraghi et al [7], reported similar intra-operative complications between laparoscopic and open anti-reflux procedures at 8%. These complications included splenctomy, esophageal or gastric perforation, hemorrhage, and pneumothorax. Postoperative complications however were higher in the open group only in the frequency of dehiscence and ventral hernia. Follow up symptoms were similar between the open and laparoscopic group with 67% of open patients and 64% of laparoscopic patients completely asymptomatic. Dysphagia, recurrent reflux, nausea, pain and gas bloat occurred in less than 7% in both groups. Using a generic quality life instrument, the SF-36, as well as symptom severity instrument, the GERD-HRQL, I showed in a nonrandomized but prospective, fashion that the symptom improvement was comparable in both the laparoscopic and the open anti-reflux surgery patients [9]. In the laparoscopic group, the total GERD-HRQL score (best score 0, worst score 50) improved form 27 to 2, while in the open group, it improve from 27 to 1. However, the laparoscopic group had better postoperative scores in the SF-36 domains of physical functioning 80 vs. 67.5 (best score 100, worst score 0) and bodily pain 64 vs. 51.5 [7]. Similarly, Rantanen et al [10] showed similar functional outcomes between the laparoscopic and the open fundoplication groups. They found no difference in persistent dysphagia, symptoms relief, bloating, and flatulence, although a higher percentage of patients reported normal belching after the open fundoplication. However, the same group in a population based study in Finland, showed that more life threatening complications occurred in the laparoscopic group compared to the open group. The patients who underwent laparoscopic fundoplication had an overall incident of 1.3% of life threatening complications, compared to the 0.6% prevalence in open surgery. The laparoscopic group also had higher incidents of nonfatal life threatening complications 1.2% vs. 0.3% in the open group. A complete cost analysis taking into account direct medical cost and indirect social cost of laparoscopic and open fundoplication was done by Blomquist et al [8] in Sweden. They found that the laparoscopic approach was more cost effective, with less sick leave (9.9 days vs. 29.9 days), less direct medical cost (27,693 SEK vs. 37,482 SEK) and less in direct medical cost (12,595 SEK vs. 37,126 SEK). Therefore, in summary these studies show that laparoscopic fundoplication has similar symptoms response rates better early quality of life and overall less cost at the expense of a slightly higher complication rates and postoperative side effects.

In reviewing the data in the randomized trials, most trails had relatively short follow-up between 6–24 months, and comparatively few patients with a total of 187 patients randomized to the open group and 188 patients randomized to the laparoscopic over the six studies (Table 2). This probably speaks to the difficulty in conducting randomized trails in this setting. In these trials the symptomatic recurrence rates varied from 0–10% with an average of 3.7% in the open group and 2.1% in the laparoscopic group. Dysphagia varied from 0–58%, with an average of 15% in the open group compared to 19% in the laparoscopic group. Bloating was similar in both groups at around 20%. However 2.6% of patients required re-operation in the laparoscopic group compared to 0.5% in the open group. Hospital stay generally favored the laparoscopic group, but by only 2 days. Average sick leave generally favored the laparoscopic group, but this was still quite variable. Importantly, there was quite a bit of variation in operative technique, including performing a hiatal repair, use of an esophageal dilator and division of the short gastric vessels. It remains unclear whether these variations lead to differences in outcome.

Overall, the outcomes of laparoscopic versus open fundoplication are similar. Symptomatic relief is similar, post-operative complications overall are similar [24]. Population based studies, however, do suggest that there is a slightly higher incident of life threatening complication in laparoscopic group. However, quality of life, at least in the short term, appears to favor the laparoscopic approach. However, it should be noted that patient satisfaction is overall mostly related to symptomatic improvement rather than to the operative approach [5], [12]. However, it appears that the quality of life advantage of the laparoscopic approach fades with time. Once a year passes quality of life scores using the SF-36 instrument are similar between patients undergoing laparoscopic and open fundoplication [25]. Therefore, the true advantage of the laparoscopic approach is in earlier recovery, less early pain, and foster return to physical functioning.

In conclusion, laparoscopic anti-reflux surgery has become a mainstay in the surgical treatment of gastroesophageal reflux disease. Symptomatic relief appears to be as good with both the laparoscopic and open approach. Short term quality of life with respect to functional recovery is superior in the laparoscopic group, however this does wan with time, as patients in the laparoscopic and open group after a year or two post-operatively appear to have similar levels of quality of life. Therefore because one approach is not decidedly superior over another approach in the long term, choice of procedures should be individualized as per the patients needs.

References

[1] Nissen R (1957) Die transpleurael resection der Kardia. Dtsch Chir 249: 311–316

[2] Dallemagen B, Weerts JM, Jehas C et al (1991) Laparoscopic Nissen fundoplication: preliminary report. Surg Laparossc Endosc 1: 178–243

[3] Peters JH, Heimbucher J, Kauer WKH et al (1995) Clinical and physiologic comparison of laparoscopic and open Nissen fundoplication. J Am Coll Surg 180: 385–393

[4] Low DE (1995) Examination of outcome and cost data of open and laparoscopic anti-reflux operations at Virginia Mason Medical Center in Seattle. Surg Endosc 9: 1326–1328

[5] Rattner DW, Brooks DC (1995) Patient satisfaction following laparoscopic and open anti-reflux surgery. Arch Surg 130: 289–294

[6] Blomquist A, Lonroth H, Dalenback J et al (1996) Quality of life assessment after laparoscopic and open fundoplication: results of a prospective clinical study. Scond J Gastreoenterol 31: 1052–1058

[7] Eshraghi N, Farahmand M, Soot SJ et al (1998) Comparison of outcomes of open versus laparoscopic Nissen fundoplication performed in a single practice. Am J Surg 175: 371–374

[8] Blomquist AM, Lonroth H, Dalenback J, Lundell L (1998) Laparoscopic or open fundoplication? A complete cost analysis. Surg Endosc 12: 1209–1212

[9] Velanovich V (1999) Comparison of symptomatic and quality of life outcomes of laparoscopic versus open anti-reflux surgery. Surgery 126: 782–789

[10] Rantanen TK, Salo JA, Salminen JT, Kellokumper H (1999) Functional outcome after laparoscopic or open Nissen fundoplication: a follow-up study. Arch Surg 134: 240–244

[11] Rantanen TK, Salo JA, Sipponen JT (1999) Fatal and life-threatening complications in antireflux surgery: analysis of 5,502 operations. Br J Surg 86: 1573–1577

[12] Streats CG, Demeester SR, DeMeester TR et al (2002) Excellent quality of life after Nissen fundoplication depends on successful elimination of reflux symptoms and not invasiveness of the surgical approach. Ann Thorac Surg 74: 1019–1025

[13] Steward GD, Watson AJ, Lamb PJ et al (2004) Comparison of three different procedures for antireflux surgery. Br J Surg 91: 724–729

[14] Laine S, Rantala A, Gullisch R et al (1997) Laparoscopic vs. conventional Nissen fundoplication. A prospective randomized trail. Surg Endosc 11: 441–444

[15] Heikkinen TJ, Hakipuro K, Kovukangus P et al (1999) Comparison of cost between laparoscopic and open Nissen fundoplication: a prospective randomized trail with 3-month follow-up. J Am Coll Surg 199: 368–376

[16] Heikkinen T, Hakipuro K, Bringman S et al (2000) Comparison of laparoscopic and open Nissen fundoplication of 2 years after operation. A prospective randomized trail. Surg Endosc 14: 1019–1023

[17] Bais JE, Bartelsman JFWM, Bonjer HJ et al (2000) Laparoscopic or conventional Nissen fundoplication for gastroesophageal reflux disease: randomized clinical trail. Lancet 355: 170–174

[18] Nilsson G, Larsson S, Johnsson F (2000) Randomized clinical trail of laparoscopic versus open fundoplication: blind evaluation of recovery and discharge period. Br J Surg 87: 873–878

[19] Werner J, Nilsson G, Oberg S et al (2001) Short-term outcome after laparoscopic and open 360° fundoplication. A prospective randomized clinical trial. Surg Endosc 15: 1124–1128

[20] Nilsson G, Larsson S, Johnsson F (2002) Randomized clinical trail of laparoscopic versus open fundoplication: evaluation of psychological well-being and changes in everyday life from a patient perspective. Scond J Gastroenterol 37: 385–391

[21] Luostorinen M, Virtanen J, Matikainen M et al (2001) Dysphasia and esophageal clearance after laparoscopic

versus open Nissen fundoplication. A randomized prospective trail. Scond J Gastroenterol 36: 565–571

[22] Chrysos E, Tsiaousis J, Athanasakis E et al (2002) Laparoscopic vs. open approach for Nissen fundoplication. Surg Endosc 16: 1679–1684

[23] Catarch M, Gentileschi P, Papi C et al (2004) Evidence-based appraisal of antireflux fundoplication. Ann Surg 239: 325–337

[24] Carlson MA, Frantzides CT (2001) Complications and results of primary minimally invasive antireflux procedures: a review of 10,735 reported cases. J Am Coll Surg 193: 428–439

[25] Velanovich V, Chowdhry SJ, Violette A (2001) Convergence of quality of life outcomes of laparoscopic and open antireflux operations. 2001 Annual Scientific Sessions of SAGES, St. Louis, MO

Chapter 16

LAPAROSCOPIC NISSEN FUNDOPLICATION

B. Dallemagne

Département de Chirurgie Digestive, CHC – Les Cliniques Saint Joseph, Liege, Belgium

Introduction

The idea of fundoplication to prevent gastroesophageal reflux was born in 1937 in Istanbul, when Rudolf Nissen performed a transpleural cardia resection and protected the anastomosis within a gastric fold. The first fundoplication without resection was performed in 1955, with a short publication appearing in 1956 [1].

Nissen's technique initially consisted of the invagination of the esophagus into a sleeve of the gastric wall obtained from the upper portion of the stomach. (*Fig. 1*). The gastrosplenic vessels and the diaphragmatic hiatus were untouched. The functional importance of the vagus trunks were ignored and neglected: many branches were transected, although without dramatic consequences.

Together with the development of modern tools to study the physiology of the foregut and review of the experience, adaptations were made to the original technique.

Marco Rossetti, coworker of Rudolf Nissen, was at the origin of these adaptations. His technique, the *anterior wall technique*, is still widely applied. The important technical changes included a more extensive mobilization of the posterior wall of the stomach from the left crus and diaphragm and use of the anterior wall of the fundus to create the total wrap. In this technique, the detachment of the fundus from the crus and diaphragm enables a complete loose wrap without the need for division of the short gastric vessels [2].

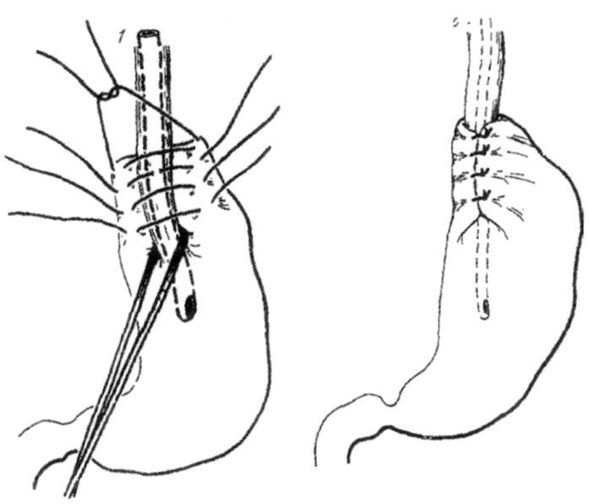

Fig. 1. Original Nissen's fundoplication (Reprint from Gastro esophageal reflux disease: back to surgery? Büchler, Farthmann (eds) Karger 1997)

The most commonly performed total wrap nowadays was introduced by Donahue and Bombeck in 1977 and validated by DeMeester in 1986. The technique involves full mobilization of the gastroesophageal junction and posterior fundus with division of the upper short gastric vessels and a crural repair [3]–[5]. Over the years, the length of the wrap has been reduced to the current 2.0 cm. This operation is commonly referred to as the *short floppy Nissen.*

Surgical technique

The short floppy Nissen

Technique

The operation is performed under general anesthesia with endotracheal intubation; the patient is placed in the lithotomy position. The surgeon stands between the legs of the patient with, at his right, the surgical assistant and on his left, the scrub nurse, or another assistant.

Pneumoperitoneum is established in normal fashion, with usual precautions. A maximal intraperitoneal pressure of 14 mmHG is allowed.

The table is maintained in a steep, head-up position: gravity displaces the abdominal viscera from the subdiaphragmatic area.

The first trocar, 10 mm caliber, is placed in the supra-umbilical midline, at the junction of the upper two-thirds and lower one-third between the umbilicus and the xyphoid process. The laparoscope is introduced through this port. Visual inspection of the entire peritoneal cavity is carried out.

Under direct vision, four other 5 mm trocars are inserted: their location is shown in (*Fig. 2*). In our set-up, the surgeon manipulates the subxyphoid and the left mid-clavicular canulas for most of the procedure.

The operation begins with retraction of the left lobe of the liver using a liver retractor introduced through the right trocar.

The remainder of the procedure follows the classical sequence of the operation performed through laparotomy.

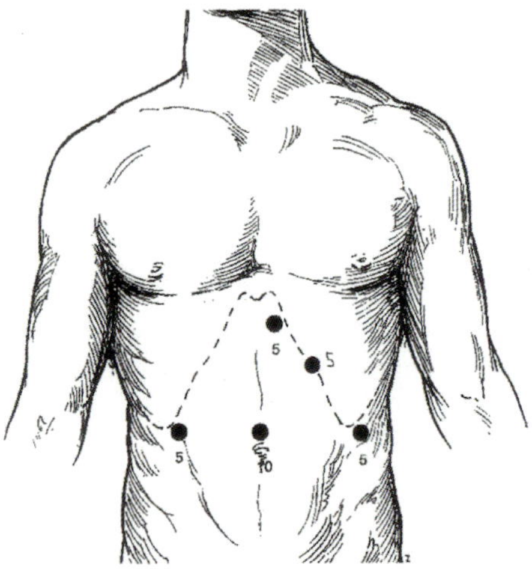

Fig. 2. Trocars placement for laparoscopic fundoplication

The GE junction is place under traction using a grasping forceps from the left lateral port. The lesser omentum is divided, beginnig above the hepatic branch of the vagus nerve to the level of the right crus (*Fig. 3*).

The phreno-esophageal membrane is then divided in a transverse direction, on the anterior aspect of the hiatal orifice. Then, along the inner side of the right crus, the right esophageal wall is freed by dissecting the cleavage plane (*Fig. 4*). This dissection is carried out using ultrasonic scissors. Attention is turned next to the left anterolateral aspect of the esophagus: at its lefts border, the left crus is identified. The clivage plane between it and the left aspect of the esophagus is freed. The gastric fundus is then pulled inferiorely and to the right. The proximal gastrophrenic ligament is divided, beginning the mobilization of the gastric pouch. Extending the dissection the length of the right diaphragmatic crus starts the liberation of the posterior aspect of the esophagus. The pars flacida of the lesser omentum is opened, preserving the hepatic branches of the vagus nerve. This allows access to the crura, left and right, the right posterior aspect of the esophagus and the posterior vagus nerve (*Fig. 5*). Careful dissection of the meso esophagus and the left crus reveals a clivage plane between this crus and the posterior gastric wall. Confirmation of having opened the correct plane is obtained by visualizing the fatty tissue of the gastrosplenic ligament or the spleen itself, when looking behind the esophagus. A drain is

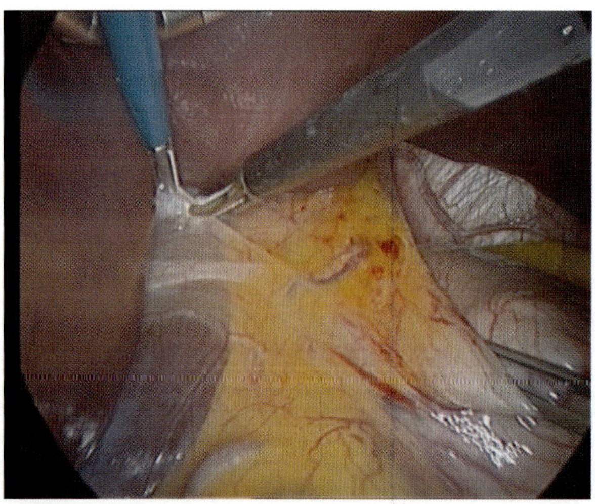

Fig. 3. Division of the pars condensa of the lesser omentum, preserving the branches of the vagus nerve and a left hepatic artery

passed through this channel and will be held by the left sided assistant and his left sub costal instrument.

This retroesophageal channel is enlarged to allow easy passage of the anti reflux valve.

With the traction on the drain at the GE junction, the mediastinal dissection of the esophagus is completed and the esophagus is free from the pleura, the aorta and the crural muscles.

At this point, one obtains an elongation of the intra-abdominal segment of the esophagus and a reduction of the hiatal hernia if one exists (*Fig. 6*).

This intramediastinal dissection must be extended to permit 2 to 3 cm of the lower esophagus to stay without traction in the abdomen, below the diaphragm. This a crucial part of the operation. If this length is not obtained, an extended mediastinal dissection should be carried out. If this is not sufficient, one should consider the possibility of a shortened esophagus and apply adequate techniques.

The following step consists of the mobilization of the gastric fundus. This requires division of the gastrosplenic ligament and the most cephalic short gastric vessels. This dissection starts on the stomach at the end of the gastro-splenic ligament, where a small fat pad is founded (*Fig. 7*). The rear cavity is opened and all the posterior attachements of the

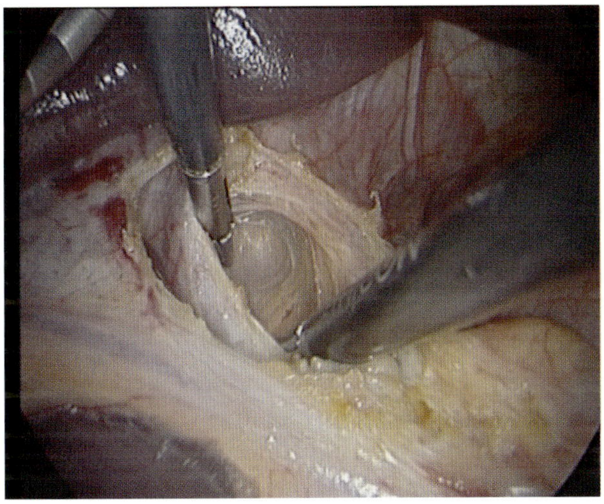

Fig. 4. Division of the phrenoesophageal membrane and identification of the right crus

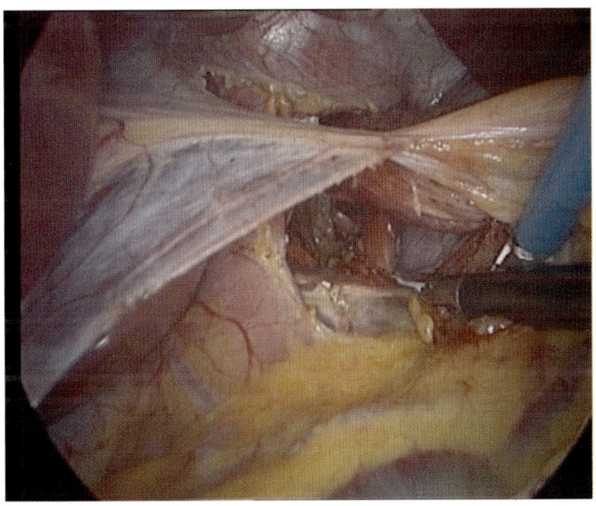

Fig. 5. Creation of the retroesophageal window

upper gastric fundus are divided, including the fundic posterior vessel that has its origin from the splenic artery on the superior border of the pancreas. This dissection ends up when the left crus is reached after division of the gastro-phrenic ligament (*Fig. 8*).

The next step involves repair of the hiatal orifice: interrupted sutures, using non-absorbable materiel are placed on the diaphragmatic crura to close the orifice. Calibration can be obtained with a 60 frenches bougie, or by modeling the crural repair on the diameter of the esophagus, without traction on the GE junction. At the end of the repair, the esophagus must be lying without compression in the repaired orifice (*Fig. 9*).

The last part of the operation consists of the passage and fixation of the antireflux valve. An atraumatic forceps is passed behind the esophagus, from right to left. It is used to grab the posterior wall of the gastric fundus to the left of the esophagus and to pull it behind, forming the wrap. At this point, a large bare bougie (50–60 frenches) can be passed down the cardia. It is used to calibrate the fundoplication.

Three interrupted stitches form and secure the wrap. A 1.5–2 cms wrap is constructed. This wrap is fixed on the anterior and left border of the esophagus by two sutures, one at the upper part and one at the lower part of the wrap (*Fig. 10*).

The peritoneum is rinsed with warm normal saline. No drains are placed. The trocars are removed and the wounds are stapled closed.

Laparoscopic Nissen-Rossetti fundoplication

Controversies still exist about the need for gastric mobilization to construct a real floppy fundoplication. Number of surgeons applies the Nissen Rossetti fundoplication, the anterior wall technique that does not need short gastric vessels division.

From the original description by Marco Rossetti, here are the main steps of the operation [2] (*Fig. 11*). Patient's positioning and trocars placement are identical to the floppy Nissen technique.

Esophageal dissection and mobilization is performed in the same manner. The gastrophrenic ligament is divided and a large retroesophageal channel is created. In the original technique, crural repair was performed only in wide hiatus. In the conventional open technique, division of the short gastric vessels was usually not necessary, but was always performed in the presence of fibrosis, adiposity, short fundic convexity and shortened esophagus.

The wrap is different: it is constructed using the anterior wall of the gastric fundus. A wide, tension free, fold of the anterior gastric fundic wall is passed behind the esophagus, grabbed on the right side of the esophagus and sutured with the anterior wall of the stomach on the left side of the esophagus, without fixation on the esophagus itself. Two additional sutures between the base of the fundic fold and the anterior wall of the stomach help to avoid eversion and "telescoping" of the junction.

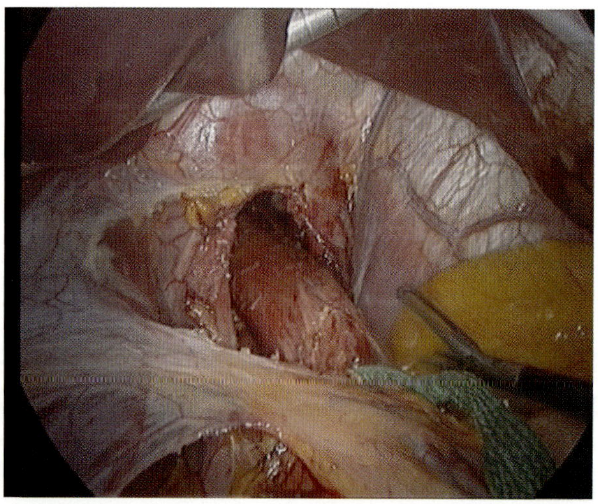

Fig. 6. Reduction of the gastroesophageal junction below the diaphragm

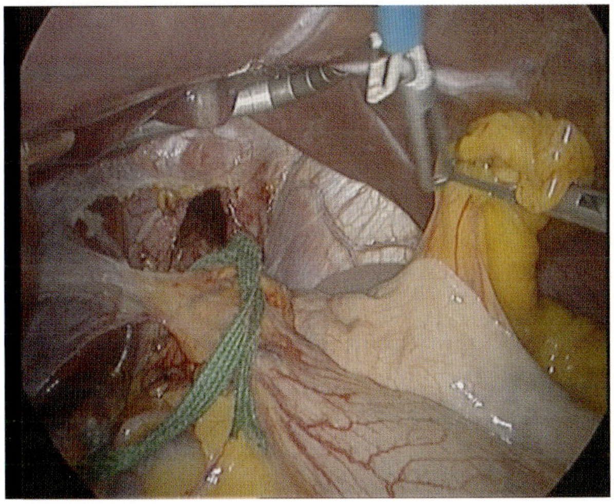

a

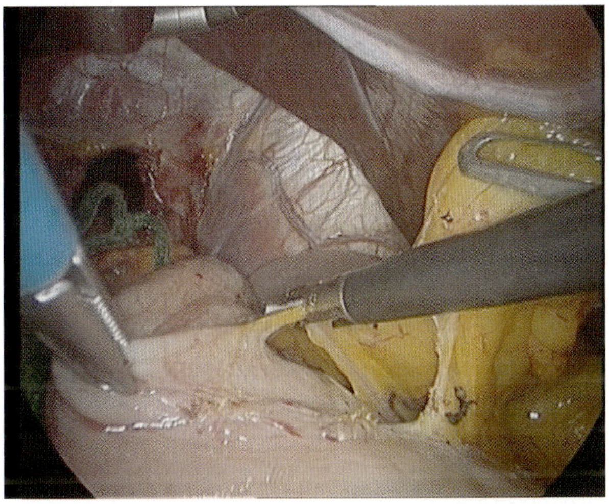

b

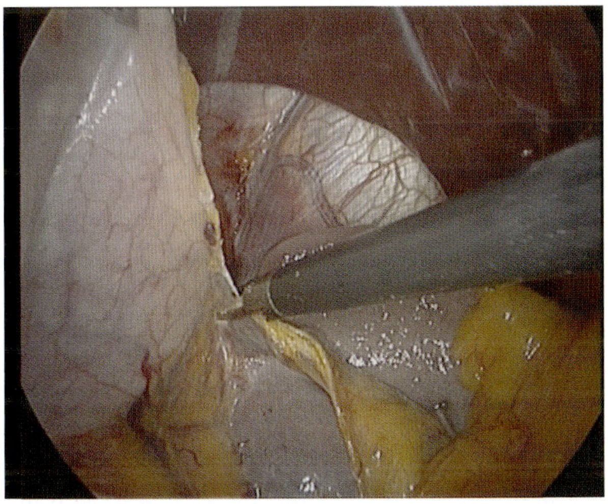

c

Fig. 7. Mobilization of the gastric fundus

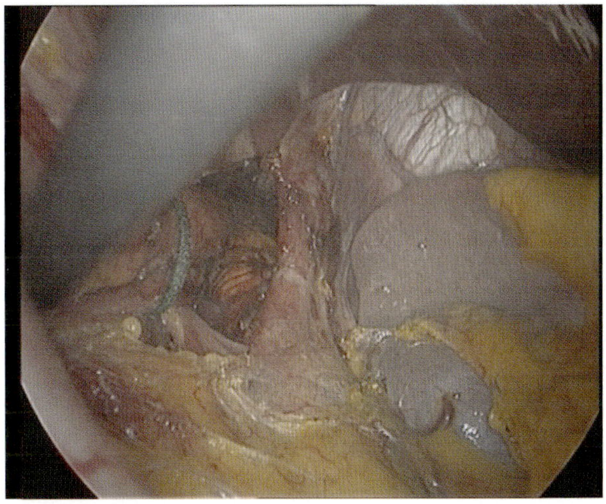

Fig. 8. End of the gastric mobilization

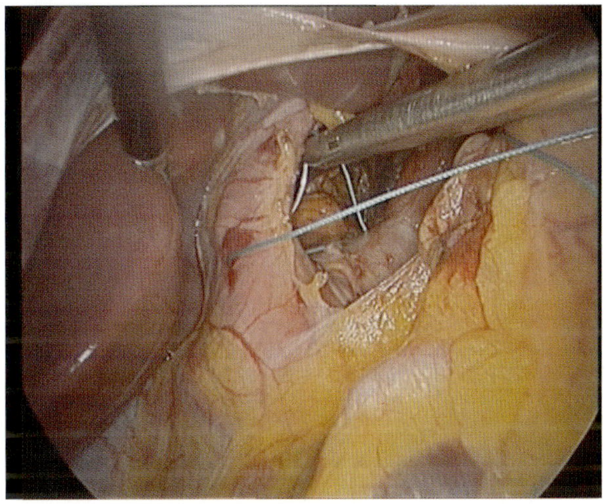

a

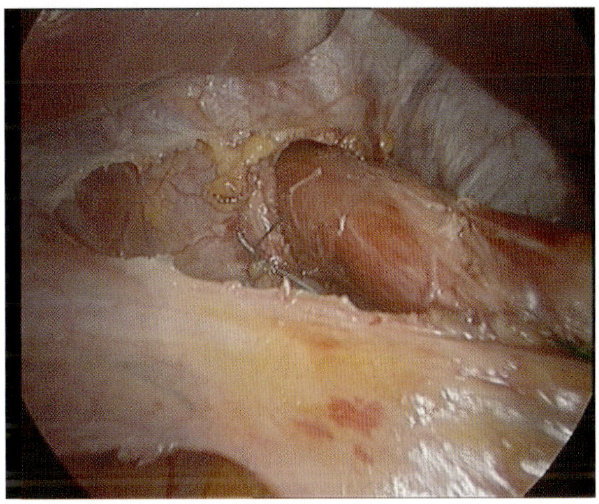

b

Fig. 9. Repair of the hiatal orifice: the esophagus is lying down on the repair without stricture

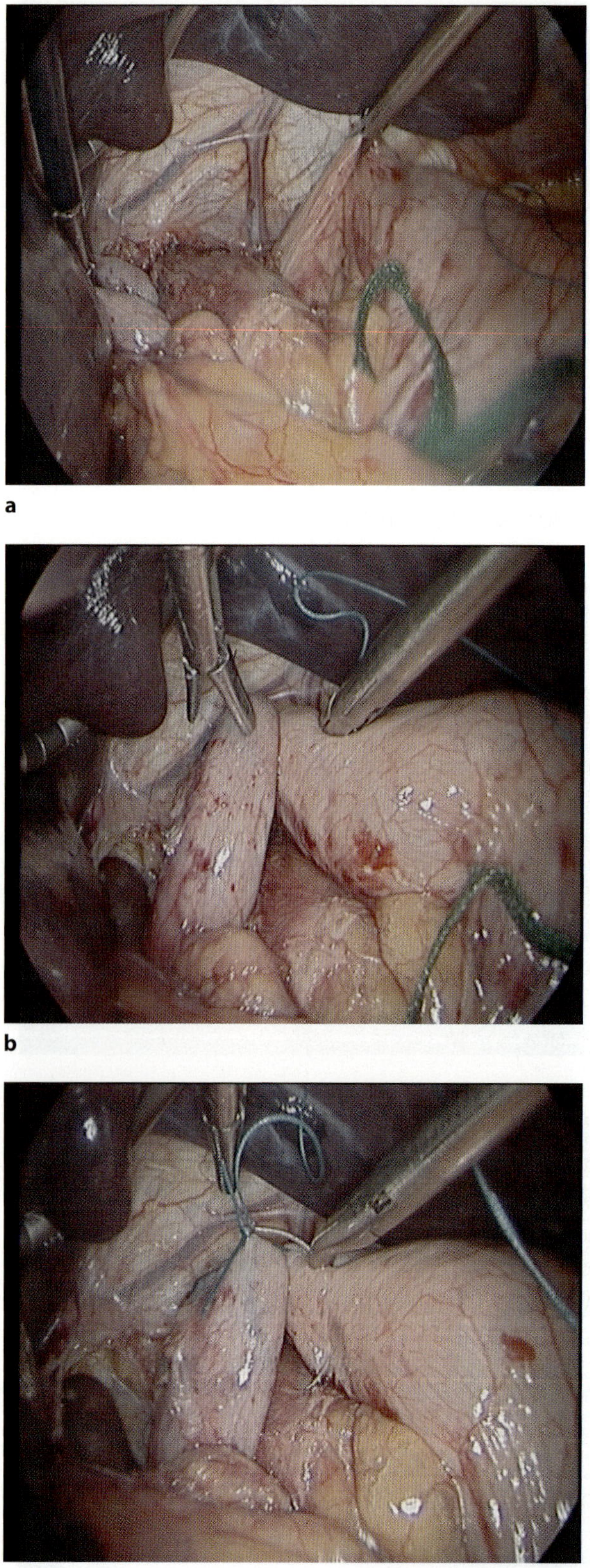

a

b

c

Fig. 10. Fundoplication with the posterior wall of the fundus on the right side of the esophagus and the anterior wall on the left side of the esophagus

From this original description, there have been a lot of adaptations. The most widely accepted is the need for crural repair in all patients. There is a general trend towards fixation of the valve on the anterior wall of the esophagus.

Some authors have described a "minimal dissection" technique, where no dissection of the lower esophagus is performed, some times no division of the phreno-esophageal membrane and the anterior gastric fundus is passed trough a small retroesophageal channel to create the valve. There is no systematic crural repair [6], [7].

Postoperative care

No naso gastric tube is left at the end of the operation.

The patient is allowed to drink on the first evening.

An intravenous line is left in place until the morning of the first postoperative day at the latest. A Gastrografin swallow is performed on the first postoperative day to verify the position and proper functioning of the antireflux valve. The patient is discharged on the second postoperative day. Dietary instructions are given to avoid the risk of food impacting in the distal esophagus during the early postoperative period.

Controversies

Floppy Nissen vs Nissen-Rossetti fundoplication

Demeesteer et al demonstrated in 1986 that fundic mobilisation and short valve, build on a large bare esophageal bougie, led to decreased incidence of side effects (dysphagia, bloating) compared to long valve and valve without gastric mobilization [5]. That concept became the "gold standard" of open fundoplication for years.

In the laparoscopic area, some authors reproduced this technique and reported excellent results [8]–[11].

Other authors defend the concept of the anterior wall technique (Nissen-Rossetti technique) without systematic division of the short gastric vessels. Randomized trials fail to demonstrate any difference between the two techniques [7], [12], [13], [14].

What can be the advantages and disadvantages of both techniques?

Difference between the short floppy Nissen and the anterior wall Nissen-Rossetti technique are not limited to the short gastric vessels division. The shape of the antireflux valve is also different. One is constructed with both the anterior and posterior wall of the gastric fundus. By definition, the other one is constructed with the anterior wall of the gastric fundus (*Fig. 12*).

Technically, we feel that the floppy Nissen fundoplication it is the most reproducible operation. Mobilization of the gastric fundus allows the surgeon to see the upper fundus in toto, and to use systematically the same landmarks to create the fundoplication. With a good fundic mobilization, the risk is to create a too floppy valve, if this idea might exist. This looseness of the valve allows also a very precise positioning of the fundoplicature on the GE junction. No traction means no tension on the sutures (risk of disrupted valve), no twist on the GE junction (risk of dysphagia).

But the fundic mobilization is not an easy step of this operation even if it has been facilitated by the new technologies (ultrasonic scissors, ligating systems...). The risk of splenic injury is present. If one mobilizes, it has to be in the good extent and not limited to the vessels of the gastro-splenic ligament. Some have advocate that gastric mobilization increases the risk of intrathoracic migration of the fundoplicature or paraesophageal acute gastric intrathoracic migration. Surgical teams who did not mobilize the stomach have reported the largest incidence of this type of complication.

The anterior wall technique appears as a more easy operation. It is not. It imposes a very precise choice of the right part of the anterior wall of the gastric fundus that has to be used for fundoplication. Bad landmarks will lead to complications such as the typical laparoscopic complication, the bilobed stomach. The stomach is divided in two pouches because the valve has been created with the body of the stomach instead of the fundus. Reoperation is unavoidable (*Fig. 13*).

Other complications include a too tight valve, a twisted fundoplication, and a gastric valve.

The defenders of this type of fundoplication argue that they can adapt their technique depending on the anatomy of the gastric fundus, that sometimes implies division of the short gastric vessels. It is not a true reproducible operation and should be reserved to well trained and experienced eso-gastric surgeons.

Crural repair

There are no randomized control trials evaluating the role of routine crural repair. Nonrandomized studies have shown an intolerable rate of intrathoracic migration and paraesophageal herniation in patients not undergoing crural repair [15]–[18]. Most surgeons use the standard posterior hiatoplasty. Controversies still exist on the use of prosthetic

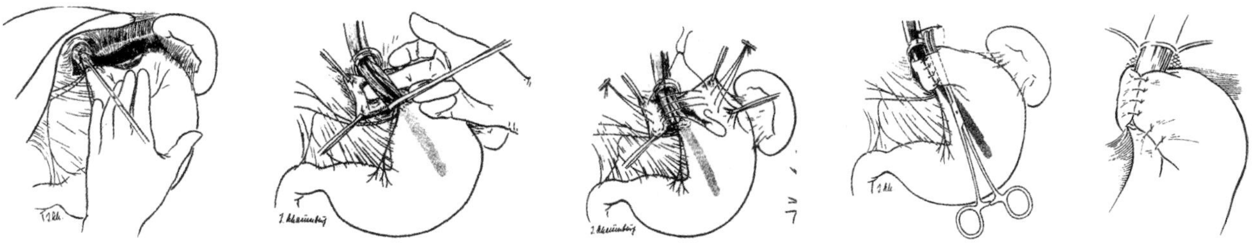

Fig. 11. Nissen-Rossetti operation: the anterior wall technique (Reprint from Gastro esophageal reflux disease: back to surgery? Büchler, Farthmann (eds) Karger 1997)

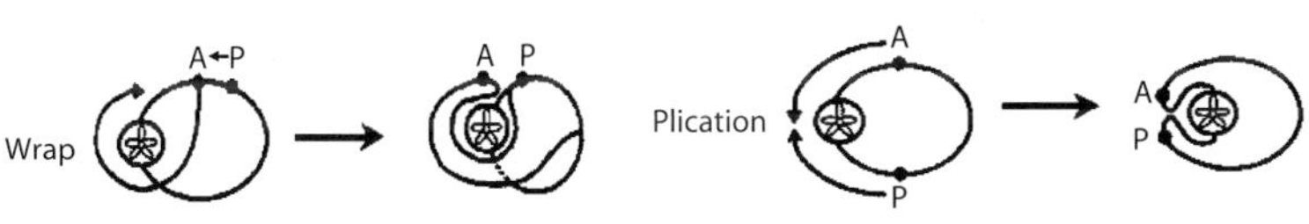

Fig. 12. Anterior fundoplication (warp) and floppy fundoplication

reinforcement for larger hiatal orifice [19]. Experience from repair of type-II-III hiatal hernia is increasing and some randomized trials demonstrate the usefulness of this concept. Long-term results are mandatory, with a special attention on the incidence of visceral injury related to the prosthesis.

Esophageal dissection-shortened esophagus

Acquired shortening of the esophagus, while still an area of controversy, is recognized by many surgeons to occur as a complication of longstanding and severe gastroesophageal reflux disease in some patients [20]–[23]. Other authors consider that the short esophagus phenomenon is overemphasized, over reported, and over treated [24], [25].

However, most surgeons agree that a critical component of the surgical management of reflux disease is successful reduction of the gastroesophageal junction below the diaphragm with a minimum of tension: a minimum of 2 cm of intraabdominal esophagus is necessary. Although this is easily accomplished in most patients, in those with a shortened esophagus it can be problematic.

The fact that the most common forms of failure after laparoscopic fundoplication are recurrent hiatal hernia, intrathoracic migration and slipped fundoplication suggests that some esophageal shortening may be present more commonly than appreciated, and that surgeons should routinely assess esophageal length and pay careful attention to the details of crural repair. There are two basic ways to reduce tension on the repair of a hiatal hernia. One is to mobilize the esophagus and the other is to add esophageal length with a Collis gastroplasty.

Mobilization should be the primary method used to achieve increased esophageal length [26]. This is a particular problem with laparoscopic antireflux surgery because several conditions conspire to mask the presence of a short esophagus with this approach. First, the laparoscopic pneumoperitoneum artificially elevates the diaphragm and gives the visual impression during the procedure that there is more abdominal length of esophagus than is actually the case. Second, the esophagus is usually pulled downward during the procedure, and because an assistant does the retraction the surgeon has little sense of the amount of force being used to pull the esophagus down into the abdomen. Both of these conditions are peculiar to the laparoscopic approach and contribute to unrecognized tension after an antireflux operation.

Although there are no absolute indicators, several abnormalities are frequently associated with a short esophagus and can be used clinically to identify patients at risk. These include an esophageal stricture, long-segment Barrett's esophagus, a paraesophageal or a large (5 cm or greater) sliding hiatal hernia that fails to reduce in the upright position, and a failed previous fundoplication [21].

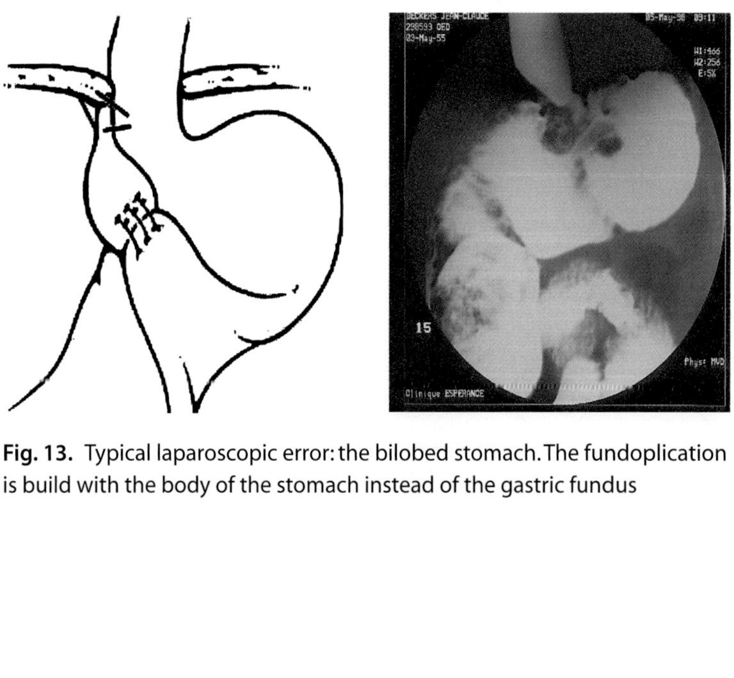

Fig. 13. Typical laparoscopic error: the bilobed stomach. The fundoplication is build with the body of the stomach instead of the gastric fundus

Conclusions

On a long-term evaluation, we feel that laparoscopic Nissen fundoplication is able to reproduce the results of open fundoplication as demonstrated in some studies. Our recent study of 100 patients at 10 years after laparoscopic fundoplication demonstrates a 90% rate of reflux control, which is comparable to the open long term results (paper submitted to publication).

Some randomized short term trials have demonstrate that after open operations, there are statistically more complains about scars. The other parameters seem to be equivalent: control of symptoms, side effects. But, we must keep in mind that these results are obtained, in the laparoscopic group, with a reduced mortality and morbidity rate, shorter hospital stay and sick leave and a lower incidence of incisional complications. There is also, a substantial reduction in the rate of incidental splenectomies, as they are reported in the open series (0–8%).

In summary, if long-term series confirm the results obtained in dedicated centres, laparoscopic Nissen fundoplication should become the "gold standard" of treatment for gastro -oesophageal reflux disease in appropriately investigated and selected patients.

References

[1] Nissen R (1956) A simple operation for control of reflux esophagitis. Schweiz Med Wochenschr 86: 590–592

[2] Rossetti M, Hell K (1977) Fundoplication for the treatment of gastroesophageal reflux in hiatal hernia. World J Surg 1: 439–443

[3] Donahue PE, Larson GM, Stewardson RH, Bombeck CT (1977) Floppy Nissen fundoplication. Rev Surg 34: 223–224

[4] Donahue PE, Samelson S, Nyhus LM, Bombeck CT (1985) The floppy Nissen fundoplication. Effective long-term control of pathologic reflux. Arch Surg 120: 663–668

[5] DeMeester TR, Bonavina L, Albertucci M (1986) Nissen fundoplication for gastroesophageal reflux disease. Evaluation of primary repair in 100 consecutive patients. Ann Surg 204: 9–20

[6] Anvari M, Allen C (1998) Laparoscopic Nissen fundoplication: two-year comprehensive follow-up of a technique of minimal paraesophageal dissection. Ann Surg 227: 25–32

[7] Watson DI, Jamieson GG, Pike GK, Davies N, Richardson M, Devitt PG (1999) Prospective randomized double-blind trial between laparoscopic Nissen fundoplication and anterior partial fundoplication. Br J Surg 86: 123–130

[8] Dallemagne B, Weerts JM, Jehaes C, Markiewicz S, Lombard R (1991) Laparoscopic Nissen fundoplication: preliminary report. Surg Laparosc Endosc 1: 138–143

[9] Hinder RA, Filipi CJ, Wetscher G, Neary P, DeMeester TR, Perdikis G (1994) Laparoscopic Nissen fundoplication is an effective treatment for gastroesophageal reflux disease. Ann Surg 220: 472–481

[10] Hunter JG, Trus TL, Branum GD, Waring JP, Wood WC (1996) A physiologic approach to laparoscopic fundoplication for gastroesophageal reflux disease. Ann Surg 223: 673–685

[11] Peters JH, DeMeester TR, Crookes P, Oberg S, de Vos SM, Hagen JA, Bremner CG (1998) The treatment of gastroesophageal reflux disease with laparoscopic Nissen fundoplication: prospective evaluation of 100 patients with "typical" symptoms. Ann Surg 228: 40–50

[12] Luostarinen ME, Isolauri JO (1999) Randomized trial to study the effect of fundic mobilization on long-term results of Nissen fundoplication. Br J Surg 86: 614–618

[13] Chrysos E, Tzortzinis A, Tsiaoussis J, Athanasakis H, Vasssilakis J, Xynos E (2001) Prospective randomized trial comparing Nissen to Nissen-Rossetti technique for laparoscopic fundoplication. Am J Surg 182: 215–221

[14] Blomqvist A, Dalenback J, Hagedorn C, Lonroth H, Hyltander A, Lundell L (2000) Impact of complete gastric fundus mobilization on outcome after laparoscopic total fundoplication. J Gastrointest Surg 4: 493–500

[15] Soper NJ, Dunnegan D (1999) Anatomic fundoplication failure after laparoscopic antireflux surgery. Ann Surg 229: 669–676

[16] Watson DI, Jamieson GG, Devitt PG, Matthew G, Britten-Jones RE, Game PA, Williams RS (1995) Changing strategies in the performance of laparoscopic Nissen fundoplication as a result of experience with 230 operations. Surg Endosc 9: 961–966

[17] Watson DI, Jamieson GG, Devitt PG, Mitchell PC, Game PA (1995) Paraoesophageal hiatus hernia: an important complication of laparoscopic Nissen fundoplication. Br J Surg 82: 521–523

[18] Dutta S, Bamehriz F, Boghossian T, Pottruff CG, Anvari M (2004) Outcome of laparoscopic redo fundoplication. Surg Endosc 18: 440–443

[19] Kamolz T, Granderath FA, Bammer T, Pasiut M, Pointner R (2004) Dysphagia and quality of life after

laparoscopic Nissen fundoplication in patients with and without prosthetic reinforcement of the hiatal crura. Surg Endosc 16: 572–577
[20] Awad ZT, Mittal SK, Roth TA, Anderson PI, Wilfley WA Jr, Filipi CJ (2001) Esophageal shortening during the era of laparoscopic surgery. World J Surg 25: 558–561
[21] Gastal OL, Hagen JA, Peters JH, Campos GM, Hashemi M, Theisen J, Bremner CG, DeMeester TR (1999) Short esophagus: analysis of predictors and clinical implications. Arch Surg 134: 633–636
[22] Horvath KD, Swanstrom LL, Jobe BA (2000) The short esophagus: pathophysiology, incidence, presentation, and treatment in the era of laparoscopic antireflux surgery. Ann Surg 232: 630–640
[23] Luketich JD, Grondin SC, Pearson FG (2000) Minimally invasive approaches to acquired shortening of the esophagus: laparoscopic Collis-Nissen gastroplasty. Semin Thorac Cardiovasc Surg 12: 173–178
[24] Madan AK, Frantzides CT, Patsavas KL (2004) The myth of the short esophagus. Surg Endosc 18: 31–34
[25] Korn O, Csendes A, Burdiles P, Braghetto I, Sagastume H, Biagini L (2003) Length of the esophagus in patients with gastroesophageal reflux disease and Barrett's esophagus compared to controls. Surgery 133: 358–363
[26] O'Rourke RW, Khajanchee YS, Urbach DR, Lee NN, Lockhart B, Hansen PD, Swanstrom LL (2003) Extended transmediastinal dissection: an alternative to gastroplasty for short esophagus. Arch Surg 138: 735–740

Chapter 17

LAPAROSCOPIC TOUPET FUNDOPLICATION

C. Zornig

Department of Surgery, Israelitisches Krankenhaus Hamburg, Germany

Summary

Toupet described his technique of fundoplication in 1963 [1]. He had little clinical experience, but saw the importance of a partial wrap to avoid postoperative dysphagia. He recommended closure of the hiatus only in case of large hernias and never divided the short gastric vessels. If we talk about a Toupet procedure today, we mean a posterior partial fundoplication. In contrary to his original technique we have learned that hiatal closure is important to avoid recurrent hernia and that the wrap can be tailored more nicely, if the short gastric vessels are divided. This modern adaptation of Toupet's operation is a very successful tool to treat gastro-oesophageal reflux disease.

Introduction

Toupet has described his technique of partial fundoplication in 1963 [1]. This technique has had an increasing success during the last years of laparoscopic surgery. Lots of technical variations have been used until today. Also in my department, in which the Toupet procedure is performed almost exclusively since 4 years, we have developed an individual technique. For a better understanding, Toupet's own technique is described first. I do this according to the original publication which followed a session at the French Academy of Surgery and according to an article of Katkhouda et al [2], which gives some further information about Toupet's work. Afterwards I will describe our technique of today after having performed about 1200 partial fundoplications out of about 1800 fundoplications that we have done on the whole.

Toupet's original technique

To avoid reflux in a patient with hiatal hernia Toupet aimed at replacing the lower oesophagus down into the abdominal cavity, at reconstructing the angle of His and at avoiding the cardia to migrate again into the chest. The operation was performed through a midline incision and consisted mainly of three steps:

(1) Mobilization of the abdominal oesophagus
(2) Mobilization of the posterior aspect of the fundus
(3) Oesophagogastroplasty with phrenogastroplasty.

After incision of the peritoneum overlying the oesophagus the lower part of the oesophagus and the crura were dissected. The two vagus nerves were identified and preserved at all steps of the operation. After incision of the lesser omentum the posterior aspect of the fundus was widely dissected. It seems to me, that Toupet has performed this dissection more intensely than we imagine today, as he has even sometimes divided the left gastric artery. Then he could easily pull the posterior wall of the fundus behind the oesophagus to the right side. This part of the fundus was fixed to the right side of the oesophagus and to the right crus with 4–5 sutures each. On the left side the fundus was then fixed to the oesophagus and the left crus.

Toupet stresses the fact that this procedure is different from the one of Nissen [3], as it does not create a total sleeve around the oesophagus. He believes, that it is preferable to leave the hemicircumference of the oesophagus free from any fundus to avoid the inability to belch, a complication that occured after the Nissen procedure, as he said. It must also be mentioned that Toupet did not divide the short gastric vessels. The extreme mobilization of the posterior aspect of the fundus allowed him to pull it easily to the right side.

Toupet recommended closure of the hiatus only when it was very enlarged. This should be done by one or two stitches in front of the oesophagus. He found, that the suturing of the crura is difficult to calibrate and was afraid of dysphagia. He could not imagine, that these sutures, which tend to cut into the muscle fibres, could create a normal oesophageal hiatus. He understands a hiatal hernia similar to a rectal prolaps. As a consequence, he aims at pulling the herniated organs (distal oesophagus, proximal stomach) back into the abdominal cavity, and of course, they should stay there. This should be managed by the fixating sutures, the obliteration of the cul-de-sac and the irritation of the serosal surfaces. He then hopes that the muscular fibres of the crura could regain tonicity, because they are not stretched anymore by the fundic prolaps (as the anal sphincter becomes better after treatment of a rectal prolaps).

Toupet published his technique after having performed a series of cadaveric operations, but with the experience of only 4 patients with limited follow-up. On the whole Toupet only performed 20 hiatal hernia operations in his career.

Our Toupet technique

We use 4 trocars (two 10 mm, two 5 mm) besides the optic trocar. The surgeon stands between the legs, the first assistent sits on the patient's left side and holds the camera and the Babcock clamp. The second assistent stands on the right side and retracts the liver. A 45° optic is our standard. If intense dissection in the mediastinum is needed, we change to a 30° optic. Dissection is performed with the ultracision scissors (Ethicon, Norderstedt, Germany). The lesser omentum is opened. If necessary vagal hepatic branches or an arterial branch from the left gastric artery to the left liver are divided. A good exposure of the operative field is more important than the questionable problems of the division of these structures. The right crus is dissected free and then the anterior part of the left. As the posterior part of the left crus is covered by fundus, we then divide the short gastric vessels. Afterwards the fundus can be pulled to the right side. The posterior part of the left crus is now nicely exposed and can be freed. Consequent dissection of the crura automatically results in a tunnel behind the oesophagus (*Fig. 1*). The oesophagus is pulled down and dissection is carried out in the mediastinum. The lower 5–8 cm of the oesophagus should finally stay in the abdominal cavity without any tension. Both vagus nerves are visualized. A posterior hiatoplasty is performed by 2 z-formed sutures with non resorbable mersilene 1 (*Figs. 2 and 3*). This thick material does not tend that much to cut into muscle fibres and the z-stitches put the tension on a large region. The polyfilament thread makes intraoperative knotting (which should be gentle) easy and probably causes more scar tissue than a monofilament suture.

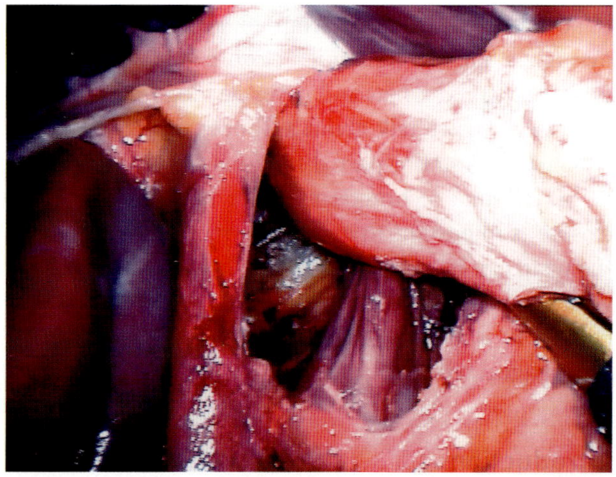

Fig. 1. Dissection of the crura and up into the mediastinum is finished. The region of the lower oesophageal sphincter is located in the abdominal cavity. The oesophagus is lifted by a Babcock clamp, which is inserted in the left lower abdomen

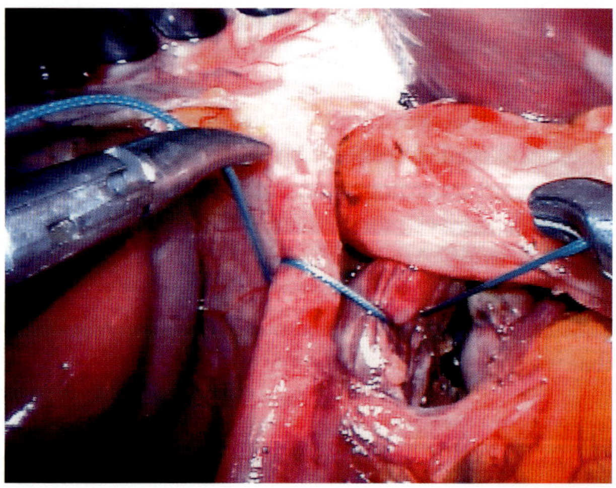

Fig. 2. The crura can nicely be approximated by the first z-formed suture with Mersilene 1

A part of the fundus is pulled behind the oesophagus to the right side. Tayloring of the wrap is controlled by the shoe shine test (*Fig. 4*). The right part of the fundus is fixed to the right crus or both with a running suture of mersilene 2/0. Another suture fixes this part of the wrap to the right side of the oesophagus. The corresponding left part of the fundus is chosen and fixed to the left side of the oesophagus (*Fig. 5*). A single suture fixes the left fundus to the diaphragm. Care is taken that the vagal nerves stay outside the sutures.

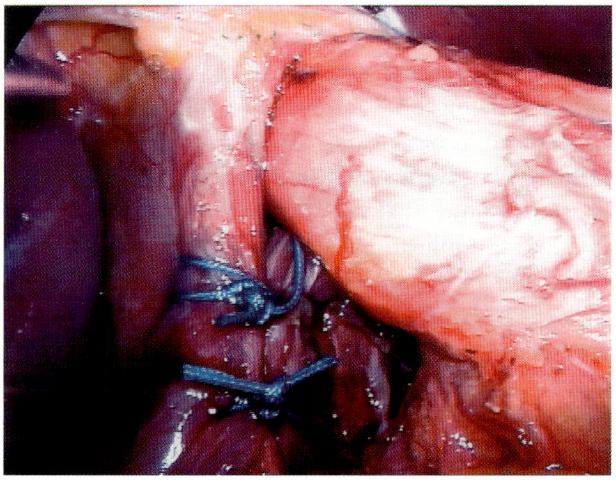

Fig. 3. The hiatus is closed sufficiently by 2 z-formed sutures. There is only an 18 ch gastric tube in the oesophagus

Our results

Between May 1999 and May 2000 we conducted a prospective randomized trial to compare the Nissen fundoplication to the one of Toupet [4], [5]. In this study we also examined the influence of preexisting oesophageal motility on the operative result in accordance to the technique. Follow-up studies were perfomed after 4 months and 2 years. Here I want to focus on the results of the 100 patients who received a Toupet fundoplication.

The mean operative time was 50 minutes. All operations were finished laparoscopically. The mean postoperative stay was 5 days. After 4 months and 2 years the overall satisfaction rate was 89% and 85%, respectively. After 2 years 12 patients complained about clinical reflux. Only half of them had objective pathological findings in a 24-h-pH-monitoring and/or endoscopically. On the other hand 22 patients had pathological findings in the 24-h-pH-monitoring and/or endoscopy. But only 6 of them had clinical symptoms. Dysphagia according to our very sensible scoring system was present preoperatively in 33 patients, whereas postoperatively only 8 patients complained about dysphagia.

Comparing the two operative techniques reflux control was equal, but the complication rate (dysphagia, need for reoperation) was higher after a Nissen fundoplication. The preoperative oesophageal motility did not influence the results with statistical significance.

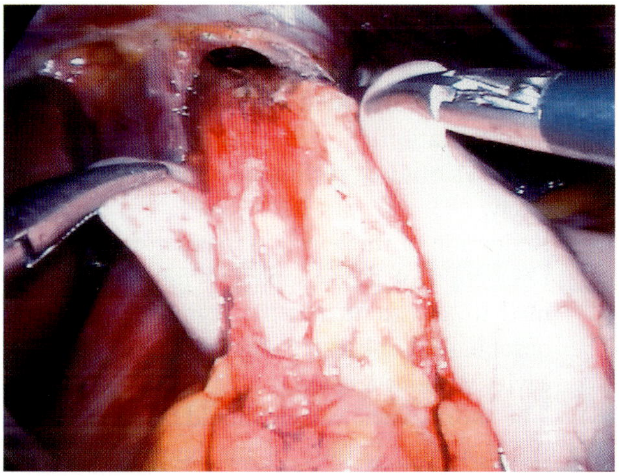

Fig. 4. Shoe shine test to chose the ideal parts of the fundus to create the wrap

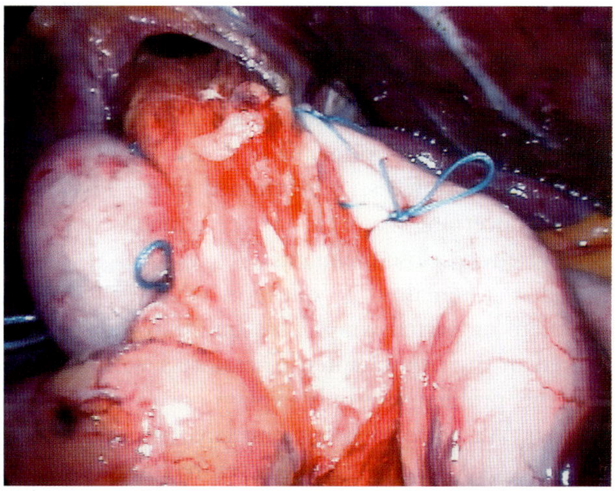

Fig. 5. The posterior partial fundoplication is completed

Discussion

I totally agree with the aims, that Toupet followed with his operation. The hernia must be reduced. The oesophagus must be dissected as far up into the mediastinum as necessary to get the segment of the lower oesophageal sphincter completely down into the abdominal cavity without any tension. The angle of His must be reconstructed. The ensemble of these operative steps with the anatomical situation (and the consecutive function) that we create avoids successfully reflux, already on the first postoperative day. As we are heading at a long-term effect, this anatomical situation must remain unchanged for the rest of the patient's life. And this effect should be connected with the lowest complication rate possible (dysphagia!).

The question is, how to achieve this aim. The reduction of the hernia and extensive dissection of the lower oesophagus is agreed by all specialists in this field. The fundoplication (whether complete or partial) certainly is the best and most stable way to reconstruct the angle of His (compared to the single suture line of Lortat-Jacob [6] or a simple gastropexy). Each sort of fundoplication creates a certain mass that should not be able to herniate up through the reconstructed hiatus. Toupet achieved a mobile fundus by extensive dissection at the posterior gastric wall. In my opinion the division of the short gastric vessels makes the tayloring of the wrap even easier. The crucial point is to avoid the recurrence of the hernia, which often is associated with recurrent reflux. In my opinion the closure of the hiatus plays an important role. Here I do not agree with Toupet. We can avoid to injure muscle fibres by suture material and technique. And by suturing the crura we create more scar tissue in this region, what Toupet principially aimed at by irritaion of the serosal surfaces, as mentioned above. His arguments concerning hiatal closure seem inconsequent to me. We always close the hiatus.

Then it remains the question whether to use a complete or partial wrap. This question will be answered in the next chapter. Therefore I will not discuss this problem but only explain our own decision making. We performed our first laparoscopic fundoplication in 1992 using the Nissen technique, which has been recognized as the leading technique since the era of conventional surgery, at least in Germany. Despite our overall success with this operation the postoperative problems remained the same as in conventional surgery – mainly dysphagia and recurrent reflux. For several years we then followed the "tailored concept". Its proponents argued that the choice between a partial or total fundoplication should depend on the presence or absence of preexisting oesophageal motility disorders [7]–[10]. Many studies had shown, that the Nissen procedure was to be the more successful in terms of reflux control [7], [11]–[14]. However it was also associated with a higher rate of postoperative dysphagia [15]–[20]. While the Nissen procedure was the preferred technique, the partial wrap was recommended for patients with motility disorders [7], [9], [21], [22].

With increasing experience in this field of surgery a growing body of evidence suggested that the concept may be invalid [16], [17], [23]–[26]. We noticed that dysphagia also developed after a Toupet procedure and that we had recurrent reflux after Nissen fundoplications and a higher rate of reoperations. Therefore we decided to evaluate the tailored concept by comparing the two operations in a prospective randomized trial [4], [5]. In conclusion, at least in our hands the Toupet procedure compared to the one of Nissen had the same success rate concerning reflux control but a lower complication rate (dysphagia and the need for reoperations). And, tailoring of the technique according to the oesophageal motility proofed not to be valid. Therefore, we principially perform the partial fundoplication.

In conclusion I would like to highlight some points that seem to be important from my personal point of view:

(1) Toupet has invented the principal of partial fundoplication.
(2) Toupet's original technique is rarely performed today.
(3) Reduction of the hernia is mandatory.
(4) Dissection of the oesophagus must be performed to an extent that the region of the lower oesophageal sphincter stays in the abdominal cavity without tension.
(5) The short gastric vessels should be divided.
(6) A (posterior) closure of the hiatus is mandatory.
(7) A posterior partial fundoplication should be performed.

References

[1] Toupet MA (1963) Technique d'oesophago-gastroplastic avec phreno-gastropexie appliquee dans la cure radicale des hernies hiatales et comme complemet de l'operation de Heller dans les cordiospasmes. Mem Acad Chir 89: 394

[2] Katkhouda N, Khalil MR, Manhas S, Grant St, Velmahos GC, Umbach TW, Kaiser AM (2002) André Toupet: Surgeon technician par excellence. Ann Surg 235: 591–599

[3] Nissen R (1995) Eine einfache Operation zur Beeinflussung der Refluxoesophagitis. Schweiz Med Wochenschr 86: 590–592

[4] Zornig C, Strate U, Fibbe C, Emmermann A, Layer P (2002) Nissen vs. Toupet laparoscopic fundoplication: a prospective randomized study of 200 patients with and without preoperative esophageal motility disorders. Surg Endosc 16: 758–766

[5] Fibbe C, Layer P, Keller J, Strate U, Emmermann A, Zornig C (2001) Esophageal motility in reflux disease before and after fundoplication: a prospective, randomized, clinicaland manometric study. Gastroenterology 121: 5–14

[6] Lortat-Jacob JL (1954) Les malpositions cardio-tuberositaires. Lyon Chir 6: 49–58

[7] DeMeester TR, Peters JH (1993) Fehler und Gefahren bei der laparoskopischen Antirefluxchirurgie. Chirurg 64: 230–236

[8] Fuchs KH, Freys SM, Heimbucher J, Thiede A (1994) Management of gastroesophageal reflux disease. Dis Esophagus 7: 250–254

[9] Hunter JG, Swanstrom L, Waring JP (1996) Dysphagia after lapasrocopic antireflux surgery: the impact of operative technique. Ann Surg 224: 51–57

[10] Hunter JG, Trus TL, Branum GD, Waring JP, Wood WC (1996) A physiologic approach to laparoscopic fundoplication for gastroesophageal reflux disease. Ann Surg 223: 673–685

[11] Cuschieri A, Hunter J, Wolfe B, Swanstrom LL, Hutson W (1993) Multicenter prospective evaluation of laparoscopic antireflux surgery: preliminary report. Surg Endosc 7: 505–510

[12] Dallmagne B, Weerts JM, Jehaes C, Markiewicz S (1996) Causes of laparoscopic antireflux operations. Surg Endosc 10: 305–310

[13] Hinder RA, Filipi CJ, Wetcher G, Neary P, DeMeester TR, Perdikis G (1994) Laparoscopic Nissen fundoplication is an effective treatment for gastroesophageal reflux disease. Ann Surg 220: 472–481

[14] Jamieson GG, Watson DI, Britten-Jones R, Mitchell PC, Anvari M (1994) Laparoscopic Nissen fundoplication. Ann Surg 220: 137–145

[15] Bell RC, Hanna P, Powers B, Sabel J, Hruza D (1996) Clinical and manometric results of laparoscopic partial (Toupet) and complete (Rosetti-Nissen) fundoplication. Surg Endosc 10: 724–728

[16] Coster CC, Bower WH, Wilson VT, Brebrick RT, Richardson GL (1997) Laparoscopic partial fundoplication vs. laparoscopic Nissen-Rosetti fundoplication: short-term results of 231 cases. Surg Endosc 11: 625–631

[17] Lundell L, Abrahamsson H, Ruth M, Rydberg L, Lonroth H, Olbe L (1996) Lonf-term results of a prospectice randomized comparison of total fundic wrap (Nissen-Rosetti) or semifundoplication (Toupet) for gastroesophageal reflux. Br J Surg 83: 830–835

[18] McKernan JB (1994) Laparoscopic repair of gastroseophageal reflux disease: Toupet partial fundoplication versus Nissen fundoplication. Surg Endosc 8: 851–756

[19] Thor KB, Silander T (1989) A long-term randomized prospective trial of the Nissen procedure versus a modified Toupet technique. Ann Surg 210: 719–724

[20] Watson A, Spychal RT, Brown MG, Peck N, Callender N (1995) Laparoscopic physiological antireflux procedure: prelimanary results of a prospective symptomatic and objective study. Br J Surg 82: 651–656

[21] Bell RC, Hanna P, Mills MR, Bowery D (1999) Patterns of success and failure with laparoscopic Toupet fundoplication. Surg Endosc 13: 1189–1194

[22] Hunter JG, Trus TL, Branum GD, Waring JP, Wood WC (1996) A physiologic approach to laparoscopic fundoplication for gastroesophageal reflux disease. Ann Surg 223: 673–685

[23] Beckingham IJ, Cariem AK, Bornman PC, Callanan MD, Louw JA (1998) Oesophageal dysmotility is not associated with poor outcome after laparoscopic Nissen fundoplication. Br J Surg 85: 1290–1293

[24] Rydberg L, Magnus R, Hasse A, Lundell L (1999) Tailoring antireflux surgery: a randomized clinical trial. World J Surg 23: 612–618

[25] Watson DI, Jamiesson GG (1998) Antireflux surgery in the laparoscopic era. Br J Surg 85: 1173–1184

[26] Watson DI, Jamiesson GG, Pike GK, Davies N, Richardson M, Devitt PG (1999) Prospective randomized double-blind trial between laparoscopic Nissen fundoplication and anterior partial fundoplication. Br J Surg 86: 123–130

Chapter 18

COMPLETE VERSUS PARTIAL FUNDOPLICATION

L. Lundell

Department of Surgery, Karolinska University Hospital, Huddinge, Stockholm, Sweden

No doubt, a total fundoplication, either modified from or constructed according to the principles originally outlined by Nissen [1], is the most frequently performed antireflux operation worldwide [2]–[4]. This surgical approach, to the long-term control of gastroesophageal reflux disease (GERD), has even further been popularised by the introduction of laparoscopy. Although the issue has been discussed quite vigorously, the current consensus is that the long-term results after laparoscopy equal that following open operations [5]–[8]. The well-known downside of a total fundoplication is the mechanical side effects which seem to occur as a consequence of an over correction of the antireflux barrier in the gastroesophageal junction (GEJ) area. This results in some degree of dysphagia, inability to belch, postprandial bloating and flatulence [9]–[13]. These issues are of crucial importance particularly so in a clinical situation where effective medical therapeutic alternatives are available and harbour documented efficacy. To circumvent at least some of these drawbacks with the total fundoplications various forms of partial fundoplications have been launched and further explored to ascertain their efficacy and mode of action [14]–[16]. In order to understand the eventual role of partial fundoplications in the surgical treatment of GERD one has to understand the essentials of pathogenetic mechanisms into which fundoplication operations interact. Furthermore, the mechanisms which cause postfundoplication complaints have to be clarified, and the degree by which partial or total fundoplications interfere with those to become relevant for the occurrence of postoperative complaints. Last but not least, this chapter will focus on the available evidence which shows that partial fundoplications truly are effective in the long-term control of GERD.

Key pathogenetic mechanisms in GERD

The interplay between aggressive and defensive mechanisms is pivotal in the causation and prevention of esophageal mucosal damage in GERD [17]. The defence against reflux is multi factorial: firstly the antireflux barrier in the gastroesophageal junction, normally prevents acid to reflux into the esophagus. Secondly an intra esophageal bolus regularly triggers esophageal primary and sometimes also secondary peristalsis resulting in esophageal clearance of refluxed material. Finally the esophageal mucosal resistance consists of acid buffering and/or dilution capacity by bicarbonate and mucus secreted by submucosal glands. Moreover, tight junctions in the basalolateral membranes can mechanically prevent the influx of hydrogen ions and thereby play an important role [18]. Apart from impaired clearance ability, lower esophageal sphincter pressure was long believed to be a key factor causing frequent reflux in GERD. The lower esophageal sphincter (LES) is a specialised part of the distal esophagus with circular and oblique smooth muscle fibre with a length of approximately 4 cm and generates a constant high-pressure zone preventing reflux [19]. The LES appears to have the following properties:

(1) The LES maintains an elevated resting pressure relative to the proximal stomach and distal esophagus
(2) The LES reduces the resting pressure to equal the intra gastric pressure response to proximal distention (i.e., swallowed food bolus).
(3) The LES contracts in response to various physiological stimuli. Although it has been recognised that in the majority of reflux patients TLESRs (see below) are the main mechanism behind reflux. A subgroup of patients have been found to have a sustained reduced LES pressure often associated with severe esophagitis [19]. In those instances reflux occurs as a consequence of steady decline and complete relaxation of the LES accompanied by a transient increase in abdominal pressure whereupon spontaneous free reflux occurs.

Subsequent work by Dent and his co-workers [20], [21] showed that virtually all reflux events in healthy subjects are associated with complete transient low esophageal sphincter relaxations (TLESRs) not associated with swallowing. Most of the acid reflux events observed in GERD patients also occurred during TLESRs. The TLESRs are manometrically defined as an abrupt LES-pressure to the level of intra gastric pressure that is not associated with a swallow. During TLESRs the activity of the crural diaphragm is also inhibited thus facilitating gastroesophageal reflux [22]–[24]. Furthermore, other phenomena, which regularly accompany a TLESR, are a common cavity reflecting venting of air from the stomach and an esophageal peristalsis after contraction. Gastric distention, particularly of the cardic region, is a major stimulus for TLESRs through activation of gastric mechano receptors [19], [25]. These receptors play a pivotal role in the occurrence of TLESRs and gastroesophageal reflux. Postprandial adaptive relaxation of the proximal stomach is also associated with an increase in TLESRs frequency and acid gastroesophageal reflux, illustrating the important relationship between gastric motor events and the occurrence of reflux [26], [27]. Intra luminal electrical impedance studies have shown that almost all TLESRs are associated with any form of reflux, being either of gas nature, mixed or liquid content in both GERD patients and controls [28]. To day it is unexplained why TLESRs in GERD patients are more frequently associated with acid reflux. Impaired gastric emptying and augmented storage of nutrients in the gastric fundus might play a role [26], [29], [30].

Postfundoplication complaints and their causation

It is likely that a fundoplication being either total, partial anterior or posterior prevents reflux through similar mechanisms. These effects involve purely mechanical consequences in addition to alterations in esophageal motor function since these procedures are effective not only when placed in the chest in vivo but also when tested in animal viscera in vivo [30], [31].

These operations have major effects on LES function. Resting pressure of the LES and the length of the abdominal portion of the high-pressure zone are increased by these operations [32]–[36]. Continued assessment of LES tone, over a longer period of time, has shown that LES pressure is considerably higher after a total fundoplication than after partial posterior one. Importantly, in the latter group pressure levels in the LES region were very close to what is seen in normal healthy controls. LES tone assessments have demonstrated that after a variety of antireflux procedures, the pressure never reaches a level at which free reflux can be considered to occur (for exceptions see below).

With a growing insight into the mechanical consequences of a total fundoplication, the adverse consequences associated with a super-competent pressure zone in the lower esophageal sphincter area have become apparent. In similar situations the LES relaxes incompletely on swallowing which is accompanied by abolition of gas reflux and therefore inability to belch. Partial fundoplication procedures seem to be associated with a lower incidence of mechanical complications but some concern has been expressed that reflux control may be suboptimal or less durable than after a total fundoplication [37]–[40]. Furthermore, in patients prospectively studied after a total fundoplication, it was suggested that compensatory mechanisms are operational within the esophageal wall to overcome an outflow obstruction in the gastro-esophageal junction, a phenomenon which is expressed in terms of increased esophageal peristaltic wave amplitude [41], [42]. It has been suggested that these mechanical adverse consequences may be counteracted by making the wrap shorter, looser and by the use of intra operative bougie [43]–[45]. In this context it is interesting to note that studies from our laboratory did not record any difference in obstructing complaints between the patients randomised to either a total or a posterior partial fundoplication even when these patients were investigated more than 10 years after the operation [13], [46]. The fact that we observed somewhat more complaints of odynophagia in those having a total wrap may be a subtle sign of an esophageal outflow obstruction.

One key mechanism behind side effects after fundoplication procedures seems to reside in the postoperative function of the LES and its capacity to relax on an appropriate stimulation. Studies have suggested that a partial posterior fundoplication normalises the LES tone but does not impair the ability of the LES to relax on proper stimulation but still counteracts the triggering of transient LES relaxations [34], [47], [48]. In fact the LES tone after a posterior partial fundoplication never reaches the level which is seen in healthy subjects after maximal inhibitory stimulation, and more importantly only exceptionally are LES pressure levels recorded which are considered to allow free reflux over the barrier. By and large, dysphagia is a transient postoperative phenomenon [49]–[51], where there seems to be a relationship between recorded basal LES tone and the magnitude of similar obstructive complaints. Both of these events seem to diminish with growing experience of the surgeon [52]. Fundoplication patients have a restricted hiatal opening and an incomplete glutative EGJ relaxation. Consequently the EGJ transit time is prolonged, the degree of which is directly related to the degree of postoperative dysphagia [26], [28].

Regarding postoperative dysphagia data have been presented to show that even a subclinical outflow obstruction in the area of the gastroesophageal junction can manometrically be assessed both in the form of increased intra bolus pressure in the distal esophagus (ramp pressure) but also expressed in terms of increased peristaltic amplitude [34]. A consistent finding in studies comparing a posterior and anterior partial fundoplication was that a higher intra bolus pressure was recorded in the Toupet group suggesting a high level of outflow obstruction exerted by the posterior fundoplication [53], [54]. Interestingly enough somewhat more patients in this group reported dysphagia like symptoms compared to those having an anterior partial wrap. It is reasonable to assume that the angulation of the gastroesophageal junction, created by the positioning of the wrap behind the esophagus constitutes a major causative factor. Apparently, we as surgeons have to master a delicate balance between offering optimal reflux control and minimising the mechanical side effects of respective reconstructive procedure.

Another important reflux promoting mechanism that antireflux procedures interfere with is the triggering of the TLESRs [55], [56]. Repeated studies have shown total and partial fundoplications to be extremely effective in more or less abolishing these relaxations. Moreover, no major differences have been found between these different type of operations. By use of well-developed experimental set-ups it has been shown that posterior partial fundoplications seemed to exert advantages over a Nissen type of total fundoplication with numerically fewer distension induced TLESRs in the latter group, tentatively explaining the differences in bloating and flatulence side effects [26], [27], [57]. When studies have been extended to the group of patients having an anterior partial wrap, the LES nadir pressure during water swallows was significantly lower than in the posterior fundoplication group both in the resting state as well as after a meal or gas distension of the stomach. Patients having an anterior partial fundoplication seemed to more easily vent air from the stomach, whereas the downside of that effect may be less effective control of reflux compared to the posterior partial fundoplication according to Toupet [40], [53], [58].

The clinical importance of reducing troubles of rectal flatulence, for example by partial fundoplication has to be recognised (*Fig. 1*). Observations of particular significance have come from a recent multicenter Nordic trial in which patients were perspectively interviewed both before and after an antireflux operation as part of a protocol comparing medical and surgical therapy. Flatulence was found to be one of the few so-called postfundoplication symptoms that indeed increased after the operation.

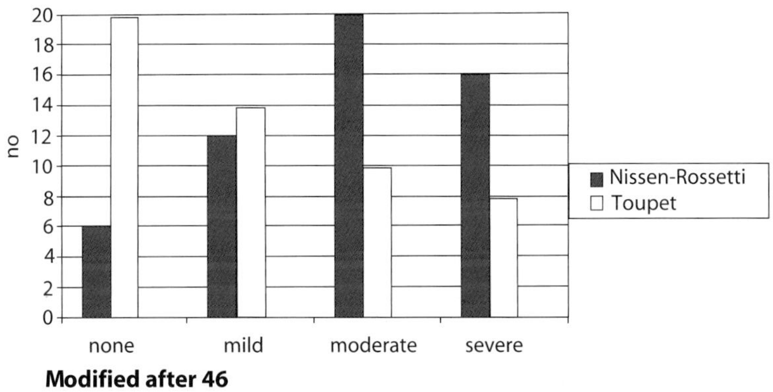

Fig. 1. Postfundoplication complaints (flatulence) after either a total or a partial posterior fundoplication

Although a laparoscopic fundoplication impairs TLESRs elicitation and renders an esophagogastric junction relaxation incomplete, the gastric accommodation to mechanical distention is not impaired [26], [27], [29], [30]. On the other hand, these operations exert an effect that leads to an attenuated accommodation of the proximal stomach followed by an increased distension of the distal stomach. This augmented distal stomach distension has to be better explored as potential causative factor behind post-fundoplication complaints. Patients having a posterior partial fundoplication exhibit a large meal induced increase in proximal stomach volume and a higher TLESRs rate than patients after a complete fundoplication [26]. The overall pressure profile across the esophagogastric junction has been demonstrated to be markedly higher after a complete fundoplication compared to partial fundoplication. The axial esophagogastric junction pressure gradient may play a crucial role in the occurrence of acid reflux during a transient lower esophageal sphincter relaxation. In patients having a complete fundoplication, meal induced proximal gastric volume increase is reduced to a greater extent compared to those having a posterior partial fundoplication. A reduced proximal gastric volume results in a diminished cardiac cross-sectional area which in turn results in increased wall elongation and thereby reducing the activation of stretch volume receptors responsible for eliciting the transient lower esophageal sphincter relaxations. A larger postprandial proximal gastric volume may therefore explain the somewhat higher rate of postprandial transient lower esophageal sphincter relaxations found after a partial fundoplication fascilitating venting of air from the stomach. In conclusion evidence are accumulating to show that a partial fundoplication to a greater and a more tuned extent normalises the physiology of the GEJ which of course is closely related to the profile and magnitude of the side effects.

Long-term reflux control

The effects of partial versus total fundoplications have been investigated in 9 randomised clinical trials. 6 were open laparotomy operations and 3 trials used laparoscopic approach and these studies have been published from 1974 to 2002. To these are also added some signle institution, preospective but uncontrolled observations [40], [58]–[71]. Concerning the partial fundoplications, the posterior partial type of operation was evaluated in 5 of these trials, the Hill repair in 2, the Lind subtotal posterior wrap in 1 and the anterior fundoplication in 1 study. The scheduled postoperative follow-up period ranged from 4 months to 8 years. No significant differences were found between partial versus total fundoplications in terms of new onset dysphagia and recurrence of gastroesohageal reflux symptoms (*Fig. 2*). Re-operations for failure were carried out in 1,5% of those having a partial fundoplication compared to 9,6% of those having a total fundoplication, a difference which was considered to be significant [72]. In the largest randomised trial comparing a posterior with a total fundoplication which covered more than 10 years of follow up, both procedures displayed the same level of reflux control. Based on the

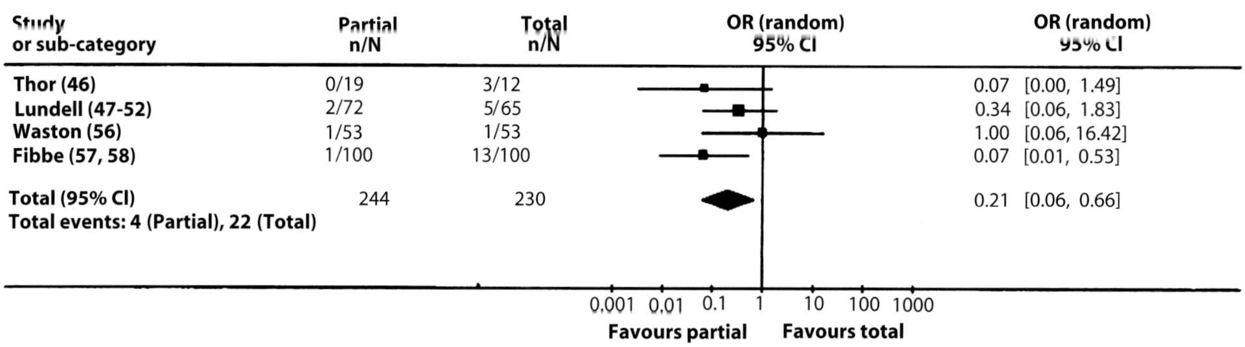

Modified after 71

Fig. 2. Pooled OR of reoperation for failure after partial vs total fundoplication

reassuring long-term follow-up data, it is difficult to understand why some investigators have found Toupet fundoplication not to be as successful as a total fundoplication, in severe cases of reflux disease particularly when performed by means of a laparoscopy [39]. It cannot be denied, of course, that some procedures are more difficult to perform when modern minimal invasive techniques are applied. In a search for factors that may have affected the outcome after the respective procedures, we have been unable to demonstrate that the severity, the duration of disease, hiatal closure by crural repair or body mass index had any impact on the level of long-term reflux control [66].

Survey of the controlled, clinical trial literature concerning posterior partial fundoplication shows that the level of clinical reflux control is not entirely similar to what can be reached by a total wrap, when studied by ambulatory 24 pH-monitoring. After the latter procedure it becomes evident that the esophageal acid exposure is reduced to near zero values. This contrast to observations made in patients having a partial wrap where corresponding values are in the ranges considered to be normal.

In 1999, Watson and his co-workers [73] reported a randomised trial comparing laparoscopic Nissen fundoplication with an anterior partial variant. The partial anterior fundopolication comprised an 180° wrap, where the wrap was anchored to the right hiatal pillar and the esophageal wall. The immediate postoperative results were very encouraging and recently the 5-year follow-up outcome was published [60]. These data have confirmed the results of the initial report showing that reflux control was somewhat better after a total fundoplication but this was reached at the prise of significantly more dysphagia, more epigastric bloating and inferior preservation of belching. This resulted in a larger proportion of patients reporting a good or excellent overall outcome at 5 years following anterior fundoplication (94 vs. 86%).

Are all partial fundoplications followed by the same results?

Since prevention is the best strategy, not the least since we lack effective treatment of established severe postfundoplication symptoms, it is important to raise the question whether all partial fundoplications are followed by the same results? It seems beyond any doubt that less troubles and complaints of rectal flatulence follows a partial fundoplication compared to a total wrap. In a recent randomised clinical trial the questions was addressed whether there are important differences between an anterior and a posterior partial fundoplication in terms of reflux control and side effects [53]. This trial incorporated almost 100 patients with a limited follow-up. Despite these drawbacks, significant differences were noted in favour of the posterior fundoplication regarding the level of reflux control. Even when only daytime acid exposure was objectively assessed, the outcome after laparoscopic anterior partial fundoplication (according to Watson) was found to be clearly inferior (*Fig. 3*). Regarding side effects it was not possible to reveal any differences in obstructive complaints between the two partial fundoplications but interestingly enough significantly more patients reported an ability to vomit after the anterior fundoplication. This observation probably reflects the efficacy of the respective repair. Why should an anterior partial

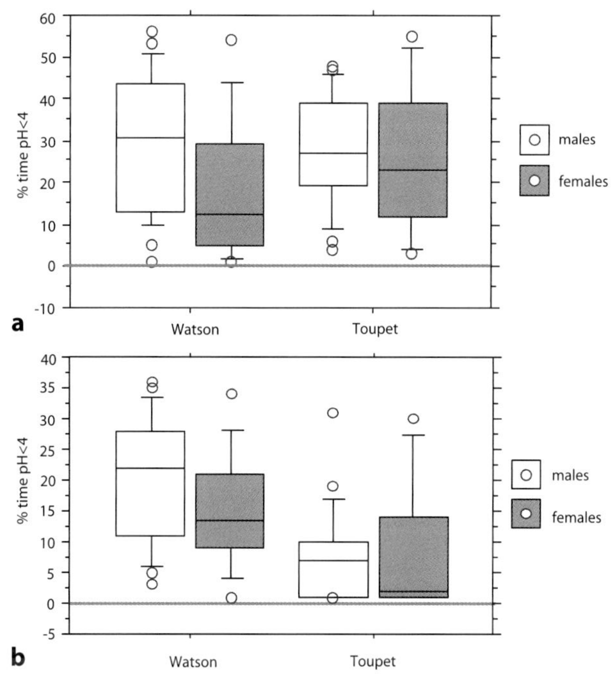

Fig. 3. Esophageal acid exposure before (**a**) and (**b**) months after an anterior (Watson) or posterior (Toupet) partial fundoplication. Adapted after [53]

fundoplication function differently from a posterior one? The extent of the distal esophageal body that is encircled by the actual wrap varies somewhat between the respective procedures. The posterior fundoplication elevates the abdominal portion of the esophagus from its native bed in the hiatus and by necessity angluates the gastroesophageal junction. The significance of this has to be better clarified but may have the potential to cause some esophageal outflow obstruction but it is totally unclear whether it contributes to a better mechanical barrier to prevent gastroesophageal reflux. The anterior partial fundoplication performed and recently validated by Watson and co-workers from Australia [60], differs somewhat from that originally described in 1991 [16]. The message is, however clear, if an anterior fundoplication is chosen it has to be a complete anterior 180° wrap but more studies are required to give firm guidance to the clinicians.

Concluding remarks

With the aim of optimising the outcome of antireflux surgery, the surgeon has to perform and master a delicate act of balance on the choice between various fundoplication procedures. On one hand we have the total fundoplication with its proved efficacy regarding reflux control but with it associated mechanical side-effects leading to symptoms relating to the relative obstruction in the gastroesophageal junction and the inability to vent air from the stomach and the sequelae that follow. The posterior partial fundoplication has obvious advantages with less postfundoplication complaints without compromising with the level of reflux control and can therefore be generally recommended. Some anterior partial fundoplication present very promising results but confirmative studies are warranted.

References

[1] Nissen R (1956) Eine einfache Operation zur Beeinflussung der Reflux Oesophagitis. Schweiz Med Wochenschr 86: 590

[2] Watson DI, Jamieson GG (1998) Antireflux surgery in the laparoscopic era. Br J Surg 85(9): 1173–1184

[3] Perdikis G, Hinder RA, Lund RJ, Raiser F, Katada N (1997) Laparoscopic Nissen fundoplication: where do we stand? Surg Laparosc Endosc 7: 17–21

[4] Peracchia A, Bancewicz J, Bonavina L et al (1995) Fundoplication is an effective treatment for gastro-oesophageal reflux disease. Gastroenterol Int 8: 1–7

[5] Anvari M, Allen C, Borm A (1995) Laparoscopic Nissen fundoplication is a satisfactory alternative to long-term omeprazole therapy. Br J Surg 82: 938–942

[6] Watson DI, Jamieson GG, Baigrie RJ et al (1996) Laparoscopic surgery for gastro-oesophageal reflux: beyond the learning curve. Br J Surg 223: 1284–1287

[7] Laine S, Rantala A, Gullichsen R, Ovaska J (1997) Laparoscopic vs conventional Nissen fundoplication. A prospective randomized study. Surg Endoscopic 11: 441–444

[8] Nilsson G, Larsson S, Johnsson F (2000) Randomized clinical trial of laparoscopic versus open fundoplication: blind evaluation of recovery and discharge period. Br J Surg 87: 873–878

[9] DeMeester, Bonavina L, Albertucci M (1986) Nissen fundoplication for gastroesophageal reflux disease. Evaluation of primary repair in 100 consecutive patients. Ann Surg 204: 9–20

[10] Luostarinen M, Isolauri J, Laitinen J, Koskinen M, Keyriläinen O, Markkula H, Lehtinen E, Uusitalo A (1993) Fate of Nissen fundoplication after 20 years. A clinical, endoscopical and functional analysis. Gut 34: 1015–1020

[11] Negre JB, Markkula HT, Keyriläinen O, Matikainen (1983) Nissen fundoplication. Results at 10-year follow-up. Am J Surg 146: 635–638

[12] Garstin WI, Hohnston GW, Kennedy TL, Spencer ES (1986) Nissen fundoplication: the unhappy 15%. Royal Coll Surg Edinburgh 31: 207

[13] Lundell L, Abrahamsson H, Ruth M, Rydberg L, Lönroth H, Olbe L (1996) Long-term results of a prospective randomised comparison of total fundic wrap (Nissen-Rossetti) or semifundoplication (Toupét) for gastro-esophageal reflux. Br J Surg 83(6): 830–835

[14] Toupét A (1963) Technique d'oesopgago- gastroplastie avec phre'nogastropexie appliquée dans la crure radicale des hernies hiatales et comme complément de l'operation d'Heller dans les cardiospasmes. Mem Acad Chir 89: 394–398

[15] Walker SJ, Holt S, Sanderson CJ, Stoddard CJ (1992) Comparison of Nissen total and Lind partial transabdominal fundoplication in the treatment of gastro-oesophageal reflux. Br J Surg 79: 410–414

[16] Watson A, Jenkinson LR, Ball CS, Barlow AP, Norris TL (1991) A more physiological alternative to total fundoplication for the surgical correction of resistant gastro-oesophageal reflux. Br J Surg 78: 1088–1094
[17] Orlando RC (1997) The pathogenesis of gastroesophageal reflux disease: the relationship between epithelial defense, dysmotility, and acid exposure. Am J Gastroenterol 92: 3S–5S
[18] Orlando RC, Bryson JC, Powell DW (1984) Mechanisms of H+ injury in rabbit esophageal epithelium. Am J Physiol 246: G718–G724
[19] Mittal RK, Balaban DH (1997) The esophagogastric junction. N Engl J Med 336: 924–932
[20] Dodds WJ, Dent J, Hogan WJ, Helm JF, Hauser R, Patel GK et al (1982) Mechanisms of gastroesophageal reflux in patients with reflux esophagitis. N Engl J Med 307: 1547–1552
[21] Dent J (1976) A new technique for continuous sphincter pressure measurement. Gastroenterology 71: 263–267
[22] Holloway RH, Hongo M, Berger K, McCallum RW (1985) Gastric distension: a mechanism for postprandial gastroesophageal reflux. Gastroenterology 89: 779–784
[23] Holloway RH, Kocyan P, Dent J (1991) Provocation of transient lower esophageal sphincter relaxations by meals in patients with symptomatic gastroesophageal reflux. Dig Dis Sci 36: 1034–1039
[24] Wyman JB, Dent J, Heddle R, Dodds WJ, Toouli J, Downton J (1990) Control of belching by the lower oesophageal sphincter. Gut 31: 639–646
[25] Martin CJ, Patrikios J, Dent J (1986) Abolition of gas reflux and transient lower esophageal sphincter relaxation by vagal blockade in the dog. Gastroenterology 91: 890–896
[26] Scheffer RCH (2004) New insights into esophago-gastric junction physiology. Thesis University of Utrecht, Febodruk BV, Enschede, The Netherlands
[27] Scheffer RC, Tatum RP, Akkermans LM, Joehl RJ, Kahrilas PJ (2003) Reduced tLESR elicitation in response to gastric distension in fundoplication patients. Am J Phys Gastrointest Liver Physiol 284: G815–G820
[28] Sifrim D, Holloway R, Silny J, Tack J, Lerut A, Janssens J (2001) Composition of the postprandial refluxate in patients with gastroesophageal reflux disease. Am J Gastroenterol 96: 647–655
[29] Lindeboom MYA, Vu MK, Ringers J, van Rijn PJJ, Neijenhuis P, Masclee AAM (2003) Function of the proximal stomach after partial *versus* complete laparoscopic fundoplication. Am J Gastroent 98(2)
[30] DeMeester TR, Stein HJ (1992) Minimizing the side effects of antireflux surgery. World J Surg 16: 335–336.
[31] Watson DI, Mathew G, Pike GK, Baigrie RJ, Jamieson GG (1998) Efficacy of anterior, posterior and total fundoplication in an experimental model. Br J Surg 85: 1006–1009
[32] Vu MK, Straathof JW, Schaar PJ, Arndt JW, Ringers J, Lamers CB, Masclee AA (1999) Motor and sensory function of the proximal stomach in reflux disease and after laparoscopic Nissen fundoplication. Am J Gastroenterol 94: 1481–1489
[33] Bjerkestet T, Nordgaard K, Schjonsby H (1980) Effect of Nissen fundoplication operation on the lower esophageal sphincter. Scand J Gastroenterol 15: 213. DeMeester TR, Wernly JA, Brian GH et al (1979) Clinical and in vitro analysis of determinants of gastroesophageal competence. A study of principles of antireflux surgery. Am J Surg 137: 39
[34] Rydberg R, Ruth M, Lundell L (1999) Mechanism of action of antireflux surgery. Br J Surg 86: 405–410
[35] Ellis FH, Crozier RE (1984) Reflux control by fundoplication: a clinical and manometric assessment of the Nissen operation. Ann Thorac Surg 38: 387–392
[36] Watson A, Spychal RT, Brown MG, Peck N, Callender N (1995) Laparoscopic "physiological" antireflux procedure: preliminary results of a prospective symptomatic and objective study. Br J Surg 82: 651–656
[37] Hunter JG, Trus TL, Branum GD, Waring JP, Wood WC (1996b) A physiologic approach to laparoscopic fundoplication for gastroesophageal reflux disease. Ann Surg 223: 673–687
[38] Laws HL, Clements RH, Swillie CM (1997) A randomised, prospective comparison of the Nissen fundoplication versus the Toupét fundoplication for gastroesophaeal reflux disease. Ann Surg 225: 647–654
[39] Horvath KD, Jobe BA, Herron DM, Swanstrom LL (1999) Laparoscopic Toupét fundoplications is an inadequate procedure for patients with severe reflux disease. J Gastrointest Surg: 583–591
[40] Jobe BA, Wallace J, Hansen PD, Swanström LL (1997) Evaluation of laparoscopic Toupét fundoplication as a primary repair for all patients with medically resistant gastroesophageal reflux. Surg Endosc 11: 1080–1083
[41] Escandell AO, DeHaro LFM, Paricio PP, Albasini JLA, Marcilla JAG, Cuencea GM (1991) Surgery improves defective esophageal peristalsis in patients with gastroesophageal reflux. Br J Surg 78: 1095–1097
[42] Rydberg L, Ruth M, Lundell L (1997) Does oesophageal motor function improve with time after successful antireflux surgery? Results of a prospective, randomised clinical study. Gut 41: 82–86

[43] Hinder A, Smith SL, Klinger PJ et al: Laparoscopic antireflux surgery – it's a wrap. Dig Surg 16: 7–11
[44] Loustarinen M, Koskinen M, Reinikainen P et al (1995) Two antireflux operations: floppy versus standard Nissen fundoplication. Ann Med 27: 199–205
[45] Patterson EJ, Herron DM, Hansen PD, Ramzi N, Standage BA, Swanström LL (2000) Effect on an esophageal bougie on the incidence of dysphagia following Nissen fundoplication. Arch Surg 135: 1055–1062
[46] Hagedorn C, Lönroth H, Rydberg L, Ruth M, Lundell L (2002) Long-term efficacy of total (Nissen-Rossetti) and posterior partial (Toupet) fundoplication: result of a randomized clinical trial. J Gastroint Surg 4: 540–545
[47] Engström C, Blomqvist A, Dalenbäck J, Lönroth H, Ruth M, Lundell L (2004) Mechanical consequences of short gastric vessel division at the time of laparoscopic total fundoplication. J Gastroint Surg 4: 442–447
[48] de Beaux AC, Watson DI, O'Boyle C, Jamieson GG (2001) Role of fundoplication in patient symptomatology after laparoscopic antireflux surgery. Br J Surg 88: 117–1121
[49] Tew S, Ackroyd R, Jamieson GG, Holloway RH (2000) Belching and bloating: facts and fantasy after antireflux surgery. Br J Surg 87: 477–481
[50] Wills VL, Hunt DR (2002) Dysphagia after antireflux surgery. Br J Surg 88: 486–499
[51] Bessell JR, Adair WD, Smithers BM, Menzies MB, Gotley DC (2002) Early reoperation for acute dysphagia following laparoscopic fundoplication. Br J Surg 89: 783–786
[52] del Pino Porres FJ, Sancho Fornos S, Benages Marinez A et al (2000) Manometric comprobation of esophagogastric junction competence after Nissen fundoplication and its relation to the length of fundic wrap. World J Surg 24: 870–873
[53] Hagedorn C, Jönsson C, Lönroth H et al (2003) Efficacy of an anterior as compared with a posterior laparoscopic partial fundoplication. Result of a randomized, controlled clinical trial. Ann Surg 238: 189–196
[54] Engström C (2004) Operations for gastro-oesophageal reflux disease – studies on mode of action and how to improve functional outcomes. Thesis, University of Göteborg, Sweden
[55] Ireland AC, Holloway RH, Toouli J, Dent J (1993) Mechanisms underlying the anti-reflux action of fundoplication. Gut 34: 303–308
[56] Johnsson F, Holloway RH, Ireland AC, Jamieson GG, Dent J (1997) Effect of fundoplication on transient lower oesophageal sphincter relaxation and gas reflux. Br J Surg 84: 686–689
[57] Lindboom MA, Ringers J, Straathof JW, van Rijn PJ et al (2003) Effect of laparoscopic partial fundoplication on reflux mechanisms. Am J Gastroenterol 98: 29–34
[58] O'Reilly MJ, Mullins SG, Saye WB, Pinto SE, Falkner PT (1996) Laparoscopic posterior partial fundoplication: analysis of 100 consecutive cases. J Laparoendosc Surg 6: 141–150
[59] Cambell KL, Munro A (1998) Efficacy and incidence of post-fundoplication symptoms at a median of 5 years following open Watson fundoplication. Br J Surg 85 (Suppl 1): 8
[60] Watson DI, Liu J, Devitt PG, Gam,e PA, Jamieson GG (2000) Outcome of laparoscopic anterior 180° partial fundoplication for gastroesophageal reflux disease. J Gastrointest Surg 4: 486–492
[61] Baxter ST, Walker SJ, Sutton R (1996) A randomised control trial of Nissen versus Lind fundoplication. Results of 10-year follow-up. In: Recent advances in diseases of the oesophagus (Perakia A, ed), pp 675–677. Monduzzi Editore
[62] DeMeester TR, Johnson LF, Kent AH (1974) Evaluation of cutrent operations for the prevention of gastroesophageal reflux. Ann Surg 180: 511–525
[63] Segol P, Hay JM, Pottier D (1989) Surgical treatment of gastroesophageal reflux: which operation to choose: Nissen, Toupet or Lotart-Jacob? Gastroenterol Clin Biol 13: 873–879
[64] Thor KBA, Silander T (1989) A long-term randomized prospective trial of the Nissen procedure versus a modified Toupet technique. Ann Surg 210: 719–724
[65] Lundell L, Abrahamsson H, Ruth M, Sandberg N, Olbe L (1991) Lower esophageal sphincter characteristics and esophageal acid exposure following partial or 360° fundoplication: results of a prospective, randomised, clinical study. World J Surg 15: 115
[66] Lundell L, Abrahamsson H, Ruth M, Rydberg L, Lönroth H, Olbe L (1996) Long-term results of a prospective randomised comparison of total fundic wrap (Nissen-Rossetti) or semifundoplication (Toupét) for gastro-esophageal reflux. Br J Surg 83(6): 830–835
[67] Rydberg L, Ruth M, Abrahamsson H, Lundell L (1999) Tailoring antireflux surgery: a randomised clinical trial. World J Surg 23(6): 612–618
[68] Walker SJ, Holt S, Sanderson CJ et al (1992) Comparison of Nissen total and Lind partial transabdominal fundoplication in the treatment of gastroesophageal reflux. Br J Surg 79: 410–414
[69] Csendes A, Burdiles P, Korn O et al (2000) Late results of a randomised clinical trial comparing total fund-

oplication versus calibration of the cardia with posterior gastropexi. Br J Surg 87: 289–297

[70] Fibbe C, Layer P, Keller J et al (2001) Esophageal motility in reflux disease before and after fundoplication: a prospective, randomized, clinical and manometric study. Gastroenterology 212: 5–14

[71] Zorning C, Strate U, Fibbe C et al (2002) Nissen vs Toupet laparoscopic fundoplication. A prospective randomized study of 200 patients with and without preoperative esophageal motility disorders. Surg Endosc 16: 758–766

[72] Catarci M, Gentileschi P, Papi C et al (2004) Evidence-based appraisal of antireflux fundoplication. Ann Surg 239: 325–337

[73] Watson DI, Jamieson GG, Pike GK et al (1999) Prospective randomized double-blind trial between laparoscopic Nissen fundoplication and anterior partial fundoplication. Br J Surg 86: 123–130

Chapter 19

ADVERSE OUTCOMES AND FAILURE FOLLOWING LAPAROSCOPIC ANTIREFLUX SURGERY

D. I. Watson

Prof. of Surgery and Head of Department, Flinders University Department of Surgery, Head of Gastrointestinal Services, Flinders Medical Centre, and Senior Consultant Surgeon, Hepatobiliary and Oesophagogastric Surgical Unit, Flinders Medical Centre, South Australia, Australia

Introduction

Since the early 1990's, laparoscopic approaches to the treatment of gastroesophageal reflux have been adopted widely, and the vast majority of surgery for reflux is now performed using a laparoscopic approach. This has reduced the overall morbidity associated with surgery for reflux, improved the willingness of patients to undergo surgical treatment, and led to an increase in the number of patients undergoing fundoplication. The reduced morbidity and excellent outcomes following laparoscopic approaches have also raised patients' expectations for a perfect outcome, and encouraged clinical research which aims to deliver this. Unfortunately, a small risk of adverse outcomes following laparoscopic fundoplication remains, and for this reason, the risk of complications following laparoscopic surgery should be balanced against the advantages of this approach. Nevertheless, the overall risk of complications is reduced following laparoscopic surgery.

Ideally, surgeons operating on patients with gastroesophageal reflux should aim to offer a risk free procedure, long term control of reflux in all patients, and no short or long term side effects. Unfortunately, even though a good or excellent outcome is achieved for the majority of patients, a small number of patients have a less than satisfactory result, either because of recurrent reflux, complications or side effects. The medium to longer term outcome following laparoscopic fundoplication has been described elsewhere. Approximately 90% of patients are free of reflux and side effects at follow-up of 5 to 8 years following laparoscopic Nissen fundoplication [1]. The cause of failure following this procedure is evenly divided between recurrent gastro-esophageal reflux and side effects. These outcomes are similar to those reported following open surgery [2]. A comparable five year success rate has also been reported following laparoscopic anterior partial fundoplication [3].

The likelihood of an adverse outcome is influenced by several factors, and these include the expertise of the operating surgeon, the type of fundoplication, and the quality of the peri-operative care. In addition, the significance of some complications can be minimized by an appropriate early management strategy [4]. When determining how to manage either side effects or recurrent reflux, it should be remembered that most patients experience some early side effects, and these will usually get better with time. For this reason, it is usually appropriate to wait up to 12 months following surgery before considering further operative intervention, unless a problem occurs within the first postoperative week. Very early problems can be corrected easily, and the morbidity of laparoscopic reintervention within one week of surgery is low [4]. Between the second postoperative week and 3 months after laparoscopic fundoplication, however, reoperation becomes more difficult, and it should be considered at this stage only if there are no other treatment options. For this reason a low threshold for relook laparoscopy in the first week following a laparoscopic fundoplication is a reasonable strategy.

In general, when dealing with a clinical problem after laparoscopic fundoplication, the management strategy will be: either conservative management, endoscopy and dilatation (Bougie versus Balloon), or further surgery – early versus late, laparoscopic versus open. The most appropriate strategy varies according to the individual patient and the particular problem, and for this reason it must be tailored to the specific situation.

Early postoperative problems

A range of complications have been reported following laparoscopic fundoplication, and these are summarized in Table 1. Fortunately, early complications are uncommon, and the more severe life threatening problems are actually quite rare. An experienced surgeon is unlikely to encounter many of these, as attention to detail will avoid the technical errors which can predispose to at least some of the adverse outcomes.

Acute hiatus hernia

Acute or early para-esophageal hiatus herniation was rarely described in the era of open fundoplication, and most patients developing a post-operative hiatus hernia following open surgery presented at late follow-up [5]. In contrast to this, a number of the early case series of laparoscopic fundoplication described a worrying incidence of para-esophageal herniation following surgery, particularly in the immediate post-operative period [6]–[10]. The incidence of this complication ranged up to 7% in some studies. The apparently greater risk following laparoscopic Nissen fundoplication, could be due to unique factors inherent in the laparoscopic approach, and these include a tendency to extend esophageal dissection further into the thorax than during open surgery, damage to the left pleura [11], reduced post-operative pain, and reduced intra-abdominal adhesions.

There is a risk of damaging the left pleural membrane when dissecting behind the esophagus from the right side, particularly when passing an instrument behind the esophagus from right to left. Breaching the barrier of the left pleura allows the stomach to slide more easily into the left hemithorax following surgery, and this can be aided by reabsorption of carbon dioxide gas from the left pleural space, which progressively reduces intra thoracic pressure, thereby generating a pressure gradient between the abdomen and the left hemithorax which can facilitate the movement of the proximal stomach into the chest.

Although reduced post-operative pain is an important advantage for laparoscopic antireflux surgery, less pain also allows a higher intra-abdominal pressure to be generated during coughing, vomiting or exertion in the early post-operative period, and hence more force can be transmitted to the hiatal area. Because the normal anatomical barriers have been disrupted by surgical dissection, less force is required to push the stomach into the thorax.

Strategies can be implemented to reduce the risk of early herniation. In prospective case series routine posterior hiatal repair to narrow the esophageal hiatus reduced the incidence by approximately 80% [8], [10]. Hence, most surgeons now agree that repairing the hiatus with sutures is mandatory during laparoscopic antireflux surgery. The magnitude of the demonstrated risk reduction is such that it is unlikely that a randomized trial will ever be conducted to compare the outcome of patients undergoing laparoscopic fundoplication with versus without hiatal repair. The reported early outcomes of a randomized trial of laparoscopic Nissen fundoplication with posterior versus anterior hiatal repair, showed that anterior hiatal repair was just as effective as posterior repair, suggesting that the actual method used for hiatal narrowing may not be important [12].

In addition to appropriate surgical technique, it makes sense to initiate measures which avoid excessive strain on the hiatal repair during the early post-operative period. Many patients who develop an acute hernia describe repeated attempts to vomit during the first 24-hours following surgery. Hence, the routine use of antiemetics, such as serotonin antagonists or droperidol, to avoid vomiting in the first few days

Table 1. Acute complications following laparoscopic antireflux surgery

Complications which are more common following laparoscopic approach
Pneumothorax
Para-esophageal hiatus hernia
Tight hiatus/Acute dysphagia
Rare events due to technical errors
Esophageal perforation
Gastric perforation
Duodenal perforation
Bowel perforation
Bilobed stomach
Cardiac laceration and tamponade
Injury to major vessels
Mesenteric thrombosis

following surgery is advised. The use of narcotic analgesia should also be minimized or avoided. In addition, all patients should avoid excessive lifting or straining for about one month following surgery. Early resumption of heavy physical work has been reported to be associated with acute herniation [10]. The use of prosthetic material to reinforce the hiatal repair when repairing a large hiatus hernia might also reduce the risk of recurrent herniation [13]. However, the potential for complications arising from the use of mesh at the hiatus also needs to be considered.

Acute dysphagia

Persistent dysphagia is well recognized as a problem for some patients at medium to late follow-up. In a small number of patients acute dysphagia occurs in the first 1 to 2 days following surgery. This occurs if a Nissen fundoplication is constructed too tightly, or if the hiatus is closed too tightly during hiatal repair [4]. The risk of these technical errors can be minimized by careful operative technique. The use of an intra-esophageal bougie to assist with calibration of the hiatal repair and construction of the fundoplication will reduce, but not eliminate the risk of this problem [14].

Acute severe dysphagia should be distinguished from the usual postoperative dysphagia experienced by most patients after antireflux surgery. This problem is usually obvious on the first postoperative day, and it should be suspected if a bowl of tissues and saliva is sitting on the patient's bed. This is due to the complete inability to swallow even saliva. A barium swallow X-ray should be performed. If contrast passes into the stomach, albeit slowly, a conservative approach can usually be followed, and swallowing will usually improve over the ensuing few days. However, if no contrast passes into the stomach, urgent intervention is necessary (*Fig. 1*).

The choice of action is between endoscopy and dilatation versus surgery. In some patients endoscopy and the passage of a large (17 mm or larger) Savary type bougie over a guide wire, is followed by improved swallowing, and further intervention is not needed. However, if this fails, it is usually straightforward to undertake a further laparoscopic procedure within the first post-operative week. At re-laparoscopy the hiatus and the fundoplication should be inspected, and a 50 to 60 Fr bougie may be passed carefully through the gastro-esophageal junction if the cause is not clear. If a tight Nissen fundoplication is present, then this is corrected by removing the uppermost suture used to construct the original fundoplication, and the fundoplication is then reinforced by placing another suture below the previous lowermost suture. This maneuver loosens the fundoplication. If, however, the fundoplication is loose, and the hiatal repair is tight when the esophagus is distended by an intra-abdominal bougie (or indeed if there is any doubt) the top hiatal repair suture, or more, should be removed, to widen the hiatal opening. If there is any concern about the risk of hiatal herniation after this, then sutures can be placed between the fundoplication and the hiatal rim. These actions should fix the problem of acute esophageal obstruction. A repeat barium swallow on the next day will confirm that treatment has been adequate (*Fig. 2*).

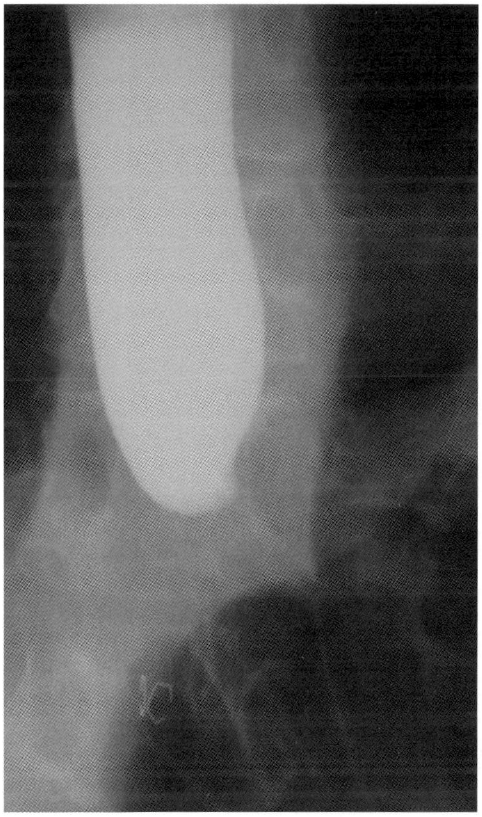

Fig. 1. Barium meal on the first postoperative day from a patient with complete esophageal obstruction

Bilobed stomach

A technical error which was described in early case series of laparoscopic Nissen fundoplication is the "bilobed stomach" [15]. It occurs when a Nissen fundoplication is constructed using too distal a piece of stomach rather than the fundus, resulting in a bilobular shaped stomach, which is best appreciated at postoperative barium meal examination (*Fig. 3*). The different angle of view provided by the laparoscope can lead to inexperienced surgeons failing to appreciate that the anterior gastric wall lies in an oblique plane, with the apex of the fundus in a more posterior position than the gastric body and antrum, and hence the gastric body can be misidentified as the fundus. Care to ensure that the actual fundus is used for construction of the fundoplication will prevent this problem from arising. Fortunately, most patients with a "bilobed stomach" are actually asymptomatic [15]. However, in the rare more extreme case, the upper part of the stomach can become obstructed at the point of constriction in the gastric body, and can cause post-prandial abdominal pain. In these patients surgical revision is necessary.

Perforation of the gastrointestinal tract

Perforations of all parts of the gastrointestinal tract during laparoscopic fundoplication have been reported. In particular, esophageal and gastric perforation are specific risks, with an incidence of approximately 0.5% to 1% reported in larger series [6], [9], [16]. Gastric perforation usually results from an avulsion injury of the gastric cardia, caused by excessive traction by the surgical assistant, or the use of inappropriate grasping instruments to retract the stomach [15], [17]. This problem is best avoided by ensuring that

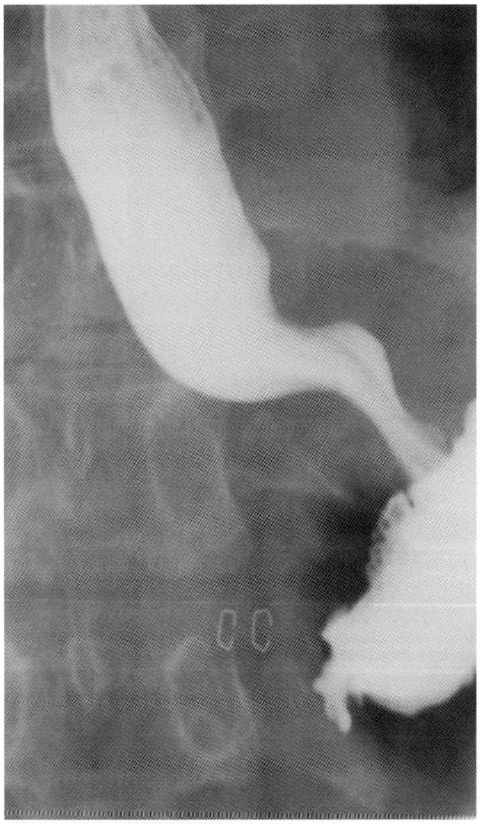

Fig. 2. Barium meal from same patient on the second postoperative day following reoperation and removal of hiatal repair suture

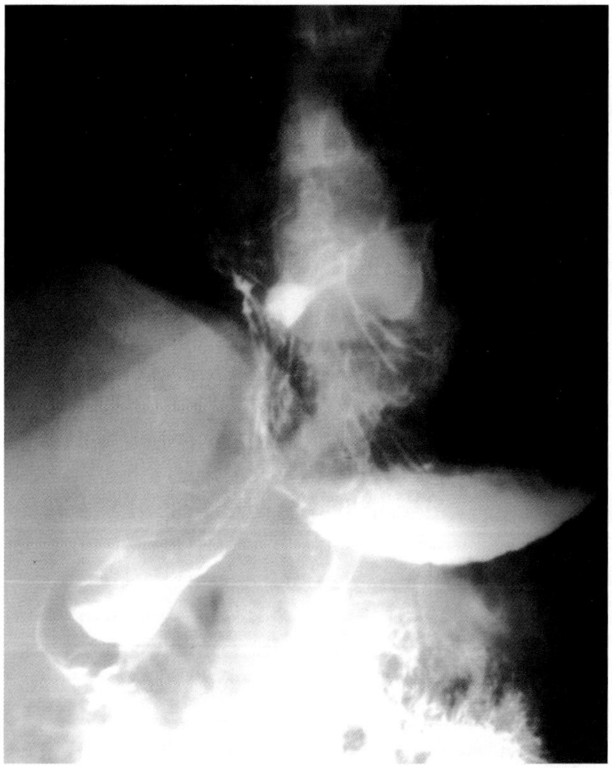

Fig. 3. Barium meal at 3 months post-operative showing "bilobed" stomach due to construction of a Nissen fundoplication using the gastric body rather than the fundus. This patient has remained asymptomatic at long term follow-up

the assistant retracts the esophago-gastric junction by grasping the fat pad which overlies the cardia, rather than the actual cardia or proximal stomach.

Perforation of the back wall of the esophagus can occur during dissection of the posterior esophagus [17], [18]. This problem is more likely to occur in patients with periesophagitis, as the usual periesophageal tissue plane can be obliterated by inflammatory changes in some of these patients. It can also occur if the surgeon is unfamiliar with the laparoscopic anatomy, and dissection is extended directly through the esophageal wall. The anterior esophageal wall is probably at greatest risk of perforation when a bougie is passed down the esophagus to calibrate the tightness of either the fundoplication or the hiatal repair [18]. Despite this risk, the results of a randomized trial of laparoscopic Nissen fundoplication calibrated with versus without an intraesophageal bougie suggest that the overall outcome is better if a bougie is used [14].

If an injury is recognized intra-operatively it should be immediately repaired by sutures, placed either laparoscopically or by an open technique. A low index of suspicion, and a willingness to re-examine the operative field laparoscopically on the first or second postoperative days will facilitate the early identification of injuries which have not been recognized at the original procedure. Delayed recognition of an esophageal or upper gastric perforation will result in more serious morbidity.

Late postoperative problems

Side effects and other adverse outcomes also occur during later follow-up following laparoscopic fundoplication. Some of these problems are present throughout the postoperative period, e.g., persistent dysphagia, and some will not occur until later, e.g., recurrent reflux or hiatus hernia. It should also be remembered that a few problems are inevitable. For example all patients with an intact fundoplication are unable to vomit, and they should be warned about this problem. Table 2 summarizes the scope of the adverse outcomes encountered at late follow-up.

Recurrent gastro-esophageal reflux

Recurrence of gastro-esophageal reflux occurs in a proportion of patients following laparoscopic fundoplication. The risk of this varies with the type of fundoplication performed. At 5 or more years follow-up, the incidence of recurrent reflux following laparoscopic Nissen fundoplication has been reported to be between 5 and 10% [1], [19]. This compares to a 5 year recurrence risk of recurrence of between 10 and 15% after laparoscopic anterior partial fundoplication [3]. The risk following posterior partial fundoplication is approximately 10% [20]. In addition, the incidence of recurrence increases as follow-up lengthens, with failure rates of 20 to 30% reported at 20 to 30 years following open surgical procedures [21], [22].

The integrity of a fundoplication requires the maintenance of close proximity between the fundus and the intra-abdominal esophagus [23], and if this physical relationship is disrupted, reflux can recur. This happens if the original fundoplication unravels, or if the gastro-esophageal junction migrates proximally through an intact fundoplication, so that the fundoplication sits around the cardia, rather than the lower esophagus – e.g., a slipped Nissen fundoplication (*Fig. 4*). When undertaking revision surgery for recurrent reflux it is actually rare to find a fundoplication which has unraveled, and the commonest cause of recurrence is proximal migration of the gastro-esophageal junction. On some occasions, there is no obvious anatomical reason for recurrent reflux. Fortunately, revision of the fundoplication in these patients is usually followed by relief of symptoms [24]. It is likely that the underlying problem is still proximal migration of the gastro-esophageal junction, even though it is not obvious at revision surgery in these patients.

Not all patients who describe symptoms of recurrent reflux actually have this problem, and for this reason all patients with recurrent symptoms should be carefully reinvestigated. Some patients experience

Table 2. Late side effects and complications following laparoscopic antireflux surgery

Recurrent reflux
Para-esophageal hiatus hernia
Persistent dysphagia
Gas bloat
Flatulence
Inability to belch

"esophageal" symptoms, due to esophageal obstruction or esophageal distension, particularly during early follow-up if they eat an inappropriate diet. An endoscopy is useful in these patients to check the integrity of the fundoplication. If this is confirmed, then these patients can be reassured that their symptoms should improve with longer follow-up. If however, recurrent reflux is likely, then the patient should be fully reassessed with endoscopy, barium meal X-ray, 24 hour ambulatory pH monitoring and esophageal manometry. Endoscopy and pH monitoring are used to confirm or refute recurrent gastroesophageal reflux. Esophageal manometry will guide any re-operative strategy, and barium meal X-ray will demonstrate any associated hiatus hernia, as well as provide some information about reflux.

If reflux has recurred, treatment should initially entail acid suppression with a proton pump inhibitor. If proton pump inhibitor therapy relieves the symptoms then it is probably not appropriate to proceed to further surgery. This is because the technical aspects of surgical revision are more difficult than a primary operation, and there is a higher risk of serious complications, including esophageal and gastric perforation, and mortality with surgical revision. Published reports of outcome following open revision antireflux surgery confirm a mortality risk of approximately 1% [24]. If the original procedure was performed laparoscopically, the real mortality of laparoscopic revision surgery might be lower than this, as there are usually less adhesions and technical difficulties following a previous laparoscopic procedure [25], [26]. However, there is insufficient published data available to either confirm or refute this statement. Proton pump inhibitor therapy will achieve satisfactory relief of symptoms in approximately 80% of patients whose fundoplication has failed because of recurrent reflux. However, in about 20% of patients with recurrent reflux medical therapy is unsatisfactory, and in these patients it is appropriate to proceed to a revision procedure [1].

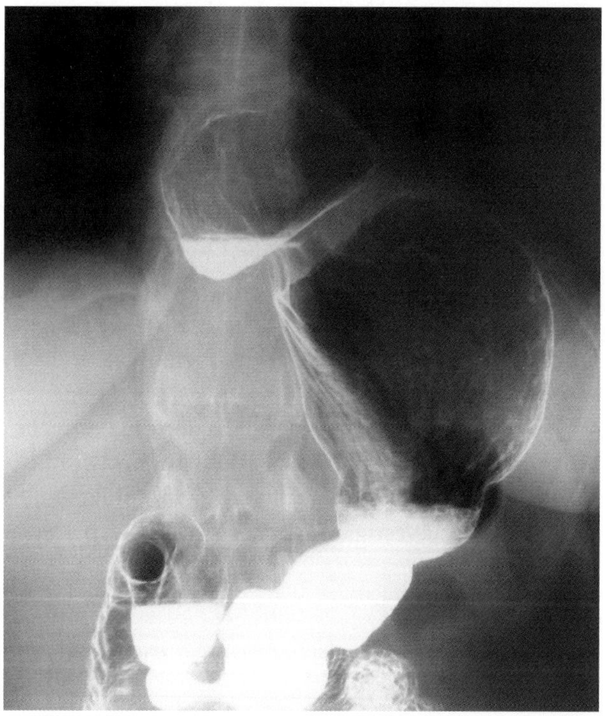

Fig. 4. Barium meal at 3 years post-operative from a patient with recurrent reflux symptoms. The fundoplication is intact and located immediately below the diaphragm. The esophagogastric junction and cardia have migrated into the lower mediastinum – i.e., a slipped Nissen fundoplication with small hiatus hernia

The operative strategy for revision surgery is to first divide all adhesions in the vicinity of the previous fundoplication to expose the old operative site [25]. The fundoplication is then divided and unraveled fully and the esophagus mobilized. Any associated hiatus hernia can then be repaired, and a new fundoplication is constructed. It is usually appropriate to perform a Nissen fundoplication, although if esophageal manometry has demonstrated very poor esophageal body peristalsis, then a partial fundoplication can be performed. The outcome for this strategy in the open surgical era was a success rate of approximately 85% [24]. Whilst there is insufficient data reported in the laparoscopic era to determine with certainty the outcome following laparoscopic revision for recurrent reflux, the success rate is likely to be similar to that of open surgery [25].

Persistent dysphagia

Although dysphagia occurs in virtually all patients in the early postoperative period following fundoplication, the majority of patients are able to swallow normally at late follow-up. Unfortunately, however, persistent dysphagia occurs in a small number of patients. It is unlikely that the risk of this problem is any greater in the laparoscopic era [2], [27]. Approximately 5% of patients at 12 or more months after laparoscopic Nissen fundoplication continue to experience dysphagia which is sufficiently severe to restrict dietary choices [1], [19]. This figure is approximately 20% at 3 months follow-up [28], [29], suggesting that whenever possible a conservative approach to the management of dysphagia should be encouraged until patients have been followed for at least 12 months. Both anterior and posterior partial fundoplications have been reported to be associated with lower risks of dysphagia [20], [29]. At 12 months follow-up, anterior 180 degree partial fundoplication is associated with an incidence of 1 to 2% of dysphagia sufficiently severe to require dietary modification [30].

A small number of patients experience dysphagia which is persistent and sufficiently severe to require further operative intervention. If nutrition is adequately maintained, then waiting 12 months before considering surgical revision should be encouraged. During this delay, dysphagia will resolve in some patients. It also allows subsequent operative intervention to be performed more easily. If nutrition is not adequate, however, and the affected patient continues to lose weight beyond the first 6 to 8 weeks, then earlier intervention will probably be needed.

Endoscopy and dilation, using a bougie passed over a guide wire can also be useful, particularly in the early follow-up period. It may achieve sufficient improvement to allow operative intervention to be avoided, although it may need to be repeated several times. If dilatation with a bougie is unsuccessful, then more vigorous dilation with a pneumatic balloon (e.g., 30 mm diameter) can be more successful. These methods should be considered before undertaking surgical revision, particularly for patients who are between 1 week and 3 months postoperative. However, if dilatation is unsuccessful, surgical revision will need to be considered.

Persistent dysphagia is associated with either a functionally tight Nissen fundoplication or a narrow diaphragmatic hiatus. Persistent dysphagia which requires operative reintervention is very uncommon after partial fundoplication procedures. Whilst the underlying cause of dysphagia may be obvious at surgical re-exploration, it can also be difficult to be certain what the problem is. A tight or narrow esophageal diaphragmatic hiatus, can be the result of either over-tightening the hiatus during initial hiatal repair, or due to excessive perihiatal scar tissue [31]. Over tightening the hiatus usually results in severe early dysphagia, and this has been discussed earlier, whereas narrowing of the esophageal hiatus due to excessive post-operative scar tissue tends to commence in the second and third post-operative weeks. The latter problem can even occur in patients who do not undergo hiatal repair [31]. Correction of a tight hiatus, irrespective of the cause, requires widening of the diaphragmatic hiatus.

A laparoscopic approach can usually be used for patients who require reoperation for post-operative dysphagia following a previous laparoscopic fundoplication [25]. At surgery the esophageal hiatus and the previous fundoplication are exposed by dividing adhesions in the region of the original fundoplication. A large (52 Fr or bigger) esophageal bougie is then used to distend the esophagus, to facilitate assessment of the fundoplication and the esophageal hiatus. If it is apparent that the fundoplication is loose, and the hiatus is tight (with the bougie in place), then widening the hiatus alone will usually restore normal swallowing. This is performed by dividing the hiatal ring and adjacent diaphragm antero-laterally to the left until the hiatus is appropriately loose. If, however, the hiatal ring is loose around the distended esophagus, conversion to a partial fundoplication is advised to improve swallowing [25]. This is done by dividing the Nissen fundoplication, and then resuturing the fundus to both sides of the esophagus as a posterior partial fundoplication, hence avoiding the need to separate the fundus from the posterior esophagus.

Often it is not clear what the actual cause of the dysphagia is, and in this situation conversion to a posterior partial fundoplication and widening of the hiatus should both be performed. This will usually improve the clinical situation. The correct operative strategy, however, can only be determined intraoperatively once the hiatal region has been exposed, and the surgeon will need to be prepared to apply a flexible strategy.

Late hiatus hernia

Some patients develop a hiatus hernia during follow-up, and this can range in extent from a minor partial slippage of the fundoplication into the thorax, to a large para-esophageal hernia which contains most of the stomach, as well as some other organs. It is difficult to know for certain what the incidence of this problem actually is, as determining the incidence would require regular barium meal X-ray examinations or endoscopy during follow-up, and this is rarely practical to do this more than once. An early report described an incidence of symptomatic hiatus hernia of approximately 10% in patients in whom the hiatus had not been repaired [10]. However, this rate declined to 2% when posterior hiatal repair was performed routinely. In one of the few studies to use barium meal examination for the follow-up of patients undergoing laparoscopic Nissen fundoplication for gastro-esophageal reflux (without a large hiatus hernia), the incidence of asymptomatic hiatus hernia at 6 months following surgery was 6% [28]. The herniae in these patients were small and did not require further surgical intervention.

The risk of late postoperative hiatus hernia following laparoscopic repair of a very large hiatus hernia has been examined by several groups. Hashemi et al reported an alarming 42% radiological recurrence rate following laparoscopic repair and Nissen fundoplication in a group of 27 patients who underwent laparoscopic repair of a very large hiatus hernia [32]. The author's own data from a longer term follow-up study of 100 patients, using barium meal examination at 2 to 8 years after laparoscopic repair of a very large hiatus hernia with hiatal sutures (rather than a mesh based technique) revealed a 30% radiological recurrence rate [33]. The symptomatic recurrence rate, however, was a much lower 7%, confirming that the majority of patients with a recurrent hiatus hernia do not have actual clinical symptoms, and therefore they might not need further surgery. Others have reported a similar rate [34]. Unfortunately, however, it will be necessary to follow the asymptomatic patients for longer to determine that they will not become symptomatic at later follow-up. The use of prosthetic material to reinforce the hiatal repair when repairing a large hiatus hernia has the potential to reduce the risk of recurrent herniation [13], [35], although this technique can be followed by other complications which are due to the use of mesh at the hiatus.

From the data discussed above, it is seems likely that approximately 2% of patients who have undergone a laparoscopic fundoplication for reflux, and 7% of those who have undergone laparoscopic repair of a large hiatus hernia using a suturing technique will develop a symptomatic recurrent hiatus hernia, and require further surgery. Symptomatic recurrence can be associated with either symptoms of recurrent reflux, or mechanical symptoms from the hernia. Patients who are being considered for further repair should be reinvestigated with endoscopy, barium meal and pH monitoring, to identify objective evidence of gastro-esophageal reflux, and to determine the size of the hernia. If reflux is occurring, then the reoperative strategy entails reversal of the previous fundoplication, reduction and repair of the hiatus hernia, and construction of a new fundoplication. If, however, there is no evidence of recurrent reflux, and the symptoms are purely mechanical, e.g., chest pain, gastric or esophageal obstruction etc, then it is usually possible to only repair the hernia, whilst leaving the previous fundoplication intact. Irrespective of the specific operative strategy, it is reasonable to aim for a laparoscopic approach for revision, although a low threshold for conversion to open surgery is advised if any difficulties are encountered.

"Wind related" side effects

"Wind-related" post-fundoplication side effects include flatulence, inability to belch and abdominal bloating, and these can be troublesome in some patients. The relative risk of one of these problems occurring is in part determined by the type of fundoplication performed. These side effects are more common in patients who have undergone a Nissen fundoplication, than following a partial fundoplication [29], [36], [37].

The results from a randomized trial which compared Nissen fundoplication with anterior 180 degree partial fundoplication revealed that at 6 months following Nissen fundoplication abdominal bloating occurred in 28% of patients, 36% could not belch normally and 49% reported increased flatus [29]. In the same trial, at 6 months after anterior partial fundoplication "wind related" side effects were less common, with 17% of patients unable to belch normally, 28% described increased flatus, and abdominal bloating was present in 19%. The incidence of post-fundoplication symptoms should, however, be compared with the preoperative incidence of the same symptoms. Indeed, 50% of patients enrolled in this trial had abdominal bloating before surgery [29].

In some patients, "wind-related" symptoms actually improve or disappear following laparoscopic fundoplication, confirming that some of these symptoms are part of the spectrum of reflux symptomatology [38]. Unfortunately, however, some patients experience at least one of these symptoms for the first time after fundoplication, and in these patients side effects can be troublesome. The likelihood of side effects which are sufficiently troublesome for patients to be dissatisfied with the overall outcome of their operation, or to request further treatment, is approximately 5% following Nissen fundoplication and 1% to 2% following an anterior partial fundoplication. The outcome following posterior partial fundoplication is probably somewhere in between.

The treatment of "wind-related" side effects is difficult. Increased flatus is to a certain extent inevitable following an otherwise successful fundoplication. Fortunately, in most patients this is not troublesome. However, occasionally it can be significant, and treatment can be difficult. If patients are unable belch, then it is necessary to avoid ingesting substances which put gas into the stomach, e.g., carbonated drinks. In addition, some patients with gastro-esophageal reflux develop the habit of air-swallowing. This entails subconscious repetitive swallowing, presumably in response to the regurgitation of gastric content into the esophagus. If air-swallowing continues following fundoplication then excessive air can enter and be trapped in the stomach by an intact fundoplication. This aggravates upper abdominal bloating. With time, this symptom will usually improve or disappear, although this will often take 12 months or longer.

There are no published reports describing the outcome of surgical revision primarily for troublesome "wind-related" side effects. In the author's personal experience, the outcome of re-operation in these patients is unpredictable and it is often poor. In the process of undertaking revision surgery, e.g., reversal of the fundoplication, it is difficult to identify the vagal nerve trunks, and inadvertent truncal vagotomy is easily performed during dissection of the esophagus. Inadvertent vagotomy will cause further disturbances of gastrointestinal function, and for this reason revision can result in worse side effects. Furthermore, the anatomy of the gastro-esophageal junction may not be returned to its original state following full reversal of the fundoplication. Hence, belching can still be a problem and bloating will often persist. A lesser strategy to complete reversal of a Nissen fundoplication is conversion to a posterior partial fundoplication, as this can be usually be achieved without dissecting the fundus away from the posterior esophagus. However, there is no certainty that this will result in a successful outcome.

In general patients should be counseled against further surgery for "wind-related" problems, and surgical revision should be reserved only for patients with troublesome symptoms of dysphagia, recurrent reflux or a recurrent hiatus hernia. Implementing changes in diet and allowing sufficient time for "wind-related" symptoms to improve will result in a satisfactory outcome in many patients. In the minority of patients in whom symptoms do not improve, further surgery can make the problem worse, and is best avoided.

Conclusions

Despite the fact that the majority of patients who undergo laparoscopic antireflux surgery have a good or excellent clinical outcome, a small proportion of patients develop a significant complication, side effect or recurrent reflux during postoperative follow-up. The management of these patients is complex. If problems occur in the immediate post-operative period, then early laparoscopic re-exploration should be considered, as many problems are easily be corrected within a week of the original procedure.

Patients who develop problems during later follow-up should be fully reinvestigated, and non-operative treatment options are initially recommended, as many of the early side effects resolve with conservative management. Endoscopy and dilatation can be helpful at this stage. If problems persist beyond 12 months, then reoperation can be considered in patients with persistent dysphagia, symptomatic recurrent hiatus hernia, or recurrent reflux which is poorly controlled with medication. However, further surgery is unlikely to be help patients with persistent "wind-related" side effects.

References

[1] Lafullarde T, Watson DI, Jamieson GG, Myers JC, Game PA, Devitt PG (2001) Laparoscopic Nissen fundoplication – 5 year results and beyond. Arch Surg 136: 180–184

[2] Nilsson G, Wenner J, Larsson S, Johnsson F (2004) Randomized clinical trial of laparoscopic versus open fundoplication for gastro-esophageal reflux. Br J Surg 91: 552–559

[3] Ludemann R, Watson DI, Game PA, Devitt PG, Jamieson GG (2005) Laparoscopic total versus anterior 180° fundoplication – five year follow-up of a prospective randomized trial. Br J Surg 92: 240–243

[4] Yau P, Watson DI, Devitt PG, Game PA, Jamieson GG (2000) Early reoperation following laparoscopic antireflux surgery. Am J Surg 179: 172–176

[5] Lundell L, Abrahamsson H, Ruth M, Rydberg L, Lonroth H, Olbe L (1996) Long-term results of a prospective randomized comparison of total fundic wrap (Nissen-Rossetti) or semifundoplication (Toupet) for gastro-esophageal reflux. Br J Surg 83: 830–835

[6] Coelho JC, Wiederkehr JC, Campos AC, Andrigueto PC (1999) Conversions and complications of laparoscopic treatment of gastroesophageal reflux disease. J Am Coll Surg 189: 356–361

[7] Collard JM, de Gheldere CA, De Cock M, Otte JB, Kestens PJ (1994) Laparoscopic antireflux surgery. What is real progress? Ann Surg 220: 146–154

[8] Gotley DC, Smithers BM, Rhodes M, Menzies B, Branicki FJ, Nathanson L (1996) Laparoscopic Nissen fundoplication – 200 consecutive cases. Gut 38: 487–491

[9] Hinder RA, Filipi CJ, Wetscher G, Neary P, DeMeester TR, Perdikis G (1994) Laparoscopic Nissen fundoplication is an effective treatment for gastroesophageal reflux disease. Ann Surg 220: 472–483

[10] Watson DI, Jamieson GG, Devitt PG, Mitchell PC, Game PA (1995) Paraoesophageal hiatus hernia: an important complication of laparoscopic Nissen fundoplication. Br J Surg 82: 521–523

[11] Joris JL, Chiche J-D, Lamy ML (1995) Pneumothorax during laparoscopic fundoplication: diagnosis and treatment with positive end-expiratory pressure. Anesth Analg 81: 993–1000

[12] Watson DI, Jamieson GG, Devitt PG, Kennedy A, Ellis T, Ackroyd R, Lafullarde T, Game PA (2001) A prospective randomized trial of laparoscopic Nissen fundoplication with anterior versus posterior hiatal repair. Arch Surg 136: 745–751

[13] Leeder PC, Smith G, Dehn TC (2003) Laparoscopic management of large paraesophageal hiatal hernia. Surg Endosc 17: 1372–1375

[14] Patterson EJ, Herron DM, Hansen PD, Ramzi N, Standage BA, Swanstrom LL (2000) Effect of an esophageal bougie on the incidence of dysphagia following Nissen fundoplication: a prospective, blinded, randomized clinical trial. Arch Surg 135: 1055–1061

[15] Jamieson GG, Watson DI, Britten-Jones R, Mitchell PC, Anvari M (1994) Laparoscopic Nissen fundoplication. Ann Surg 220: 137–145

[16] Collet D, Cadiere GB (1995) Conversions and complications of laparoscopic treatment of gastroesophageal reflux disease. Am J Surg 169: 622–626

[17] Schauer PR, Meyers WC, Eubanks S, Norem RF, Franklin M, Pappas TN (1996) Mechanisms of gastric and esophageal perforations during laparoscopic Nissen fundoplication. Ann Surg 223: 43–52

[18] Cadiere GB, Himpens J, Bruyns J (1995) How to avoid esophageal perforation while performing laparoscopic dissection of the hiatus. Surg Endosc 9: 450–452

[19] O'Boyle CJ, Watson DI, Jamieson GG, Myers JC, Game PA, Devitt PG (2002) Division of short gastric vessels at laparoscopic Nissen fundoplication – a prospective double blind randomized trial with five year follow-up. Ann Surg 235: 165–170

[20] Hagedorn C, Lonroth H, Rydberg L, Ruth M, Lundell L (2002) Long-term efficacy of total (Nissen-Rossetti) and posterior partial (Toupet) fundoplication: results of a randomized clinical trial. J Gastrointest Surg 6: 540–545

[21] Luostarinen M, Isolauri J, Laitinen J, Koskinen M, Keyrilainen O, Markkula H, Lehtinen E, Uusitalo A (1993) Fate of Nissen fundoplication after 20 years. A clinical, endoscopical, and functional analysis. Gut 34: 1015–1020

[22] Allison PR (1973) Hiatus hernia: a 20-year retrospective survey. Ann Surg 178: 273–276

[23] Watson DI, Mathew G, Pike GK, Jamieson GG (1997) Comparison of anterior, posterior and total fundoplication using a viscera model. Dis Esoph 10: 110–114

[24] Rieger NA, Jamieson GG, Britten-Jones R, Tew S (1994) Reoperation after failed antireflux surgery. Br J Surg 81: 1159–1161

[25] Watson DI, Jamieson GG, Game PA, Williams RS, Devitt PG (1999) Laparoscopic reoperation following failed antireflux surgery. Br J Surg 86: 98–101

[26] Curet MJ, Josloff RK, Schoeb O, Zucker KA (1999) Laparoscopic reoperation for failed antireflux procedures. Arch Surg 134: 559–563

[27] Ackroyd R, Watson DI, Majeed AW, Troy G, Treacy PJ, Stoddard CJ (2004) Randomized clinical trial of laparoscopic versus open fundoplication for gastro-esophageal reflux disease. Br J Surg 91: 975–982
[28] Watson DI, Pike GK, Baigrie RJ, Mathew M, Devitt PG, Britten-Jones R, Jamieson GG (1997) Prospective double blind randomized trial of laparoscopic Nissen fundoplication with division and without division of short gastric vessels. Ann Surg 226: 642–652
[29] Watson DI, Jamieson GG, Pike GK, Davies N, Richardson M, Devitt PG (1999) A prospective randomized double blind trial between laparoscopic Nissen fundoplication and anterior partial fundoplication. Br J Surg 86: 123–130
[30] Watson DI, Liu JF, Devitt PG, Game PA, Jamieson GG (2000) Outcome of laparoscopic anterior 180 degree partial fundoplication for gastro-esophageal reflux disease. J Gastrointest Surg 4: 486–492
[31] Watson DI, Jamieson GG, Mitchell PC, Devitt PG, Britten-Jones R (1995) Stenosis of the esophageal hiatus following laparoscopic fundoplication. Arch Surg 130: 1014–1016
[32] Hashemi M, Peters JH, DeMeester TR, Huprich JE, Quek M, Hagen JA, Crookes PF, Theisen J, DeMeester SR, Sillin LF, Bremner CG (2000) Laparoscopic repair of large type III hiatal hernia: objective followup reveals high recurrence rate. J Am Coll Surg 190: 553–560
[33] Aly A, Munt J, Jamieson GG, Gabb M, Ludemann R, Devitt PG, Watson DI (2005) Large hiatal hernia: recurrence after laparoscopic repair. Br J Surg 92: 648–653
[34] Jobe BA, Aye RW, Deveney CW, Domreis JS, Hill LD (2002) Laparoscopic management of giant type III hiatal hernia and short esophagus. Objective follow-up at three years. J Gastrointest Surg 6: 181–188
[35] Carlson MA, Richards CG, Frantzides CT (1999) Laparoscopic prosthetic reinforcement of hiatal herniorrhaphy. Dig Surg 16: 407–410
[36] Watson DI, Jamieson GG, Lally C, Archer S, Bessell JR, Booth M, Cade R, Cullingford G, Devitt PG, Fletcher DR, Hurley J, Kiroff G, Martin C, Martin IJG, Nathanson LK, Windsor J (2004) Multicentre prospective double blind randomized trial of laparoscopic Nissen versus anterior 90 degree partial fundoplication. Arch Surg 139: 1160–1167
[37] Hagedorn C, Jonson C, Lonroth H, Ruth M, Thune A, Lundell L (2003) Efficacy of an anterior as compared with a posterior laparoscopic partial fundoplication: results of a randomized, controlled clinical trial. Ann Surg 238: 189–196
[38] de Beaux A, Watson DI, O'Boyle C, Jamieson GG (2001) Role of fundoplication in patient symptomatology after laparoscopic antireflux surgery. Br J Surg 88: 1117–1121

LAPAROSCOPIC REFUNDOPLICATION: SURGICAL INTERVENTION AFTER FAILED ANTIREFLUX OPERATIONS

R. Pointner

Department of General Surgery, Public Hospital of Zell am See, Zell am See, Austria

Introduction

The progress of laparoscopic surgery and a more profound understanding of the pathophysiological conditions leading to gastroesophageal reflux disease have resulted in a revival of antireflux surgery. Since 1991 [1] the laparoscopic Nissen and Toupet fundoplication and their modifications have emerged as the surgical alternative for treatment of GERD. The reduced morbidity and an approximately cero per cent mortality rate in combination with excellent outcomes following laparoscopic approaches have encouraged surgeons to a more liberal indication to surgery and have also raised patient's expectations for a perfect outcome. Success and failure rates depend on a precise indication to surgery and on the frequency how often the procedure is performed in the institution and by a single surgeon [2]. As the "learning curve" for laparoscopic antireflux procedures even in centers is low, redo procedures require surgeons experienced in GERD and in laparoscopy, too. With the increase in laparoscopic antireflux procedures the debate has ceased whether redo fundoplications should be done open or laparoscopically. There is no doubt, that the standard for redo procedures after failed antireflux surgery is the minimal invasive technique for both, primary open and primary laparoscopic surgery, even if there are usually more adheasions and technical difficulties following a previous open procedure.

Diagnosis

Antireflux surgery is failed, if the patient is not able to swallow undisturbed, reports about epigastric pain or shows the same symptoms of reflux disease which were the initially reasons for primary antireflux surgery. In addition to persisting or new onset symptoms the quality of life in these patients is typically lower than before primary surgery [3]. The analysis of the underlying failures which are responsible for the reported symptoms is essential for a successful treatment. Possible failures and adverse outcomes following laparoscopic antireflux surgery are discussed in the chapter before. Reviewing the literature, 5 to 20 per cent of all patients who underwent antireflux procedures have to be treated again because of new onset or persistent reflux symptoms [4]. These symptoms are either dysphagia, recurring or persistent reflux or a combination of both, reflux and dysphagia. Aim of the diagnostic procedure is to clarify the morphologic changes that are responsible for the above mentioned symptoms. Patients description of the kind, intensity and beginning of new or recurrent symptoms after primary antireflux procedures are essential comments for a further analysis. In combination with a distinct anamnesis, the evaluation has to clarify whether the wrap is open or too loose, whether the hiatus or the wrap is too tight and to define the position of the wrap with regard to the diaphragm or the fundus. The most important tool is a barium X-ray swallow using a videographic or kinematographic technique. For both, a skilled radiologist and an experienced antireflux surgeon, it should be possible to define the position of the former constructed wrap in relation to the diaphragm and the crura.To confirm or exclude a radiologically suspected diagnosis upper GI endoscopy is emphasized in every patient. Beneeth the visualisation and histologic documentation of obvious leasons or strictures, the location of the gastroesophageal junction must be defined above or below the diaphragmatic crura. Further more, the typical "Nissen nipple" can be seen in the so called inversion of the scope and clearyfies whether the plication is in the right position or not. To exclude functional problems it makes sense to examine the body motility as well as the emptying of the stomach.

Early reintervention

Only in rare cases, reintervention is indicated in an early stage after primary surgery. Fortunately severe life threatening problems following laparoscopic fundoplication are quite rare. They are caused by injury of the gastric wall, esophagus, or parts of the intestinal tract, leading to perforation or peritonitis. In these cases, when suspicion arouses that a perforation could have taken place, earliest reintervention is advocated. If an esophageal leak is the reason for early reintervention, this leak has to be identified exactly. For a definite identification an endoscope or tube in the esophagus can help to find the leak. In case of a small damage of the esophageal wall the leak can be oversewn with a few stiches but should be covered by a part of the fundoplication. If the leakage is bigger or more than a quarter of the circumference conversion to open and distal esophageal resection is advocated. There is no doubt, that the procedure has to begin with breaking down the sutures of the fundoplication for a better visualisation of the complete area. Perforations following laparoscopy of the intestine are handled as perforations following open surgery.

Specifically fundoplication related early complications are uncommon. Beneeth the life threatening problems of perforations, acute dysphagia is the most troublesome early complication. The reason for early dysphagia may be an acute postoperative re-hiatal herniation with a slipping wrap which possibly can lead to incarceration intrathoracically. It should be mentionend, that in the early postoperative stage less force is required to push the stomach into the thorax, since the normal anatomical barriers have been disrupted by surgical dissection. If the wrap has been constructed too tight or the hiatus was closed too tight, dysphagia occurs within the first two days resulting in complete inability to swallow even saliva. In this case a swallow X-ray with a soluble contrast should be performed. If no contrast passes from the esophagus into the stomach early reoperation is advocated. The reintervention should be done within the first week. At the beginning of the second postoperative week reoperation becomes more difficult and should therefore be done only after three months again. At reintervention the wrap and the hiatus have to be inspected to make clear, what the cause for dysphagia is. In every case the fundoplication has to be taken down for having a good look at the hiatus. If the hiatus was too tight, the uppermost suture has to be removed, followed by recreating a loose Nissen or Toupet fundoplication. A fifty french bougie can be passed carefully into the stomach to clarify whether the hiatus is wide enough or another suture has to be opened.

As just mentioned reintervention should be avoided between the second week and third month after surgery and patients should be treated conservatively in this period if ever possible.

Late reoperation

Late postoperative problems are recurrent gastroesophageal reflux, dysphagia or a combination of both. In case of recurrent reflux, patients can be managed conservatively in most cases. Only if quality of life is lower than before the primay surgical procedure, reintervention is indicated. A reason for recurrent reflux is either a too loose wrap or the suspected brake down of the primary intact original fundoplication. As mentioned in the chapters before, recurrent reflux occurs more often following a Toupet than a Nissen procedure. Fortunately the fundoplication in these patients can easily be reconstructed. At first, all adheasions from the stomach to the surrounding liver, diagphragm or fat have to be dissected. The preparation has to be done in a way, that the fundus becomes as mobile as it should have been at primary surgery. Whether a Nissen or Toupet fundoplication is reconstructed does not depend on the former constructed wrap, but should be a result of the body motility at the moment of redo surgery.

Beneeth recurrent reflux redo surgery is indicated in patients with the symptom of persistent dysphagia over months in combination with a decreased quality of life. These cases are rare, since dysphagia solely related to the wrap or the diaphragm has either to be operated on in the early stage or becomes better and disappears within one year in the majority of patients. Therefore a very cautious proceeding is advocated and if nutrition is adequately maintained, waiting for almost a year before considering surgical revision should be encouraged. Redo surgery should then be performed more easily. Whilst it is difficult to be certain what the underlying cause of dysphagia is, a reexploration before surgical intervention should be done. The investigation of joice is a diagnostic pneumatic dilatation in general anesthesia. The figure of the dilated balloon on X-ray control shows, whether the stenosis is related to the wrap or the diaphragm. A hiatal related stenosis shows the typical radiological pricture of a sand-glas form. Laparoscopic reintervention contains not only the dissection of all adheasions with the break down of the wrap but the complete exposition of the hiatus with the preparation of the distal and intrathoracically positioned part of the esophagus too. Then the crural sutures have to be opened until a fifty french bougie slides unhindered into the stomach. If the stenosis is related to excessive parahiatal scar tissue this has to be removed, followed by the reconstruction of a normal wide hiatus. If the underlying problem of persistant dysphagia is a primary too tight wrap the fundoplication has to be devided and unravelled fully. A new and loose wrap has to be constructed and it is appropriate to perform a posterior 270° or 180° Toupet fundoplication even if an esophageal manometry demonstrates normal esophageal body peristalsis. In cases when the actual cause of dysphagia is not clear, widening of the hiatus and conversion to a Toupet fundoplication should both be performed.

The most frequent symptom leading to late redo surgery is the combination of reflux and dysphagia. This combined problem can occur as a result of a rehiatal hernia with the consecutive migration of a part or the total wrap intrathoracically, the so called "Slipping Nissen". These patients experience dysphagia as a result of a beginning strangulation of the wrap or the upper part of the stomach in between the crural branches with gastric mucosa above the stenosis resulting in peptic reflux. The symptoms in patients with a herniation of a part of the fundus through an intact wrap, the so called "telescoping" are the same, recurrent reflux and dysphagia. A telescope phenomenon can occur with or without a rehiatal hernia.

Indication for redo surgery in these patients is a decreased quality of life compared to the quality of life score before primary surgery. The operative strategy is always the same: deviding the adheasions from the stomach to the liver, the diaphragm and the fat, unravelling the previous fundoplication and exposing the diaphragmatic crura and the esophageal hiatus. It is essential to lengthen the esophagus by extensive preparation of its distal intrathoracically part. Only if the complete unravelled fundus and the distal esophagus lay loose without tension intraabdominally the reconstruction of the new hiatus and refundoplication can start.

Although for every patient undergoing redo surgery, the kind of the fundoplication can be predicted preoperatively the correction of the hiatus can only be established intraoperatively. The strategy there is according to the individual patient and his particular hiatal problem. It has to be decided whether the crura should be adapted only with sutures or armed by a small or circular prosthetic material. In contrast to this kind of closure of the hiatus with tension on the crura the hiatus can be closed in a tension free technique using a special mesh. As mentioned in a chapter before, there is no doubt, that the use of prosthetic material in repairing a large hiatal hernia reduces the risk of recurrent herniation.

Results

According to the literature, mortality for laparoscopically done refundoplications is not higher than for primary procedures. It can be estimated that the complication rates are even lower since redo procedures generally are done more in centers with surgeons more skilled in antireflux surgery and in laparoscopy. Open reoperation after open failed antireflux surgery is associated with a mortality of about 2 per cent and a morbidity of 20 to 40 per cent [4], [5]. Even in centers excellent to good results can only be expectet in 85 per cent of patients after open redo surgery. In the literature, there are only a few articles available dealing with a greater number of patients having undergone redo fundoplication [6]. The reported mortility in these papers is zero as it is in our serie of more than 150 redo procedures too. Morbidity and reported complications are unessential higher than in case of primary laparoscopic fundoplication. Data from the literature emphasize that patients assess the result of redo surgery as excellent to good in 65 to 85 per cent [7]. In case of a poor result (in 10 to 20 per cent), with persisting or new onsert symptoms a second or even third reintervention can be done without more problems than at the first refundoplication. Even in these patients in our series the success rates are as high as they are after the first reintervention. The quality of life in redo patients evaluated by means of the gastrointestinal quality of life index [8] is not much worse compared to those after successfully done primary surgery but much more better than before primary laparoscopic fundoplication. Laparoscopic revisional surgery in patients having undergone open fundoplication is feasible too with the restriction that adheasions from the stomach to the liver, to diaphragm and to the adominal wall are much more pronounced compared to patients with previous laparoscopic surgery.

References

[1] Dallemagne B, Weerts JM, Jehaes C, Markiewicz S, Lombard R (1991) Laparoscopic Nissen fundoplication: preliminary report. Surg Laparosc Endosc 1: 138–143

[2] Watson DI, Baigrie RJ, Jamieson GG (1996) A learning curve for laparoscopic fundoplication. Definable, avoidable, or a waste of time? Ann Surg 224: 198–203

[3] Kamolz T, Granderath PA, Bammer T, Pasiut M, Wykypiel H Jr, Herrmann R, Pointner R (2002) Mid- and long-term quality of life assessments after laparoscopic fundoplication and refundoplication: a single unit review of more than 500 antireflux procedures. Dig Liver Dis 34: 470–476

[4] Stein HJ, Feussner H, Siewert JR (1996) Failures of antireflux surgery: causes and management strategies. Am J Surg 171: 36–40

[5] Little AG, Ferguson MH, Skinner DB (1986) Reoperations for failed antireflux operations. J Thorac Cardiovasc Surg 91: 511–519

[6] Pohl D, Eubanks TR, Omelanczuk PE, Pellegrini CA (2001) Management and outcome of complications after laparoscopic antireflux operations. Arch Surg 136: 399–404

[7] Granderath FA, Kamolz T, Schweiger UM, Pointner R (2002) Long-term follow-up after laparoscopic refundoplication for failed antireflux surgery: quality of life, symptomatic outcome and patient satisfaction. J Gastrointest Surg 6: 812–818

[8] Eypasch E, Williams JI, Wood-Dauphinee S, Ure BM, Schmülling C, Neugebauer E, Troidl H (1995) Gastrointestinal quality of life index: development, validation and application of a new instrument. Br J Surg 82: 216–222

Chapter 21

HIATAL CLOSURE – NEW TRENDS IN LAPAROSCOPIC ANTIREFLUX SURGERY

F. A. Granderath[1] • C. T. Frantzides[2] • M. A. Carlson[3]

1 Department of General Surgery, Hospital Zell am See, Austria
2 Minimally Invasive Surgery Center, Evanston Northwestern Healthcare, Evanston, Il, USA
3 Department of Surgery, University of Nebraska Medical Center, Omaha, NE, USA

Introduction

Gastroesophageal reflux disease (GERD) has proven to be the most common upper gastrointestinal disorder in the western world with 10% of patients having daily symptoms [1], [2]. In many patients, GERD is associated with the presence of a hiatal hernia. The differences between the three traditional types of hiatal hernia regarding their morphological characteristics as well as the symptomatic correlation with GERD have to be considered. The most comprehensive classification recognizes three types of hiatal hernias. Type-I hiatal hernias, the classical sliding hiatal hernias, are characterized by transdiaphragmatic migration of the gastroesophageal junction and the proximal stomach toward the mediastinum. Type-I hiatal hernias are proven to be most common (80–90% of all types), particularly when the hernia is small. In type-II hiatal hernias or paraesophageal hernias, the gastroesophageal junction remains below the diaphragm in its normal position and the gastric fundus herniates alongside the esophagus into the mediastinum. The type-III hiatal hernias are a combination of both type-I and -II hernias. The gastroesophageal junction is above the diaphragm, and the gastric fundus herniates alongside the esophagus (*Figs. 1–3*). More than 80% of all paraesophageal hernias are considered to be type-III hiatal hernias.

Depending on these morphological entities, these three types show several symptomatic and clinical differences. A type-I hiatal hernia often causes characteristic GERD symptoms such as heartburn and regurgitation. Considerations regarding surgical therapy for this hernia type depends on the presence of GERD symptoms; therefore, the most common indication for surgery in type-I hiatal hernia is persistent GERD symptoms recalcitrant to medical therapy. A type-II hiatal hernia also can be accompanied by GERD symptoms, but this hernia type is typically associated with chest pain, dysphagia, pulmonary problems, nausea or bleeding, which are caused by the gastric herniation. Although paraesophageal hernia is a rare condition, it is associated with a rather high incidence of complications.

In case of axial rotation of the gastric fundus, the risk for intrathoracic strangulation and gastric volvulus with eventual incarceration and necrosis is increased. Therefore, most authors recommend a surgical management of paraesophageal hernia, even in patients without symptoms. The minimally invasive approach to paraesophageal hernia repair has become the standard of care for surgical management of this problem. Several studies have shown that laparoscopic paraesophageal hernia repair is associated with a lower incidence of morbidity, a shorter hospital stay, and a shorter recovery period compared to open repair [3]. Additionally, most authors agree that the laparoscopic

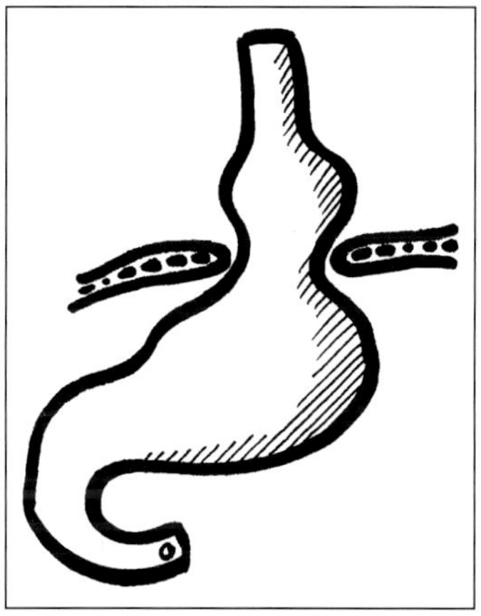

Fig. 1. Type-I hiatal hernia

approach allows better visibility and higher dissection of the intrathoracic esophagus. Whether performed open or laparoscopically, however, paraesophageal hernia repair is associated with a high recurrence rate. Recent reports have shown the laparoscopic approach in particular has a higher recurrence rate than the open approach, with recurrence rates in the former up to 42% [4]. Due to this high recurrence rate, several technical details have been considered to minimize the rate of recurrent hiatal herniation. Some of these details are still a matter of controversy; for example the complete removal of the hernia sac, the need to perform an antireflux procedure, or the performance of a gastropexy are frequent topics of discussion [5], [6]. The main question, however, has to be whether to perform the hiatoplasty with simple interrupted sutures or with prosthetic material.

During the past few years it has been shown that hiatal closure also has become a central point in laparoscopic antireflux surgery for GERD [7]. The causes of failure of an antireflux procedure are multiple, but the most frequent cause has proven to be the recurrent hiatal hernia with consecutive intrathoracic herniation of the fundic wrap into the mediastinum [8]. Typical symptoms of an intrathoracic wrap herniation are persistent or recurrent reflux, dysphagia, or the combination of both. The combination of these symptoms and this anatomic complication leads to redo-surgery in most of these patients [9]. In a large review of more than 10.000 laparoscopic antireflux procedures, it was documented that postoperative intrathoracic wrap herniation was the most common intraoperative finding during redosurgery for the failed antireflux procedure [10].

Some possible patient-related and procedure-related mechanisms for postoperative intrathoracic wrap migration include inappropriate postoperative activities of the patients immediately after surgery, inadequate mobilization of the esophagus, inadequate crural closure secondary to widely spaced crura sutured under tension, or a postoperative rupture of the cruroplasty due to continuous excursion of the diaphragm.

Crural closure has become a relevant problem in laparoscopic antireflux surgery, as well as during laparoscopic paraesophageal hernia repair. To solve this problem, some authors have advocated the use of prosthetic material for crural closure in both laparoscopic paraesophageal hernia repair and laparoscopic antireflux surgery. The concept of using prosthetic meshes is based upon the lessening of tension on the hiatal crura or the reinforcement of simple sutured crura to prevent postoperative hiatal disruption. Since the first description of prosthetic hiatal closure by Kuster in 1993 [5], a number of techniques have been published. There has debate regarding the shape of the mesh, the material of the mesh, the position and placement of the mesh, and especially whether a prosthetic hiatal reinforcement has to be tension-free. Additionally, there is no agreement regarding the question of selective versus routine use of mesh. Some authors recommend the routine use of prosthetic mesh in order to prevent tension on the hiatal crura and therefore decrease hiatal hernia recurrence. Other authors use mesh selectively, e.g., in patients in whom a

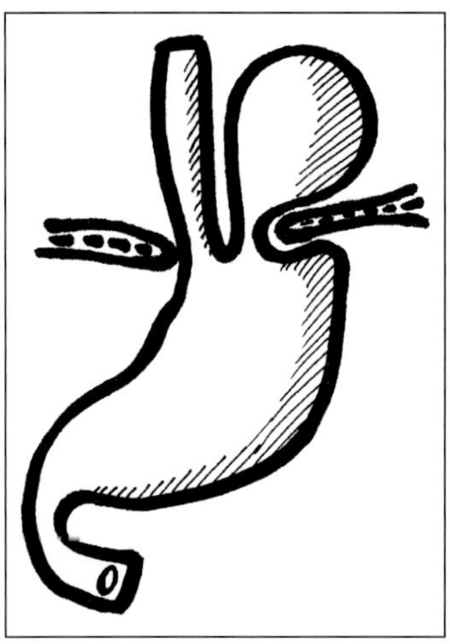

Fig. 2. Type-II hiatal hernia

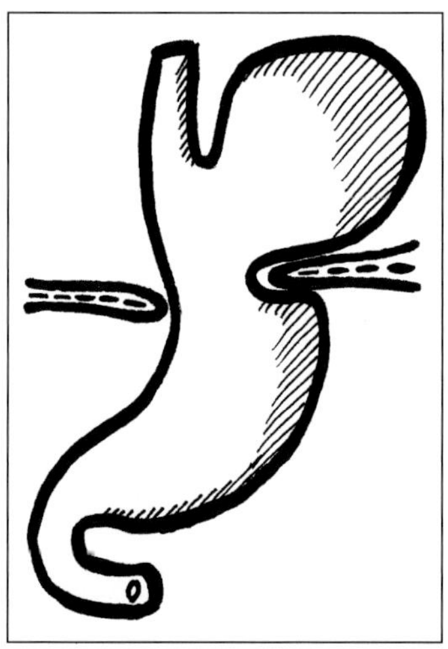

Fig. 3. Type-III hiatal hernia

sufficient tension-free hiatal closure cannot be achieved with simple sutures.

For some authors, the indication for reinforcement of the hiatal crura with prosthetic material depends on the size of the hiatal defect. Another point of controversy focuses on the shape and material of the prosthetic mesh. Some authors routinely use polypropylene meshes for hiatal closure, believing that polypropylene rapidly incorporates and that the developing scar tissue strengthens the muscular fibers of the hiatal crura. Other authors discourage the use of polypropylene due to the development of visceral adhesions and the risk of intestinal fistula [11]. On the other hand polytetrafluoroethylene (PTFE) has been recommended for hiatal closure because of its low adhesive potential.

Techniques and results of prosthetic meshes for closure of the esophageal hiatus

Several techniques have been described for prosthetic closure of the hiatal crura. Basically, two different approaches have to be differentiated: mesh repair without primary sutured crura ("tension-free") or mesh repair with primary cruroplasty.

The first study regarding laparoscopic large hiatal hernia repair with hiatal mesh prosthesis was published by Kuster and Gilroy in 1993 [5]. These authors preferred tension-free anterior repair of the hiatal defect. In 6 patients with large paraesophageal hernia, the hiatal crura could not be sutured anterior to the esophagus without significant tension. Therefore a Mersilene® mesh was placed on the hiatus as an anterior onlay patch, overlapping the hiatal crura about 2 cm in all directions. The mesh was secured to the crural edges with staples. No intraoperative or postoperative mesh-related complications occurred during a follow-up period of 8–22 months. Postoperative gastrointestinal series showed no evidence of postoperative hernia recurrence; however, 2 patients had slippage of a small part of the posterior segment of the fundus. None of these patients developed postoperative mesh-related dysphagia or GERD symptoms during the follow-up period.

A similar technique has been used by Paul et al [12] in 3 elderly patients. A 5 × 10 cm Gore-tex® mesh (PTFE) was cut to cover the hiatal defect, and then was placed as an anterior onlay patch. The mesh was secured at the lower mesh edges, and then sutured in a running fashion up to the top of the mesh (*Fig. 4*). In this small series there were no complications, and for a mean follow-up period of 10 months there were no hernia recurrences.

Another technique of tension-free hiatal closure has been avocated by Basso and colleagues [13]. In 65 patients who underwent laparoscopic Nissen fundoplication with simple sutured hiatal closure the authors experienced a hiatal hernia recurrence rate of 13.8% during a mean follow-up period of 48.3 months. After reviewing the videotapes of these patients, it became clear that the crural sutures were under tension, and that hiatal disruption led to postoperative intrathoracic migration of the fundic wrap. Due to these findings, the authors began using a 3 × 4 cm polypropylene mesh for posterior hiatal reinforcement.The mesh was secured with staples on the upper side and on the lateral sides of both crura as a tension free hiatoplasty (*Fig. 5*). This technique was used in a subsequent group of 67 patients who underwent laparoscopic Nissen fundoplication for GERD. During a mean follow-up period of 22.5 months, the authors saw no complication related to the prosthetic mesh nor hiatal hernia recurrence.

An interesting technique to achieve a tension-free hiatal closure has been described by Huntington et al [14]. If a tension-free crural closure with simple sutures was nor possible, then a relaxing incision on the

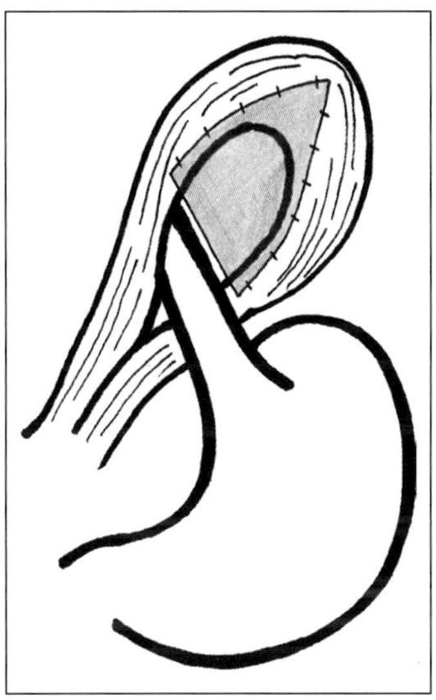

Fig. 4. Tension-free anterior repair

diaphragm was performed to gain crural mobility for a simple sutured hiatoplasty. The diaphragmatic defect of the relaxing incision then was closed with a polypropylene patch (*Fig. 6*). This technique was used successfully in 8 patients with paraesophageal hernia; there was no recurrence during a follow-up period of 8 months.

Champion et al [15] preferred prosthetic reinforcement of primarily sutured crura. Similar to Basso et al [13], these authors used a 3 × 5 cm polypropylene mesh for posterior hiatal closure. After placing interrupted permanent sutures posteriorly to the esophagus, the polypropylene mesh was placed as an onlay prosthesis, and then fixed with a hernia stapler along the crural edges. The mesh was secured further with a centrally placed permanent mattress suture; this ensured that the upper edge of the mesh was positioned at least 1 cm below the upper edge of the crural repair (*Fig. 7*). This technique was performed in 52 consecutive patients with symptomatic GERD and a large hiatal/paraesophageal hernia. During a mean postoperative follow-up period of 25 months, only one patient developed a postoperative intrathoracic wrap migration; this was caused by violent retching in the recovery room after surgery. Later on, this patient underwent redo-surgery due to recurrent GERD symptoms. Importantly, no mesh migrations or visceral erosion occurred in this series of patients.

In a recently published article by Keidar and Szold [16], the authors use a circular mesh in a similar shape as Frantzides et al [17]. Out of a sample of 33 patients, a group of 10 patients with large paraesophageal hernias underwent laparoscopic prosthetic hiatal repair. The simple cruroplasty then was reinforced with Gore-tex® mesh in six patients and Prolene® mesh in four patients. The mesh was precut to an oval sheet, placed around the esophagus and then fixed to the diaphragm using a hernia stapler (*Fig. 8*). During a follow-up period of 46–76 months, the satisfaction score was good to excellent in the majority of patients. Only 1 patient of the mesh-repaired patients developed a hiatal hernia recurrence in contrast to 4 patients who underwent repair without mesh. No complications related to the use of the mesh were seen in this study.

Casaccia et al [18] published their experience with an innovative physiological composite "A" – shaped mesh. The authors first performed a physical and geometrical analysis of the esophageal hiatus with a theoretical model. Based on their findings regarding the physiological strengths of the hiatal crura with or without direct sutures, they performed an anatomical study on 20 cadavers to verify the anatomical findings of their theoretical model. As a result, they developed a special "A" shaped PTFE – mesh (BARD® Composix mesh)

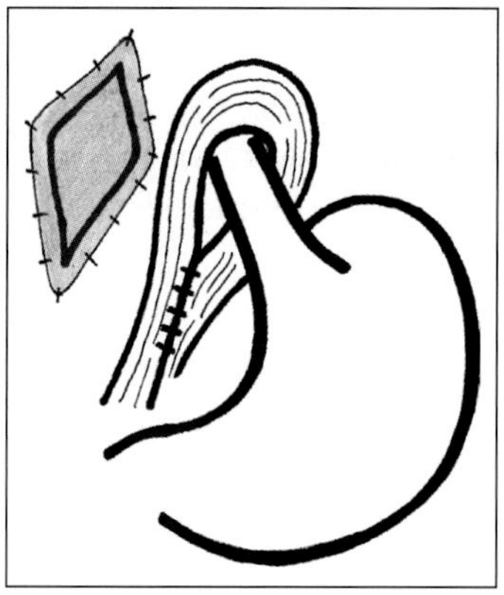

Fig. 6. Tension-free sutured repair

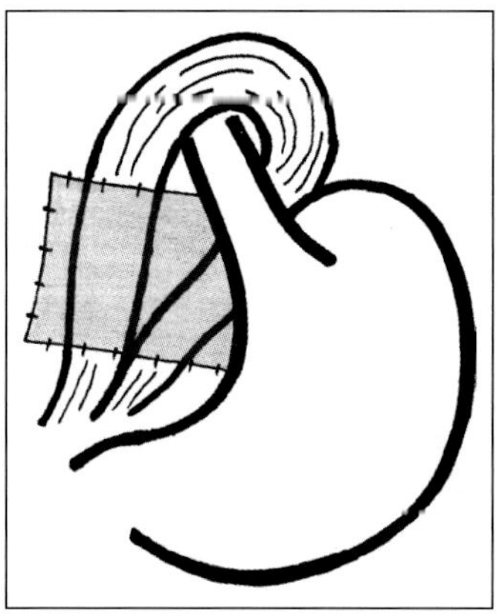

Fig. 5. Tension-free posterior repair

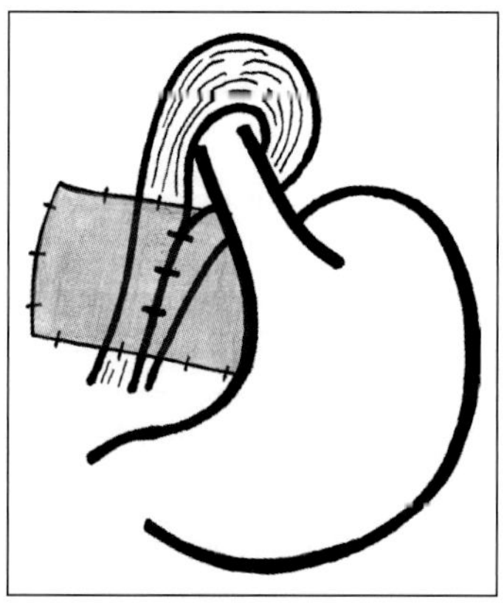

Fig. 7. Sutured crura and posterior mesh repair

which, when positioned over the hiatal defect, was intended to effect closure similar to the physiological condition (*Fig. 9*). In 8 patients with large type-II and type-III hiatal hernia, laparoscopic repair was performed with this composite "A" shaped PTFE mesh. Intraoperatively, the authors found that the mesh fit well in the hiatal region, with good handling and easy placement on the diaphragm. Postoperative dysphagia occurred in 2 patients for up to 3 months after surgery, but no recurrence was observed during an average follow-up period of 8 months.

Based on the possibility of mesh-related complications such as esophageal stricture, mesh migration, or visceral erosion, Oelschlager et al [19] advocated the use of a new type of mesh made from porcine small intestine submucosa (SIS) for laparoscopic repair of paraesophageal hernias. The authors closed the hiatal crura with interrupted 2−0 silk sutures, and then positioned a U-shaped 7 × 10 cm four-ply Surgisis® mesh posteriorly so that the mesh covered the crural repair. The mesh was secured with interrupted silk sutures to the diaphragm (*Fig. 10*). This technique has been used in 9 patients with large paraesophageal hernias that could not be closed without tension. In 8 patients who were available for follow-up, only 1 had a small (2 cm) recurrent hiatal hernia on barium esophagram; this recurrence was asymptomatic. Another patient had to undergo pneumatic dilatation for persistent mild dysphagia, but without signs of anatomic failure on endoscopy or barium swallow. There were no other complications in this series.

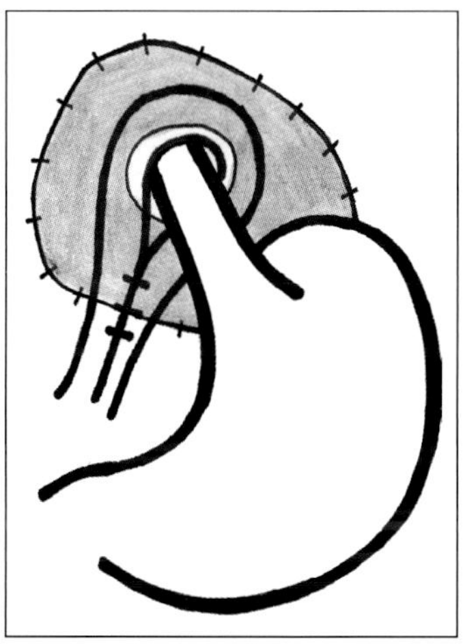

Fig. 8. Simple cruroplasty and circular mesh repair

Another approach to crural closure with biomaterial has been described by Varga et al [20]. In this study, the hiatoplasty was performed with the ligamentum teres in addition to simple sutures. After closing the hiatal crura with nonabsorbable interrupted sutures, the mobilized ligamentum teres was pulled between the closed crura and posterior esophagus, and then sutured to the crura. This created a U-shaped hiatal onlay reinforcement (*Fig. 11*). This technique was performed in 4 patients with type-III hiatal hernia. There were no perioperative complications related to this kind of hiatoplasty. One patient had minor episodic epigastric pain postoperatively; otherwise, all patients relieved of symptoms. No recurrent hiatal hernia occurred during follow-up of 3–11 months.

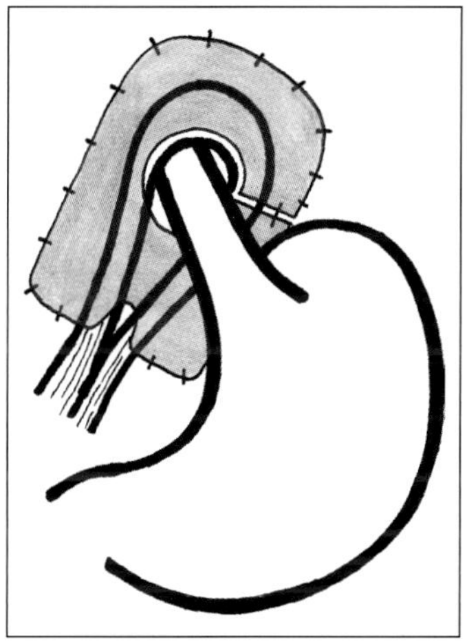

Fig. 9. Simple cruroplasty and "A"-shaped mesh repair

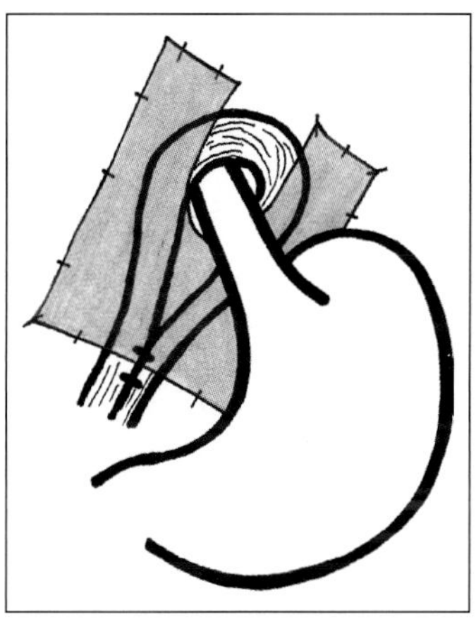

Fig. 10. Simple cruroplasty and SIS® mesh repair

Own experience

The high rate of postoperative intrathoracic wrap migration after laparoscopic antireflux surgery prompted us to use prosthetic meshes for crural closure in December 1998. In all patients who underwent laparoscopic antireflux surgery at our surgical unit, hiatal hernia recurrence with intrathoracic wrap migration was the most common cause of anatomic failure after primary laparoscopic antireflux surgery. In over 70% of patients who underwent laparoscopic refundoplication after primary failed antireflux surgery, intrathoracic wrap migration was found as the reason for failure.

In a prospective non-randomized trial [21] we compared 361 patients with GERD who underwent laparoscopic Nissen or Toupet fundoplication with simple crural closure to 170 GERD patients who underwent laparoscopic antireflux surgery with simple hiatal closure reinforced with polypropylene mesh. In the group of patients who underwent primary cruroplasty, the number of sutures depended on the size of hiatal hernia; in these patients, the crura were approximated with 2–4 interrupted nonbasorbable polyfilament sutures (*Figs. 12* and *13*).

In the cruroplasty and mesh group, the crura were approximated with simple interrupted sutures as above. Additionally, a 1 × 3 cm section of polypropylene mesh (cut from a 10 × 15 Prolene® mesh for groin hernia repair) was placed on the sutured crura as a posterior onlay and sutured with one stitch on the lateral sides of both the right and the left crus (*Figs. 14* and *15*).

Follow-up examinations were performed 6 weeks, 3 months and 1 year after surgery. After 1 year of follow-up, a significant difference in the postoperative occurrence of intrathoracic wrap migration was found. In the initial group with non-mesh hiatoplasty, a postoperative intrathoracic wrap migration occurred in 6.1% of patients compared to 0.6% of patients who underwent cru-

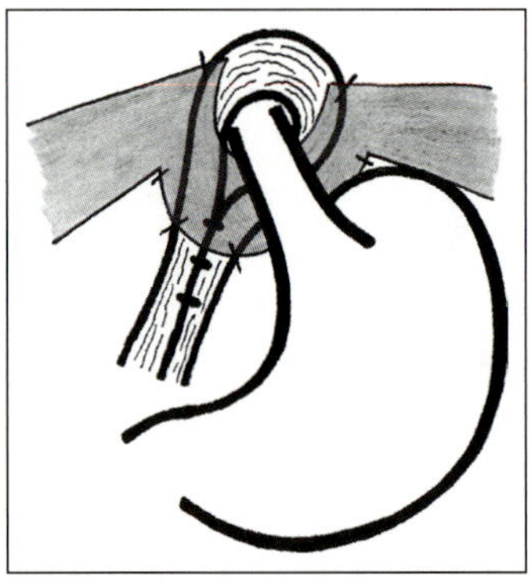

Fig. 11. Simple cruroplasty and ligamentum teres repair

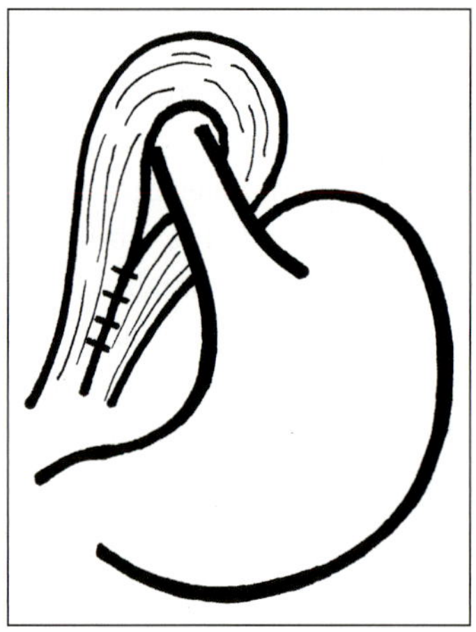

Fig. 12. Simple cruroplasty

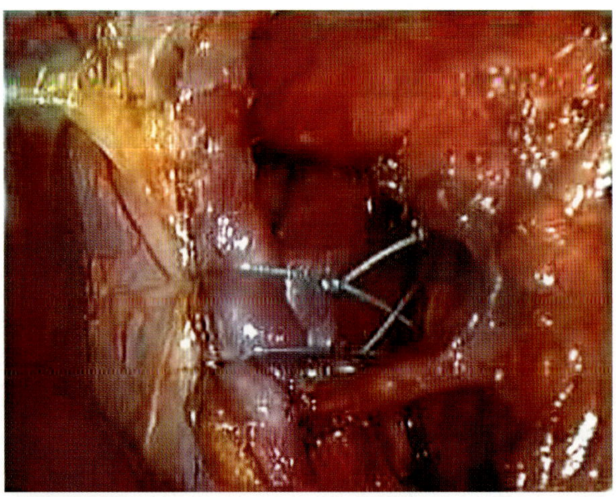

Fig. 13. Simple cruroplasty

ral closure with polypropylene mesh onlay. A significant difference also occurred in the incidence of postoperative dysphagia. Patients with mesh-cruroplasty had a dysphagia rate of 35.3% compared to 19.8% in the non-mesh group 3 months after surgery; however, the dysphagia rate resolved at the 1 year visit and was not different between the two groups.

These findings were re-evaluated in another non randomized trial [22], in which 100 GERD patients with simple crural closure were compared to 100 GERD patients with simple closure reinforced with the 1 × 3 cm polypropylene mesh hiatoplasty. The postoperative dysphagia rate and its impact on quality of life was evaluated for a period of 12 months after surgery. The postoperative dysphagia rate was significantly higher in the mesh-group at 3 month follow-up, but again decreased to comparable values at 1 year follow-up. Apart from these results, patients quality of life (GQLI) significantly improved after surgery in both groups. This improvement remained stable up to one year postoperatively, was comparable between the two groups, and similar to values from a healthy control group.

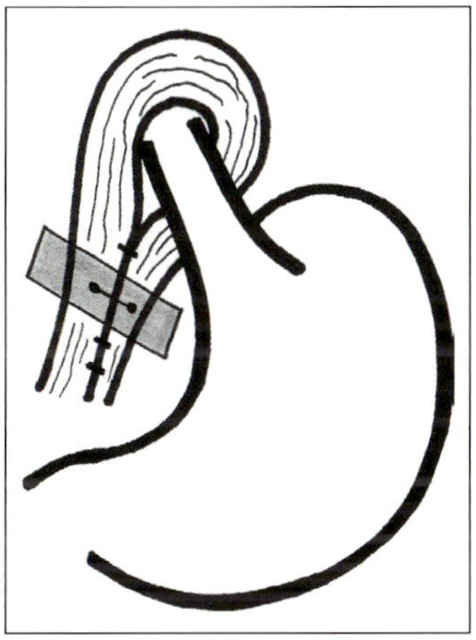

Fig. 14. Simple cruroplasty and posterior 1 × 3 cm polypropylene mesh repair

To verify these findings, a prospective randomized study was performed on 100 GERD patients scheduled for laparoscopic Nissen fundoplication [23]. Fifty patients were prospectively randomized to laparoscopic 360° floppy Nissen fundoplication with simple hiatoplasty, and fifty were randomized to laparoscopic 360° floppy Nissen fundoplication with 1 × 3 cm polypropylene mesh onlay. Follow-up of 12 months was obtained in all patients. Three months after surgery, a significant difference in postoperative intrathoracic wrap migrations was observed. Five patients (10%) of the non-mesh group had a recurrence compared to 1 patient (2%) of the mesh-group. Twelve months after surgery, the recurrence rates increased to 4 patients (8%) in the mesh-group and 13 patients (26%) in the non-mesh-group. In addition, patients with prosthetic hiatal closure again had a higher dysphagia rate at the 3 months visit, as previously observed.

A different type of prosthetic mesh was used in 24 patients who underwent laparoscopic refundoplication in our surgical unit for a failed primary antireflux surgery. The cause of failure in all of these patients was a symptomatic intrathoracic wrap mig-ration [24]. The failed hiatal repair was primarily approximated with interrupted nonabsorbable sutures and then reinforced with a circular precut polypropylene mesh. The mesh was cut out with a 3–4 cm "keyhole" as described by

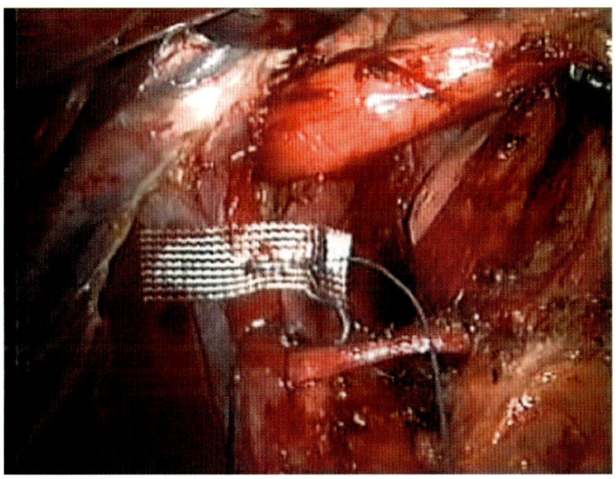

Fig. 15. Simple cruroplasty and posterior 1 × 3 cm polypropylene mesh repair

Frantzides and Carlson [25]. The mesh was placed around the esophagus and secured to the diaphragm and crura with a hernia stapler (*Figs. 16* and *17*). All patients were followed for 12 months after surgery, and no one had a hiatal hernia recurrence. We have had no evidence of any mesh-related complications such as erosion, migration, or visceral perforation in our patients.

We also are working on other alternatives for hiatal closure. The higher dysphagia rate in patients with hiatal mesh prosthesis has led us to use a special "V" shaped Composix mesh (Crurasoft®, BARD) for large hiatal hernia repair. After dissection of the hiatal crura, the mesh is brought into the abdomen and positioned on to the crura as a tension-free posterior onlay. The mesh is fixed with interrupted sutures on the edges of the mesh and secured with staples on the lateral side of the mesh (*Figs. 18* and *19*). The advantages of this mesh type have been ascribed to the combination of two clinically proven materials: BARD® mesh on the one side for maximum tissue ingrowth and ePTFE on the other side for minimal visceral adhesions.

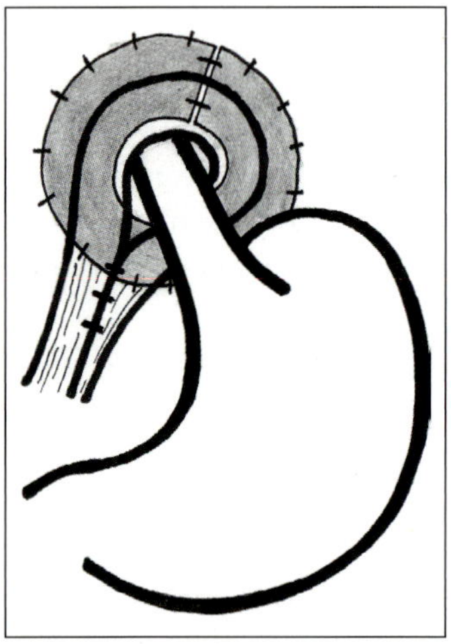

Fig. 16. Simple cruroplasty and circular polypropylene mesh repair

In addition, we are participating in a multicenter study regarding the use of PARIETEX®, a newer mesh, which, similar to the Composix mesh, combines two different materials. Parietex® composite mesh has a three-dimensional weave of polyester on the one side with a hydrophilic collagen material on the other side. The resorbable collagen side has been designed for the prevention of intrabdominal adhesions to the mesh in the early postoperative period. The polyester side guarantees rapid tissue ingrowth with permanent reinforcement. In conjunction with the participating colleagues and the manufacturer, we have designed a special "V" shape of this mesh particularly for laparoscopic closure of the hiatal crura. The mesh is used both for tension-free hiatal closure (*Figs. 20* and *21*) and as an additional reinforcement of primary sutured hiatal crura. Positioned as a posterior onlay prosthesis, the mesh is secured to the diaphragm with a hernia stapler.

Based on our previous findings and experiences, we are developing a new kind of prosthetic mesh which specifically will be for hiatal closure. During laparoscopic refundoplication for primary failed hiatal closure, the fundic wrap often does not slip posterior to but also anterior to the esophagus. Therefore, in addition to posterior closure, the mesh should also cover the anterior diaphragmatic region to prevent postoperative anterior slippage. Circular meshes have proven

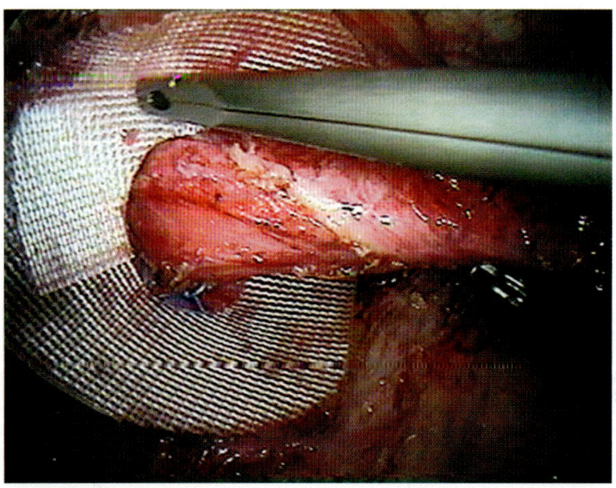

Fig. 17. Simple cruroplasty and circular polypropylene mesh repair

to be an effective method to prevent hiatal hernia recurrence in some studies. We have employed a "heart" shaped modification of this mesh with large anterior and posterior portions which completely cover the hiatal crura behind the esophagus. The esophagus lies in a 3–4 cm central keyhole, which is protected by a PTFE collar to prevent esophageal erosion by the mesh (*Fig. 22*).

Experience of Drs. Frantzides and Carlson

Our initial results with laparoscopic mesh-reinforced diaphragmatic hernia repair

To our knowledge, Dr. Robert Condon of the Medical College of Wisconsin (Milwaukee, Wisconsin, USA) was the first to address the problem of unacceptably high recurrence rate after (open) sutured hiatal herniorrhaphy by using a mesh-reinforced cruroplasty. Beginning in the latter 1970's, this surgeon (who was our mentor) instituted a policy of polypropylene onlay to the diaphragm for patients with large hiatal hernia with intrathoracic stomach [26]. His technique consisted of a sutured posterior cruroplasty onto which a sheet of Marlex® was placed, followed by a gastrostomy. In order to accommodate passage of the esophagus, a "keyhole" was cut in the center of the mesh. Over a fifteen year period, 44 patients with intrathoracic stomach were treated in such a manner. After a mean follow-up period of 52 months (range 2 months to 15 years), the clinical recurrence rate was zero [26]. At the time of its publication in 1998, this manuscript represented one of the largest series of prosthesis-reinforced diaphragmatic hernia repairs, either open or laparoscopic.

Encouraged with the result of open mesh repair of diaphragmatic hernia, we elected to perform the repair with a minimally invasive approach. We did have a concern with using a stiff prosthetic mesh (such as Marlex®) at the hiatus, because this mesh did erode into the esophagus in one patient from the open series [26]. Polypropylene mesh erosion into exposed bowel has been a frequent enough problem in mesh repair of anterior abdominal wall defects, especially in the presence of acute inflammation [27]. We believed that the use of PTFE at the hiatus might lessen the risk for erosive complications, since only a handful of cases have been published documenting PTFE as the cause or suspected cause of a bowel fistula (at the time we were contemplating such repairs, no reports of erosive complications

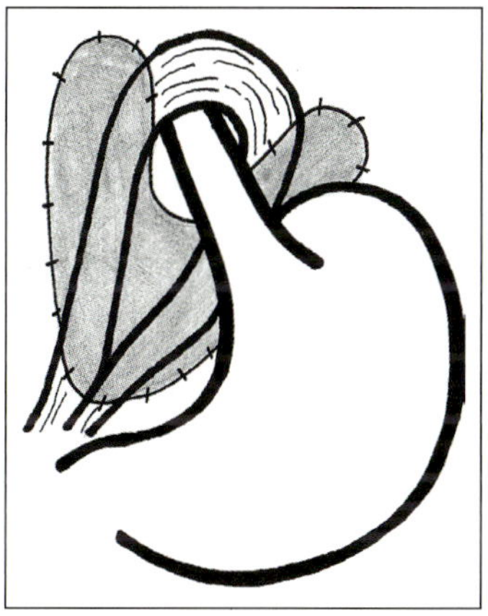

Fig. 18. Tension-free posterior Crurasoft® mesh repair

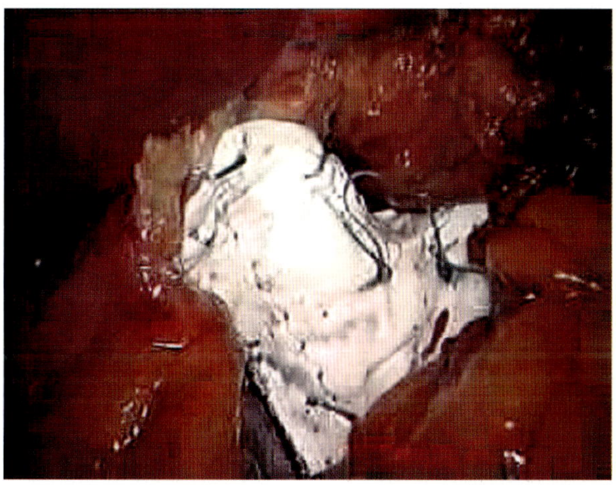

Fig. 19. Tension-free posterior Crurasoft® mesh repair

from PTFE could be found). Another theoretical concern we had was whether the use of mesh actually would be of benefit in the repair of diaphragmatic hernia. Our retrospective series suggested that utilization of mesh decreased hernia recurrence rate, but we did not have any controlled data that confirmed this. Therefore, after a small number of cases to demonstrate the feasibility of minimally invasive hiatal herniorrhaphy with PTFE onlay reinforcement [17], we embarked on a randomized controlled trial to test whether mesh placement reduced the recurrence rate after laparoscopic diaphragmatic hernia repair.

We hypothesized that a benefit from mesh placement most likely would be seen in patients with a large hiatal defect (which we defined as ≥ 8 cm). Seventy-two patients with gastroesophageal reflux disease and large defect hiatal hernia were enrolled into this trial [25]. The study population consisted of a subset of all patients (> 600) undergoing primary minimally invasive antireflux surgery under the care of Dr. Frantzides. The decision whether to enroll a patient into the study was made after intraoperative measurement of the hiatal defect. If the defect diameter was ≥ 8 cm, then the subject was randomized, and a simple posterior cruroplasty with or without PTFE onlay reinforcement (see below) followed by a floppy Nissen fundoplication was performed. After a mean follow-up period of 3.3 years, the recurrence rate in the cruroplasty-only group was 22% (i.e., 8 of 36), and the rate in the cruroplasty plus PTFE group was zero. There were no mesh-related complications. We concluded that PTFE reinforcement of posterior cruroplasty was indicated for hiatal defects ≥ 8 cm.

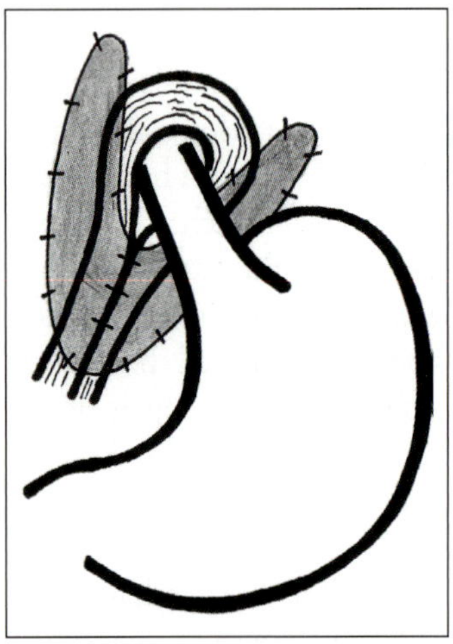

Fig. 20. Parietex® mesh repair

Our technique of laparoscopic mesh-reinforced hiatal hernia repair

Our technique of minimally invasive hiatal hernia repair has been described in detail elsewhere [28]. The patient is placed in a modified lithotomy position with 15–20° of reverse-Trendelenburg tilt, and the surgeon stands between the patient's legs. We employ five 10 mm ports; this gives us maximum flexibility in instrument choice, including atraumatic 10 mm tissue graspers (atraugrip grasper – Pilling and Weck Surgical, Ft. Washington, PA). The liver is retracted with an inflatable nontraumatic balloon retractor (Soft Wand atraumatic balloon, Southborough, MA). The contents of the hiatal

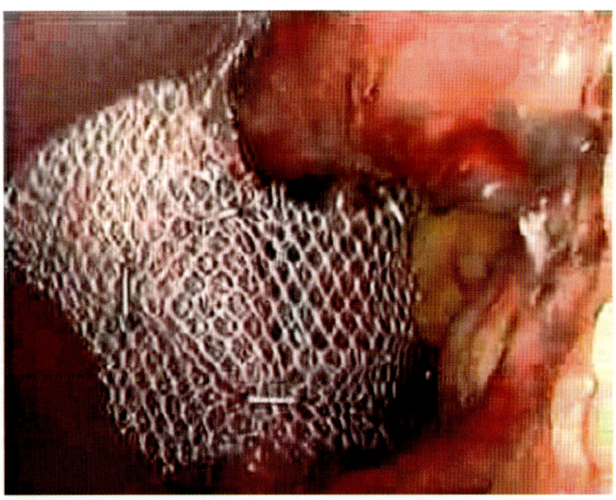

Fig. 21. Parietex® mesh repair

hernia (stomach, omentum, transverse colon, etc.) are reduced using the atraumatic grasper. The lesser omentum is then entered at the avascular area above the caudate lobe and the incision extended to the anterior arch of the crura. The hernia sac is reduced and excised. This dissection of the sac should be done meticulously so that pneumothorax is avoided. We advocate routine excision of the hernia sac; without such excision, the subsequent dissection can be difficult and confusing. The esophagus should be mobilized such that the distal 5 cm lies within the abdomen without tension. We prefer to employ a lighted esophageal bougie during this part of the procedure; this can aid in the identification of the esophagus, which can be a difficult task.

After the esophagus is fully mobilized, a posterior cruroplasty is performed with nonpledgeted, interrupted sutures of braided polyester. If an anterior hiatal defect is present at this point, then we also will a employ a 1–2 stitch anterior cruroplasty. A PTFE patch then is custom-cut from a larger sheet of mesh (see *Fig. 23*); a "keyhole" (3.5 cm circular defect) is cut into the center of the mesh to accommodate the esophagus (*Fig. 23*). The patch is introduced into the abdomen through a trocar (avoiding contact with the skin), and then applied as an onlay to the diaphragmatic repair, ensuring that the macroporous (rough) surface of the mesh faces the diaphragm. The prosthetic is anchored in place with a rigid laparoscopic hernia stapler (see *Fig. 24*). This 10 mm instrument fires titanium staples; we have found its performance optimal for securing PTFE to the diaphragm. The procedure is completed with a floppy 3-stitch, 2 cm-long Nissen fundoplication, performed over a 50–60 Fr bougie.

There are issue regarding the technique of mesh fixation to the diaphragm; specifically, whether to apply the mesh as on onlay, or to perform a "tension-free" repair. We have preferred the former; that is, to complete a primary cruroplasty first, and then to cover the cruroplasty with an onlay patch. In this situation, the mesh acts as a buttress for the sutured cruroplasty, relieving the tissue repair from the forces of intraabdominal pressure, respiratory excursion, and so forth. In the tension-free repair, the crura are not approximated; the mesh bridges the native defect. At this point in time there is no evidence from the field of mesh hiatal herniorrhaphy to support the use of onlay repair over tension-free repair (or *visa versa*). Our preference for the onlay repair has been our practice pattern, and we have had and continue to have salutary results from this practice. Practically speaking, it is easier to staple the mesh in place around the esopha-

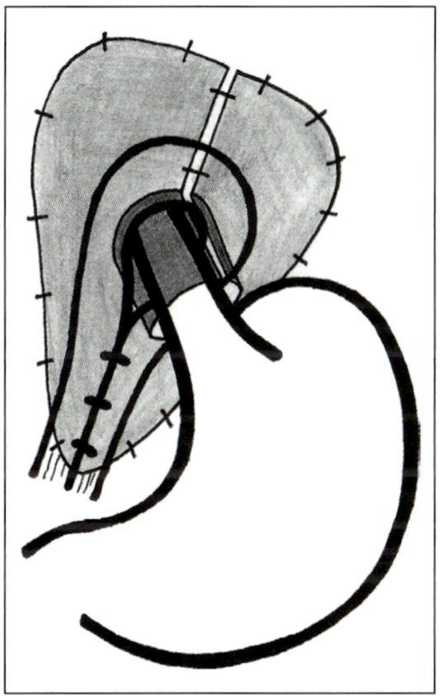

Fig. 22. The "Zell" mesh

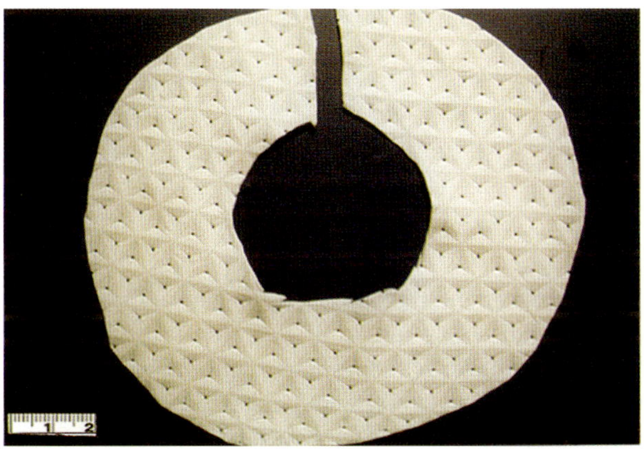

Fig. 23. PTFE onlay patch is constructed to have an oval shape with a horizontal diameter of 12 cm and anterior-posterior dimension of 10 cm. A 3.5 cm "keyhole" is made in the center of the mesh in order to accommodate passage of the esophagus

gus when it is surrounded by the sutured crura. In a small number of cases, it will be impossible to suture the crura together secondary to excessive tension, poor tissue, or other reasons. In these situations a tension-free application of the prosthetic should be employed. In the final analysis, it likely is the presence of the mesh itself (and not whether it is applied as an onlay or a bridge) which prevents hernia recurrence.

We believe that in order for the mesh to have an optimal effect (i.e., producing the lowest possible recurrence rate), the mesh should cover the repair with a large "overlap". That is, the mesh should extend beyond the crural margins by as much as the local anatomy will allow (see *Fig. B*). Practically speaking, extension of the mesh in this location is limited to the right by the inferior vena cava, anteriorly by the left lobe of the liver, posteriorly by retroperitoneal structures and to the left by the spleen. Thus caution should be taken to avoid injury to any of these structures. The importance of several centimeters of mesh extension beyond the entire circumference of a hernial defect has been borne out by a large amount of retrospective data from underlay repair of ventral herniorrhaphy, both open and laparoscopic [29], [30] For example, if a surgeon is faced with a 4 cm round-shaped ventral hernia, then the diameter of the mesh used in an underlay repair typically should be 8–10 cm, which permits a 2–3 cm extension of the mesh beyond the entire circumference of the defect. While it is difficult to satisfy these same criteria for mesh coverage of a hiatal defect, the precept of mesh overlap of the hernial defect should be kept in mind when applying this technique to a hiatal hernia.

The actual firing of the stapler can be a "tricky" maneuver, because unfortunate stapler deployment can injure the heart, which can result in fatal outcomes [31]. The precise technical details in stapling PTFE to the diaphragm with proximity of the heart are difficult to convey in written form. The surgeon must use enough pressure on the stapler to ensure that the staple penetrates the prosthesis and secures an adequate tissue bite, but not so much pressure that the staple penetrates the diaphragm and breaches the pericardium. The attainment of this skill is facilitated with training, anatomic knowledge, and experience.

Recent results with laparoscopic mesh-reinforced diaphragmatic hernia repair

Since the conclusion of our randomized trial [25] we have routinely employed PTFE mesh reinforcement during minimally invasive repair of large hiatal hernia. We have decreased our threshold for mesh usage to hiatal defects whose diameter is in the range of 5–6 cm. Our original indication for the utilization of PTFE reinforcement during hiatal herniorrhaphy was a defect size of ≥ 8 cm; this cut-off size is relatively large. Since we had an impressive difference in outcome between the control and mesh groups in our randomized trial [25] we felt justified in broadening the indication for mesh usage. Since 2000, we have performed 63 minimally invasive hiatal hernia repairs; PTFE was employed in 28 (44%) of these herniorrhaphies. Since 1992 sixty four patients have undergone laparoscopic large hiatal hernia repairs with placement of PTFE prosthesis. We have yet

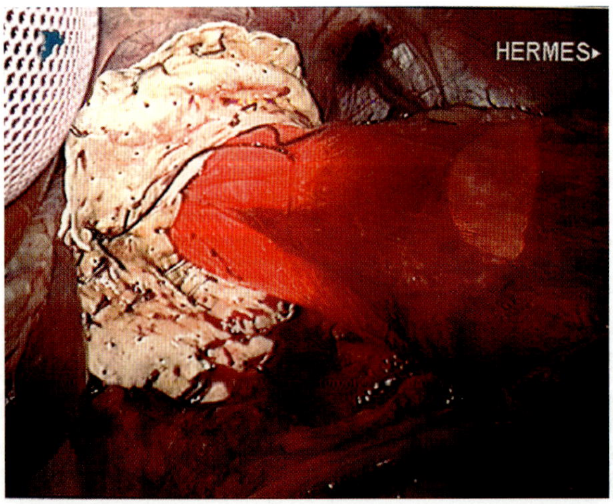

Fig. 24. Completed mesh repair of a hiatal hernia. The crura first were closed with simple sutures of 2–0 braided polyester, and then a patch as shown in the previous figure was applied to the cruroplasty (i.e., as an onlay) and stapled circumferentially in place. Note the extensive overlap of the repair by the mesh

to document a recurrence after mesh reinforcement of minimally invasive hiatal hernia repair with our technique described above. In addition, no patient has been documented to have mesh infection, erosion, or contraction ("mesh shrinkage" [32]). We have noted in the literature a few reported cases reports of PFTE erosion into a gastrointestinal lumen (see below), but this has not dissuaded us from using PTFE-onlay reinforcement of sutured cruroplasty for the repair of the large hiatal defect.

Complications of prosthetic hiatal repair

The use of prosthetic materials in surgery for gastroesophageal reflux disease and/or large hiatal hernia repair is accompanied by alow incidence of foreign body complications. For instance, the use of Teflon-pledgets in fundoplication has been associated with visceral erosion, foreign body migration, or gastroesophageal fistula after surgery [33]–[35].

In particular, a risk for complications related to the use of prosthetic materials for closure of the hiatal crura has been predicted by some authors. The focus is on the possibility of erosion or migration of the mesh into the esophagus or stomach, as well as complications due to severe mesh adhesions, infection, or the development of fibrotic strictures in the hiatal area. In a study by Carlson et al [26], one patient (2.3%) out of 44 who underwent open prosthetic hiatal closure for large hiatal hernia repair developed a mesh erosion into the esophagus 29 months after surgery. Edelman et al [36] reported one patient out of 5 who had to undergo revisional surgery after primary laparoscopic paraesophageal hernia repair with mesh. This patients had severe dysphagia due to esophageal stenosis secondary to mesh-induced fibrosis. Likewise, Trus et al [37] also saw one patient who had undergone primary laparoscopic mesh repair for paraesophageal hernia who then suffered from refractory postoperative dysphagia. During re-laparotomy the authors found a circular scar at the distal esophagus caused by the hiatal mesh. The mesh had to be excised, a myotomy was performed, and then the crura were approximated. Persistent postoperative dysphagia refractory to dilatations was reported by Van der Peet et al [38]. One patient who underwent laparoscopic hiatal hernia repair with Dacron mesh reinforcement had a significant fibrotic reaction to the mesh; This had to be removed during a reoperation. Another two patients with mesh-related complications were reported by Casabella et al [39]. One patient developed fibrotic damage at the hiatus postoperatively; the other patient had a mesh erosion into the esophagus. Both of these patients underwent redo-surgery and required distal resection of the esophagus because of the mesh intrusion into the lumen. Coluccio et al [40] also reported about one case who required resection of the distal esophagus due to a mesh-related complication. This patient underwent large hiatal hernia repair with the use of a PTFE prosthesis which subsequently migrated into the cardial lumen. During reoperation the mesh had to be removed, and the patient required a distal esophageal resection. A fatal complication was described by Kemppainen et al [31]. This patient had a large paraesophageal hernia with acute thoracic herniation and incarceration of the stomach, and underwent laparoscopic hiatal hernia repair with tension-free hiatoplasty using PTFE. Fixation of the mesh was undertaken with a hernia stapler. After surgery, this patient developed a cardiac tamponade caused by a stapler laceration of a coronary vein.

Although there has been a limited number of complications related to prosthetic mesh after laparoscopic antireflux surgery or large hiatal hernia repair, some authors recommend the use of biomaterials or autologous tissue to avoid any risk of complication secondary to prosthetic mesh. Varga et al [20] advocated the use of ligamentum teres for reinforcement of the hiatal crura in four patients with a hiatal hernia ≥ 6 cm. In a similar way, the successful use of biomaterial has been described by Oelschlager et al [19]. Nine patients underwent laparoscopic paraesophageal hernia repair with the use of a porcine small intestine submucosa (SIS) mesh for crural closure to avoid mesh-related esophageal or gastric injury.

Conclusion and future perspectives

In general, hiatal reinforcement with the use prosthetic meshes has proven to be a safe and effective procedure to prevent postoperative hiatal hernia recurrence and/or postoperative intrathoracic migration of the fundic wrap in both laparoscopic surgery for hiatal or paraesophageal hernia repair as well as in laparoscopic antireflux surgery for gastroesophageal reflux disease. A few comparative studies and trials of laparoscopic hiatal closure with simple sutures versus mesh-hiatoplasty have shown, that patients with a prosthetic hiatal closure had a lower rate of postoperative hiatal hernia recurrences in comparison to patients with simple hiatal repair. Some patients with prosthetic hiatal closure, however, suffer from prolonged postoperative symptoms like dysphagia or chest pain; Fortunately, this resolves in most of the patients without further treatment. A true complication related to the use of prosthetic material for hiatal closure is a rare condition when the procedure is performed properly.

A consensus regarding a standard indication for the use of prosthetic mesh for hiatal closure does not exist at this time. Some authors advocate the use of prosthetic meshes empirically only in patients in whom a tension-free crural closure with simple sutures seems impossible. Some authors, however, employ prosthetic hiatoplasty in a more liberal matter. These authors agree that the primary indication for prosthetic hiatal closure should be the size of the hiatal defect. Dr. Frantzides (Chicago, USA) and Dr. Carlson (Omaha, USA) have reduced their original indication of hiatal defect $\geq$ 8 cm to a typical cut-off point of 5–6 cm. Other factors like body mass index or sociodemographic aspects may influence the indication somewhat, but the primary indication for them has remained the size of the hiatus. Dr. Szold (Tel Aviv, Israel) recommends the use of meshes in all patients with paraesophageal hernias, in all hiatal hernias $>$ 4 cm, or in patients in whom the crura seem weak or damaged.

Regarding the characteristics of the mesh, most authors agree that the ideal mesh has to be easy to handle during laparoscopy, able to adhere to the diaphragmatic surface on the one side, and be benign to the visceral surface on the other side. It should be resistant to infection and to long-term contraction.

The shape of the mesh is still a matter of controversy. Most authors recommend a posterior onlay repair; others have advocated the use of circular prostheses with good results. This topic will be a matter of future research, especially when long-term results of published series are available. An overview of experts recommendations is shown in Table 2.

Table 1. Results of laparoscopic hiatal hernia repair with mesh prosthesis

Author (Ref.)	Publication (year)	Patients (n)		Mesh type	Repair	Follow-up (months)	Recurrence rate	
		Mesh	*Non-mesh*				*Mesh*	*Non-mesh*
Kuster [5]	J Laparoendosc Surg (1993)	6	–	Mersilene	LPEHR	8–22	0	–
Pitcher [42]	Arch Surg (1995)	2	10	PTFE	LPEHR(4), LARS(8)	–	0	0
Odsdottir [43]	Surg Endsoc (1995)	10	–		LARS	8.9	0	
Edelman [37]	Surg Laparosc Endosc (1995)	5	–	Surgipro	LARS	–	0	
Behrns [44]	J Laparoendosc Surg (1996)	2	10		LPEHR(5), LARS(7)	6	0	0
Trus [38]	J Gastrointest Surg (1997)	1	75		LPEHR(5), LARS(71)	≤ 16	5(7%)	
Huntington [14]	J Am Coll Surg (1997)	8	–	Prolene		8	0	
Paul [12]	Surg Endosc (1997)	3	–	PTFE	LPEHR(2), LARS(1)	10	0	
Willekes [45]	Ann Surg (1997)	30		PTFE	LARS		0	
Frantzides [17]	Surg Endosc (1997)	3	–	PTFE	LARS	≤ 11	0	
Medina [46]	JSLS (1998)	2	18	Goretex	LPEHR(6), LARS(14)	6–48	0	0
Hawasli [47]	Am Surg (1998)	27		Prolene	LARS	1–56	0	
Carlson [36]	J Am Coll Surg (1998)	44	–	Prolene	PEHR	52	0	–
Simpson [48]	Am Surg (1998)	38	–	Dacron	LARS	15	0	
Schulz [49]	Abstract (1998)	161	157	Prolene	LARS		2 (1.2%)	12 (7.1%)
Horgan [50]	Am J Surg (1999)	5	36		LARS		0	0
Wu [51]	Surg Endosc (1999)	6	–	Marlex	LARS			
Carlson [52]	Dig Surg (1999)	15	16	PTFE	LARS	12–36	0	3 (18.8%)
Frantzides [53]	Surg Endosc (1999)	17	18	PTFE	LARS	36	0	3 (16.6%)
Basso [13]	Surg Endosc (2000)	67	65	Prolene	LARS	22.5–48.3	0	9 (13.8%)
Hui [54]	Am Surg (2001)	12	12	Goretex(8), Marlex(2), Prolene(2)	LARS	24–48	0	0

(continued)

Table 1 (*continued*)

Author (Ref.)	Publication (year)	Patients (n)		Mesh type	Repair	Follow-up (months)	Recurrence rate	
		Mesh	*Non-mesh*				*Mesh*	*Non-mesh*
Lambert [55]	Pediatr Surg Int (2001)	7		Prolene	LARS	12	0	
Livingston [56]	Am Surg (2001)	10	22	Composix	LARS	1–72	0	3 (13.6%)
Athanasakis [3]	Endoscopy (2001)	3	7	PTFE	LARS	12	0	0
Frantzides [25]	Arch Surg (2002)	36	36	PTFE	LARS	6–72	0	8 (22%)
Meyer [57]	Ann Chir (2002)	10		PTFE(5), Prolene(5)	LARS	8–40	0	
Kamolz [22]	Surg Endosc (2002)	100	100	Prolene	LARS	12	1 (1%)	9 (9%)
Casaccia [18]	Surg Endosc (2002)	8		PTFE		8	0	
Granderath [21]	J Gastrointest Surg (2002)	170	361	Prolene	LARS	12	1 (0.6%)	22 (6.1%)
Morales [58]	Springer (2002)	9	55	PTFE	LARS		1 (1.1%)	3 (5.4%)
Champion [15]	Surg Endosc (2003)	52	–	Prolene	LPEHR	7–60	1 (1.9%)	–
Leeder [59]	Surg Endosc (2003)	14	39	Prolene	LARS	6–89	2 (14%)	3 (7.6%)
Diaz [60]	J Gastrointest Surg (2003)	9	107	Polene, SIS	LARS	30 ± 25	2 (33%)	19 (21%)
Oelschlager [19]	Am J Surg (2003)	9	–	SIS	LARS	3–16	1	
Granderath [24]	Arch Surg (2003)	24	–	Prolene	RELARS	12	0	
Ponsky [61]	Surg Endosc (2003)	1				21	0	
Keidar [16]	Surg Lap End Per Tech (2003)	10	23	Goretex(6), Prolene(4)	LARS	46–76	1 (10%)	4 (18%)
Granderath [23]	Arch Surg (2005)	50	50	Prolene	LARS	12	4 (8%)	13 (26%)

Table 2. Experts experience and recommendations

Surgeon	Mesh type	Recur-rences	Redo-procedures for failed hiatal closure	Mesh related complications (erosion, migration, infection)	Indication for prosthetic hiatal closure	Tension-free vs. additional sutures	Ideal mesh?
Filipi	Gore Dual mesh (PTFE)	0	0	0	(1) Weight >100 lbs (2) Physical jobs (3) Tearing crura introperatively	Simple sutures + Onlay mesh	"C"-shaped with 4 cm inner hole
Basso	Polypropylene	1	1	2 migrations	(1) Hiatal defect >3 cm (2) Weak pillars (3) Stretching pillars	Tension-free	3 × 4 cm polypropylene 6 × 6 cm polypropylene for large hernias
Szold	Goretex, Polypropylene, Composite	3	3	0	(1) All paraesophageal hernias (2) Hiatal defect >4 cm (3) Weak crura	Simple sutures + Onlay mesh	"U" shaped covering the posterior repair
Carlson	Polypropylene, PTFE	0	0	1 esophageal erosion (Polypropylene)	(1) Hiatal defect ≥6 cm	Tension-free	(1) easy to handle (2) benign to visceral surfaces (3) resistant to long-term contraction (4) inexpensive (5) able to adhere to diaphragma (6) noncarcinogenic
Frantzides	PTFE	0	0	0	(1) Hiatal defect >5 cm (2) poor muscle crura quality	Tension-free	Oval shape with 3.5 cm keyhole

References

[1] Dent J, Jones R, Kahrilas P, Talley NJ (2001) Management of gastro-oesophageal reflux disease in general practice. BMJ 322: 344

[2] Spechler SJ (1992) Epidemiology and natural history of gastro-oesophageal reflux disease. Digestion 51: 24

[3] Athanasakis H, Tzortzinis A, Tsiaoussis J, Vassilakis JS, Xynos E (2001) Laparoscopic repair of paraesophageal hernia. Endoscopy 33: 590–594

[4] Hashemi M, Peters JH, DeMeester TR, Huprich JE, Quek M, Hagen JA, Crookes PF, Theisen J, DeMeester SR, Sillin LF, Bremner CG (2000) Laparoscopic repair of large type-III hiatal hernia: objective followup reveals high recurrence rate. J Am Coll Surg 190(5): 553–560; Discussion 560–561

[5] Kuster GG, Gilroy S (1993) Laparoscopic technique for repair of paraesophageal hiatal hernias. J Laparoendosc Surg 3: 331–338

[6] Perdikis G, Hinder RA, Filipi CJ, Walenz T, McBride PJ, Smith SL, Katada N, Klingler PJ (1997) Laparosopic paraesophageal hernia repair. Arch Surg 132: 586–590

[7] Hunter JG, Smith CD, Branum GD et al (1999) Laparoscopic fundoplication failures: patterns of failure and response to fundoplication revision. Ann Surg 230: 595–604

[8] Soper NJ, Dunnegan D (1999) Anatomic fundoplication failure after laparoscopic antireflux surgery. Ann Surg 229: 669–677

[9] Granderath FA, Kamolz T, Schweiger UM, Pointner R (2004) Quality of life, patients satisfaction and surgical outcome after laparoscopic refundoplication: experiences with 100 laparoscopic redo-procedures. Surg Endosc (Suppl 18): O212

[10] Carlson MA, Frantzides CT (2001) Complications and results of primary minimally invasive antireflux procedures: a review of 10,735 reported cases. J Am Coll Surg 193: 428–439

[11] Ponce JF, Barriga R, Martin I, Morales Conde S, Morales S (1998) Prosthetic materials in incisional hernia. Experimental study. Cir Esp 63: 189–194

[12] Paul MG, De Rosa RP, Petrucci PE, Palmer ML, Danovitch SH (1997) Laparoscopic tension-free repair of large paraesophageal hernias. Surg Endosc 11: 303–307

[13] Basso N, DeLeo A, Genco A et al (2000) 360° laparoscopic fundoplication with tension – free hiatoplasty in the treatment of symptomatic gastroesophageal reflux disease. Surg Endosc; 14: 164–169

[14] Huntington TR (1997) Laparoscopic mesh repair of the oesophageal hiatus. J Am Coll Surg 184: 399–401

[15] Champion JK, Rock D (2003) Laparoscopic mesh cruro plasty for large paraesophageal hernias. Surg Endosc 17: 551–553

[16] Keidar A, Szold A (2003) Laparoscopic repair of paraesophageal hernia with selective use of mesh. Surg Laparosc Endosc 13: 149–154

[17] Frantzides CT, Carlson MA (1997) Prosthetic reinforcement of posterior cruroplasty during laparoscopic hiatal herniorraphy. Surg Endosc 11: 769–771

[18] Casaccia M, Torelli P, Panaro F, Cavaliere D, Ventura A, Valente U (2002) Laparoscopic physiologic hiatoplasty for hiatal hernia: new composite "A" shaped mesh. Surg Endosc 16: 1441–1445

[19] Oelschlager BK, Barreca M, Chang L, Pellegrini CA (2003) The use of small intestine submucosa in the repair of paraesophageal hernias: initial observations of a new technique. Am J Surg 186(1): 4–8

[20] Varga G, Cseke L, Kalmar K, Horvath OP (2004) Prevention of recurrence by reinforcement of hiatal closure using ligamentum teres in laparoscopic repair of large hiatal hernias. Surg Endosc 18: 1051–1053

[21] Granderath FA, Schweiger UM, Kamolz T et al (2002) Laparoscopic antireflux surgery with routine mesh-hiatoplasty in the treatment of gastroesophageal reflux disease. J Gastrointest Surg 6: 347–353

[22] Kamolz T, Granderath FA, Bammer T, Pasiut M, Pointner R (2002) Dysphagia and quality of life after laparoscopic Nissen fundoplication in patients with and without prosthetic reinforcement of the hiatal crura. Surg Endosc 16(4): 572–577

[23] Granderath FA, Schweiger UM, Kamolz T, Asche KU, Pointner R (2005) Laparoscopic Nissen fundoplication with prosthetic hiatal closure reduces postoperative intrathoracic wrap herniation: Preliminary results of a prospective randomized functional and clinical study. Arch Surg 140: 40–48

[24] Granderath FA, Kamolz T, Schweiger UM et al (2003) Laparoscopic refundoplication with prosthetic hiatal closure for recurrent hiatal hernia after primary failed antireflux surgery. Arch Surg 138: 902–907

[25] Frantzides CT, Madan AK, Carlson MA et al (2002) A prospective, randomized trial of laparoscopic polytetraflouroethylene (PTFE) patch repair vs simple cruroplasty for large hiatal hernia. Arch Surg 137: 649–653

[26] Carlson MA, Condon RE, Ludwig KA, Schulte WJ (1998) Management of intrathoracic stomach with polypropylene mesh prosthesis reinforced transabdominal hiatus hernia repair. J Am Coll Surg 187(3): 227–230

[27] Voyles CR, Richardson JD, Bland KI et al (1981) Emergency abdominal wall reconstruction with polypropylene

mesh: short-term benefits versus long-term complications. Ann Surg 194(2): 219–223
[28] Frantzides CT, Carlson MA (2001) Paraesophageal herniation. In: Mastery of surgery, vol. 1 (Baker RJ, Fischer JE, eds). Philadelphia: Lippincott Williams & Wilkins, pp 721–736
[29] Wantz GE (1991) Atlas of hernia surgery. New York: Raven Press
[30] Heniford BT, Park A, Ramshaw BJ, Voeller G (2003) Laparoscopic repair of ventral hernias: nine years' experience with 850 consecutive hernias. Ann Surg 238(3): 391–399; Discussion 399–400
[31] Kemppainen E, Kiviluoto T (2000) Fatal cardiac tamponade after emergency tension-free repair of a large paraesophageal hernia. Surg Endosc 14(6): 593
[32] Amid PK (2004) Shrinkage: Fake or Fact? In: Meshes: benefits and risks (Schumpelick V, Nyhus LM, eds). Berlin: Springer, pp 198–206
[33] Baladas HG, Smith GS, Richardson MA, Dempsey MB, Falk GL (2000) Esophagogastric fistula secondary to teflon pledget: a rare complication following laparoscopic fundoplication. Dis Esophagus 13: 72–74
[34] Arendt T, Stuber E, Monig H, Folsch UR, Katsoulis S (2000) Dysphagia due to transmural migration of surgical material into the esophagus nine years after Nissen fundoplication. Gastrointestinal Endosc 51: 607–610
[35] Dally E, Falt GL (2004) Teflon pledget reinforced fundoplication causes symptomatic gastric and esophageal lumenal penetration Am J Surg 187: 226–229
[36] Carlson MA, Condon RE, Ludwig KA, Schulte WJ (1998) Management of intrathoracic stomach with polypropylene mesh prosthesis reinforced transabdominal hiatus hernia repair. J Am Coll Surg 187: 227–230
[37] Edelman DS (1995) Laparoscopic paraesophageal hernia repair with mesh. Surg Laparosc Endosc 5: 32–37
[38] Trus TL, Bax T, Richardson WS, Branum GD, Mauren SJ, Swanstrom LL, Hunter JG (1997) Complications of laparoscopic paraesophageal hernia repair. J Gastrointest Surg 1: 221–228
[39] Van der Peet DL, Klinkerberg-Knol EC, Alonso A, Sietses C, Eijsbouts QAJ, Cuesta MA (2000) Laparoscopic treatment of large paraesophageal hernias. Surg Endosc 14: 1015–1018
[40] Casabella F, Sinanan M, Horgan S, Pellegrini CA (1996) Systematic use of gastric fundoplication in laparoscopic repair of paraesophageal hernias. Am J Surg 171: 485–489
[41] Coluccio G, Ponzio S, Ambu V, Tramontano R, Cuomo G (2000) Dislocation into the cardial lumen of a PTFE prosthesis used in the treatment of voluminous hiatal sliding hernia, a case report. Minerva Chir 55: 341–345
[42] Pitcher DE, Curet MJ, Vogt DM, Mason J, Zucker KA (1995) Successful repair of praesophageal hernia. Arch Surg 130: 590–596
[43] Oddsdottir M, Franco AL, Laycock WA, Waring JP, Hunter JG (1995) Laparoscopic repair of paraesophageal hernia. New access, old technique. Surg Endosc 9: 164–168
[44] Behrns KE, Schlinkert RT (1996) Laparoscopic management of paraesophageal hernia: early results. J Laparoendosc Surg 6: 311–317
[45] Willekes CL, Edoga JK, Freeza EE (1997) Laparoscopic repair of paraesophageal hernia. Ann Surg 225: 31–38
[46] Medina L, Peetz M, Ratzer E, Fenoglio M (1998) Laparoscopic paraesophageal hernia repair. JSLS 2: 269–272
[47] Hawasli A, Zonca S (1998) Laparoscopic repair of paraesophageal hiatal hernia. Am Surg 64: 703–710
[48] Simpson B, Ricketts RR, Parker PM (1998) Prosthetic patch stabilization of crural repair in antireflux surgery in children. Am Surg 64: 67–70
[49] Schulz HG (1998) Rezidivrate nach laparoskopischer Antirefluxoperation mit und ohne Prolenenetzplastik bei 318 Fällen – erste Ergebnisse. 7. Jahreskongress der Gesellschaft für Gastroenterologie Westfalen
[50] Horgan S, Eubanks TR, Jacobsen G, Omelanczuk P, Pellegrini CA (1999) Repair of paraesophageal hernias. Am J Surg 177: 354–358
[51] Wu JS, Dunnegan DL, Soper NJ (1999) Clinical and radiologic assessment of laparoscopic paraesophageal hernia repair. Surg Endosc 13: 497–502
[52] Carlson MA, Richards CG, Frantzides CT (1999) Laparoscopic prosthetic reinforcement of hiatal herniorrhaphy. Dig Surg 16: 407–410
[53] Frantzides CT, Richards CG, Carlson MA (1999) Laparoscopic repair of large hiatal hernia with polytetrafluoroethylene. Surg Endosc 13: 906–908
[54] Hui TT, David T, Spyrou M, Phillips EH (2001) Mesh crural repair of large paraesophageal hiatal hernias. Am Surg 67: 1170–1174
[55] Lambert AW, Huddart SN (2001) Mesh hiatal reinforcement in Nissen funduplication. Pediatr Surg Int 17: 491–492
[56] Livingston CD, Lamar Jones H, Askew RE, Victor BE, Askew RE (2001) Laparscopic hiatal hernia repair in patients with poor esophageal motility or paraesophageal herniation. Am Surg 67: 987–991
[57] Meyer C, Bufffler A, Rohr S, Lima MC (2002) Le traitement laparoscopique des hernies hiatales de gran taille avec mise en place d'une prothese. A propos de dix cas. Ann Chir 127: 257–261

[58] Morales Conde S, Ponce JF, Morales Mendez S (2002) Paraesophageal hernia: technique and method of fixation a mesh by laparoscopy. In: Laparoscopic ventral hernia repair (Morales-Conded S, ed). Springer

[59] Leeder PC, Smith G, Dehn TC (2003) Laparoscopic management of large paraesophageal hiatal hernia. Surg Endosc 17: 1372–1375

[60] Díaz S, Brunt M, Klingensmith ME, Frisella PM, Soper NJ (2003) Laparoscopic paraesophageal hernia repair, a challenging operation: medium-term outcome of 116 patients. J Gastroint Surg 7: 59–67

[61] Ponsky J, Rosen M, Fanning A, Malm J (2003) Anterior gastropexy may reduce the recurrence after laparoscopic paraesophageal hernia repair. Surg Endosc 17: 1036–1041

Chapter 22

RADIOLOGIC IMAGING OF GASTROESOPHAGEAL REFLUX DISEASE

M. S. Levine

Gastrointestinal Radiology, Department of Radiology, Hospital of the University of Pennsylvania,
University of Pennsylvania School of Medicine, Philadelphia, PA, USA

Introduction

Gastroesophageal reflux disease (GERD) is a ubiquitous problem in modern medical practice; 20% of Americans experience heartburn on a weekly basis [1]. In the past, barium studies have been advocated for patients with reflux symptoms primarily to document the presence of a hiatal hernia or gastroesophageal reflux (GER), to detect complications such as deep ulcers or strictures, and to rule out other organic or motor abnormalities in the esophagus. By permitting a more detailed assessment of the esophageal mucosa, however, double-contrast radiographic techniques have made it possible to detect superficial ulceration and other changes of mild or moderate esophagitis before the development of deep ulcers or strictures. Double-contrast esophagography is also a useful screening examination for Barrett's esophagus to determine the relative need for endoscopy and biopsy in these patients. With double-contrast techniques, barium studies therefore have a major role in the evaluation of patients with known or suspected GERD.

Gastroesophageal reflux

Ambulatory 24-hour esophageal pH monitoring is currently accepted as the gold standard for the detection of GER, with a sensitivity and specificity of greater than 95% [2], [3]. In contrast, barium studies have been found to have relatively limited value in detecting GER, with a reported overall sensitivity of only about 35% [4]. The frequent inability to demonstrate reflux at fluoroscopy in patients with GERD is at least partly related to the observation that reflux often results from transient relaxations of the lower esophageal sphincter rather than from a sustained decrease in sphincter pressure [5], [6]. Provocative tests such as the water siphon test have been shown to increase the sensitivity of the barium study for the detection of GER, but these techniques also result in a lower specificity, compromising the overall accuracy of the radiologic examination [7], [8].

Despite the limitations of barium studies in detecting GER, a recent study found that virtually all patients with massive GER at fluoroscopy (defined as reflux of barium to or above the thoracic inlet with the patient in the recumbent position) had pathologic acid reflux on 24-hour esophageal pH monitoring in the recumbent position [9]. In this study, patients with massive GER on barium studies also had an abnormally low pH for a significantly greater percentage of time than those in a control group. Such work suggests that patients with massive reflux on barium studies are so likely to have pathologic acid reflux in the recumbent position that these individuals can be further evaluated and treated for their reflux disease without need for pH monitoring.

Hiatal hernias

Sliding hiatal hernias occur with greater frequency in older patients as a result of a degenerative process in which there is progressive weakening and laxity of the ligaments that anchor the gastroesophageal junction to the surrounding esophageal hiatus of the diaphragm [10]. There is considerable controversy about the relationship between hiatal hernias and the development of GERD. Because most patients with clinically significant reflux disease have evidence of a hiatal hernia, it has been postulated that a hernia predisposes to the development of GER and that it has a permissive role in the development of reflux esophagitis [11], [12]. Nevertheless, many patients with a hiatal hernia have no evidence of GER, and many patients with GER have no evidence of a hiatal hernia [13]–[15]. Investigators therefore believe that intrinsic dysfunction of the lower esophageal sphincter is probably the major factor in the development of GER, independent of the anatomic location of the sphincter above or below the diaphragm [14], [16]–[18].

Reflux esophagitis

Conventional single-contrast esophagography has been considered to be an unreliable technique for detecting reflux esophagitis, with an overall sensitivity of only 50–75% [19]–[22]. On the other hand, the use of double-contrast esophagography has increased the radiographic sensitivity to almost 90% [20], [22], [23]. A major advantage of the double-contrast technique is that it permits a detailed assessment of the esophageal mucosa for superficial ulceration or other changes of mild or moderate esophagitis that cannot be detected on single-contrast barium studies. Nevertheless, single-contrast technique (with the patient ingesting barium in the prone position) is best for demonstrating areas of decreased distensibility resulting from lower esophageal rings or strictures. A biphasic examination with upright double-contrast views and prone single-contrast views of the esophagus therefore appears to be the best radiologic technique for evaluating patients with suspected reflux disease.

Abnormal esophageal motility

Between 25 and 50% of patients with reflux esophagitis have abnormal esophageal motility, manifested by intermittently decreased or absent primary peristalsis in the middle or lower thirds of the thoracic esophagus [24]–[26]. In this author's experience, such esophageal dysmotility is rarely associated with nonperistaltic contractions, whereas esophageal dysmotility in the elderly is usually characterized by decreased primary peristalsis with multiple nonperistaltic contractions (the latter condition has been called "presbyesophagus") [27]. Thus, in young patients, the presence of intermittently weakened or absent primary peristalsis without nonperistaltic contractions should be highly suggestive of GERD on barium studies.

Much less frequently, esophageal aperistalsis may be the only radiographic finding in patients with reflux disease [28]. Abnormal motility may be secondary to neuronal damage in Auerbach's plexus caused by direct extension of the inflammatory process into the esophageal wall [28]. Conversely, pre-existing esophageal dysmotility (such as that associated with esophageal involvement by scleroderma) may predispose patients to the development of reflux esophagitis by impairing clearance of refluxed peptic acid from the esophagus. In either case, the combination of abnormal motility and GER produces a vicious cycle, often leading to progressively severe esophagitis [17].

Mucosal nodularity

Early reflux esophagitis may be manifested on double-contrast studies by a finely nodular or granular appearance caused by mucosal edema and inflammation in the distal third or half of the thoracic esophagus (*Fig. 1*) [29]–[31]. This granularity is characterized by tiny radiolucencies with poorly defined borders that fade peripherally into the adjacent mucosa. Less frequently, reflux esophagitis may be manifested by coarse nodularity of the mucosa. In almost all cases, the granularity or nodularity extends proximally from the gastroesophageal junction as a continuous area of disease.

More advanced reflux esophagitis may occasionally be associated with inflammatory exudates or pseudomembranes that resemble the plaquelike lesions of *Candida* esophagitis (*Fig. 2*) [32]. However, these patients usually present with reflux symptoms rather than odynophagia. A single large pseudomembrane can also be mistaken for a plaquelike carcinoma, particularly an adenocarcinoma arising in Barrett's mucosa [32]. However, pseudomembrane formation may be suggested by the presence of other satellite lesions or by a change in the size and shape of the lesions at fluoroscopy.

Ulceration

Shallow ulcers and erosions associated with reflux esophagitis may be seen on double-contrast studies as tiny collections of barium at or near the gastroesophageal junction (*Fig. 3*) [29], [30], [33]. The ulcers can have a punctate, linear, or stellate configuration and are often associated with surrounding halos of edematous mucosa, radiating folds, or sacculation of the adjacent esophageal wall [29], [30], [33]. When superficial ulceration is detected in patients with reflux esophagitis, the correct diagnosis is almost always suggested by the distal location of the ulcers, the presence of a hiatal hernia or gastroesophageal reflux, and the clinical presentation. Some patients may have relatively diffuse ulceration of the distal third or even half of the thoracic esophagus (*Fig. 4*). However, ulceration in reflux esophagitis tends to occur as a continuous area of disease extending proximally from the gastroesophageal junction, so the presence of one or more ulcers in the middle third of the esophagus with sparing of the distal third should suggest another cause for the patient's disease.

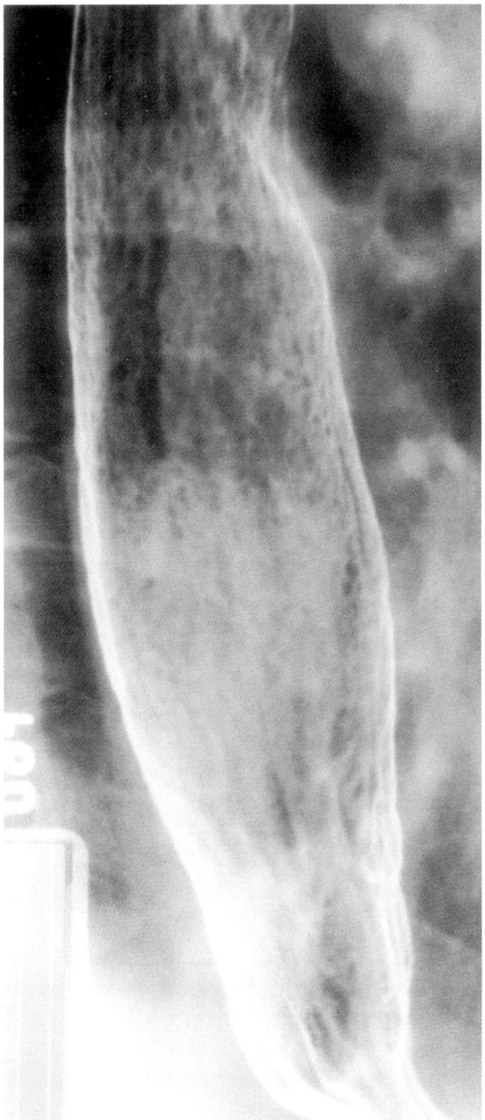

Fig. 1. Reflux esophagitis with granular mucosa. Note finely nodular or granular appearance in the lower third of the esophagus with poorly defined radiolucencies that fade peripherally as a result of mucosal edema and inflammation

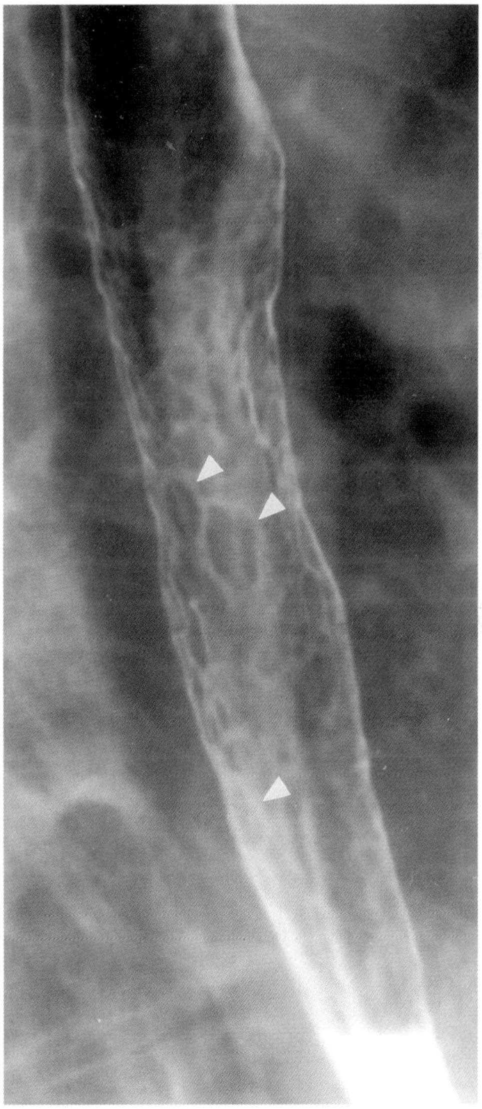

Fig. 2. Reflux esophagitis with pseudomembranes. There are multiple discrete plaquelike lesions (arrowheads) representing pseudomembranes and exudates associated with severe reflux esophagitis. The plaquelike lesions of *Candida* esophagitis could produce similar radiographic findings

Other patients with reflux esophagitis may have solitary ulcers in the distal esophagus at or adjacent to the gastroesophageal junction (*Fig. 5*) [34]. These "marginal" ulcers can be recognized en face as discrete collections of barium but are best visualized when the ulcers are projected in profile beyond the normal contour of the esophagus. In one study, about 70% of these ulcers were found to be located on the posterior esophageal wall [34]. Because GER often occurs dur-ing sleep, it has been postulated that patients who sleep primarily in the supine position are more likely to develop posterior wall ulcers as a result of prolonged exposure to refluxed acid that pools by gravity on the dependent or posterior esophageal wall, causing maximal injury in this location [34].

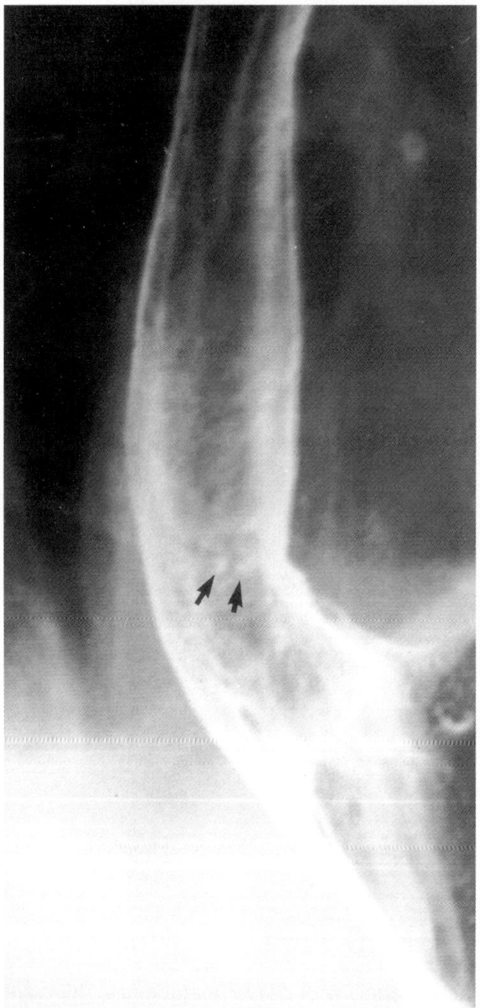

Fig. 3. Reflux esophagitis with ulceration. Several tiny ulcers (arrows) are seen in the distal esophagus above the gastroesophageal junction

Thickened folds

Reflux esophagitis may also be manifested on barium studies by thickened longitudinal folds as a result of edema and inflammation that extend into the submucosa (*Fig. 6*) [29]. These folds may have a smooth or irregular contour, occasionally mimicking the appearance of esophageal varices [35]. In general, thickened folds should be recognized as a nonspecific finding of esophagitis resulting from a host of causes. Other patients with chronic reflux esophagitis may have a single prominent fold that arises in the region of the gastric cardia and extends upward into the distal esophagus as a smooth, polypoid protuberance, also known as an inflammatory esophagogastric polyp (*Fig. 7*) [36]–[38]. Because these lesions have no

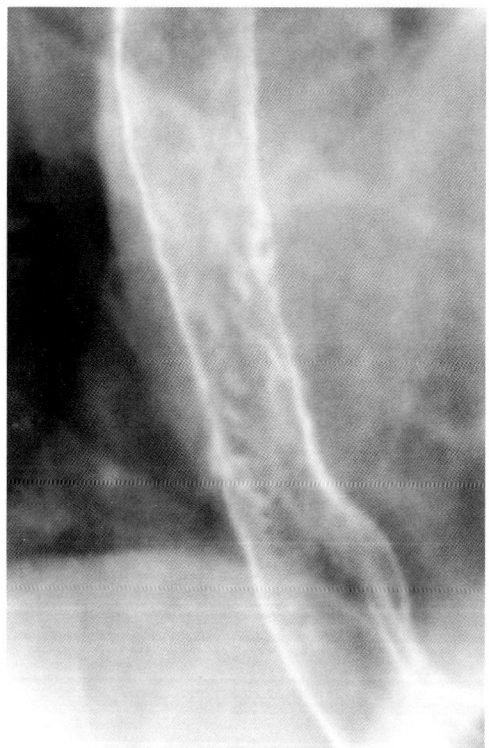

Fig. 4. Reflux esophagitis with extensive ulceration. Multiple ulcers of varying sizes are seen throughout the distal third of the esophagus (Reproduced with permission from [33])

malignant potential, endoscopy is not warranted when barium studies reveal typical findings of an inflammatory polyp in the distal esophagus at or abutting the gastroesophageal junction.

Multiple transverse folds may also be found in patients with GERD, an appearance also known as the "feline" esophagus because transverse esophageal folds are normally found in cats [39], [40]. The folds tend to be closely spaced and completely traverse the circumference of the esophagus (*Fig. 8*). These delicate transverse striations occur as a transient phenomenon resulting from contraction of the longitudinally oriented muscularis mucosae [41]. Transverse folds are often observed in patients with GER, but this finding alone does not indicate the presence of esophagitis [40].

Advanced findings

In advanced reflux esophagitis, extensive ulceration, edema, and spasm may cause the esophagus to have a grossly irregular contour with serrated or spiculated margins and loss of distensibility (*Fig. 9*). Occasionally, the narrowing and deformity associated with

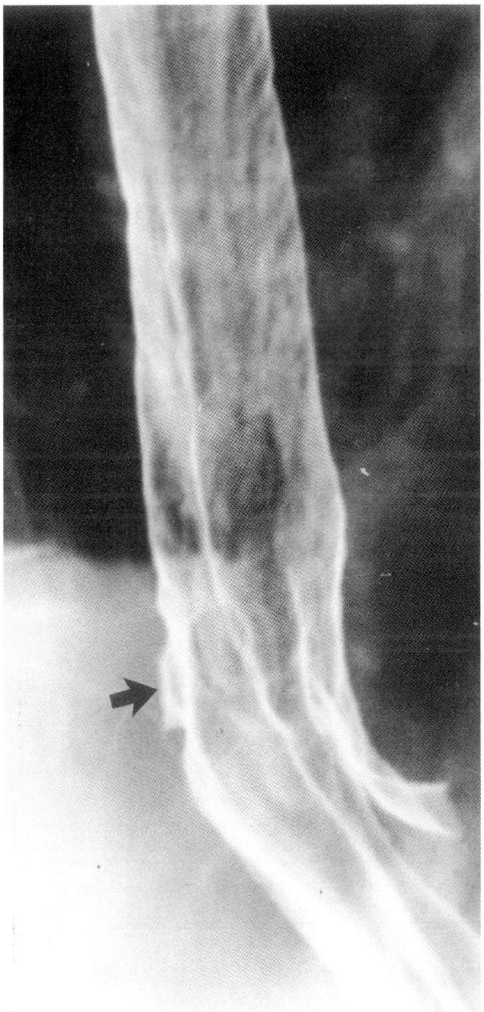

Fig. 5. Reflux esophagitis with a solitary ulcer. A large, relatively flat ulcer (arrow) is present on the right posterolateral wall of the distal esophagus (Reproduced with permission from [33])

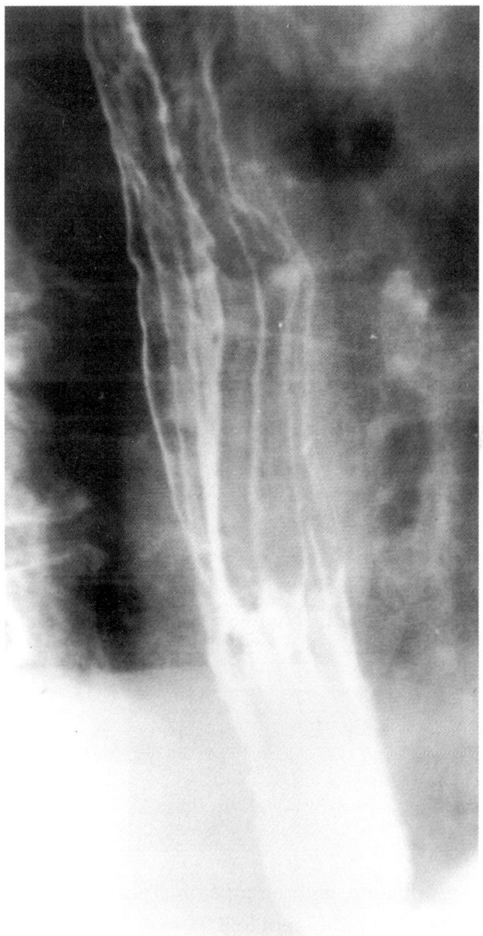

Fig. 6. Reflux esophagitis with thickened folds. Diffusely thickened folds are seen in the thoracic esophagus. This is a nonspecific finding of esophagitis due to a host of causes (Reproduced with permission from [33])

severe esophagitis can mimic the appearance of an infiltrating esophageal carcinoma, so endoscopy and biopsy may be required for a definitive diagnosis.

Peptic scarring

Strictures

As the esophagitis heals, localized scarring may be manifested on barium studies by flattening, puckering, or sacculation of the adjacent esophageal wall, often associated with the development of radiating folds (*Fig. 10*). Further scarring can lead to the development of circumferential strictures, also known as "peptic" strictures. The vast majority of these strictures are located in the distal esophagus above a hiatal hernia. Because many patients with GER or mild reflux esophagitis do not have an associated hiatal hernia, it has been postulated that scarring from reflux esophagitis leads not only to circumferential narrowing of the distal esophagus but also to longitudinal scarring and shortening with subsequent hernia formation [16]. Whatever the explanation, a

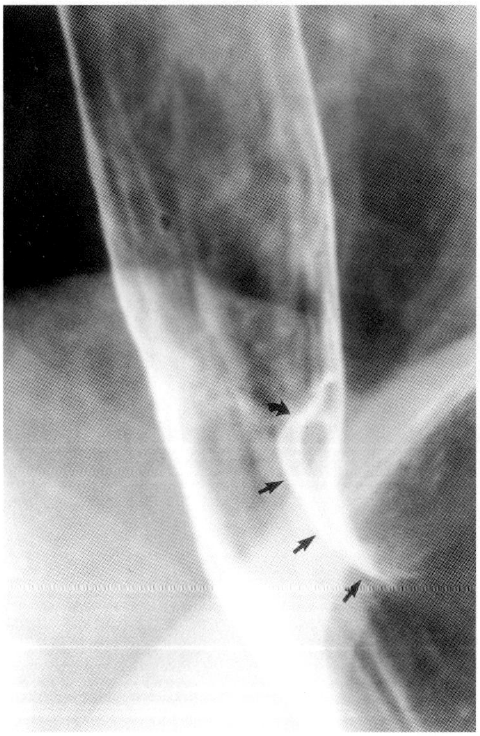

Fig. 7. Reflux esophagitis with an inflammatory esophagogastric polyp. There is a prominent fold (straight arrows) that extends from the gastroesophageal junction into the distal esophagus, terminating as a smooth polypoid protuberance (curved arrow). This lesion has the typical appearance and location of an inflammatory esophagogastric polyp (Reproduced with permission from [33])

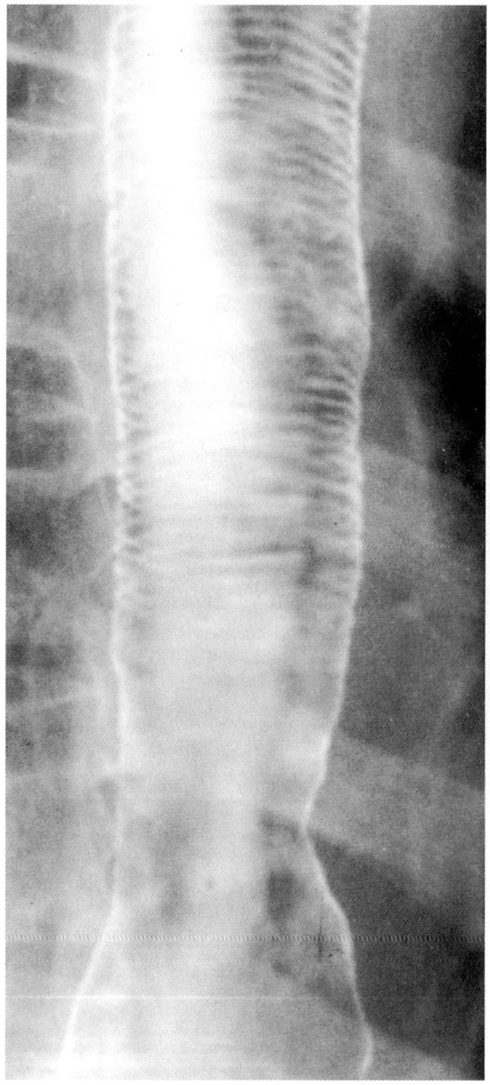

Fig. 8. Feline esophagus. Multiple transverse folds or striations are seen in the esophagus. Note how the folds are closely spaced and extend completely across the circumference of the esophagus. This appearance should be differentiated from the fixed transverse folds associated with scarring from reflux esophagitis, as shown in *Fig. 15* (Reproduced with permission from [33])

hiatal hernia is found on barium studies in more than 95% of patients with peptic strictures [42]. When a hiatal hernia is not present in patients with distal esophageal strictures, the possibility of malignant tumor therefore should be considered as a possible cause of these strictures.

Peptic strictures often appear as concentric areas of smooth, tapered narrowing (*Fig. 11*), but some patients can have short, ringlike strictures (*Fig. 12*) that are difficult to differentiate from Schatzki rings at the gastroesophageal junction (see later section on Schatzki rings). Asymmetric scarring can also lead to asymmetric narrowing with focal sacculation or ballooning of the esophageal wall between areas of fibrosis (*Fig. 13*). Finally, peptic strictures can be associated with the development of esophageal intramural pseudodiverticula (*Fig. 14*) [43]. The pseudodiverticula typically appear as tiny collections of barium "floating" outside the wall of the esophagus without any apparent communication with the lumen, whereas true ulcers are almost always seen to communicate directly with the lumen. When there is marked irregularity, flattening, or nodularity of one or more walls of the stricture, endoscopy and biopsy should be performed to rule out malignant tumor as the cause of these findings.

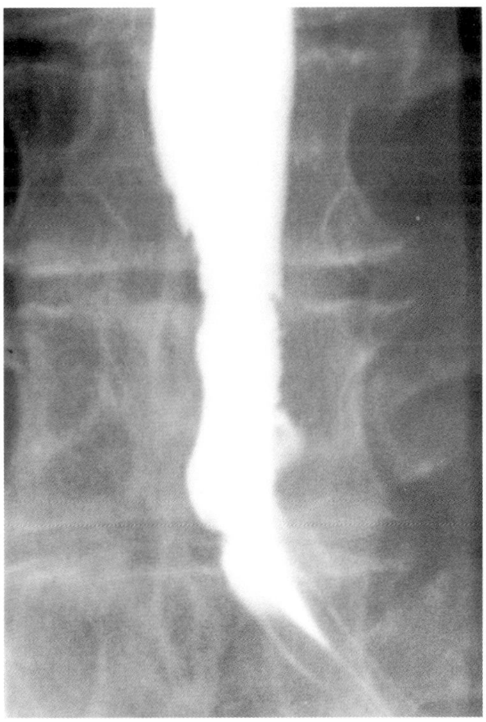

Fig. 9. Advanced reflux esophagitis. The distal esophagus has an irregular, serrated contour and loss of distensibility as a result of ulceration, edema, and spasm associated with severe reflux esophagitis

Accurate detection of peptic strictures on barium studies requires continuous drinking of low-density barium in the prone position to optimally distend the lower esophagus and demonstrate subtle areas of narrowing that cannot be visualized on upright double-contrast views. With careful biphasic technique, esophagography has a sensitivity of almost 95% in detecting peptic strictures and my even reveal strictures that are missed at endoscopy [44], [45].

Scarring from reflux esophagitis can also lead to longitudinal shortening of the esophagus and the development of fixed transverse folds, producing a characteristic "stepladder" appearance caused by pooling of barium between the folds (*Fig. 15*) [46]. These fixed transverse folds should be differentiated on barium studies from the thin transverse folds (also known as the "feline" esophagus) often seen as a transient finding in patients with GER (see *Fig. 8*) [39], [40].

Schatzki rings

A Schatzki ring was originally described by Schatzki himself as a symptomatic lower esophageal ring that caused dysphagia [47]. The pathogenesis of these rings is uncertain. Some investigators favor a congenital origin, but the rarity of symptoms before 50 years of age tends to refute this theory [48]. Others believe that a Schatzki ring represents an annular, ringlike stricture caused by scarring from reflux esophagitis [49], [50]. This theory is supported by a study showing that Schatzki rings progressed or underwent transformation into true peptic strictures on serial radiologic examinations [49].

A Schatzki ring usually appears on barium studies as a thin (1–3 mm in height), weblike (less than 13 mm in diameter) constriction at the gastroesophageal junction, almost always above a hiatal hernia (*Figs. 16A* and *17A*) [47], [51], [52]. Except for its smaller caliber, a Schatzki ring therefore has the same appearance and location as an asymptomatic mucosal ring. Almost all rings less than 13 mm in diameter cause dysphagia [52], so they may be classified as

Schatzki rings on the basis of the radiographic findings. However, some rings between 13 and 20 mm in diameter may also cause symptoms [52], so the diagnosis of a Schatzki ring requires some knowledge of the clinical history in these patients.

Like other types of narrowing in the distal esophagus, Schatzki rings are visualized on barium studies only if the lumen above and below the ring is distended beyond the caliber of the ring. As a result, single-contrast views of the distal esophagus with the patient in the prone position may demonstrate rings that are not visible, even in retrospect, on upright double-contrast views from the same examination (*Fig. 16B*). In fact, studies have shown that when biphasic barium examinations are performed, prone single-contrast views of the esophagus are more sensitive for detecting Schatzki rings than upright double-contrast views [53] and may even detect rings that are missed at endoscopy [54].

Another potential pitfall in the detection of Schatzki rings on barium studies results from overlap of the distal esophagus and adjacent hiatal hernia tangential to the X-ray beam. This overlap phenomenon may obscure the region of the gastroesophageal junction on esophagrams performed with the patient in the prone position, preventing visualiza-

A

B

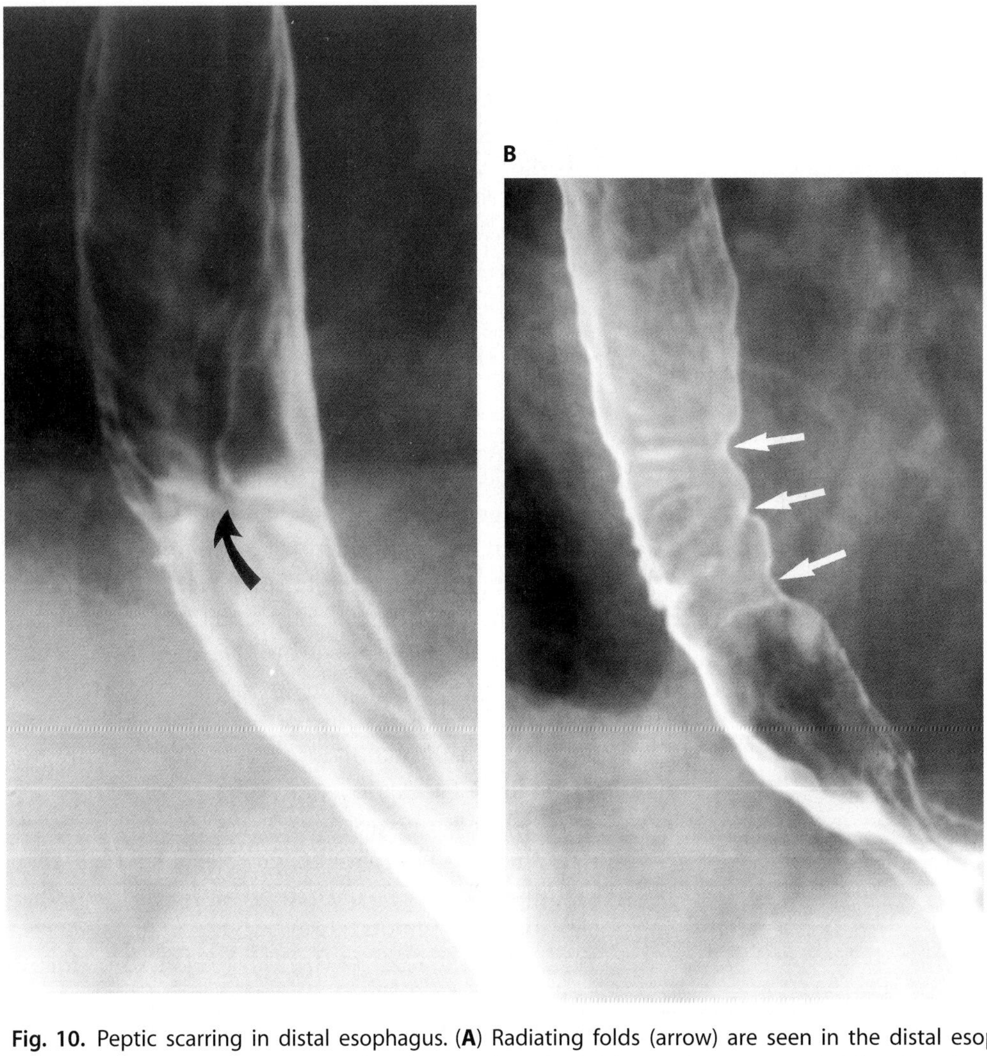

Fig. 10. Peptic scarring in distal esophagus. (**A**) Radiating folds (arrow) are seen in the distal esophagus without associated luminal narrowing. (Reproduced with permission from [30]); (**B**) Note flattening and deformity of one wall (arrows) of the distal esophagus with folds radiating toward the site of scarring in another patient

tion of symptomatic lower esophageal rings (*Fig. 17B*) [55]. When this phenomenon occurs, additional images should be obtained when minimal or no overlap of the distal esophagus and adjacent hiatal hernia is present, improving detection of these rings (see *Fig. 17A*).

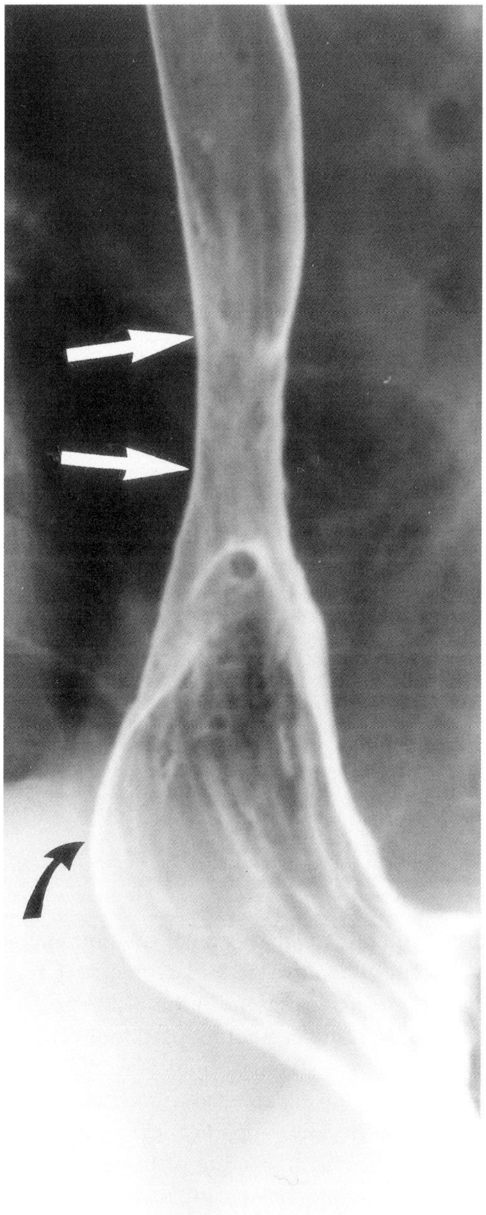

Fig. 11. Peptic stricture. A smooth, tapered area of concentric narrowing (white arrows) is seen in the distal third of the esophagus above a hiatal hernia (black arrow) (Reproduced with permission from [33])

Barrett's esophagus

Barrett's esophagus is a well-recognized entity in which there is progressive columnar metaplasia of the lower esophagus due to long-standing gastroesophageal reflux and reflux esophagitis [56]. This condition is important because it is associated with an increased risk of developing esophageal adenocarcinoma via a well-established dysplasia-carcinoma sequence [57]. During the past decade, revised histopathologic criteria have been developed for this condition in which patients with Barrett's esophagus are classified as

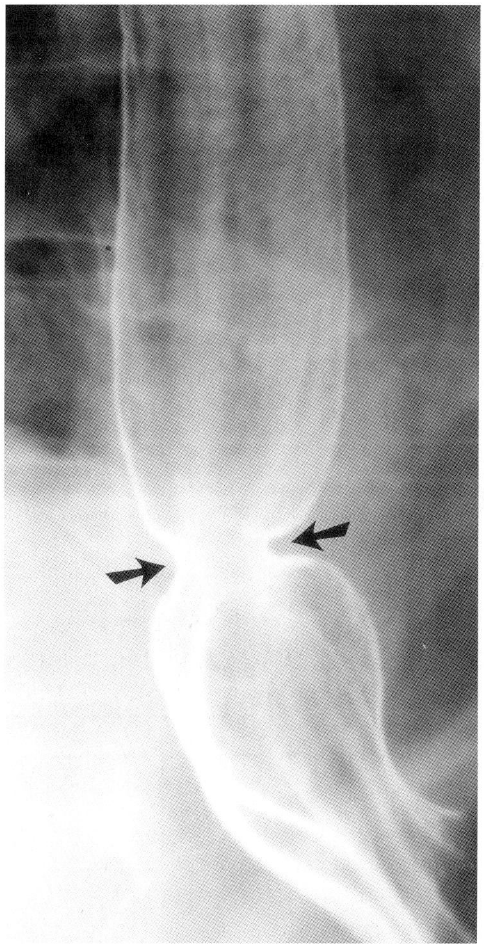

Fig. 12. Ringlike peptic stricture. A short segment of ringlike narrowing (arrows) is seen in the distal esophagus directly above a hiatal hernia. The narrowed segment closely resembles the Schatzki rings shown in *Figs. 16A* and *17A*. However, note asymmetry and slightly greater length of the ringlike peptic stricture in *Fig. 12*

having either "long-segment" (i.e., extending more than 3 cm from the gastroesophageal junction) or "short-segment" (i.e., extending 3 cm or less from the gastroesophageal junction) disease based on the extent of columnar metaplasia in the distal esophagus [58], [59]. Long-segment Barrett's esophagus is thought to be associated with a greater risk of developing esophageal adenocarcinoma and, hence, a greater need for endoscopic surveillance [57], [60], [61]. The radiographic findings in long-segment and short-segment Barrett's esophagus are considered separately in the following sections.

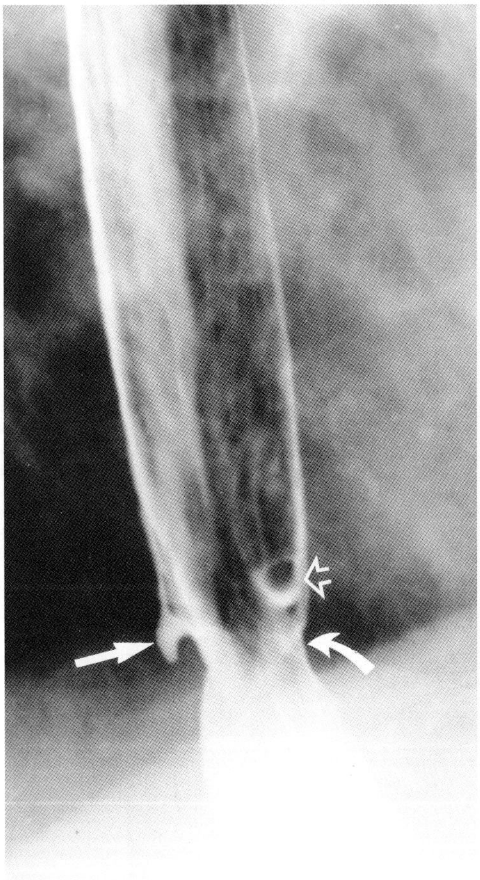

Fig. 13. Peptic stricture with sacculations. There is asymmetric narrowing (curved arrow) of the distal esophagus with focal outpouchings or sacculations en face (open arrow) and in profile (straight arrow) due to outward ballooning of the wall between areas of fibrosis. Note how these sacculations have a more rounded appearance than true ulcers

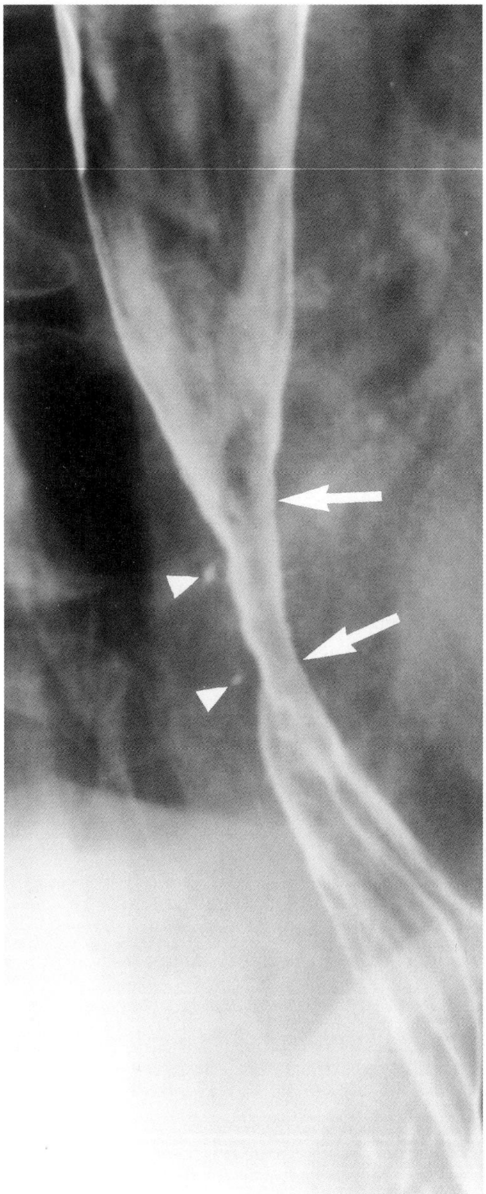

Fig. 14. Peptic stricture with esophageal intramural pseudodiverticulosis. A smooth, tapered segment of concentric narrowing (arrows) is present in the distal esophagus. Barium is also seen in several tiny pseudodiverticula (arrowheads) abutting the stricture. Note how the pseudodiverticula appear to be "floating" outside the wall of the esophagus without any apparent communication with the lumen, a characteristic feature of these relatively innocuous structures (Reproduced with permission from [30])

Long-segment Barrett's esophagus

The classic radiologic features of long-segment Barrett's esophagus consist of a midesophageal stricture (*Fig. 18*) or ulcer, often associated with a sliding hiatal hernia and gastroesophageal reflux [62]–[64]. These strictures or ulcers are thought to be located in the proximal zone of columnar metaplasia at or near the transposed squamocolumnar mucosal junction [63]. However, strictures are actually more common in the distal esophagus in patients with Barrett's esophagus, so most cases do not fit the classic description of a high stricture or ulcer [65]–[67]. A reticular mucosal pattern has also been described as a relatively specific sign of long-segment Barrett's esophagus on double-contrast esophagrams, particularly if located adjacent to the distal aspect of a midesophageal stricture (*Fig. 19*) [68]. This reticular pattern is characterized by innumerable tiny, barium-filled grooves, resembling the areae gastricae found on double contrast studies of the stomach. However, a reticular mucosal pattern is present on barium studies in only 5–30% of all patients with long-segment Barrett's esophagus [64], [66]–[69].

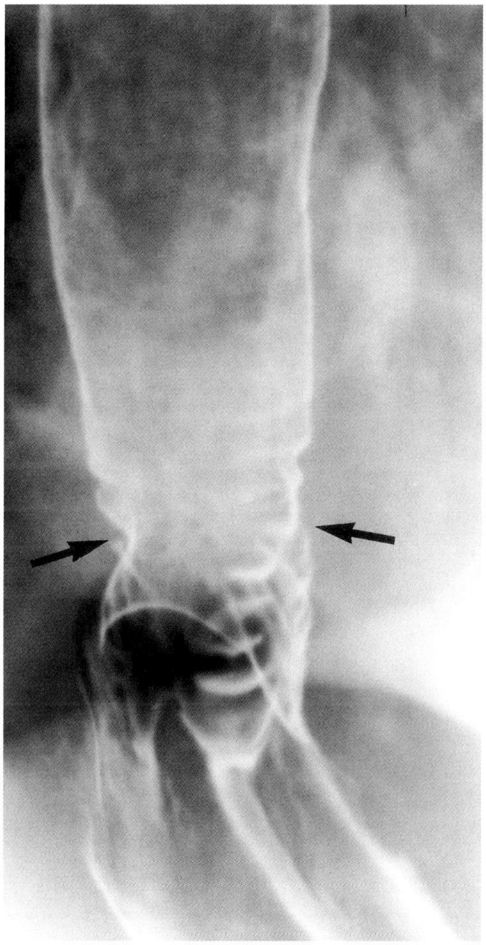

Fig. 15. Peptic stricture with a "stepladder" sign. A mild peptic stricture (arrows) is present in the distal esophagus above a hiatal hernia. In addition, horizontal collections of barium are seen trapped between multiple fixed transverse folds, producing a characteristic stepladder appearance. These folds are further apart and less circumferential than the delicate transverse striations of the feline esophagus shown in *Fig. 8* (Reproduced with permission from [46])

Other morphologic findings of reflux disease, such as hiatal hernias, gastroesophageal reflux, reflux esophagitis, and peptic strictures, can be detected on double-contrast studies in the vast majority of patients with long-segment Barrett's esophagus [69], [70], but these findings frequently occur in patients with uncomplicated reflux disease. Thus, those radiographic findings that are relatively specific for Barrett's esophagus are not sensitive, and those findings that are more sensitive are not specific. As a result, double-contrast esophagography has traditionally been thought to have limited value for diagnosing Barrett's esophagus in patients with known or suspected gastroesophageal reflux disease.

In 1988, Gilchrist et al [70] introduced a novel approach for the diagnosis of Barrett's esophagus on double-contrast esophagography by stratifying patients based on the following radiologic criteria: patients were classified at high risk for Barrett's esophagus if double-contrast images revealed a high stricture or ulcer or a reticular mucosal pattern; patients were classified at moderate risk if the images revealed a distal stricture or reflux esophagitis; and patients were classified at low risk if the images revealed a normal-appearing esophagus. The vast majority of patients classified at high risk and approximately 15% classified at moderate risk for Barrett's esophagus on double-contrast esophagrams were found to have this condition [70]. Conversely, less than 1% of patients classified at low risk for Barrett's esophagus because of the absence of esophagitis or strictures were found to have this condition [70]. Other investigators have also found morphologic evidence of reflux esophagitis and/or peptic strictures on double-contrast esophagrams in 97% of all patients with long-segment Barrett's esophagus [69]. Thus, esophagitis or peptic scarring severe enough to cause Barrett's esophagus can almost always be detected on technically adequate double-contrast examinations.

On the basis of such data, it seems reasonable to conclude that patients who are found to be at high risk for Barrett's esophagus on double-contrast esophagrams because of a midesophageal stricture or ulcer or a reticular mucosal pattern should undergo endoscopy and biopsy for a definitive diagnosis. A larger group of patients are found to be at moderate risk for Barrett's esophagus because of reflux esophagitis or peptic strictures in the distal esophagus, so clinical judgment should be used regarding the decision for endoscopy in this group based on the severity of symptoms as well as the age and overall health of the patients (i.e., whether they are reasonable candidates for endoscopic surveillance). However, most patients are found to be at low risk for Barrett's esophagus because of the absence of esophagitis or strictures, and the risk of Barrett's esophagus is so low in this group that endoscopy does not appear to be warranted. Thus, the major value of double-contrast esophagography is its ability to separate patients into these various risk groups for Barrett's esophagus to determine the relative need for endoscopy and biopsy [70].

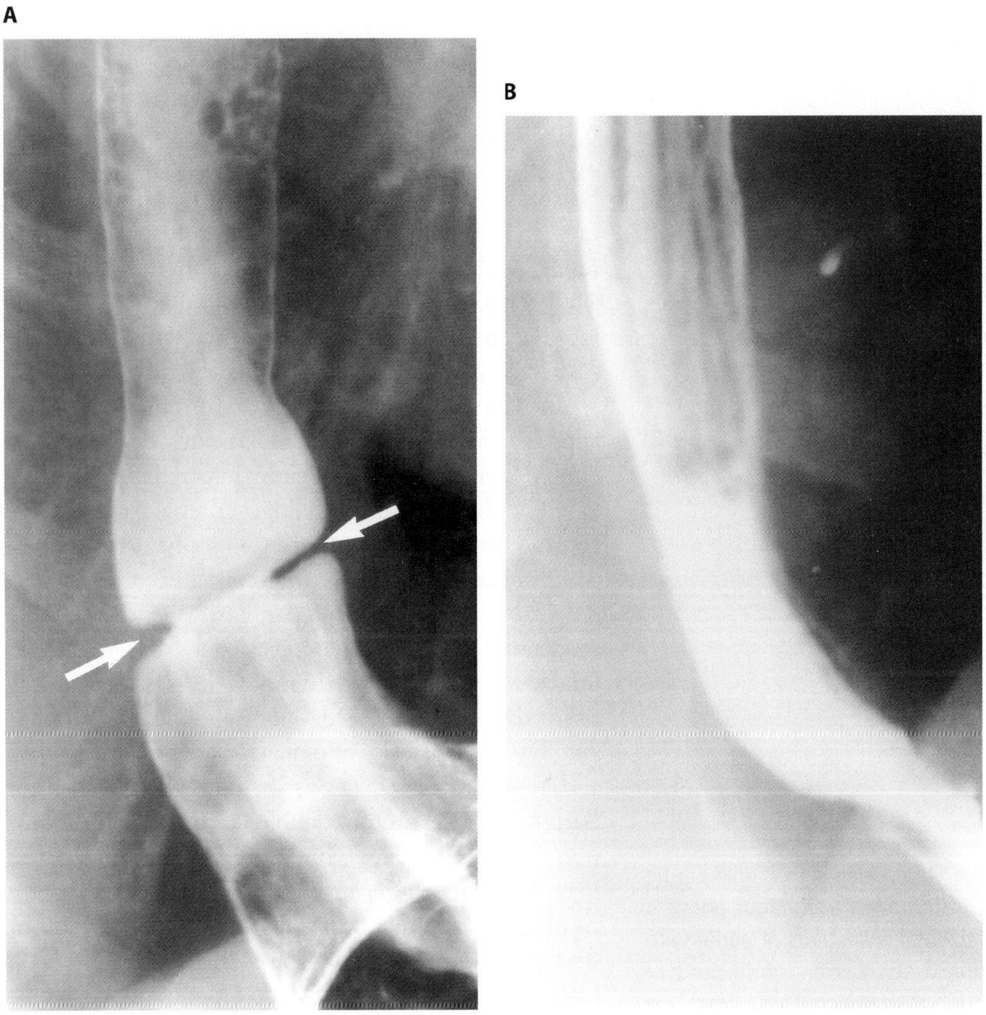

Fig. 16. Schatzki ring seen on prone view of esophagus. (**A**) Prone single-contrast view shows a smooth, symmetric ringlike constriction (arrows) (also known as a Schatzki ring) in the distal esophagus above a hiatal hernia; (**B**) Upright double-contrast view from the same examination shows no evidence of a ring in the distal esophagus because of inadequate distention of this region

Short-segment Barrett's esophagus

Although the radiographic features of long-segment Barrett's esophagus have been well documented [62]–[70], much less is known about the findings in short-segment Barrett's esophagus. In a recent study by Yamamoto et al [71], 70% of patients with short-segment Barrett's esophagus had morphologic evidence of esophagitis and/or peptic scarring or strictures in the distal esophagus on double-contrast esophagrams (*Figs. 20* and *21*). In this study, all of the patients had disease confined to the distal third of the esophagus on barium studies. In contrast, long-segment Barrett's esophagus may be manifested by the development of strictures, ulcers, or a reticular mucosal pattern in the midesophagus (see earlier section on long-segment Barrett's esophagus). Thus, patients with long-segment Barrett's esophagus have more specific radiographic findings for this condition than those with short-segment Barrett's esophagus. It should also be recognized that the length of involvement of the distal esophagus by esophagitis or peptic scarring may extend more than 3 cm above the gastroesophageal junction in patients with short-segment Barrett's esophagus [71], so the diseased segment on esophagography does not necessarily correspond to the vertical extent of columnar metaplasia in the esophagus.

Although 70% of patients with short-segment Barrett's esophagus had reflux esophagitis and/or peptic scarring or strictures on double-contrast esophagrams in the study by Yamamoto et al, the remaining 30% had hiatal hernias or gastroesophageal reflux as the only radiographic findings [71]. The absence of reflux esophagitis or peptic strictures on

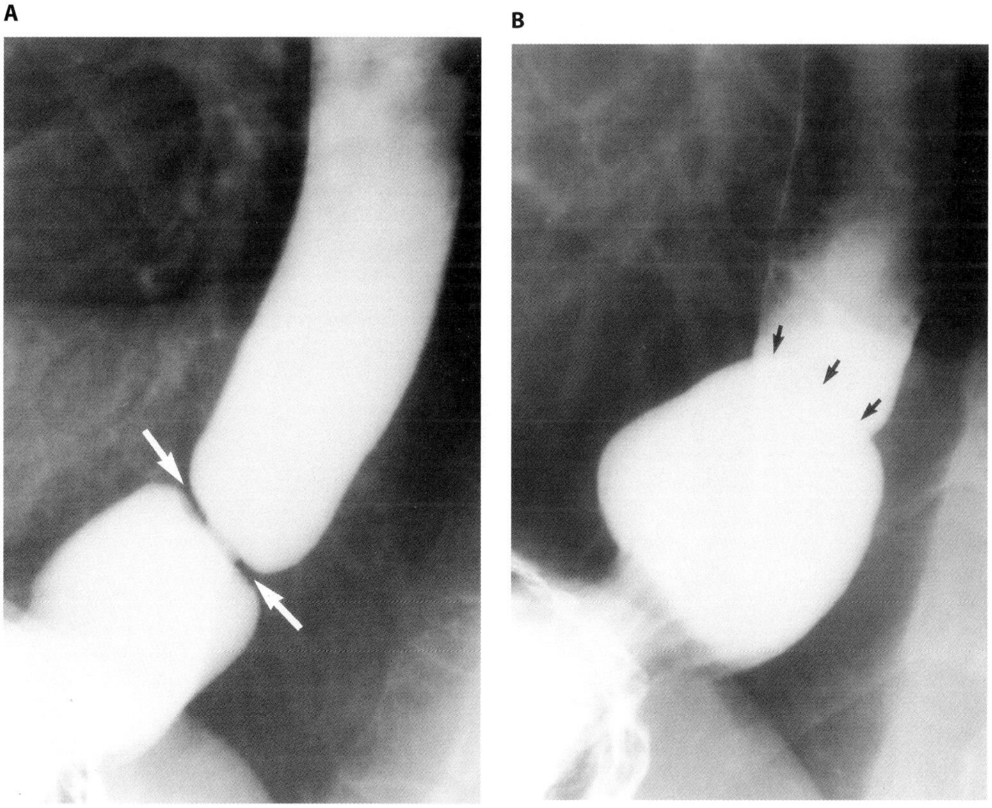

Fig. 17. Schatzki ring obscured by overlap phenomenon. (**A**) Prone single-contrast view shows a tight Schatzki ring (arrows) in the distal esophagus above a hiatal hernia; (**B**) The ring is no longer visible on another prone view from the same examination because of overlap of the distal esophagus and hiatal hernia (arrows) obscuring the region of narrowing. (*Figs. 17A* and *B* reproduced with permission from [55])

double-contrast barium studies therefore does not exclude the possibility of short-segment Barrett's esophagus. In contrast, morphologic findings of reflux disease (reflux esophagitis or peptic strictures) or Barrett's esophagus (midesophageal strictures or ulcers or a reticular mucosal pattern) have been found on double-contrast esophagography in 97–99% of patients with long-segment Barrett's esopha-

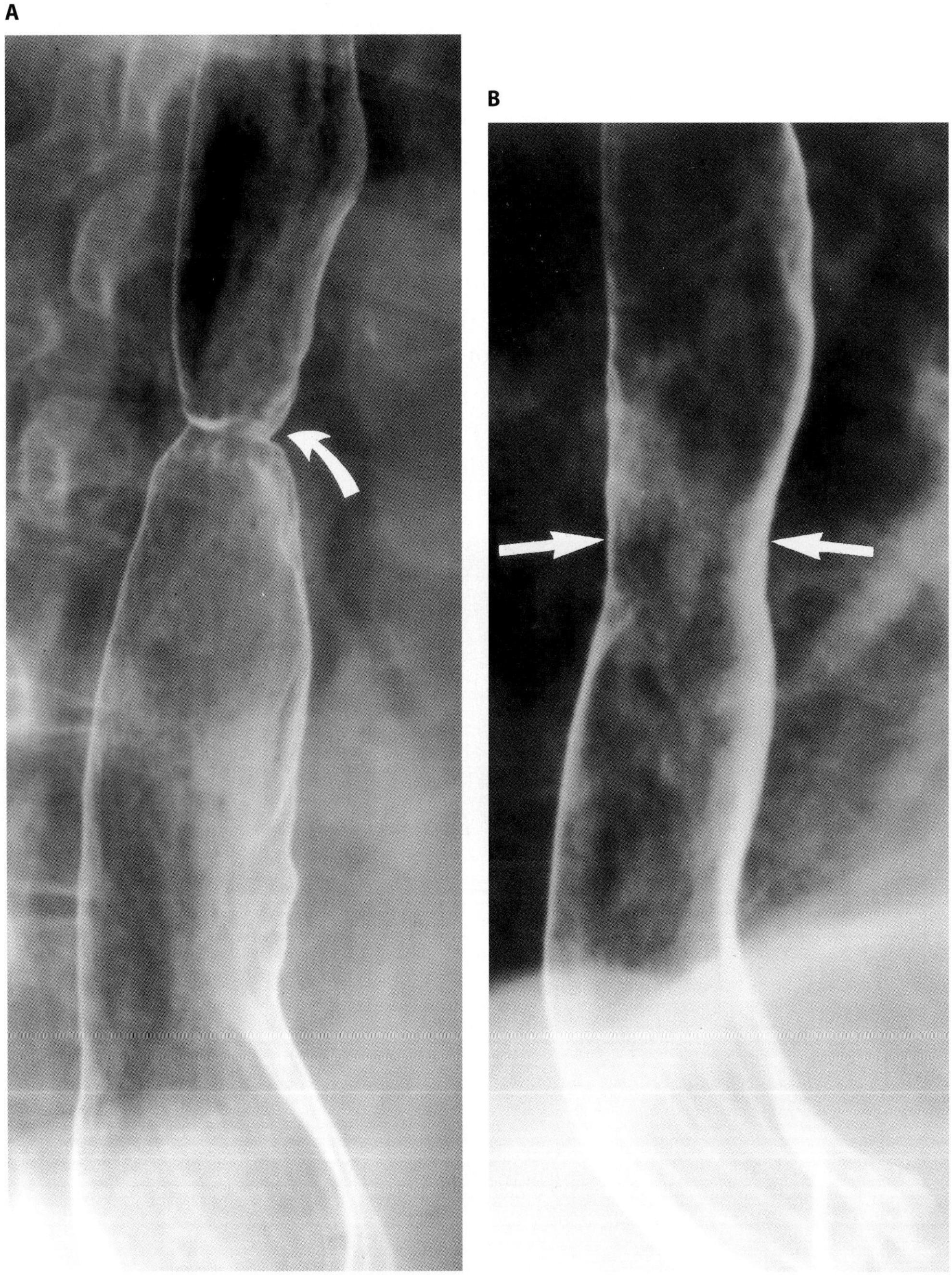

Fig. 18. Long-segment Barrett's esophagus with midesophageal strictures. (**A**) A focal stricture (arrow) is seen in the midesophagus at a considerable distance from the gastroesophageal junction. In the presence of a hiatal hernia and gastroesophageal reflux, this finding is virtually pathognomonic of Barrett's esophagus (Reproduced with permission from [33]); (**B**) A subtler stricture (arrows) is seen in the midesophagus in another patient with Barrett's esophagus

gus [69], [70], so these individuals rarely have a normal-appearing esophagus on double-contrast studies. Thus, patients with short-segment Barrett's esophagus are far more likely to have a normal-appearing esophagus on double-contrast esophagrams than those with long-segment disease. Nevertheless, the clinical importance of this observation remains uncertain because of the lower cancer risk of short-segment Barrett's esophagus compared to that associated with long-segment disease [72]–[74].

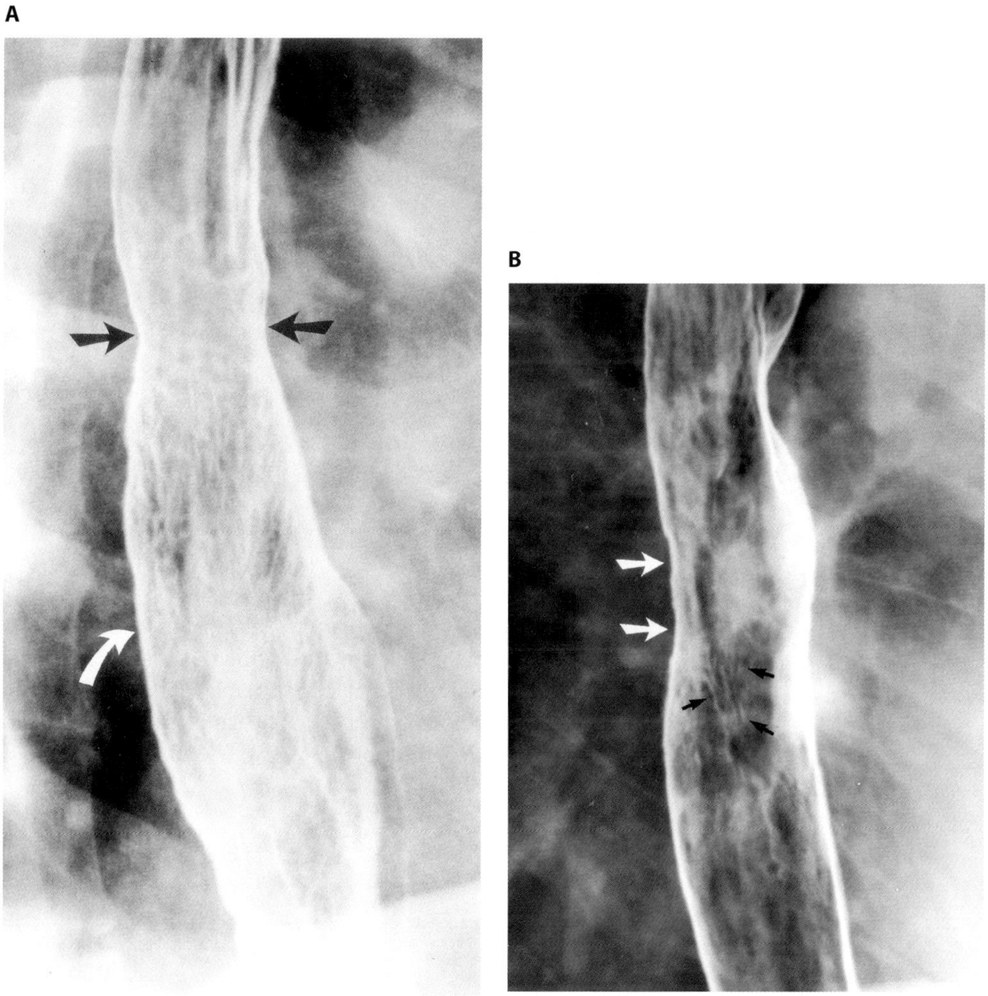

Fig. 19. Long-segment Barrett's esophagus with a reticular pattern of the mucosa. (**A**) A distinctive reticular pattern of the mucosa is seen extending distally a considerable distance (to level of white arrow) from a midesophageal stricture (black arrows) in a patient with Barrett's esophagus; (**B**) There is an early stricture in the midesophagus manifested by slight flattening and retraction of one wall (white arrows) in another patient with Barrett's esophagus. Note the delicate reticular pattern (black arrows) abutting the distal aspect of the stricture (*Figs. 19A* and *B* reproduced with permission from [68])

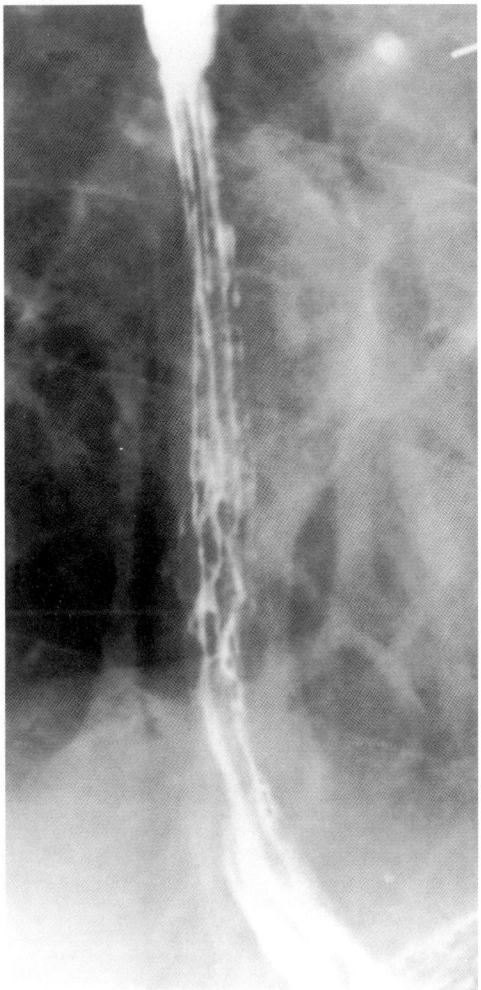

Fig. 20. Short-segment Barrett's esophagus with reflux esophagitis. Thickened, irregular folds are seen in the distal half of the thoracic esophagus due to reflux esophagitis. Endoscopic biopsy specimens confirmed the presence of esophagitis with short-segment Barrett's esophagus (Reproduced with permission from [71])

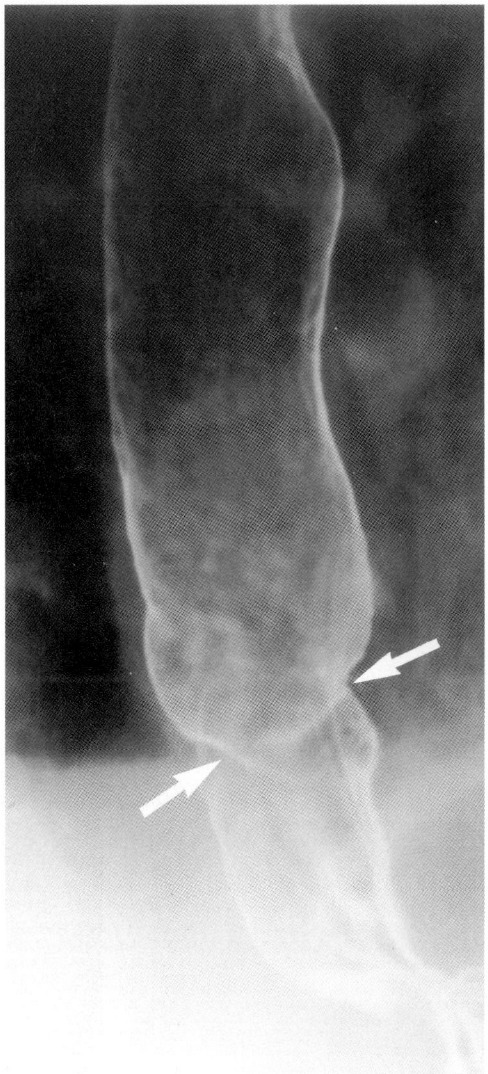

Fig. 21. Short-segment Barrett's esophagus with a peptic stricture. A mild peptic stricture (arrows) is seen in the distal esophagus above a small hiatal hernia. Endoscopic biopsy specimens revealed short-segment Barrett's esophagus (Reproduced with permission from [71])

References

[1] Locke GR, Talley NJ, Fett SL, Zinsmeister AR, Melton LJ (1997) Prevalence and clinical spectrum of gastroesophageal reflux: a population-based study in Olmsted county. Minnesota Gastroenterol 112: 1448–1456

[2] Wiener GJ, Morgan TM, Copper JB et al (1988) Ambulatory 24-h esophageal pH monitoring: reproducibility and variability of pH parameters. Dig Dis 33: 1127–1133

[3] Mattox HE, Richter JE (1990) Prolonged ambulatory esophageal pH monitoring in the evaluation of gastroesophageal reflux disease. Am J Med 89: 345–356

[4] Ott DJ (1994) Gastroesophageal reflux: what is the role of barium studies? AJR 162: 627–629

[5] Schoeman MN, Tippett MD, Akkermans LMA, Dent J, Holloway RH (1995) Mechanisms of gastroesophageal reflux in ambulant healthy human subjects. Gastroenterology 108: 83–91

[6] Mittal RK, Holloway RH, Penagini R, Backshaw LA, Dent J (1995) Transient lower esophageal sphincter relaxation. Gastroenterology 109: 601–610

[7] Sellar RJ, De Caestecker JS, Heading RC (1987) Barium radiology: a sensitive test for gastro-esophageal reflux. Clin Radiol 38: 303–307

[8] Thompson JK, Koehler RE, Richter JE (1994) Detection of gastroesophageal reflux: value of barium studies compared with 24-h pH monitoring. AJR 162: 621–626

[9] Pan JJ, Levine MS, Redfern RO, Rubesin SE, Laufer I, Katzka DA (2003) Gastroesophageal reflux: comparison of barium studies with 24-h pH monitoring. Eur J Radiol 47: 149–153

[10] Cohen S (1976) The diagnosis and management of gastroesophageal reflux. Adv Intern Med 21: 47–75

[11] Wright RA, Hurwitz AL (1979) Relationship of hiatal hernia to endoscopically proved reflux esophagitis. Dig Dis Sci 24: 311–313

[12] Ott JD, Gelfand DW, Chen YM et al (1985) Predictive relationship of hiatal hernia to reflux esophagitis. Gastrointest Radiol 10: 317–320

[13] Hiebert CA, Belsey R (1961) Incompetency of the gastric cardia without radiologic evidence of hiatal hernia: the diagnosis and management of 71 cases. J Thorac Cardiovasc Surg 42: 352–359

[14] Cohen S, Harris LD (1971) Does hiatus hernia affect competence of the gastroesophageal sphincter? N Engl J Med 284: 1053–1056

[15] Ellis FH (1972) Current concepts: esophageal hiatal hernia. N Engl J Med 287: 646–649

[16] Behar J (1976) Reflux esophagitis: pathogenesis, diagnosis, and management. Arch Intern Med 136: 560–566

[17] Dodds WJ, Hogan WJ, Helf JM et al (1981) Pathogenesis of reflux esophagitis. Gastroenterology 81: 376–394

[18] Mittal RK, Balaban DH (1997) The esophagogastric junction. N Engl J Med 336: 924–932

[19] Ott DJ, Gelfand DW, Wu WC (1979) Reflux esophagitis: radiographic and endoscopic correlation. Radiology 130: 583–588

[20] Koehler RE, Weyman PJ, Oakley HF (1980) Single- and double-contrast techniques in esophagitis. AJR 135: 15–19

[21] Ott DJ, Wu WC, Gelfand DW (1981) Reflux esophagitis revisited: prospective analysis of radiologic accuracy. Gastrointest Radiol 6: 1–7

[22] Creteur V, Thoeni RF, Federle MP et al (1983) The role of single and double-contrast radiography in the diagnosis of reflux esophagitis. Radiology 147: 71–75

[23] Graziani L, De Nigris E, Pesaresi A et al (1983) Reflux esophagitis: radiologic-endoscopic correlation in 39 symptomatic cases. Gastrointest Radiol 8: 1–6

[24] Dodds WJ (1977) Current concepts of esophageal motor function: clinical implications for radiology. AJR 128: 549–561

[25] Ott DJ, Dodds WJ, Wu WC et al (1982) Current status of radiology in evaluating for gastroesophageal reflux disease. J Clin Gastroenterol 4: 365–375

[26] Kahrilas PJ, Dodds WJ, Hogan WJ et al (1986) Esophageal peristaltic dysfunction in peptic esophagitis. Gastroenterology 91: 897–904

[27] Hollis JB, Castell DO (1974) Esophageal function in elderly men- a new look at "presbyesophagus." Ann Intern Med 80: 371–374

[28] Simeone JF, Burrell M, Toffler R et al (1977) Aperistalsis and esophagitis. Radiology 123: 9–14

[29] Kressel HY, Glick SN, Laufer I et al (1981) Radiologic features of esophagitis. Gastrointest Radiol 6: 103–108

[30] Levine MS (2000) Gastroesophageal reflux disease. In: Textbook of gastrointestinal radiology (Gore RM, Levine MS, eds). Philadelphia: W. B. Saunders, pp 329–349

[31] Graziani L, Bearzi I, Romagnoli A et al (1985) Significance of diffuse granularity and nodularity of the esophageal mucosa at double-contrast radiography. Gastrointest Radiol 10: 1–6

[32] Levine MS, Cajade AG, Herlinger H et al (1986) Pseudomembranes in reflux esophagitis. Radiology 159: 43–45

[33] Levine MS (1989) Reflux esophagitis. In: Radiology of the esophagus (Levine MS, ed). Philadelphia: W. B. Saunders, pp 15–48

[34] Hu C, Levine MS, Laufer I (1977) Solitary ulcers in reflux esophagitis: radiographic findings. Abdom Imaging 22: 5–7

[35] Rabin M, Schmaman IB (1979) Reflux oesophagitis resembling varices. S Afr Med J 55: 293–295
[36] Bleshman MH, Banner MP, Johnson RC et al (1978) The inflammatory esophagogastric polyp and fold. Radiology 128: 589–593
[37] Ghahremani GG, Fisher MR, Rushovich AM (1984) Prolapsing inflammatory pseudopolyp-fold complex of the oesophagogastric region. Eur J Radiol 4: 47–51
[38] Styles RA, Gibb SP, Tarshis A et al (1985) Esophagogastric polyps: radiographic and endoscopic findings. Radiology 154: 307–311
[39] Gohel VK, Edell SL, Laufer I et al (1978) Transverse folds in the human esophagus. Radiology 128: 303–308
[40] Williams SM, Harned RK, Kaplan P et al (1983) Transverse striations of the esophagus: association with gastroesophageal reflux. Radiology 146: 25–27
[41] Furth EE, Rubesin SE, Rose D (1995) Feline Esophagus. AJR 164: 900
[42] Ho CS, Rodrigues PR (1980) Lower esophageal strictures, benign or malignant? J Can Assoc Radiol 31: 110–113
[43] Levine MS, Moolten DN, Herlinger H, Laufer I (1986) Esophageal intramural pseudodiverticulosis: a reevaluation. AJR 147: 1165–1170
[44] Ott DJ, Gelfand DW, Lane TG et al (1982) Radiologic detection and spectrum of appearances of esophageal strictures. J Clin Gastroenterol 4: 11–15
[45] Ott DJ, Chen YM, Wu WC et al (1985) Endoscopic sensitivity in the detection of esophageal strictures. J Clin Gastroenterol 7: 121–125
[46] Levine MS, Goldstein HM (1984) Fixed transverse folds in the esophagus: a sign of scarring from reflux esophagitis. AJR 143: 275–278
[47] Schatzki R, Gary JE (1953) Dysphagia due to a diaphragm-like localized narrowing in the lower esophagus ("lower esophageal ring"). AJR 70: 911–922
[48] Friedland GW (1978) Historical review of the changing concepts of lower esophageal anatomy: 430 B.C.–1977. AJR 131: 373–388
[49] Chen WM, Gelfand DW, Ott DJ, et al (1987) Natural progression of the lower esophageal mucosa ring. Gastrointest Radiol 12: 93–98
[50] Marshall JB, Kretschmar JM, Diaz-Arias AA (1990) Gastroesophageal reflux as a pathogenic factor in the development of symptomatic lower esophageal rings. Arch Intern med 150: 1669–1672
[51] Schatzki RE (1963) The lower esophageal ring: long term follow-up of symptomatic and asymptomatic rings. AJR 90: 805–810
[52] Ott DJ, Gelfand DW, Wu WC, Castell DO (1984) Esophagogastric region and its rings. AJR 142: 281–287
[53] Chen YM, Ott DJ, Gelfand DW, Munitz HA (1985) Multiphasic examination of the esophagogastric region for strictures, rings, and hiatal hernia: evaluation of the individual techniques. Gastrointest Radiol 10: 311–316
[54] Ott DJ, Chen YM, Wu WC, Gelfand DW, Munitz HA (1986) Radiographic and endoscopic sensitivity in detecting lower esophageal mucosal ring. AJR 147: 261–265
[55] Hsu WC, Levine MS, Rubesin SE (2003) Overlap phenomenon: a potential pitfall in the radiographic detection of lower esophageal rings. AJR 180: 745–747
[56] Spechler SJ, Goyal RK. Barrett's esophagus (1986) N Engl J Med 315: 362–371
[57] Naef AP, Savary M, Ozzello L (1975) Columnar-lined lower esophagus: an acquired lesion with malignant predisposition: report on 140 cases of Barrett's esophagus with 12 adenocarcinomas. J Thorac Cardiovasc Surg 70: 826–835
[58] Sharma P, Morales TG, Sampliner RE (1998) Short segment Barrett's esophagus- the need for standardization of the definition and of endoscopic criteria. Am J Gastroenterol 93: 1033–1036
[59] Spechler SJ (2002) Barrett's esophagus N Engl J Med 346: 836–842
[60] Hamilton SR, Smith RRL (1987) The relationship between columnar epithelial dysplasia and invasive adenocarcinoma arising in Barrett's esophagus. Am J Clin Pathol 87: 301–312
[61] Hameeteman W, Tytgat GNJ, Houthoff HJ et al (1989) Barrett's esophagus: development of dysplasia and adenocarcinoma. Gastroenterology 96: 1249–1256
[62] Missakian MM, Carlson HC, Andersen HA (1967) The roentgenologic features of the columnar epithelial-lined lower esophagus. AJR 99: 212–217
[63] Robbins AH, Hermos JA, Schimmel EM, Friedlander DM, Messian RA (1977) The columnar-lined esophagus: analysis of 26 cases. Radiology 123: 1–7
[64] Chen YM, Gelfand DW, Ott DJ, Wu WC (1985) Barrett esophagus as an extension of severe esophagitis: analysis of radiologic signs in 29 cases. AJR 145: 275–281
[65] Robbins AH, Vincent ME, Saini M, Schimmel EM (1978) Revised radiologic concepts of Barrett esophagus. Gastrointest Radiol 3: 377–381
[66] Shapir J, DuBrow R, Frank P (1985) Barrett oesophagus: analysis of 19 cases. Br J Radiol 58: 491–493
[67] Agha FP (1986) Radiologic diagnosis of Barrett's esophagus: critical analysis of 65 cases. Gastrointest Radiol 11: 123–130
[68] Levine MS, Kressel HY, Caroline DF, Laufer I, Herlinger H, Thompson JJ (1983) Barrett esophagus: reticular pattern of the mucosa. Radiology 147: 663–667

[69] Chernin MM, Amberg JR, Kogan FJ, Morgan TR, Sampliner RE (1986) Efficacy of radiologic studies in the detection of Barrett's esophagus. AJR 147: 257–260

[70] Gilchrist AM, Levine MS, Carr RF et al (1988) Barrett's esophagus: diagnosis by double-contrast esophagography. AJR 150: 97–102

[71] Yamamoto AJ, Levine MS, Katzka DA, Furth EE, Rubesin SE, Laufer I (2001) Short-segment Barrett's esophagus: findings on double-contrast esophago-graphy in 20 patients. AJR 176: 1173–1178

[72] Sharma P, Morales TG, Bhattacharyya A, Garewal HS, Sampliner RE (1997) Dysplasia in short-segment Barrett's esophagus: a prospective 3-year follow-up. Am J Gastroenterol 92: 2012–2016

[73] Weston AP, Krmpotich PT, Cherian R, Dixon A, Topalosvki M (1997) Prospective long-term endoscopic and histological follow-up of short-segment Barrett's esophagus: comparison with traditional long-segment Barrett's esophagus. Am J Gastroenterol 92: 407–413

[74] O'Connor B, Falk FW, Richter JE (1999) The incidence of adenocarcinoma and dysplasia in Barrett's esophagus. Am J Gastroenterol 94: 2037–2042

Chapter 23

LONG-TERM OUTCOME AND PERSPECTIVES OF LAPAROSCOPIC FUNDOPLICATION

B. Hugl and R. A. Hinder

Mayo Clinic, Jacksonville, FL, USA

Introduction

The ability to perform a fundoplication laparoscopically since 1991 has changed the surgical approach to patients with gastroesophageal reflux disease (GERD). Laparoscopic antireflux surgery remains an excellent option in patients with severe GERD.

Laparoscopic Nissen fundoplication offers less morbidity and mortality than the open procedure with at least the same short-term outcome and better results compared to medical therapy. The rate of conversion to an open procedure is now close to zero.

Appropriate preoperative investigation, patient selection and adequate discussion of risks are important in securing a good outcome and long-term patient satisfaction.

Some patients have continuing symptoms, but more than 90% of patients remain satisfied with their decision to undergo surgery. This excellent success rate is maintained for up to 20 years after open fundoplication and indications are that this should be the same after the laparoscopic procedure [1], [2].

Long-term results of laparoscopic fundoplication will be discussed under various headings.

1. Overall satisfaction with surgery-quality of life

When a new procedure or technology is introduced the most important outcome measurements are mortality, morbidity, recurrence rate and long-term survival. However, from the patient's point of view symptom relief, duration of convalescence, satisfaction, well-being and quality of life are of great importance.

Recently, a number of studies have evaluated the quality of life of patients with GERD-related symptoms [3]. These have shown that quality of life in GERD patients is significantly impaired when compared to that of healthy individuals [4]. Therefore, improvement of quality of life is one of the major goals of GERD treatment. During recent years, laparoscopic antireflux surgery has shown itself to be effective at improving the long-term quality-of-life in the treatment of patients with GERD [5]–[7]. Several authors have used quality-of-life assessments to compare the results of different surgical treatments and medical versus surgical treatment, respectively. Antireflux surgery, open or laparoscopically performed, led to a significant improvement of quality-of-life in a 5- to 8-year follow up [5], and even after laparoscopic redo fundoplication [8]–[10]. This applied to all domains including physical functioning (how patients perceive their ability to perform physical tasks), role-physical (how patients perceive their ability to fulfill their life role physically), role-emotional (how patients perceive their ability to fulfill their life role emotionally), bodily pain (how patients perceive their level of pain), vitality (how patients perceive their level of "energy"), mental health (how patients perceive their emotional and psychological well-being), social functioning (how patients perceive their ability to participate in social activities), and general health (how patients perceive their overall health and well-being). Kamolz et al [11] showed that patients without Barrett esophagus undergoing laparoscopic antireflux surgery achieve a better quality-of-life improvement than those with Barrett esophagus. However, after surgery the Gastrointestinal Quality-of-Life Index of both groups was comparable to the mean value of the general population.

Nevertheless, some appropriately selected patients will not be satisfied with the result of antireflux surgery [5], [12]. This dissatisfaction may be due to failure of the fundoplication including misdiagnosis of esophageal disorders, complications or side effects of surgery or to symptoms of non-esophageal disease. There remains a percentage of patients who are dissatisfied with antireflux surgery without physiologically demonstrable reason. Vélanovich [13] recently showed that 68% of dissatisfied patients had no physiological or anatomic problem with their surgery. The median scores of the 36-Item Short-Form Health Survey (SF-36) for dissatisfied patients with unexplained dissatisfaction were generally lower than those for patients with documented surgical failure. Patients who were dissatisfied with surgery had statistically significantly worse median preoperative scores in 6 domains (role-physical, role-emotional, bodily pain, mental health, social functioning, and general health) compared with patients who were satisfied with surgery and worse postoperative scores in all domains, statistically significant in 2 domains (role-emotional and vitality). Postoperative scores were statistically significantly better in all 8 domains for the satisfied group compared with the dissatisfied group. Patients with lower preoperative quality of life are more likely to be dissatisfied despite successful antireflux surgery.

This is another reason why both physician and surgeon should be very sensitive to how GERD affects each patient's quality-of-life before making treatment recommendations.

2. Dysphagia

Transient dysphagia occurs in 40% to 70% of patients after Nissen fundoplication [14]–[16]. Dysphagia is reported by Anvari et al in up to 72% of patients after surgery with a mean dysphagia score of 4.3 ± 4.8 decreasing to 2.6 ± 3.8 ($p < 0.001$) 6 months after surgery and remaining stable at 2 years (2.2 ± 3.4) and 5 years (2.4 ± 3.4) after surgery [17]. This may be secondary to postoperative edema at the gastroesophageal junction or transient esophageal hypomotility with most symptoms resolving in a few weeks [14], [17], [18]. Most of these patients have mild symptoms and postoperative dilatation was required in 3.5% of 2068 reported patients [19].

In our experience dilation shortly after fundoplication is safe and successful in most patients with dysphagia. Symptoms other than dysphagia were found not to respond well to dilation. Dilation was performed in 29 of 233 (12%) patients after laparoscopic antireflux surgery. This was required in 6 patients within the first week after surgery. Dysphagia resolved in 67% after dilation and in an additional 17% after reoperation [20]. Severe or persistent dysphagia, however occurs in 3% to 43% of patients after Nissen fundoplication [16], [17], [19], [21], [22] and is usually related to the tightness of the fundic wrap around the esophagus, fibrosis at the esophageal hiatus or hiatal herniation with or without migration of the wrap into the chest. Redo surgery to achieve hiatal closure with or without prosthetic material will frequently cure this problem [23]–[25].

Some feel that avoidance of dividing the short gastric vessels contributes to dysphagia with a rate of dysphagia of 4.7% compared to 2.6% when the short gastric vessels are taken down [26]. Others feel that this is only selectively required during the Nissen fundoplication and never needed during a partial fundoplication.

Inability to belch is an expected outcome after fundoplication and most patient learn to compensate.

Patients with an esophageal stricture prior to surgery usually have dysphagia. The need for dilation was found to be 252 dilations in 102 patients over 26 months prior to surgery and 29 dilations in 24 months after surgery [27].

3. Barrett esophagus

Barrett esophagus is associated with chronic gastroesophageal reflux disease and represents the severest form of GERD with malignant potential.

There is no well-defined therapy for patients with this disease. Barrett esophagus is unlikely to regress with medical or surgical therapy, and progression to cancer in not prevented by either [28]. Most studies show no difference in cancer risk after medical or surgical therapy for Barrett. Our own meta-analysis shows a cancer risk in Barrett of 1:294 patient years after anti-reflux surgery and 1:145 patient years during medical therapy [29].

Spechler et al [30] showed that 4 of 166 patients developed adenocarcinoma during long-term follow-up in a medically treated group and none of 82 patients after fundoplication, however El-Serag and

Sonnenberg [31] reported that fundoplication did not protect patients, with either complicated or uncomplicated esophagitis, against esophageal adenocarcinoma.

As it is hypothesized that adenocarcinoma develops among a subset of patients who have acquired genomic instability in Barrett epithelium and takes up to 6 years for developing from low-grade dysplasia, the genetic alteration may have occurred before antireflux surgery was performed [32]. Thus, development of adenocarcinoma in the first few years after antireflux surgery may not represent progression of disease after surgery [33]. This is supported by the fact that a Mayo analysis showed that all cancers occurred within 3 years of the fundoplication. The development of Barrett esophagus is rare after an effective procedure [34]–[36]. This was also shown by Wetscher et al [37] who found that progression to Barrett was frequently seen when patients were on medical therapy and that this was halted after surgery.

Bammer et al [29], in a review, showed that antireflux surgery seems to result in a lower incidence of new cancers and less progress in length or dysplasia. They suggest that surgery may be superior to medical therapy to prevent progression of Barrett esophagus and the development of carcinoma. Nevertheless, surveillance is required, irrespective of the treatment modality.

Patients with severe dysplasia on a biopsy specimen of the esophagus have a high incidence of coexisting carcinoma and are candidates for esophagectomy.

Surgical therapy for Barrett esophagus should be reserved for patients who are resistent to medical therapy or who develop complications of GERD.

4. Bowel dysfunction and diarrhea

Postoperative bowel dysfunction after laparoscopic antireflux surgery, particularly diarrhea, has not received wide recognition. Klaus et al [38] found that 35% of patients had bowel dysfunction before surgery. Swanstrom et al noted that as many as 66% who underwent antireflux surgery had pre-existing irritable bowel syndrome. In the series of Klaus et al [38] 43% of patients undergoing laparoscopic antireflux surgery did not experience any bowel problems before or after surgery and, in 21% the same symptom was experienced before and after surgery. However, new-onset bowel dysfunction occurred in 36% of the patients with 14% having new onset diarrhea.

Diarrhea is an uncommon complication after antireflux surgery but has been reported to be persistent in 8% of patients. The diarrhea seen is most commonly postprandial, resembling the dumping syndrome. The cause of the diarrhea is unclear and possible causes include an increased rate of gastric emptying, bacterial overgrowth or vagus nerve injury resulting in postvagotomy diarrhea.

5. Abdominal bloating

Temporary, mild bloating occurs in up to 100% of patients. The inability to belch and reduced fundic volume can predispose patients to the development of gasbloat after fundoplication. The habit of frequent swallowing of spit and aerophagy contribute to the problem. On the other hand, gastric emptying particularly of liquids has been shown to be accelerated after fundoplication. While in the majority this symptom improves after surgery, few patients develop severe symptoms of bloating after fundoplication.

The treatment can be frustrating, and includes avoidance of carbonated beverages, gas trapping medications and promotility agents.

6. Recurrence of GERD after surgery

In our experience, the cumulative failure rate of surgery is about 1% per year. Continuing symptoms such as abdominal bloating, excess flatus, nausea, diarrhea, dysphagia and chest pain are not uncommon after surgery and were frequently present before surgery.

Carlson et al [26] in a review of 41 papers reporting 9,433 procedures showed a reoperation rate of 2.77% (individual reoperation rate ranging from 0% to 15.4%). The most common indications for reoperation after a primary minimally invasive antireflux procedure were reflux (43%), followed by dysphagia (24%) and wrap herniation (18%).

We have found that only 0.7% of all patients require revisional surgery and the remainder are easily controlled by medical therapy. In our experience of 46 patients requiring reoperation after previous fundoplication, the most common causes of failure were hiatal herniation (67%), fundoplication breakdown (43%), fundoplication slippage (20%), tight fundoplication (4%), misdiagnosed achalasia (4%), and displaced Angelchik prosthesis (4%). Twenty-two patients (48%) had more than 1 cause [39]. There was no mortality and a conversion rate to the open procedure of 20% after previous laparoscopy.

Antireflux reoperation with the open technique has a higher mortality than the initial procedure, with an average mortality of 2.8% and success rate of 79% [40]. Our 0% mortality attests to the safety of doing these procedures laparoscopically. The cause of most deaths is an unsuspected esophageal or gastric perforation with ensuing sepsis. The presence of severe fibrosis makes dissection difficult and dangerous leading to a high conversion rate [41].

7. Need for further medical therapy

Patients with GERD are known to have associated functional bowel symptoms that will persist after antireflux surgery and generally cannot be expected to improve on antireflux medication given before or after surgery. In a recent study, 62% of patients were given antireflux medications after antireflux surgery and 32% of patients were using proton pump Inhibitors (PPI) [42]. Lord et al showed that 14% of patients who had undergone fundoplication were found to be using PPIs for abdominal and chest symptoms, but 79% of these were using the medication for symptoms unrelated to gastroesophageal reflux [43]. Bammer et al found 39% of patients 2 years after laparoscopic antireflux surgery to be on acid suppressive or promotility agents. Eighty-four percent of these subjects reported a good surgical outcome despite continuing on medication [44].

This is an unexpectedly high need for antireflux medication, but an evaluation of postoperative use of medication showed that the indication for proton pump inhibitors is often for vague, nonspecific symptoms. Only 6% had evidence of GERD requiring therapy; therefore the high postoperative use of PPI is questionable. The appropriateness of prescribing antireflux medications in patients with nonspecific symptoms after antireflux surgery must be carefully considered by the prescribing physician.

8. Who should not have had surgery?

Patients who present with atypical symptoms (gastric, respiratory, chest pain) and with a normal LES pressure have a 56% failure rate after antireflux surgery [45].

The Nissen fundoplication will reliably replace the gastroesophageal junction into the abdomen and restore LES barrier function. Little benefit is likely to occur if the patient's symptoms are not caused by a transient or permanent loss of this barrier. Thus, in large part the predictability of success following laparoscopic fundoplication is directly proportional to the degree of certainty that gastroesophageal reflux is the underlying cause of the patient's complaints. It is therefore important to identify patients less likely to benefit from antireflux surgery and to avoid surgery in these cases. The presence of an abnormal 24-hour pH score, typical primary symptoms, and a significant response to acid suppression therapy predicts a successful outcome after Nissen fundoplication [46]. Twenty-four-hour pH monitoring provides the strongest predictor, which is based more on the correct identification of the disease than on its severity. Campos et al [46] showed that excellent and good symptomatic outcome occurred in those who satisfied these criteria, and a fair or poor outcome occurred in those who did not. The most common pattern of failure seemed to be inadequate patient selection with atypical symptoms or a normal 24-hour pH study prior to surgery.

9. Delayed gastric perforation

Gastric perforation in a fundoplication is a rare event. Our series of 1600 laparoscopic fundoplications resulted in six delayed gastric perforations at the fundoplication in 3 patients 13 to 84 months after fundoplication. All had been taking Celexobid. One possible cause of the full thickness ulceration could be the suture material or Teflon pledgets used to secure the fundoplication. Another possibility is that entrapment of tablets caught in the folds of the fundoplication may have produced severe, local injury with transmural gastric perforation.

10. Vagus nerve dysfunction

Mechanical changes in the cardia with lack of accommodation to liquids may be related to some symptoms such as bloating and diarrhea, but vagus nerve injury during the fundoplication has been proposed as an etiological factor.

DeVault et al found vagus nerve dysfunction in 30% of patients prior to antireflux surgery rising to 42% after surgery. But, most importantly, dysfunction did not correlate with worsening or development of new symptoms in these patients [47].

In conclusion, laparoscopic Nissen fundoplication is an excellent long-term treatment for selected patients with severe GERD with good success for several years. It provides an excellent alternative to patients requiring long-term medical therapy. There is a low morbidity and mortality similar to medical treatment, and it is cost-effective.

Side effects and complications can occur and patients should be aware of this. Some patients have continuing symptoms and remain on therapy, but more than 90% of patients remain satisfied with their decision to undergo surgery.

Careful patient selection, preoperative evaluation, and correct choice of operation are necessary for successful surgical outcome and long-term results.

References

[1] DeMeester TR, Stein HJ (1992) Minimizing the side effects of antireflux surgery. World J Surg 16: 335–336

[2] Grande L, Toledo-Pimentel V, Manterola C, Lacima G, Ros E, Garcia-Valdecasas JC, Fuster J, Visa J, Pera C (1994) Value of Nissen fundoplication in patients with gastro-esophageal reflux judged by long-term symptom control. Br J Surg 81: 548–550

[3] Korolija D, Sauerland S, Wood-Dauphinée S, Abbou CC, Eypasch E, García Caballero M et al (2004) Evaluation of quality of life after laparoscopic surgery. Surg Endosc 18: 879–897

[4] Dimenäs E, Glise H, Hallerbäck B et al (1995) Wellbeing and gastrointestinal symptoms among patients referred to endoscopy owing to suspected doudenal ulcer. Scand J Gastroenterol 30: 1046–1052

[5] Bammer T, Hinder RA, Klaus A, Klingler PJ (2001) Five to eight year outcome of the first laparoscopic Nissen fundoplications. J Gastrointest Surg 5: 42–48

[6] Kamolz T, Granderath FA, Bammer T, Pasiut M, Wykypiel H Jr, Herrmann R, Pointner R (2002) Mid- and long-term quality of life assessments after laparoscopic fundoplication and refundoplication: a single unit report of more than 500 antireflux procedures. Dig Liver Dis 34: 470–476

[7] Trus TL, Laycock WS, Waring JP, Branum GD, Hunter JG (1999) Improvement in quality of life measures after laparoscopic antireflux surgery. Ann Surg 229: 331–335

[8] Kamolz T, Bammer T, Pasuit M et al (2000) Health-related and disease-specific quality of life assessment after laparoscopic refundoplication. Chirurg 71: 707–711

[9] Kamolz T, Bammer T, Pasuit M et al (2002) Failed antireflux surgery: surgical outcome of laparoscopic refundoplication in the elderly. Hepato Gastroenterol 49: 865–868

[10] Granderath F, Kamolz T, Schweiger UM, Pointner R (2003) Failed antireflux surgery: quality of life and surgical outcome after laparoscopic refundoplication. Int J Colorectal Dis 18: 248–253

[11] Kamolz T, Granderath F, Pointer R (2003) Laparoscopic antireflux surgery: disease related quality-of-life assessment before and after surgery in GERD patients with and without Barrett's esophagus. Surg Endosc 17: 880–885

[12] Anvari M, Allen C (2003) Five-year comprehensive outcomes evaluation in 181 patients after laparoscopic Nissen Fundoplication. J Am Surg 196: 51–57

[13] Vélanovich V (2004) Using quality-of-life measurements to predict patient satisfaction outcomes for antireflux surgery. Arch Surg 139: 621–626

[14] DeMeester TR, Bonavina L, Albertucci M (1986) Nissen fundoplication for gastroesophageal reflux disease. Evaluation of primary repair in 100 consecutive patients. Ann Surg 204: 9–20

[15] Hinder RA, Perdikis G, Klingler PJ, DeVault KR (1997) The surgical option for gastroesophageal reflux disease. Am J Med 103: 144S–148S

[16] Sato K, Awad ZT, Filipi CJ, Selima MA, Cummings JE, Fenton SJ, Hinder RA (2002) Causes of long-term dysphagia after laparoscopic Nissen fundoplication. JSLS 6: 35–40

[17] Anvari M, Allen CJ (1996) Prospective evaluation of dysphagia before and after laparoscopic Nissen fundoplication without routine division of short gastrics. Surg Laparosc Endosc 6: 424–429

[18] Gott JP, Polk HC Jr (1991) Repeat operation for failure of antireflux surgery. Gastroenterol Clin North Am 71: 13–32

[19] Perdikis G, Hinder RA, Lund RJ, Raiser F, Katada N (1997) Laparoscopic Nissen fundoplication: where do we stand? Surg Laparosc Endosc 7: 17–21

[20] Malhi-Chowla NM, Gorecki P, Bammer T, Achem SR, Hinder RA, DeVault KR (2002) Dilation after

Fundoplication: timing, frequency, indications, and outcome. Gastro Intest Endosc 55: 219–223
[21] Luostarinen M (1993) Nissen fundoplication for reflux esophagitis. Long-term clinical and endoscopic results in 109 of 127 consecutive patients. Ann Surg 217: 329–337
[22] Guarner V (1997) 30 years experience with posterior fundoplasty in the treatment of gastroesophageal reflux. Chirurgie 122: 443–448
[23] Granderath FA, Schweiger UM, Kamolz T et al (2002) Laparoscopic antireflux surgery with routine mesh-hiatoplasty in the treatment of gastroesophageal reflux disease. J Gastrointest Surg 6: 347–353
[24] Basso N, De Leo A, Genco A et al (2000) 360° laparoscopic fundoplication with tensionfree hiatoplasty in the treatment of gastroesophageal reflux disease. Surg Endosc 14: 164–169
[25] Granderath FA, Kamolz T, Schweiger UM, Pointner R (2003) Laparoscopic refundoplication with prosthetic hiatal closure for recurrent hiatal hernia after primary failed antireflux surgery. Arch Surg 138: 902–907
[26] Carlson MA, Frantzides CT (2001) Complications and results of primary minimally invasive antireflux procedures: A review of 10,735 reported cases. J Am Coll Surg 193(4): 428–439
[27] Klingler PJ, Hinder RA, Cina RA, DeVault KR, Floch NR, Branton SA, Seelig MH (1999) Laparoscopic antireflux surgery for the treatment of esophageal strictures refractory to medical therapy. Am J Gastroenterol 94: 632–636
[28] Hinder RA, Smith SL, Branton SA et al (1999) Laparoscopic antireflux surgery – it's a wrap! Dig Surg 16: 7–11
[29] Bammer T, Hinder RA, Klaus A, Trastek VF, Achem SR (2001) Rationale for surgical therapy of Barrett esophagus. Mayo Clin Proc 76: 335–342
[30] Spechler S, Lee E Ahnen D et al (2000) Long-term outcome of medical and surgical therapies for GERD: effects on survival. Gastroenterology 118(2 Pt 1): A489. Abstract 2635
[31] El-Serag HB, Sonnenberg A (1999) Outcome of erosive reflux esophagitis after Nissen fundoplication. Am J Gastroenterol 94: 1771–1776
[32] McArdle JE, Lewin KJ, Randall G, Weinstein W (1992) Distribution of dysplasia and early invasive carcinoma in Barrett's esophagus. Hum Pathol 23: 479–482
[33] Hameeteman W, Tytgat GN, Houthoff HJ, van den Tweel JG (1989) Barrett's esophagus: development of dysphagia and adenocarcinoma. Gastroenterology 96(5 Pt 1): 1249–1256
[34] Luostarinen M, Isolauri J, Laitinen J et al (1993) Fate of Nissen fundoplication after 20 years: a clinical, endoscopical, and functional analysis. Gut 34: 1015–1020
[35] Thor KB, Silander T (1989) A long-term randomized prospective trial of the Nissen procedure versus a modified Toupet technique. Ann Surg 210: 719–724
[36] Johansson J, Johnsson F, Joelsson B, Floren CH, Walther B (1993) Outcome 5 years after 360 degree fundoplication for gastro-oesophageal reflux disease. Br J Surg 80: 46–49
[37] Wetscher GJ, Profanter C, Gadenstädter M, Perdikis G, Glaser K, Hinder RA (1997) Medical treatment of gastroesophageal reflux disease does not prevent the development of Barrett's metaplasia and poor esophageal body motility. Langenbecks Arch Chir 382: 95–99
[38] Klaus A, Hinder RA, DeVault KR, Achem AR (2003) Bowel dysfunction after laparoscopic antireflux surgery: incidence, severity, and clinical course. Am J Med 114: 6–9
[39] Floch NR, Hinder RA, Klingler PJ, Branton SA, Seelig MH, Bammer T, Filipi CJ (1999) Is laparoscopic reoperation for failed antireflux surgery feasible?. Arch Surg 134: 733–737
[40] Jamieson GG (1993) The result of antireflux surgery and reoperative antireflux surgery. Gullet 3: 41–45
[41] O'Reilly MJ, Mullins S, Reddick EJ (1997) Laparoscopic management of failed antireflux surgery. Surg Laparosc Endosc 7: 90–93
[42] Spechler SJ, Lee A, Ahnen D et al (2001) Long-term outcome of medical and surgical therapies for gastroesophageal reflux disease: follow-up of a randomized controlled trial. JAMA 285: 2331–2338
[43] Lord RV, Kaminski A, Ölberg S et al (2002) Absence of gastroesophageal reflux disease in a majority of patients taking acid suppression medications after Nissen fundoplication. J Gastrointest Surg 6: 3–9
[44] Bammer T, Achem SR, DeVault KR, Napoleillo DA, Rodriguez JA, Lukens FJ, Hinder RA (2000) Use of acid suppressive medications after laparoscopic antireflux surgery: prevalence, clinical indications and causes. Gastroent 118: A478
[45] Ritter MP, Peters JH, DeMeester TR et al (1998) Outcome after laparoscopic fundoplication is not dependent on a structurally defective lower esophageal sphincter. J Gastrointest Surg 6: 567–571
[46] Campos G, Peters Joffrey H, DeMeester TR, Oberg S, Crookes PF, Tan S, DeMeester SR, Hagen JA, Bremner CG (1999) Multivariate analysis of factors predicting outcome after laparoscopic Nissen fundoplication. J Gastroint Surg 3: 292–300
[47] DeVault KR, Swain JM, Wentling GK, Floch NR, Achem SR, Hinder RA (2004) Evaluation of vagus nerve integrity before and after antireflux surgery. J Gastroint Surg 8: 881–887

Chapter 24

TELEROBOTIC-ASSISTED ANTIREFLUX SURGERY: NISSEN FUNDOPLICATION

G. B. Cadière • J. Himpens • G. Dapri

Department of Gastrointestinal Surgery, Saint-Pierre University Hospital, Brussels, Belgium

Introduction

In open surgery, the flexibility of the surgeon's wrist and the hands inside the abdomen permits movement of all kinds and in every direction. In laparoscopy, however, the fact that the surgeon must work through a fixed opening means that the number of degrees of freedom is limited. The degrees of freedom that are allowed involve movement in and out, up and down and rotational and oscillatory, although oscillation is limited by the presence of the entrance port. Because the surgeon has to adapt his or her position relative to the location of the port, the operation often has to be performed from a difficult position [1]. The ideal solution to this problem would be to have an additional articulation inside the abdomen so the degrees of freedom that have been lost may be regained.

When one has an articulation inside and outside the abdomen, on both sides of a fixed point, it is logical and natural to introduce the concept of robotics, even more so because it is extremely difficult to manipulate two articulations with the same tool. The human brain is not up to the task. Robotics allows the surgeon to work at a distance from the operating table in an ergonomically correct position, instead of having to bend awkwardly above the patient [2].

Prototype for robotic-assisted abdominal surgery

In robotic-assisted surgery, the robot is positioned at the patient's side. It holds and activates surgical instruments, obeying the orders of the surgeon who is removed from the patient and is seated in front of a console in a perfectly comfortable position. The surgeon manipulates handles under the control panel of a three-dimensional monitor; three-dimensional vision is permitted by means of special glasses worn by the surgeon. The surgeon's movements are transmitted to the computer at the patient's side. These movements are actually improved by the computer. At the patient's side are the anesthesiologist, the engineer, the surgeon's assistant and the scrub nurse.

At the surgeon's side there is only a console and the computer, which is under control of two engineers. In the future the computer will be incorporated in the console. The patient's station and the surgeon's station are united by a cable. This is only a few yards long, but there is no practical limit to its length. The cable could be several kilometers long, or the impulses could be transmitted by satellite, which implies surgery from a distance.

After obtaining authorization from the Ethics Committee of Centre Hospitalier Universitaire Saint-Pierre in March 1997, one of the Authors (JH) performed the first laparoscopic cholecystectomy ever performed on a human being using the prototype described here [3]. Following that experience, we worked to improve the various components of the system: the surgical cart, the computer and the console. The most significant innovation was changing the shape of the clinical laparoscopic tools to handles that look like joysticks. In May 1998, one of the authors (GBC) performed the first two Nissen fundoplications procedures entirely performed by robot, in the Broussais hospital in Paris [4].

Mona robot system

In this new Mona setup (Intuitive Surgical, Inc., Mountain View, CA), the surgeon sits comfortably with his or her arms resting on a support. Manipulation of the articulated instruments is done by activating handles that are mounted just underneath a three-dimensional video screen, thereby eliminating the problem of hand-eye coordination. Impulses coming from the handles are transmitted to a computer that activates the robotic arms mounted on the operating table. The computer interface can translate large deflections of the handles into minute motions on the operative field (a process called downscaling). Minor involuntary motions such as physiologic tremor can be eliminated. The number of degrees of freedom is increased because the tips of instruments can move in a different plane from that of the instrument shaft. This device perfectly mimics the surgeon's wrist and fingers movements, bringing to fruition the concept of a master-slave robotic system.

After performance of the two first Nissen fundoplication procedures by robotic laparoscopic surgery, we realized that a comparison of this procedure with the classic laparoscopic procedure was necessary. We performed 24 robotically-assisted laparoscopic procedures in humans, including 12 Nissen fundoplications, we assumed we had completed the learning curve associated with this novel technique. We decided to compare, in a randomized prospective trial, the advantages and disadvantages of using a robot (Mona), with those of the conventional laparoscopic approach.

Materials and method

We performed a randomized, prospective trial on a group of 21 patients who are candidates for laparoscopic Nissen fundoplication. Eleven patients were treated by conventional laparoscopy and ten by telesurgery. The location of the trial was Mexico city (Department of Surgery, headed by Dr. Cabral). All procedures were performed by the same surgeon (GBC) who had an experience with more than over 400 laparoscopic Nissen fundoplications.

Patient characteristics

All patients suffered from operable, pathological, gastro-esophageal reflux as documented by 24-hour blood gas, gastroscopy, barium swallow and esophageal manometry. All patients were determined to have low operative risk (ASA 1). There were 11 controls in trial group: three female and eight male patients; median age, 38 years (range, 18 to 52); median body mass index, 27.3 kg/m^2 (range, 22.3 to 29.7). In the telesurgery group there were ten patients: three females and seven males patients; median age, 40 years (range, 29 to 62); median body mass index 28.5 kg/m^2 (range, 24.6 to 41.7).

Robot description

Use of the robot (Mona) in humans had been approved by the local Ethics Committee of the hospital. All patients had signed a document of informed consent. For surgery, the robot was placed to the left of the patient. It held and manipulated articulated surgical tools (*Figs. 1* and *2*). The surgeon was located at a distance of 12 feet from the patient and was not scrubbed. He was seated at a console, manipulating two handles that commanded three robotic arms (*Fig. 3*). The surgeon's movements corresponded to three-dimensional images of the operative field, which he observed with binoculars. Five trocars had been placed in the patient's abdomen. The optical trocar (12 mm) and two operative trocars (8 mm) were snapped onto the robot's arms. Two additional trocars were placed for exposure: one (5 mm) housed the liver retractor that was attached to a fixed, rigid retraction system; and the other (10 mm) housed a grasping forceps that was held by the surgeon's assistant who was scrubbed and waiting on standby. The position of the

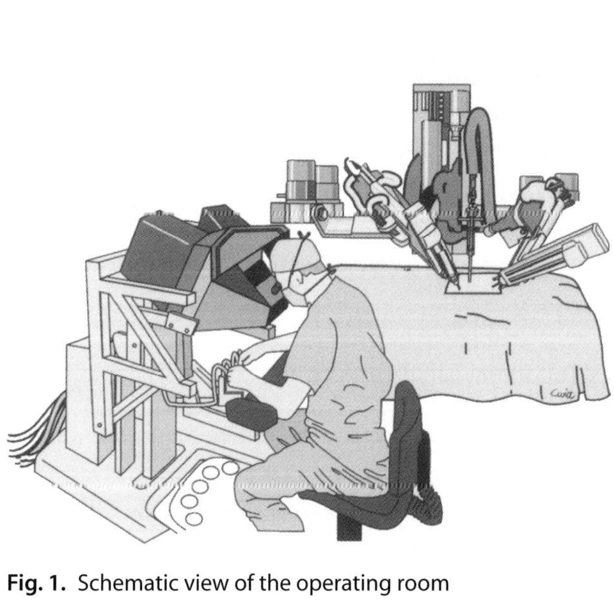

Fig. 1. Schematic view of the operating room

trocars, which were introduced by the assistant, varied slightly with the positions used previously [5]. This modification was necessary in order to accomodate the considerable bulk of the robotic arms.

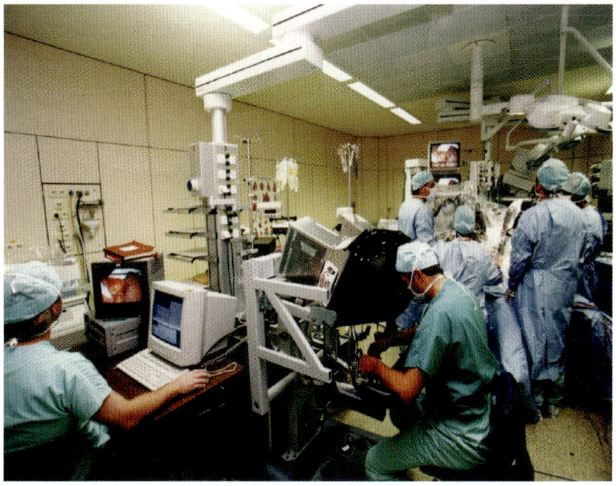

Fig. 2. Photografic view of the operating room

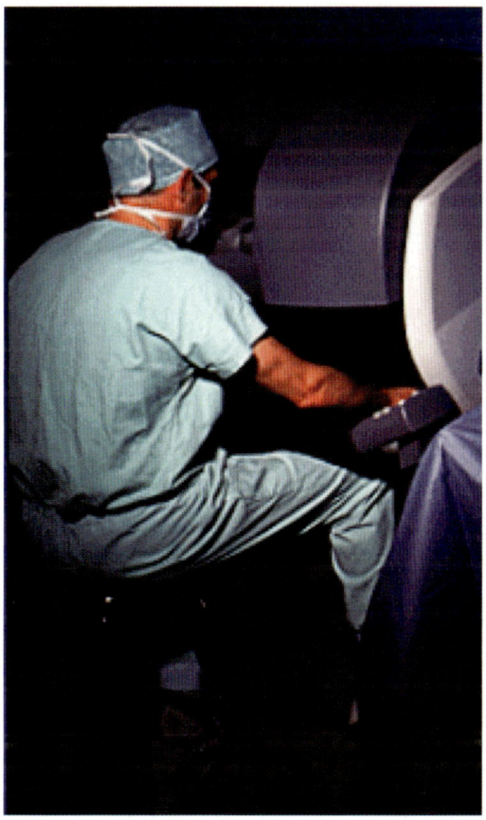

Fig. 3. Surgeon at the console

Manipulation of the console handles created electrical impulses that were transmitted to the computer. This information was digitized and translated into impulses that commanded the robotic arms and the tools (effectors) attached to them. In this setup, the right handle was also in control of the optical system as soon as tool manipulation was deactivated. Translation by the computer of the motions coming from the console accomplished the necessary downscaling on the effector side. Thus, deflections of 5 cm at the surgeon's site resulted in a smaller deflection at the patient's side (by a factor of 5 to 1 or 3 to 1). For this reason, physiological trembling could be virtually eliminated. The robotic arms were connected to disposable tools of different shapes, featuring an articulation 2 cm from their distal tip. They were introduced inside the abdomen by means of trocars that were also attached to the mechanical arms.

Nissen fundoplication procedure

The laparoscopic version of the Nissen procedure has been described extensively [5]. For this procedure, five trocars were used; however, placement of the trocars was slightly different in the groups of patients undergoing telesurgery (see the previous robot description). The first step in the procedure for both groups was the freeing of the greater curvature by the Harmonic scalpel (Autosonic, Autosuture Norwalk, Conn.). In the laparoscopic group, this was done with the aid of a 30 degree angled scope. In the robot group, a three-dimensional camera was used for this maneuver and for the rest of the procedure. The robot was activated only after full mobilization of the greater curvature. Hiatal dissection was performed along the pillars at a distance from the esophagus. The wrap, 4 cm long and fixed to the esophagus by three stitches, was subsequently sutured to the hiatus.

Postoperatively, the patients were discharged after a satisfactory gastrograph recorded contrast study had been performed and adequate positioning of the wrap, as well as patency of the gastric inlet, had been documented.

Statistical analysis was done using Student's t test. The study protocol was designed in accordance with Food and Drugs Administration (FDA) regulations.

Results

Operative time was 52 minutes (range, 45 to 62) in the control group and 76 minutes (range, 59 to 130) in the telesurgery group (*Fig. 4*). The difference was significant ($p < 0.01$).

The mean time for dissection of the greater curve was 12 minutes (range, 5 to 23) in the control group and 15.5 minutes (range, 9 to 32) in the telesurgery group ($p = 0.139$) (*Fig. 5*).

The mean time for hiatal dissection time was 9 minutes (range, 5 to 14) in the control group and 15 minutes (range, 8 to 27) in the telesurgery group ($p < 0.05$) (*Fig. 6*).

The mean hiatal pillar closure time was 2.5 minutes (range, 1 to 5) in the control group and 4 minutes (range, 2 to 8) in the telesurgery group ($p < 0.05$) (*Fig. 7*).

The mean suturing time of the wrap was 6.5 minutes (range, 4 to 12) in the control group and 8 minutes (range, 6 to 13) in the telesurgery group ($p = 0.151$) (*Fig. 8*).

Postoperative blood loss was evaluated at less than 10 ml in both groups. Median hospital stay was 1 day in the telesurgery group (range 1 to 4 days) and 1 day in the control group (range, 1 to 18). There were no conversions to open surgery in either group. There were no deaths.

There were two complications, one in each group. Immediately after induction of anesthesia, one patient in the control group vomited forcefully, causing intrathoracic migration of the wrap and of the entire gastric fundus. The patient suffered acute

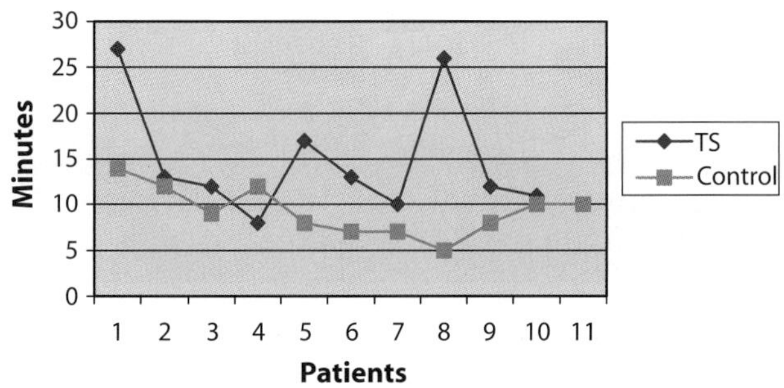

Fig. 6. Hiatal dissection time

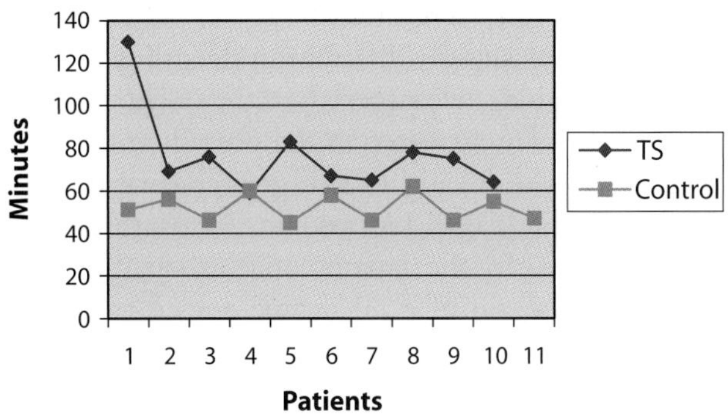

Fig. 4. Operative time

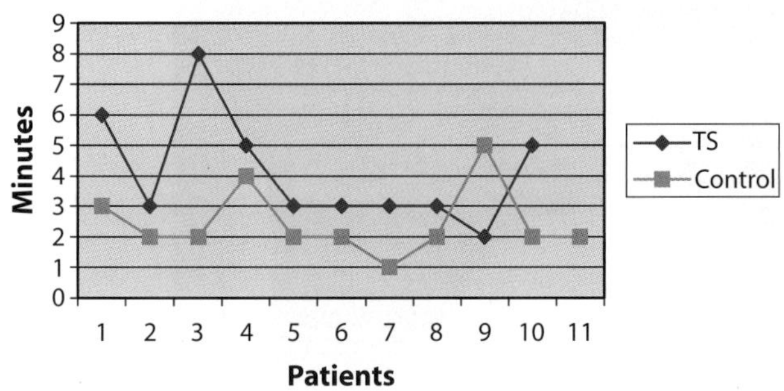

Fig. 7. Hiatal pillar closure time

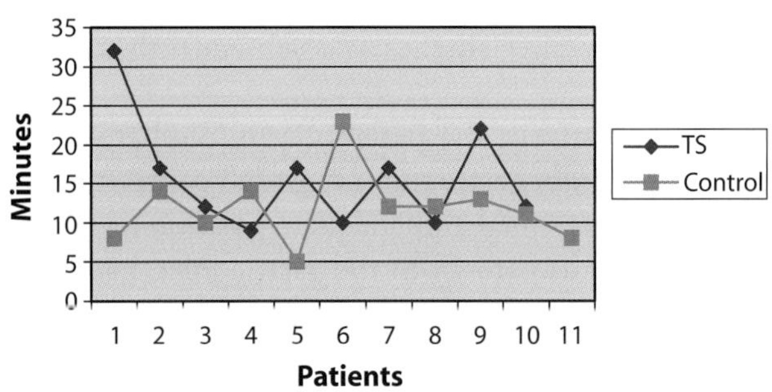

Fig. 5. Time for dissection of the great curve

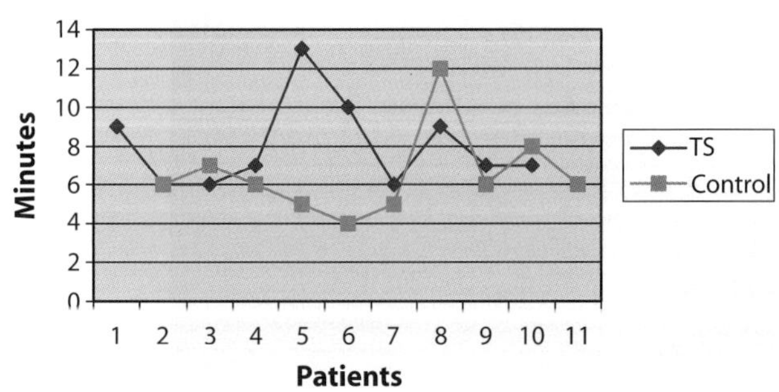

Fig. 8. Suturing time of the wrap

gastric dilation; the wrap perforated in the mediastinum and into both pleural spaces. At laparoscopic reexploration, the perforated fundus was resected and bilateral chest tubes were inserted. The patient left the hospital on the fourth post-operative day. The complication for the patient in the robot group occurred when there was a stomach perforation at the insertion of the first trocar. The perforation was immediately recognized and treated by laparoscopic suturing. The patient was allowed to leave the hospital on the fourth postoperative day.

The absence of morbidity directly related to this new technology is reassuring and encourages us to continue operating in this manner.

The *da Vinci* robot system

Experience with the robotic system led us to see the need for incorporating the computer in the surgeon's console, thus abolishing the need of an engineer. After many improvements in robotic systems, we began performing the Nissen fundoplication with a new prototype, *da Vinci*, which was installed in our hospital.

Major differences between Mona and *da Vinci*

(1) Overall, the Mona system was an early version of the *da Vinci* system. Mona had manually initiated mode transitions, inferior optics, and a reduced set of tools, compared with *da Vinci*.

(2) Control of the Mona system was done by an intuitive engineer through a graphical user interface. In other words, every mode transition (master of robot clutch, camera control, tool change, etc.) had to be voiced by the surgeon and then activated with a push button on a computer screen. This was slow and laborious, compared with the current setup where transitions are fast, seamless, and intuitive.

(3) Camera control for Mona was performed by a force-controlled joystick, whereas we now have a navigator algorithm. This arrangement was analogous to the mouse button on a laptop computer: the harder you push, the faster the pointer moves, as opposed to the action of the regular hand-held mouse. With Mona, it was difficult for the surgeon to go in the desired direction, and the transition time into camera control was slow because of the need to move the right master handle. The *da Vinci* provides intuitive and seamless navigator control.

(4) The procedures in Mexico City were done with a low-quality, single optical, three-dimensional system. This visual system did not provide the stereo separation or the resolution of our current insight visual system.

(5) The Mona system had no self-starting capabilities. As a result, a whole battery of tests had to be performed manually every morning prior to surgery.

(6) The set of instruments for Mona consisted of only rudimentary graspers and low-force needle drivers. Various types of graspers and more forceful needle drivers are now available to us. The instruments have since been adapted to Nissen fundoplication (*Figs. 9* and *10*).

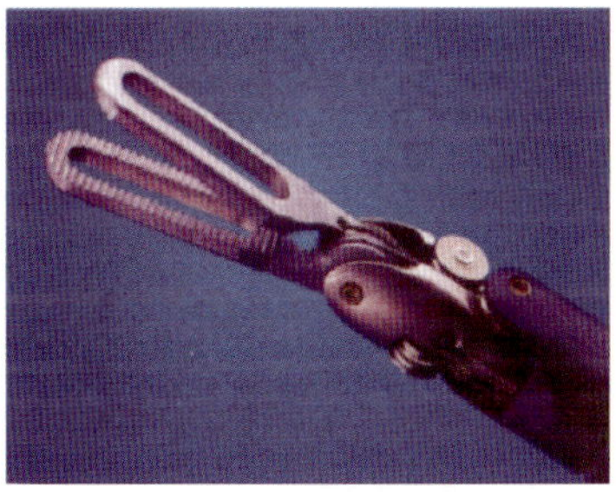

Cadiere Forceps

Fig. 9. Cadière Forceps

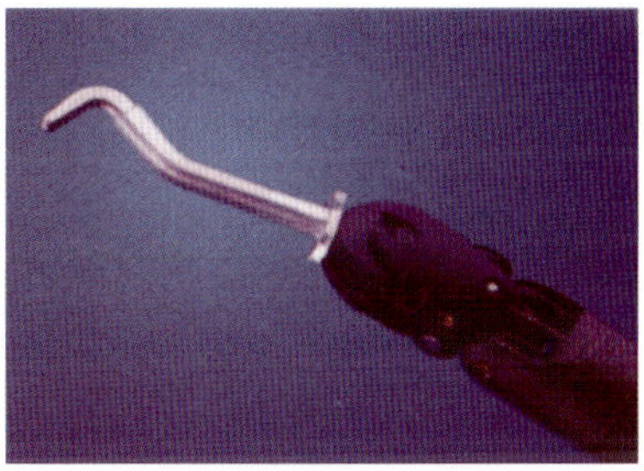

Electrocautery
with Hook

Fig. 10. Electrocautery with hook

We performed 39 procedures for gastroesophageal reflux (36 Nissen fundoplications and 3 Toupet procedures). In these procedures, we found that the ideal position for the robot was with the surgical cart located to the patient's right, at the level of the patient's head, at a 45-degree angle with the operating table axis. Three trocars are used for the robotic instruments and scope, another trocar is used for the liver retractor and a fifth trocar is used by the assistant (*Figs. 11* and *12*).

The median system time of the 21 Saint-Pierre Hospital patients was 82 minutes (range, 54 to 125). We had two complications: one perforation of the stomach by a trocar, which was repaired by robotic suturing; and one bleeding at the greater curvature, which was treated laparoscopically. The median hospital stay was 2 days (range, 1 to 4) (*Fig. 13*).

Discussion of global results

We believe that all procedures performed with a telemanipulated robot were actually world premieres for this type of surgery. Because of the novel character of the procedures, we were obliged to fully inform our patients on all possible implications of this new technology. It was also necessary to promptly determine if there was any morbidity specifically connected to the use of the robotic technique.

The operating times of the Nissen fundoplication for gastroesophageal reflux disease correlated with several parameters: (a) different operating locations (Paris, Brussels, Mexico City), (b) training of the entire team of doctors, nurses and technicians for this new technology, (c) surgeon's learning curve, as for any new operation, and (d) ongoing improvements in the system in terms of ergonomics, console setup, computer performance and tool development. Operative time depended not only on the surgical dissection, but also on installation of the system; it was comparable to that reported by the Academic Robotics Group (6). The procedure time, including all the setup, depended on the intensive training results of

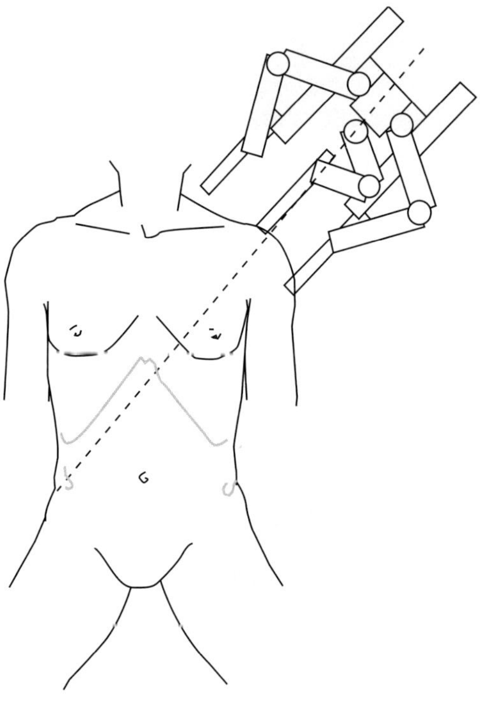

Fig. 11. Positioning of the robot

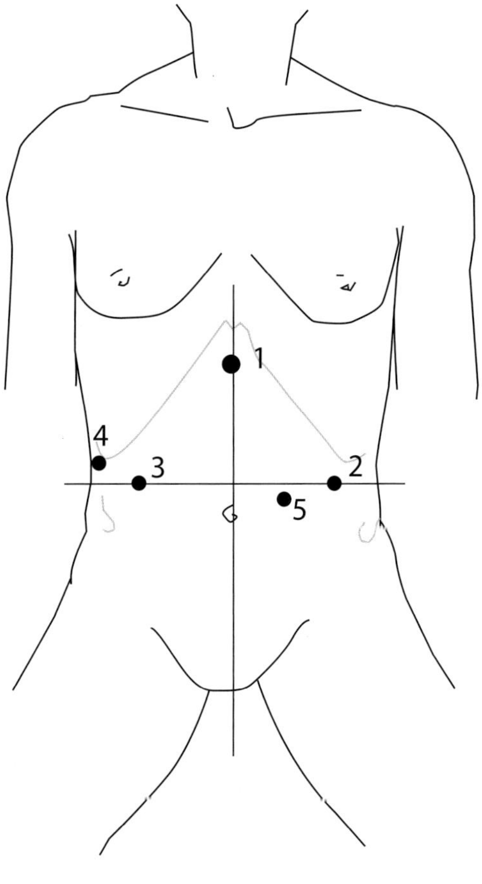

Fig. 12. Placement of the trocars

the surgical team. This novel type of surgery indeed created the need for a new team, a person dedicated exclusively to the well functioning of the robot during the procedure. We chose to call this person a clinical technician. This person needs a clinical as well as a technical background. His or her competence influences the time and the safety of the procedure. We encountered no morbidity specifically related to the use of robotics and the length of hospitalization was comparable with that of the conventional laparoscopic approach. Same results were also confirmed by the Academic Robotics Group [6].

The placement of the trocar was slightly different from that used in conventional laparoscopy because of the space occupied by the articulating robotic arms. Operative times compared favorably with our first 80 conventional laparoscopic procedures. Dissection behind and around the esophagus was clearly improved with the use of articulated tools. This finding suggests that may be possible in the future to perform a less extended dissection of the gastric cardia at the level of the peritoneal attachments. This dissection is performed only in the laparoscopic approach and only for reasons of safety. The articulated tools make the procedure easier, safer and more like open technique.

Another phase of the operation in which the articulation tools proved valuable was in the dissection of the short gastric vessels, facilitated by the fact that the tools could always be brought perpendicular to the vessels. On the other hand, we did become aware of a significant drawback of the robotic system in its present configuration: the three-dimensional optical system has a very narrow field of vision. Because of this, we had to continually interrupt dissection to reposition the optics. These frequent interruptions, as well as the absence of a general view of the operative field, may have been responsible for the bleeding we encountered while dissecting the greater curvature with the robotic system. This complication prompted the conversion to conventional laparoscopy.

The articulated tools made suturing the wrap a more straightforward procedure because it was easier to follow the curve of the needle while driving the suture through tissues. We also noticed a decided improvement in tying the knots. On the other hand, evaluating the tension on the knots is more difficult because there is no tactile feedback. The theoretical advantage gained by downscaling in the robotic technique we found to be insignificant [7].

Conclusion

We used robotic-assisted surgery and demonstrated the feasibility of having a standard robotic laparoscopic surgery without specific morbidity and within acceptable operative times. In its present configuration, the system seems to provide the greatest benefit for microsuturing within the abdomen or in very confined spaces. Improved ergonomic conditions and improved instrument dexterity at the level of the distal articulation appear to be of value in routine abdominal procedures. More research is needed for further improvement in tool design and optics arrangement. The robotic approach requires new operative strategies and modification of the pattern of trocar placement.

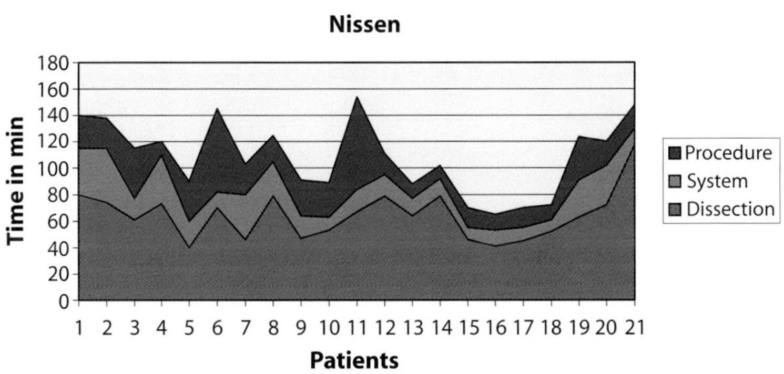

Fig. 13. Operative time for the latest 21 Nissen fundoplication procedures

References

[1] Berguer R, Rab GT, Abu-Ghaida H et al (1997) A comparison of surgeons' posture during laparoscopic and open surgical procedures. Surg Endosc 11: 139–142

[2] Wappler M (1995) Medical manipulators, a realistic concept? Minim Invas Ther Allied Technol 4: 261–266

[3] Himpens J, Leman G, Cadière GB (1998) Telesurgical laparoscopic cholecystectomy. Surg Endosc 12: 1091

[4] Cadière GB, Himpens J, Vertruyen M et al (1999) Nissen fundoplication done by remotely controlled technique. Ann Chir 53: 137–141

[5] Cadière GB, Houben JJ, Bruyns J et al (1994) Laparoscopic Nissen fundoplication technique and preliminary results. Br J Surg 81: 400–403

[6] Talamini MA, Chapman S, Horgan S, Melvin WS (2003) A prospective analysis of 211 robotic-assisted surgical procedures. Surg Endosc 17: 1521–1524

[7] Garcia-Ruiz A, Smedira NG, Loop FD et al (1997) Robotic surgical instruments for dexterity enhancement in thoracoscopic coronary artery bypass graft. J Laparoendosc Adv Surg Tech A 7: 277–283

SYMPTOMS, HEALTH-RELATED QUALITY OF LIFE AND PATIENT SATISFACTION: USING THESE PATIENT-REPORTED OUTCOMES IN PEOPLE WITH GASTROESOPHAGEAL REFLUX DISEASE

S. Wood-Dauphinee[1] and D. Korolija[2]

1 School of Physical and Occupational Therapy, Department of Epidemiology and Biostatistics, Department of Medicine, McGill University, Montreal, Quebec, Canada
2 University Surgical Clinic, Clinical Hospital Center Zagreb, Zagreb, Croatia

Introduction

Patient-reported outcomes, defined as any report coming directly from the person whose life is affected by a health problem, are becoming increasingly important in helping professionals determine the impact of their treatments. This represents a change in focus. Traditionally, clinicians and researchers were primarily interested in outcomes related to morbidity and mortality. This approach was consistent with the biomedical model of disease that relied on tests to identify pathology or changes in physiological processes. A treatment was judged to be successful if the biologic test returned to normal, as was often the case for acute conditions. A more recent approach, termed an outcomes model [1], suggests that medical care is designed to focus on how people feel and how they are able to function as well as how long they live. Measures of symptoms, health-related quality of life (HRQL) and patient satisfaction are considered to be appropriate outcomes. While there is clearly overlap between the models, the outcomes model focuses attention on the determinants of patient outcomes and relies primarily on reports by patients to judge the result of the treatment. It is particularly appropriate for diseases that are chronic in nature. Currently, it is believed that both types of outcomes are important. The physiological measures reflect the value system of the professionals and provide information that helps confirm their clinical impression. The patient-reported measures reflect the subjective evaluation and reporting of the illness experience and its treatment [2]. These measures reflect their value system.

A recent study from Austria [3] illustrates the different points of view of clinicians and patients in rating the importance of different outcomes. This study examined the expectations of patients with gastroesophageal reflux disease (GERD) in terms of the outcomes of laparoscopic anti-reflux surgery. Responses of 70 patients to open-ended questions provided the following information. Relief of GERD symptoms was expected by 92.8%; 84.3% anticipated a return to usual daily and work-related activities; and for 72.9% an improved quality of life was important. Successful surgery without complications was named by 52.9% of patients and protection from a future Barrett's esophagus or cancer was noted by 48.6%. Only two patients expected normalization of pH values and healing of the esophagus.

These results demonstrate that patients' expectations are generally different from those of the clinician. In fact, patients primarily seek medical care because of bothersome symptoms. It should, thus, be anticipated that symptom relief would be their top expectation. The ability to assume usual patterns of daily activities including work, as well as customary roles were also important. These latter factors are well-accepted components of quality of life as it relates to health, in other words HRQL, and this was also a priority of the patients. Satisfaction with the process and end result of surgery is another patient-reported outcome that reflects their expectations and degree to which they were met.

The purposes of this chapter are to describe the rational for using these patient-reported outcomes, the criteria by which the measures should be selected and how they can be used in both clinical research and daily surgical practice. Information will also be provided about available measures to assess these constructs in individuals with GERD.

Why are patient-reported outcomes useful in the care of individuals with GERD and in clinical studies of GERD?

Including patient-reported outcomes in clinical practice and in clinical studies of GERD provides several important benefits. First, as noted previously, it allows the clinician or the investigator to characterize the impact of GERD and its treatment in terms that are of value to and understood by the patients. In fact, patient-reported measures specifically reflect their point of view, as most often, patients provided input as to the content of the measures. Second, certain components of these patient-reported measures may be independent predictors of surgical outcomes. For example, measures of HRQL usually contain a component that assesses mental health in terms of anxiety and depression. It has been shown that people with these problems are less satisfied with the outcome of surgery than those without such psychiatric comorbidity [4], [5]. A change in symptoms may forecast increasing severity and this information may provide insight into the progression of GERD, or decreasing symptoms may denote treatment adherence or recovery. For instance, the resolution of heartburn is highly correlated with post-operative return to normal 24-h pH monitoring [6]. Thirdly, measures *of* symptoms are excellent indicators of the severity of the disease, and those assessing HRQL portray the impact on functioning, engagement in daily activities and participation in life events. Finally, data specifically related to patient satisfaction provide information on the quality of care provided. A well-developed measure of patient satisfaction will indicate both the patients' perceptions of the process of care and the outcomes of treatment. Surgeons in particular, have long been concerned with the results of surgical care that reflect the patient's subsequent health state [7]. This information is also useful to administrators and payers concerned with the quality of care.

Which patient-reported outcomes are important to measure?

Symptoms

Prior to surgery for GERD, patients undergo a number of objective tests including 24-hr pH monitoring, esophageal manometry, esophagastric duodenoscopy with a biopsy and histological examination of the gastroesophageal junction, as well as a careful history and assessment of symptoms. Traditionally, these pre-operative tests were repeated post-operatively at various points in time, and physiologic changes demonstrating normalization of pH values and lower esophageal sphincter pressure, along with the elimination of reflux that signified esophagitis healing, were used as indicators of operative success. Today, while the evaluations are similar, the overt surgical objective is mainly focussed on the alleviation of symptoms.

Symptoms have been defined by the Patient-reported Outcomes Harmonization Group in 2002 as "the subjective experience of abnormal function, sensations, or appearance, generally indicating disorder or disease" [8]. Surgeons aim to decrease the presence, severity, frequency and duration of symptoms, as they portray the sensory changes perceived by the patient [9]. Operative success is often judged by patient reports of few remaining or new symptoms, negligible complications and a limited need for further medications [10], [11].

A number of findings have led to this focus on symptoms. First, severity of the symptoms has not been found to be strongly associated with the pathological extent of the reflux or other physiological parameters. For example, studies of esophageal pH monitoring or manometry are not highly correlated with reported symptom severity [12], [13]. Symptoms and esophageal lesions do not always correlate strongly [14]. There are few differences in symptoms between patients with Barrett's esophagus, erosive and non-erosive GERD [15]. Some studies have found that surgery is of value for people with severe symptoms regardless of the endoscopic appearance of the esophageal mucosa [16], [17]. Finally, as mentioned previously, stress-related symptoms and psychiatric diagnoses are independent predictors of the surgical outcome [4], [5], [18], [19].

GERD may be associated with many symptoms but the primary one is heartburn. Others, including acid regurgitation, epigastric pain, belching, bloating, nausea, vomiting and dysphagia, may range from causing mild impairment to severe disability [20]. Despite the long standing interest in symptoms and the resent reaffirmation of their importance as outcomes, there appears to be no unified approach to the assessment of symptoms or an in-depth knowledge of the best way to do so, either in daily practice or research [21]. There is some agreement that self-report is the most appropriate approach [8], [22], partially because there is no strong correlation between patient and clinician reporting. In some circumstances, clinicians tend to underestimate the presence of symptoms and their severity compared to those who actually have GERD [23], and at other times, particularly when estimating treatment response, investigators report more positive results than do the patients [24].

Self-completed symptom questionnaires have been developed and validated and some examples will be presented later in the Chapter. There is, however, a tendency in the literature to use traditional, clinical, ordinal scales asking questions about the presence, frequency and severity of common symptoms, rather than standardized measures. In fact, surgical investigators frequently report the use of a "standard scale" but the meaning of the term is unclear. Information about the origin and psychometric properties is seldom provided.

In a recent international, multidisciplinary workshop [21], the issue of symptom reporting in trials was extensively addressed. Using heartburn as an example of a common, salient symptom in GERD, Bytzer [22] discussed issues related to its assessment that ranged from problems in defining heartburn itself, its severity, and frequency, to when, how and by whom heartburn and other symptoms should be measured. While a large number of symptom-response measures have been reported in the literature, there is little consistency of approach and a general lack of validation studies. In connection to this workshop, Wrywich and Staebler Tardino [25] provided a blueprint for creating symptom scales that uses a cognitive psychology framework approach to development. They also gave general information about developing optimal scales and interpreting their results.

In sum, there is considerable evidence that relief of symptoms caused by GERD is at times more complex than simply correcting the pathologic lesion. How patients perceive the sensations and respond to them must be taken into consideration. Because of the lack of physiological and pathologic markers for differentiating disease severity, an individual's description of his or her symptoms is a predominant source of information for the surgeon in making a diagnosis, monitoring a patient and assessing the outcomes of surgery [8], [21], [26]. Given the increasing importance of their use in outcomes assessment, increased attention to the development and validation of symptom scales is warranted.

Health-related quality-of-life

Patients seek medical care because of symptoms. Often, however, it is not because of their presence, or even their severity, but to the distress they cause the patient by intruding on daily activities and life in general. In other words, it is how the symptoms impact on their HRQL. In GERD it is evident how problems related to eating, drinking, sleeping, pain, and reduced vitality impair life's quality. In fact, it has been well documented that people with GERD have a lower quality of life than those without this disorder [27], [28].

While no one definition has received universal acceptance, there is a general consensus that measures of HRQL are multi-dimensional and should assess physical, mental, social and role-functioning, a person's perception of overall well-being and symptoms to a greater or lesser extent depending on the type of measure [29]. As noted by Guyatt and colleagues [30], HRQL is concept that embraces the World Health Organization's definition of health [31] by incorporating both personal health status and social well-being. It reflects peoples' subjective perceptions of how they feel and function.

There are two main types of HRQL measures [32]. Generic measures cover the full range of domains and can be used across different patient populations to compare the impact of various diseases. Some generic measures have normative data, by age and sex, from ostensively healthy populations. When available, these data make it possible to compare people with GERD, for example, to those without the condition, perhaps prior to and after surgery. Moreover, because generic measures are broad in scope, they sometimes help identify previously undisclosed problems that are not tapped by a measure specifically for people with GERD. This latter type of measure, known as disease-specific, focuses on the specific feelings, dysfunctions and symptoms associated with a given condition. They, therefore, are able to detect treatment effects and mirror changes in patient status.

Generic and disease-specific measures may be health profiles, which usually yield sub-scales for each domain allowing the assessment of interventions on the different components of HRQL, or utility measures, derived from economic and decision theory. These measures have preference weights incorporated in their scoring. Utility measures provide a single numerical estimate of HRQL that includes patient choices about both duration of life and its quality. Some profiles also generate a single number for analysis. Today, many studies use a combination of a generic and a disease-specific measure so that response to change is captured, but no important aspect of the person's HRQL is missed.

Finally, clinicians and investigators also use a single item to evaluate HRQL. While common, particularly in clinical practice, these single-item ratings have not usually been tested for their measurement properties, and are known not to be very reliable. Moreover, they provide no help in explaining why patients respond the way they do.

Patient satisfaction

Patient satisfaction is the patient's perceptions of both the quality of treatment provided and its effectiveness. A measure of satisfaction is one that documents patients' assessments or affective responses to different dimensions of the treatment experience [33]–[35]. Typically, it compares the process and outcomes of the treatment experience with prior expectations that may or may not have been met or surpassed [36], [37]. Although individual patients may have different expectations for the distinct components of treatment or care, their individual expectations and satisfaction with the various components are independent predictors of overall satisfaction [38].

Different conceptual frameworks for understanding patient satisfaction have been proposed [37], [39], and used as a basis for the development of measures. In general terms, the frameworks include sociodemographic, personal, medical and functional characteristics of the patients, their values, preferences and expectations of treatment outcome, prior experiences with treatment for the current and other disorders, the way treatment is delivered and experienced, as well as its impact on symptoms, function and HRQL. In some models, access, cost and convenience are incorporated. There has been at least one suggestion that satisfaction with the treatment process should be assessed separately from that of the outcome of the treatment [33].

In recent years, most surgical investigators evaluating the impact of various surgical procedures and approaches in GERD have selected patient satisfaction as one of the outcomes. In the majority of studies, the degree of satisfaction reported one to five years after the surgery was high. A few reports were not as glowing. For example, Bessell and colleagues [40] found that 27% of those patients who replaced severe preoperative heartburn preoperatively for severe dysphasia after the surgery would not have the surgery again.

Another study [41], assessing surgical outcomes in routine clinical practice rather than in a referral centre reported similar overall outcomes in the face of less positive data about complications, symptoms, and medication use after surgery as well as the need for post-surgical dilatation or repeat operations. These investigators attributed the positive global response regarding satisfaction to a type of measure that fails to include specific components of the process or outcomes of care [42]. This is not an uncommon finding. Global ratings of satisfaction tend to be positively skewed [43]. Patients rate high levels of satisfaction in the face of other negative information [43], [44]. Additionally, they tend to be less satisfied if asked about specific areas [44]. In fact, there are many problems with global single item ratings, although they are easy to use and intuitively appealing. Because the dimensions within the satisfaction construct are not named, it is not known what factors the patient took into consideration or excluded when making the rating, why elements received the assigned ratings, or how they were combined [45].

Other investigators [17], [46] used "standard" series of questions about such areas as the success of the surgery, whether or not the patient would again decide to undergo the surgery, and difficulties experienced since the operation. Each question was treated individually and provided descriptive information about the patients' responses. While somewhat more informative it is unknown if all salient aspects that are important to patients were included, and it is still difficult to form a concrete picture of the patient's judgement of the process and outcomes of care.

In summary, the single item ratings or questionnaires with only a few items used in surgical studies to assess patient satisfaction have not been carefully developed and examined for their psychometric properties. In other words, they have not been developed in the currently accepted rigorous manner [39].

To the best of our knowledge, only one group of researchers [47] has developed and validated a measure of patient satisfaction for GERD patients, the Treatment Satisfaction Questionnaire for Gastroesophageal reflux disease (TSQ-G). The measure was developed using input from patient focus groups, physicians and the literature and it was tested appropriately for reliability and validity. Unfortunately, the measure is targeted for GERD patients being managed by medications and, thus, is not appropriate as an outcome of surgery. Nonetheless, it is a model for the development of such a measure for use with patients undergoing surgery.

Our concerns about the assessment of treatment satisfaction mirror those of Revicki [48]. He pointed out that considerable attention needs to be given to the psychometric properties of satisfaction measures including the theoretical model that underpins the instrument, reliability, all types of validity and the interpretability of the numerical scores.

It should be noted that surgical investigators working in GERD are not alone in their difficulty assessing satisfaction. A few years ago an analysis of 195 studies found that little attention had been given to the development of satisfaction measures and this its self cast doubt on the credibility of the satisfaction findings [49]. It is an area that needs immediate attention. Specifically, we need to develop measures of satisfaction that reflect the components of global satisfaction such as personal expectations, indicators of quality of treatment as well as the outcomes of care as judged by the patients.

Issues in selecting patient-reported outcomes for use in clinical practice and research

First, we are interested in selecting standardized measures that are "evaluative" in purpose [50]. A standardized measure is one that has been published along with information about its psychometric properties, and instructions as to with whom, when and how it is to be administered, scored and interpreted. Conversely, "ad hoc" measures, most often created by clinicians, are those without formal testing or established measurement properties. An evaluative measure is designed to assess an individual at a baseline point, and again at one or more points later in time, principally to determine if change has occurred. Evaluative measures may also discriminate between different groups and predict future events as well.

The content if the instrument is of primary interest. While content may be influenced by the literature and information from clinicians, as alluded to previously, most content should come directly from patients and reflect their issues and concerns. There is a growing consensus that the "content" validity or the adequacy with which the items sample the construct being assessed by the measure, can only be judged by the persons being evaluated [2]. It is, thus, important that patients with the specific health problem have had major input. Assuring that this is the case is an early step in the selection process.

In general terms, validity refers to the ability of an instrument to measure what it is supposed to measure. Beyond "content", information on criterion and construct validity may be available. Criterion validity evaluates the relationship between the measure of interest and a criterion measure or "gold standard", concurrently or in the future. For concurrent criterion validity a new disease-specific measure of HRQL for people with GERD should correlate moderately with a well-known disease-specific measure of HRQL. While the criterion measure may not be "gold" it should at least be "silver"! For predictive criterion validity one may test if the score on a measure of HRQL taken two weeks after surgery will forecast return to work. Given the difficulty of finding gold standards for patient-reported measures, construct validity is more often reported. Construct validation examines if the measure performs according to theoretical expectations by examining the direction and magnitude of relationships with other variables. For example, one might hypothesize and test if a generic measure of HRQL can discriminate among groups of patients who have different levels of symptoms, or if it will negatively correlate with measure of pain. A measure of patient satisfaction following an anterior partial fundoplication for GERD should be positively correlated with the degree of symptom resolution or an objective outcome such as results from a 24-hr gastric pH monitoring.

Reliability reflects the extent to which a measure is free from random error and it refers to the reproducibility or stability of the measure over time. This is termed test-retest reliability. It also includes estimates of internal consistency, or how well the items in a scale relate to each other and to the total score. While there are several test statistics to assess reliability, the reliability coefficients are interpreted similarly. A coefficient of 0.89 means that 89% of the variance is true variance, related to the patients in the sample, and 11% is the amount of random error. For groups, as in research, a coefficient of 0.70 is the minimum level, but for use in clinical practice the minimum has been set between 0.85 and 0.90 [51].

The last psychometric property is responsiveness, or the ability of the measure to accurately detect patient change when it has occurred [52]. Most approaches to test responsiveness depend on assessing patients periodically over time during a period of anticipated change, and evaluating the change that occurs [53], [54]. While various approaches to quantifying responsiveness exist, clinical studies primarily report one of the variants of "effect size". Coined by Cohen [55], this term simply means a standardized, unitless measure of change. Today such variants are termed "effect sizes" [56], "standardized response means" [57] or "responsiveness statistics" [58].

Potential users of measures also need direction in how to interpret the score. By "interpretability" we mean the capacity to assign a qualitative meaning to a quantitative score [59]. One approach to the interpretation of change that is "distribution based" employs effect sizes [60]. Cohen [55] suggested that 0.2, 0.5 and 0.8 represent small, medium and large effect sizes. While these values are somewhat arbitrary [61], they are used in the literature. The second approach, termed "anchor-based" [60], examines the relationship between the change score on the instrument being tested to that on another measure that is well-known, associated with the test measure and clinically meaningful [61]. Population norms, severity classifications, symptom scores and global ratings of change by patients or physicians as well as the minimum important difference (MID) have all been used. The MID, the smallest change that patients perceive as beneficial [62], is another useful piece of information for potential users of a measure as it not only has implications for sample size in investigations, but it can provide some direction about how an individual patient is doing. Readers wishing more information on the psychometric properties of measures are referred to work by the Scientific Advisory Committee of the Medical Outcomes Trust [63].

In addition to knowledge about psychometric properties, the potential user of an instrument needs other information before making a choice. For example, does the timeframe associated with the questions or items fit the intended use? Patients can be asked to consider their responses in terms of the past 24 hours, a week, month or even a year. The choice depends on the typical illness or recovery trajectory of the patients or on the design of the study. Which response options are provided for the patient? Are they dichotomous (yes/no), made up of several ordinal categories (poor – fair – good – excellent) or presented as a visual analog scale? Are population norms available for the country of the study which can be used for comparison purposes? This is particularly useful for generic measures of HRQL so clinicians or investigators can compare their patients' or study subjects' scores to age- and sex-matched population values. What is the burden on subjects? More specifically, how long does the instrument take to complete, and does it include questions that are potentially upsetting for the patient? What is the burden on the professional? How easily is the measure scored? Can the scoring be automated? Does one have to obtain permission to use the measure, and if so, is there an associated cost? All of this information needs to be ascertained prior to selecting a measure.

Moreover, today, clinical research is conducted in countries around the world, and thus, the demand for instruments that can be used internationally has risen dramatically. By now many instruments have been culturally adapted, translated into different languages and then retested psychometrically to insure that the language, meaning and performance of the instrument remain consistent. There are different methods to enhance cross-cultural comparability, and while guidelines are available, [64]–[66] it is a time consuming process. Investigators or clinicians planning to use a patient-reported measure in their clinical practice or research project should determine if the measure they select has undergone such a process and is available for use.

Brief information about the psychometric properties of patient-reported measures used in people with

GERD and answers to some of the questions raised in this section of the Chapter are presented in Table 1, but such information accumulates over time, and so a potential user should refer to recent literature.

Patient-reported outcomes currently used in people with GERD

A number of articles have reviewed the development, psychometric performance and applications of patient-reported measures of symptoms and HRQL for people with GERD [67]–[71]. Table 1 revisits this information and presents those measures appearing in the surgical literature, along with information on the different domains tapped in each measure, the number of items per domain, the time-frame within which patients are to consider their responses and how the measures are scored. Additional information is provided about the approach to content development (specifically if patient input had been sought), other aspects of validity, estimates of reliability and how responsiveness has been examined. Some measures have information about the minimal important difference in score that patients can detect as well. When known, the languages in which the measure is available are stated in the text. It is acknowledged, however, that other language versions, unknown to the authors, may exist in the international literature.

The Gastrointestinal Symptom Rating Scale (GSRS) [72] and the Gastroesophageal Reflux Disease Health-related Quality of Life (GERD-HRQL) scale [73] have been available for a number of years and appear frequently in surgical investigations. Both these measures were recently recommended for use by the European Association for Endoscopic Surgery [74]. The GSRS has been used in Scandinavian, UK and US samples. The Symptom Questionnaire for Gastroesophageal Reflux Disease [75] is more recent and has been employed in one study of the long-term follow-up of patients after laparoscopic Nissen fundoplication [76].

The gastrointestinal-specific and the GERD-specific measures of HRQL have also been widely used in surgical studies. Both the Gastrointestinal Quality of Life Index (GIQLI) [77] and the Quality of Life in Reflux and Dyspepsia (QOLRAD) [78] were recommended by the European Association for Endoscopic Surgery [74], and the GIQLI [77] was recommended specifically for outcome assessment by the European Study Group for Antireflux Surgery [79]. It is available in English [77], French [80], German [81] and Spanish [82]. The QOLRAD was developed in French and English [78].

In terms of generic HRQL measures, people with GERD have mainly been assessed using two well-known measures – the Psychological General Well Being Index (PGWB Index) and the Medical Outcomes Study Short Form-36 (SF-36). These measures were recommended by the European Association for Endoscopic Surgery [74] partially because individuals with GERD score lower on these measures than ostensibly healthy individuals and their scores decrease as symptoms become more severe [83]–[85].

The PGWB Index was developed as a measure of subjective well-being or distress [86]. The Index is comprised of six domains, including anxiety, depressed mood, positive well-being, self control, general health and vitality. The domains contain 3–5 items, each of which is scored on a 6-point ordinal scale. Domain scores and a total score can be calculated. Higher values denote better quality of life. Internal consistency and test-retest reliability as well as construct and criterion validity were moderate to strong [86]–[89]. PGWB total scores were able to discriminate between individuals with and without heartburn [83]. Moreover, sensitivity to change in response to treatment has been demonstrated in patients with upper gastrointestinal symptoms [88]–[91] and a change of 4 points on the Index is a clinically meaningful difference in people with GERD [83]. Swedish norms are available [89].

The SF-36 is a generic measure of perceived health status that incorporates behavioural functioning, subjective well-being and perceptions of health, by assessing eight health concepts: limitations in physical activities due to health problems; limitations in role activities due to physical health problems; pain; limitations in social activities due to health problems; general mental health; limitations in usual role activities due to emotional problems; vitality; and general health perceptions [92]. The questionnaire is made up of 36 items that are divided into the 8 scales. The scores on all scales range from 0–100, with higher scores reflecting better health. There is also a computerized method of scoring two major components, physical and mental health. Each component has been standardized

Table 1. Patient-reported measures of symptoms and health-related quality of life used in surgical studies of people with GERD

1 Symptoms

Instrument	Domains	# of items	Time frame	Scoring	Reliability	Validity	Responsiveness
Gastrointestinal Symptom Rating Scale (GSRS) [72]	Reflux syndrome Abdominal pain Indigestion Diarrhea Constipation	2 3 4 3 3	Past 1–2 weeks	7-point ordinal scale [1–7] No Discomfort – Severe Discomfort Sum domain scores Calculate domain means Higher score → greater severity	Internal consistency: Alphas – Moderate to Moderately High [115]–[116] Test-retest: ICCs – Moderate to Moderately High [116]–[117]	Content: Developed using literature and professional input [72] Construct: Adequate; with SF-36 & PGWB Scales [116], [118] Discriminative Adequate; between different symptom severities & responses to treatment [83], [115], [116]	Effect Sizes and Standardized Response Means: Adequate [115]–[118] Minimal Important Difference: 0.5 per Item [117]
Gastroesophageal Reflux Disease Health-related Quality of Life Scale (GERD-HRQL) [73]	Heartburn Dysphagia Bloating Medication impact Satisfaction with condition	6 2 1 1 1	Current	6-point ordinal scale [0–5] No symptoms – Incapacitating Symptoms Sum 10 symptom items Higher score → greater severity 3-point categorical scale (Satisfied – Neutral – Unsatisfied)		Content: Face validity judged by clinicians Construct: Adequate; Correlates with degree of esophagitis [12] Discriminative Adequate; between satisfied/unsatisfied patients and medical/surgical treatments [73]	Pre-post treatment changes evident on symptom scale [73]
Symptom Questionnaire for Gastroesophageal Reflux Disease [75]	Heartburn Regurgitation Epigastric / chest pain Epigastric fullness	1 1 1 1	Current	4-point ordinal scale [0–3] Severity 5-point ordinal scale [0–4] Frequency Severity × Frequency =	Test-retest ICC – High [75]	Content: Face validity judged by clinicians Construct: Adequate Correlates with	Responsiveness Index: Adequate [75] Minimal Important

Table 1 (*continued*)

	Dysphagia Cough	1 1		[0–12] points per item Total Score = [0–72] Higher score → greater symptom impact		disease activity measures and SF36 cross-sectionally and longitudinally [75]	Difference = [5–10] points [75]
2 Health-related quality of life: gastrointestinal and disease-specific							
Gastrointestinal Quality of Life Index (GIGLI) [77]	Symptoms Emotional status Physical status Social activities Treatment stress	19 5 7 4 1	Past 2 weeks	5-point ordinal scale [0–4] Severity or frequency of symptoms, dysfunctions Total score [0–144] Higher score → Better HRQL	Internal Consistency Alpha – High [77] Test-retest ICC – high [77]	Developed by interviews with patients and clinicians and from the literature [77] Construct: Adequate; Correlates with measures of QOL & well-being [77] Data on normal people available [77]	Demonstrated expected gradient pre-pos surgery and follow-up [119], [120]
Quality of Life in Reflux and Dyspepsia (QOLRAD) [78]	Emotional distress Sleep disturbance Food/drink problems Physical/social functioning Vitality	5 5 6 5 4	Past week	7-point ordinal scale [1–7] Severity: none at all – a great deal Frequency: none of the time – all of the time Total score and domain scores Higher score → better HRQL	Internal Consistency Alphas – High (total and domain scores) [78] Test-retest ICC – Moderately High [117]	Developed by focus groups with patients (N.A., Australia and Europe), clinicians, and a literature review [78] Construct: Adequate; Correlates with SF-36 and GSRS [78] Discriminative Adequate; Better with symptom severity than frequency [78]	Effect Sizes and Standardized Response means Adequate [117] Minimal Important Difference: 0.5 per Item [15]

Abbreviations: ICC = Intraclass Correlation Coefficient; Alpha = Cronbach's alpha; QoL = Quality of Life
Reliability coefficients: 0.80+ = high; 0.60–0.79 = moderately high; 0.40–0.59 = moderate

to have a mean of 50 and a standard deviation of 10 [93]. One version of the SF-36 asks people to think about their health over the past four weeks and another version uses a one-week recall period.

Good to excellent internal consistency and test-retest reliability have been demonstrated in diverse patient groups including those with GERD [88], [94]. Subscales of the SF-36 (pain and general health perceptions) and the component summary scores were able to discriminate between people with GERD reporting no heartburn and those reporting heartburn symptoms [83]. Responsiveness to treatment has also been demonstrated in people with GERD [83], [88]. As part of an international initiative that used a standard protocol, the SF-36 has been translated, culturally adapted and revalidated in over 50 languages. Norms for many countries are available [95].

Issues in using patient-reported outcomes in clinical research

Using measures of symptoms, HRQL and patient satisfaction in surgical studies requires additional considerations in both the planning and execution of the investigation. Specific guidelines for selecting measures have already been discussed. This section will focus on the successful use of these measures in a study.

When stating the objectives in the study protocol it is important to identify that symptom resolution, improved HRQL or high satisfaction with the treatment are defined outcomes, each with a hypothesis attached to them and that they will be as rigorously evaluated as the more traditional outcomes. This is crucial in a multi-centered study so that these outcomes are not considered as "add-ons" by co-investigators who may treat them with less rigour than used with traditional assessments.

When patients are asked to participate in a study and informed consent is sought, they should also be told about the study and what participation will entail [96]. In studies using patient-reported outcomes this means that patients should agree to complete questionnaires or be interviewed face-to-face or over the telephone at specific points in time. Some trials have actually asked patients to complete a set of forms as part of the eligibility criteria. Providing this information up front and making sure that patients understand the commitment will help insure continued involvement. Moreover, patient-reported measures rely on the ability of the patient to provide the answers. The patient must, therefore, have sufficient reading ability or someone must read the questions to him or her to obtain the response. This is an acceptable practice, but ad hoc translating the question by a family member, a researcher or even a qualified translator is not permitted, as a bias may be introduced by the way the question is translated and asked [96]. While the use of proxy respondents has a place in research they are not patient-reported measures [2].

When designing the study, the timing of the assessments should be planned within the context of the surgery and the recovery trajectory [97]. Baseline assessments of symptoms and HRQL are essential in both observational and controlled studies. In both types, one comparison will be between pre-surgery and post-surgery at various points in the recovery trajectory. In a controlled trial the baseline assessment should be administered prior to randomization so as to eliminate any possible bias resulting from knowledge of the allocation either on the part of the patient or the individual administering the measure. This baseline assessment in a controlled situation also provides data for group comparisons at study entry as well as allowing between-group comparisons over time.

From the previous paragraph it is obvious that preoperative assessments are clearly important to provide baseline data. Yet, asking patients to complete questionnaires as they are waiting for imminent surgery is probably not the best time to have them provide reflective responses. Completion at an earlier point in time, perhaps at the last visit to the doctor, or through a telephone interview a few days prior to surgery might yield more considered answers.

Another issue to think about in terms of appropriate timing is that the immediate effects, particularly when an open approach to surgery for GERD is used, will be negative on most HRQL domains. Moreover, there will be after-effects and possibly new symptoms with which the patients must deal. However, by four weeks after the operation, patients will likely associate positive changes in eating, or level of pain with an improved quality of life. If one wants information on the patient's perceptions of the care process, assessments of treatment satisfaction are best made directly after discharge when details are fresh in patients' minds.

Satisfaction with the outcome of the operation, however, must wait a sufficient time until the person is fully recovered from the surgery itself and probably until the long-term effects are apparent.

The investigators should also plan where and how the assessments will be made. Where might be in the doctor's office, in a clinic or hospital or in the home [96]. Ideally it should take place in a consistent location but often this is impractical. A professional setting provides a milieu in which conditions are more controllable and personnel responsible for administering the questionnaires can make sure that the patient completes it without input from family or friends [96]. Telephone interviews, however, are widely used, provide data similar to face-to-face interviews [98] and control for timing and patient completion. If an external person is involved in administering the questionnaire, that individual should not be part of the treatment team and preferably should be unaware of the objective of the study and the group assignment if it is a controlled trial. Providing questionnaires for patients to complete at a later date, or mailing questionnaires for completion are other accepted approaches but ones that often result in considerable missing data.

Several points are important to remember. We know that data obtained from self-completed forms are slightly different for those obtained through interviews so it is preferable to select one approach [99]–[101]. Feasibility may dictate, however, that administrative modes are mixed. In any case, detailed instructions must be provided to personnel responsible for collecting the data and procedures should be established that facilitate compliance with questionnaire completion. It is also essential to clarify what should be done with the questionnaire when completed. Most often direct entry using computers and electronic transmission is used. Sometimes patients respond directly on a computer. Instructions on preserving confidentiality are also essential.

Detailed descriptions of analytic methods are clearly beyond the scope of this chapter, and so only a few general points will be made. First, it is important to have statistical expertise when the study is being planned. HRQL or symptom scores are seldom the primary endpoints upon which sample size is calculated, and therefore, investigators need to be sure that they have sufficient subjects to make the comparisons they plan. Moreover, most HRQL measures are multidimensional and made up of subscales. This again may increase the number of endpoints. Not only do we select one or more multidimensional measures, but we make measures at several points in time. An outline for data analysis should, thus, be made in the planning stages. All these issues are within the purview of the statistician or someone very familiar with multi-level and multivariate analyses.

Finally, procedures to contend with missing items within measures, or missing data forms need to be defined. Missing data within a measure are generally dealt with according to the following process. If at least 50% of the questions or items in a subscale have been completed, a mean score calculated for that subscale can be imputed to replace the missing values. While this may decrease the variance in the data, it will probably not have a major impact on the results [102], [103]. Missing forms are more of a problem. If they are missing at random because someone forgot to mail the questionnaire to the patient or the patient missed a follow visit because he or she was on a holiday, it is not too serious. Forms not missing at random, which is the more common scenario, may be telling us that the patient is sicker (or healthier) or perhaps more upset with the results of treatment than the average patient. In other words there may be a health-related reason that the questionnaire was not completed. For these cases it is important that a protocol is developed to handle the situation. Several options are available and all rely on statistical expertise and use of appropriate statistical packages [103].

In clinical practice

While symptoms have traditionally been assessed, advocates of patient-reported outcomes have supported the use of other such measures in daily clinical practice. In particular, the assessment of HRQL has been seen as an aid to screening for unidentified problems, making decisions about treatment, monitoring patient status and response to treatment, as well as a mechanism for quality assurance [104]. Barriers, however, were identified to routine use for conceptual, methodological, practical and attitudinal reasons [105]. Scepticism about the importance of the measures was voiced. Practitioners preferred traditional, pathologic or physiologic tests and did not understand the usefulness of information from both types of measures. They cited time and resource constraints, and were concerned about the costs of administering the tools, collecting the information, compiling it rapidly, interpreting and using it.

Over the years a number of these concerns have been addressed. Studies have shown that assessing HRQL in different practice settings is feasible and is easily incorporated into the office or clinic routine [106]. Briefer and more precise disease-specific measures have been developed and computer-assisted technology is available to provide instant scoring and feedback to the clinicians. Information about population values and the amount of change in patient status required to reflect an important difference, as perceived by the patient, have added ease to the interpretation of the scores.

A number of studies, both controlled trials and other designs, have investigated the impact of the use of HRQL information on the doctor-patient communication. To summarize, the provision of information to the clinician seems to have an impact on the process of care. It increases the identification of previously unrecognized problems [107]–[109], improves doctor-patient communication and facilitates more emotional support for patients [107], [110], and increases physicians' awareness of their patients' problems and concerns [106], [107]. Moreover, the process was perceived as useful by most physicians and it was acceptable to patients and office and clinic staff [108], [109]. Finally, it did not significantly increase the time of the doctor-patient interaction [110]. The impact of providing HRQL information to the clinicians appears to have had less impact on the outcomes of care. With the exception of the systematic review by Espallargues and colleagues [109], there was no reported impact on patient satisfaction, which was generally high [107], [111]. There was also little evidence of change in management decisions as the result of HRQL knowledge [107], [111], and most studies did not find that it influenced health-related quality of life. There is, however, some recent evidence in people with cancer that providing HRQL information to the clinician, positively impacted the patient's HRQL particularly in mental health and role performance areas [112].

The studies referenced in the previous paragraph were all conducted using patients with problems other than GERD. While the use of patient-reported outcomes in follow-up after an operation was often reported in the GERD literature, articles related to the value of these tools in clinical decision-making was very scarce. One study conducted in Montreal [113], had been presented at the 58th Annual Meeting of the Central Surgical Association in 2001. The ensuing discussion included questions to the presenting author and these questions and their answers were provided at the end of the article. One question was about the practical use of continued assessment of HRQL and why a simple satisfaction rating scale was not sufficient. Her responses indicated that the 5-point satisfaction measure varied little across patients and this was not sufficient as a sole endpoint, but that the HRQL scores yielded practical information. For example, if there were unexpected responses on the questionnaire, patients were asked to return to the clinic for re-studies. As was pointed out by the author, after you start to use HRQL questionnaires and "you get a feel for what is normal and abnormal, they help drive decision-making in a practical way". Hopefully, patient-reported measures will be seen as an adjunct to traditional care in the future. Their use can be seen as formalizing what clinicians have been implicitly doing for ever when they ask a patient "How are you?"

Conclusions

Patient reported outcomes have been advocated following surgery for GERD for the past several years [114]. Those outlined in this chapter, as well as others such as "adherence to treatment", are important for measuring the impact of GERD and its treatment. Clinicians and researchers who use these measures should select them carefully according to their reliability, validity and responsiveness, as well as to information about how the score is interpreted. It is also important to think about how traditional, objective tests are related to patient-reported measures, and to use each type as appropriate. Objective tests and measures provide information about the medical status of the patient that is essential for management of the disease. Patient-reported measures give information about the individual's perception of the symptoms and dysfunctions and how they impact on the quality of their lives before and in response to treatment. Both are important.

References

[1] Kaplan RM (2002) Quality of life: An outcomes perspective. Arch Phys Med Rehabil 83 (Suppl 2): S44–S50

[2] Patrick DL (2003) Patient-reported outcomes (PROs): an organizing tool for concepts, measures and applications. Qual Life Newsletter 31: 1–5

[3] Kamolz T, Pointer R (2002) Expectations of patients with gastroesophageal reflux disease for the outcome of laparoscopic antireflux surgery. Surg Laparosc Endo Percutan Tech 12: 389–392

[4] Velanovich V, Karmy-Jones R (2001) Psychiatric disorders affect outcomes of antireflux operations for gastroesophageal reflux disease. Surg Endosc 15: 171–175

[5] Velanovich V (2003) The effect of chronic pain syndromes and psychoemotional disorders in symptomatic and quality of life outcomes of antireflux surgery. J Gastrointest Surg 7: 53–58

[6] Eubanks TR, Omelanczuk P, Richards C et al (2000) Outcome of laparoscopic antireflux procedures. Am J Surg 179: 391–395

[7] Codman EA (1914) The product of a hospital. Surg Gyn Obst 18: 491–496

[8] McColl E (2004) Best practice in symptom assessment: a review. Gut 53 (Suppl IV): IV49–IV54

[9] Price DD, Harkins SW, Baker C (1987) Sensory-affective relationships among different types of clinical and experimental pain. Pain 28: 297–307

[10] Stein HJ, Feussner H, Siewert JR (1998) Antireflux surgery: a current comparison of open and laparoscopic approaches. Hepatogastroenterology 45: 1328–3337

[11] Pope CE II (1992) The quality of life following antireflux surgery. World J Surg 16: 355–358

[12] Velanovich V, Karmy-Jones R (1998) Measuring gastroesophageal reflux disease: relationship between health-related quality-of-life scores and physiologic parameters. Am Surg 64: 649–653

[13] Shi G, Tatum RP, Joehl RJ et al (1999) Esophageal sensitivity and symptom perception in gastroesophageal reflux disease. Curr Gastroenterol Rep 1: 214–219

[14] Katzka DA (1999) Digestive system disorders: gastroesophageal reflux disease. Clin Evidence 1: 145–153

[15] Kulig M, Leodolter A, Vieth M et al (2003) Quality of life in relation to symptoms in patients with gastro-oesophageal reflux disease – an analysis based on the ProGERD initiative. Aliment Pharmacol Ther 18: 767–776

[16] Watson DI, Foreman D, Devitt PG (1997) Preoperative endoscopic grading of esophagitis versus outcome after laparoscopic Nissen fundoplication. Am J Gastroenterol 92: 222–225

[17] Bammer T, Freeman M, Shabriari A et al (2002) Outcome of laparoscopic antireflux surgery in patients with nonerosive reflux disease. J Gastointest Surg 6: 730–737

[18] Kamolz T, Bammer T, Granderath FA et al (2001) Laparoscopic antireflux surgery in gastro-oesophageal reflux disease patients with concomitant anxiety disorders. Dig Liver Dis 33: 659–664

[19] Kamolz T, Granderath FA, Pointner R (2003) Does major depression affect the outcome of laparoscopic antireflux surgery? Surg Endosc 17: 55–60

[20] Falk GW (2001) Gastroesophageal reflux disease and Barrett's esophagus. Endoscopy 33: 109–118

[21] Dent J, Armstrong D, Delaney B et al (2004) Symptom evaluation in reflux disease: workshop background, processes, terminology, recommendations and discussion outputs. Gut 53 (Suppl IV): IV1–IV24

[22] Bytzer P (2004) Assessment of reflux symptom severity: methodological options and their attributes. Gut 53 (Suppl IV): IV28–IV34

[23] Stephens RJ, Hopwood P, Girling DJ et al (1997) Randomized trials with quality of life end-points: are doctors' ratings of patients' physical symptoms interchangeable with patients self-ratings? Qual Life Res 6: 225–236

[24] Sandmark S, Carlsson R, Fausa O et al (1988) Omeprazole or ranitidine in the treatment of reflux esophagitis. Results of a double-blind, randomized Scandinavian multicenter study. Scand J Gastroenterol 23: 625–632

[25] Wyrwich KW, Staebler Tardino VM (2004) A blueprint for symptom scales and responses: measurement and reporting. Gut 53 (Suppl IV): IV45–IV48

[26] Shaw M (2004) Diagnostic utility of reflux disease symptoms. Gut 53 (Suppl IV): IV25–IV27

[27] Revicki DA, Wood M, Maton PN et al (1998) The impact of gastroesophageal reflux disease on health-related quality of life. Am J Med 104: 252–258

[28] Eloubeidi MA, Provenzale D (2000) Health-related quality of life and severity of symptoms in patients with Barrett's esophagus and gastroesophageal reflux disease patients without Barrett's esophagus. Am J Gastroenterol 95: 1881–1887

[29] Berzon RA, Hays RD, Shumaker SA (1993) International use, application and performance of health-related quality of life instruments. Qual Life Res 2: 367–368

[30] Guyatt GH, Feeny DH, Patrick DL (1993) Measuring health-related quality of life. Ann Intern Med 118: 622–629
[31] World Health Organization (1948) WHO Constitution. Geneva WHO
[32] Guyatt G, Veldhuyzen Van Zanten S, Feeny D et al (1989) Measuring quality of life in clinical trials: a taxonomy and review. Can Med Assoc J 140: 1441–1448
[33] Hudak PL, Wright JG (2000) The characteristics of patient satisfaction measures. Spine 25: 3167–3177
[34] Linder-Pelz S (1982) Toward a theory of patient satisfaction. Soc Sci Med 16: 577–582
[35] Ware JE, Davies-Avery A, Stewart AL (1978) The measurement and meaning of patient satisfaction. Health Med Care Serv Rev 1: 13–15
[36] Kravitz RL (1996) Patients' expectations for medical care: an expanded formulation based on review of the literature. Med Care Res Review 53: 3–27
[37] Patrick DL, Martin ML, Bushnell DM et al (2003) Measuring satisfaction with migraine treatment: expectations, importance, outcomes and global ratings. Clin Ther 25: 2920–2935
[38] Locker D, Dunt D (1978) Theoretical and methodological issues in sociological studies of consumer satisfaction with medical care. Soc Sci Med 12: 283–292
[39] Weaver M, Patrick DL, Markson PD et al (1997) Issues in the measurement of treatment satisfaction. Am J Manag Care 3: 579–594
[40] Bessell JR, Finch R, Gotley DC et al (2000) Chronic dysphagia following laparoscopic fundoplication. Br J Surg 87: 1341–1345
[41] Vakil N, Shaw M, Kirby R (2003) Clinical effectiveness of laparoscopic fundoplication in a U.S. community. Am J Med 114: 1–5
[42] Cleary P, McNeil B (1998) Patient satisfaction as an indicator of quality of care. Inquiry 22: 25–36
[43] Patrick DL, Erickson P (1993) Health status and health policy: quality of life in health care evaluation and resource allocation. Oxford University Press, New York
[44] Dougall A, Russel A, Rutin G et al (2000) Rethinking patient satisfaction: patient experiences of an open access flexible sigmoidoscopy service. Soc Sci Med 50: 53–62
[45] Feinstein AR (1987) Global indexes and scales. In: Clinimetrics. Yale University Press, New Haven, pp 91–103
[46] Granderath FA, Kamolz T, Schweiger M et al (2002) Long term follow-up after laparoscopic refundoplication for failed antireflux surgery: quality of life, symptomatic outcome, and patient satisfaction. J Gastrointest Surg 6: 812–818
[47] Coyne KS, Wiklund I, Schmier J et al (2003) Development and validation of a disease-specific treatment satisfaction questionnaire for gastro-oesophageal reflux disease. Ailment Pharmacol Ther 18: 907–915
[48] Revicki DA (2004) Patient assessment of treatment satisfaction: methods and practical issues. GUT 53 (Suppl IV): IV40–IV44
[49] Sitzia J (1999) How valid and reliable are patient satisfaction data? An analysis of 195 studies. Int J Qual Health Care 11: 319–328
[50] Kirshner B, Guyatt G (1985) A methodological framework for assessing health indices. J Chron Dis 38: 27–36
[51] Portney LG, Watkins MP (2000) Reliability. In: Foundations of clinical research: applications to practice (2nd ed), Prentice Hall Health, New Jersey, pp 61–77
[52] de Bruin AF, Diederiks JPM, de Witte LP et al (1997) Assessing the responsiveness of a functional status measure: the Sickness Impact Profile versus the SIP68. J Clin Epidemiol 50: 529–540
[53] Husted JA, Cook RJ, Farewell VT et al (2000) Methods for assessing responsiveness: a critical review and recommendations. J Clin Epidemiol 53: 459–468
[54] Terwee CB, Dekker FW, Wiersinga WM et al (2003) On assessing responsiveness of health-related quality of life instruments: guidelines for instrument evaluation. Qual Life Res 12: 349–362
[55] Cohen J (1988) Statistical power analysis for the behavioral sciences. 2nd ed. Hillsdale: Laurence Erlbaum
[56] Kazis L, Anderson J, Meenan R (1989) Effect sizes for interpreting changes in health status. Med Care 27 (Suppl): 178–189
[57] Liang MH, Fossel AH, Larson MG (1990) Comparisons of five health status instruments for orthopaedic evaluation. Med Care 28: 632–642
[58] Guyatt G, Walter S, Norman G (1987) Measuring change over time: assessing the usefulness of evaluative instruments. J Chron Dis 40: 171–178
[59] Ware JE, Keller SD (1996) Interpreting general health measures. In: Quality of life and pharmacoeconomics in clinical trials (Spilker B, ed). Philadelphia: Lippencott-Raven, pp 445–460
[60] Lydick EG, Epstein RS (1993) Interpretation of quality of life changes. Qual Life Res 2: 221–226
[61] Guyatt G, Osoba D, Wu A et al (2002) Methods to explain the clinical significance of health status measures. Mayo Clin Proc 77: 371–383

[62] Jaeschke R, Singer J, Guyatt GD (1989) Measurement of health status: ascertaining the minimal clinically important difference. Control Clin Trials 10: 407–415

[63] Scientific Advisory Committee of the Medical Outcomes Trust (2002) Assessing health status and quality of life instruments: attributes and review criterion. Qual Life Res 11: 193–205

[64] Acquadro C, Jambon B, Ellis D et al (1996) Language and translation issues. In: Quality of life and pharmacoeconomics in clinical trials (Spilker B, ed). Philadelphia: Lippencott-Raven, pp 575–585

[65] Guillemin F, Bombardier C, Beaton D (1993) Cross-cultural adaptation of health-related quality of life measures: literature review and proposed guidelines. J Clin Epidemiol 46: 1417–1432

[66] Bullinger M, Power MJ, Aaronson NK et al (1996) Creating and evaluating cross-cultural instruments. In: Quality of life and pharmacoeconomics in clinical trials (Spilker B, ed). Philadelphia: Lippencott-Raven, pp 659–668

[67] Yacavone RF, Locke R, Provenzale DT et al (2001) Quality of life measurement in gastroenterology: what is available? Am J Gastroenterol 96: 285–297

[68] Eisen GM, Locke GK, Provenzale D (1999) Health-related quality of life: a primer for gastroenterologists. Am J Gastro Enterol 94: 2017–2021

[69] Kamolz T, Pointer R, Velanovich V (2003) The impact of gastroesophageal reflux disease on quality of life. Surg Endosc 17: 1193–1199

[70] Irvine EJ (2004) Quality of life assessment in gastro-oesophageal reflux disease. GUT 53 (Suppl IV): IV35–IV39

[71] Borgaonkar MR, Irvine EJ (2000) Quality of life measurement in gastrointestinal and liver disorders. GUT 47: 444–454

[72] Svedlund J, Sjödin I, Dotevall G (1988) GSRS – A clinical rating scale for gastrointestinal symptoms in patients with irritable bowel syndrome and peptic ulcer disease. Dig Dis Sci 33: 129–134

[73] Velanovich V, Vallance SR, Gusz JR et al (1996) Quality of life scale for gastro-esophageal reflux disease. J Am Coll Surg 183: 217–224

[74] Korolija D, Sauerland S, Wood-Dauphinee S et al (2004) Evaluation of quality of life after laparoscopic surgery. Evidence-based guidelines of the European Association of Endoscopic Surgery. Surg Endosc 18: 879–897

[75] Allen CJ, Parameswaran K, Belda J et al (2003) Reproducibility, validity and responsiveness of a disease-specific symptom questionnaire for gastroesophageal reflux disease. Dis Esophagus 13: 265–270

[76] Anvari M, Allen C (2003) Five-year comprehensive outcomes evaluation in 181 patients after laparoscopic Nissen fundoplication. Am Coll Surg 196: 51–59

[77] Eypasch E, Williams J, Wood Dauphinee S et al (1995) Gastrointestinal Quality of Life Index: development, validation and application of a new instrument. Br J Surg 82: 216–222

[78] Wiklund IK, Junghard O, Grace E et al (1998) Quality of life in reflux and dyspepsia patients. Psychometric documentation of a new disease-specific questionnaire (QOLRAD). Eur J Surg 164 (Suppl 583): 41–49

[79] Fuchs KH, Feussner H, Bonavina L et al (1997) Current status and trends in laparoscopic anti-reflux surgery: results of a consensus meeting. Endoscopy 29: 298–308

[80] Slim K, Bousquet J, Kwiatkowski F et al (1999) First validation of the French version of Gastrointestinal Quality of Life Index (GIQLI). Gastroenterol Clin Biol 23: 25–31

[81] Eypasch E, Wood Dauphinee S, Williams JI et al (1993) Der Gastrointestinale Lebensqualiitäts-Index (GLQI). Der Chirurg 64: 264–274

[82] Quintana JM, Cabriada J, De Lòpez Tejada I et al (2001) Translation and validation of the Gastrointestinal Quality of Life Index (GIQLI). Rev Esp Enferm Dig 93: 693–706

[83] Revicki DA, Crawley JA, Zodet MW et al (1999) Complete resolution of heartburn symptoms and health-related quality of life in patients with gastro-oesophageal reflux disease. Aliment Pharmacol Ther 13: 1621–1630

[84] Kaplan-Machlis B, Spiegler GE, Revicki DA (1999) Health-related quality of life in primary care patients with gastrointestinal reflux disease. Ann Pharmacother 33: 1032–1036

[85] Ofman JJ (2003) The economic and quality-of-life impact of symptomatic gastroesophageal reflux disease. Am J Gastroenterol 98: S9–S14

[86] Dupuy HJ (1984) The Psychological General Well-Being (PGWB) Index. In: Wegner NK, Mattson ME, Furberg CF, Elinson J (eds) Assessment of quality of life in clinical trials of cardiovascular therapies. Le Jadq Publishing Inc., pp 170–183

[87] Nilsson G, Larsson S, Johnsson F (2002) Randomized clinical trial of laparoscopic versus open fundoplication. Scand J Gastroenterol 37: 385–391

[88] Rothman M, Farup C, Stewart W et al (2001) Symptoms associated with gastroesophageal reflux disease: Development of a questionnaire for use in clinical trials. Dig Dis Sci 46: 1540–1548
[89] Dimenäs E, Carlsson G, Glise H et al (1996) Relevence of norm values as part of the documentation of quality of life instrument for use in upper gastrointestinal disease. Scand J Gastroenterol 31 (Suppl 221): 8–13
[90] Glise IT, Halterbach B, Johansson B (1995) Quality of life assessment in the evaluation of gastrointestinal reflux and peptic ulcer disease before, during and after treatment. Scand J Gastroenterol 30 (Suppl 208): 133–135
[91] Revicki DA, Leidy NK, Howland L (1996) Evaluating the psychometric characteristics of the Psychological General Well-Being Index with a new response scale. Qual Life Res 5: 417–423
[92] Ware JE, Sherbourne CD (1992) The MOS 36-item short-form health survey (SF-36). I. Conceptual framework and item selection. Med Care 30: 473–483
[93] Ware JE, Kosinski M, Keller SD (1994) SF-36 Physical and Mental Health Summary Scales: A user's manual. The Health Institute, New England Medical Center, Boston
[94] McHorney CA, Ware JE Jr, Lu JF et al (1994) The MOS 36-item Short-Form Health Survey (SF-36): III. Tests of data quality, scaling assumptions, and reliability across diverse patient groups. Med Care 32: 40–66
[95] Gandek B, Ware JE (1998) Translating functional health and well-being: International Quality of Life Assessment (IQOLA) project studies of the SF-36 health survey. J Clin Epidemiol 51: 903–1214
[96] Osoba D (1998) Guidelines for measuring health-related quality of life in clinical trials. In: Quality of life assessment in clinical trials (Staquet MJ, Hays RD, Fayers PM, eds). Oxford: Oxford University Press, pp 19–35
[97] Osoba D (1996) Rationale for the timing of health-related quality-of-life (HQL) assessments in oncological palliative therapy. Can Treat Rev 22 (Suppl A): 69–73
[98] Korner-Bitensky N, Wood-Dauphinee S, Williams JI et al (1994) Eliciting health related information post-discharge: telephone versus face-to-face interviewing. Arch Phys Med Rehabil 75: 1286–1296
[99] Cook D, Guyatt G, Juniper E et al (1993) Interviewer versus self-administered questionnaires in developing a disease-specific, health-related quality of life instrument for asthma. J Clin Epidemiol 46: 529–534
[100] Weinburger M, Oddone EZ, Sainsa G et al (1996) Are health related quality of life measures affected by the mode of administration? J Clin Epidemiol 49: 135–140
[101] Chambers LW, Haight M, Norman G et al (1987) Sensibility to change and the effect of mode of administration. Med Care 21: 551–567
[102] Fairclough DL (1998) Methods of analysis for longitudinal studies of health-related quality of life. In: Quality of life assessment in clinical trials (Staquet MJ, Hays RD, Fayers PM, eds). Oxford: Oxford University Press, pp 227–247
[103] Fairclough DL (2004) Patient reported outcomes as endpoints in medical research. Stat Meth Med Res 13: 115–138
[104] Lohr KN (1992) Application of health status assessment measures in clinical practice. Med Care 30: MS1–MS14
[105] Deyo RA, Patrick DL (1989) Barriers to the use of health status measures in clinical investigation of patient care and policy research. Med Care 27: S254–S267
[106] Kazis LE, Callahan LF, Meenan RF et al (1990) Health status reports in the care of patients with arthritis. J Clin Epidemiol 43: 1243–1253
[107] Detmar SB, Muller MJ, Schornagel JH et al (2002) Health-related quality-of-life assessments and patient-physician communication. JAMA 288: 3027–3034
[108] Wagner AK, Ehrenberg BL, Tran TA et al (1997) Patient-based health status measurement in clinical practice: a study of its impact on epilepsy patients' care. Qual Life Res 6: 329–341
[109] Espallargues M, Valderas JM, Alonso G et al (2000) Provision of feedback on perceived health status to healthcare professionals. Med Care 38: 175–186
[110] Detmar SB, Aaronson NK (1998) Quality of life assessment in daily clinical oncology practice: a feasibility study. Eur J Cancer 34: 1181–1186
[111] McLachlan S-A, Allenby J, Wirth A et al (2001) Randomized trial of coordinated psychosocial intervention based on patient assessments versus standard care to improve social functioning of patients with cancer. J Clin Oncol 19: 4117–4125
[112] Velikova G, Brown JM, Booth L et al (2002) A randomized study of using regular quality of life measurement in the care of individual cancer patients. Qual Life Res 11: 631

[113] Feldman LS, Mayrand S, Stanbridge D et al (2001) Laparoscopic fundoplication: a model for assessing new technology in surgical procedures. Surgery 130: 686–695

[114] Eypasch E, Neugebauer E, Fisher F et al (1997) Laparoscopic antireflux surgery for gastroesophageal reflux disease (GERD). Results of a Consensus Development Conference. Surg Endosc 11: 413–426

[115] Dimenäs E, Glise H, Hallerback B et al (1995) Well-being and gastrointestinal symptoms among patients referred to endoscopy owing to suspected duodenal ulcer. Scand J Gastroenterol 30: 1046–1052

[116] Revicki DA, Wood M, Wiklund I et al (1998) Reliability and validity of the gastrointestinal symptom rating scale in patients with gastroesophageal reflux disease. Qual Life Res 7: 75–82

[117] Talley NJ, Fullerton S, Junghard O et al (2001) Quality of life in patients with endoscopy-negative heartburn: reliability and sensitivity of disease-specific instruments. Am J Gastroenterol 96: 1998–2004

[118] Dimenäs E, Glise H, Hallerback B et al (1993) Quality of life in patients with upper gastrointestinal symptoms. An improved evaluation of treatment regimens? Scand J Gastroenterol 28: 681–687

[119] Mobius C, Stein HJ, Feith M et al (2001) Quality of life before and after laparscopic Nissen fundoplication. Surg Endosc 15: 353–356

[120] Granderath FA, Kamolz T, Schweiger UM et al (2002) Quality of life, surgical outcome and patient satisfaction three years after laparoscopic Nissen funoplication. World J Surg 26: 1234–1238

THE IMPACT OF DISEASE AND TREATMENT ON HEALTH-RELATED QUALITY OF LIFE IN PATIENTS SUFFERING FROM GERD

T. Kamolz[1] and V. Velanovich[2]

1 Division of Clinical Psychology, Public Hospital of Zell am See, Zell am See, Austria
2 Division of General Surgery, Department of Surgery, Henry Ford Hospital, Detroit, USA

Introduction

The increasing interest in measuring patients' health-related quality of life (HRQOL) as an outcome reflects an increasing awareness that traditional physiological endpoints often do not correlate with patients' functional status, general well being, and satisfaction with therapy. It has been shown that gastroesophageal reflux disease (GERD) has a significant impact on patients' HRQOL. Therefore, improvement of HRQOL should be one of the major goals of any GERD treatment. This improvement can be achieved by medical, endoscopic as well as surgical treatment. Finally, quality of life data help us also in a more selective selection of our patients concerning to the treatment regimen we may offer.

Reflux esophagitis was first recognized in the early 1930's [1]. Since then, much has been learned about gastroesophageal reflux disease (GERD). Presently, GERD is recognized as the most common acid-related disorder. Heartburn, the primary manifestation of GERD, occurs in approximately 20% of the western adult population on a weekly basis. Other symptoms include regurgitation, epigastric pain, chest pain. The severity of GERD symptoms range from mild, infrequent, and merely bothersome to severe, frequent and debilitating. Similarly, the spectrum of endoscopic findings in patients with GERD-related symptoms ranges from normal appearing mucosa to ulcerative esophagitis, stricture, or Barrett's metaplasia. Unfortunately, symptom severity may not be directly related to objective physiologic or endoscopic findings [2], [3].

However, an illness per se affects more than a patient's physical functioning – it may also affect a patient's emotional, social and occupational functioning. Recognizing that traditional objective clinical variables are not sufficient to assess the overall effect of disease, interest has shifted to patient-reported aspects in disease assessment. In the last two decades, health-related quality of life (HRQOL) assessments have become recognized and established medical endpoints in clinical research. A large number of different instruments have been developed, for generic, disease-specific, and symptom severity uses. Instruments for HRQOL evaluation are still being developed especially for international use, thereby making data comparable worldwide. However, HRQOL is a concept which is not directly measurable and exists primarily in our subjective perception. In fact, the robustness of HRQOL data suffers due to variation in definition.

Although there is no universally agreed on scope of HRQOL, several aspects include the psychological, physical, social, spiritual, personal role, and general well-being dimensions of a patient's health. These concepts are based on the WHO definition in 1948 that health is a complete state of physical, psychological, and social health, and not merely the absence of disease [4]. This WHO definition of health has become a common starting point for discussion and research of health status, HRQOL and to develop a biomedical model of health and disease which included aspects of a bio-psycho-social model of human existence.

Dent et al [5] emphasized HRQOL in defining GERD stating GERD "is likely present when heartburn occurs on two or more days a week, on the basis of the negative impact of this symptom frequency on health-related well being (quality of life)". Therefore, the goal of GERD treatment is to relieve symptoms, prevent complications, minimize adverse side-effects of treatment, and to improve patients HRQOL. Treatment options for those diagnosed with GERD include medications, endoscopic or surgical interventions. HRQOL has been assessed in all three. The primary objective of this chapter is to examine the impact of disease on HRQOL and the effects of treatment on HRQOL on patients living with GERD.

The impact of gastroesophageal reflux disease on patients quality of life

There have been a number of studies evaluating HRQOL of patients with GERD-related symptoms. These have shown that quality of life in GERD patients is significantly impaired when compared to healthy individuals [6]. Using the generic SF-36, Revicki et al [7] have shown that GERD patients have significantly worse scores in all 8 domains of the SF-36 (physical functioning, role-physical, role-emotional, bodily pain, vitality, mental health, social functioning and general health) when compared with the general population of the United States. These results were found in all age groups, independent of gender. GERD patients are more impaired compared to health controls with regard to pain, emotional distress, vitality, and are more limited in social and physical functioning. Compared with patients with major depression, GERD patients were as impaired in the domain of bodily pain, but less impaired in the emotional or physical functioning domains. In contrast, GERD patients experienced worse pain, emotional states, and social functioning than patients with hypertension or diabetes, and are comparable to patients suffering from irritable bowel syndrome [8]. Kaplan-Machlis et al [9] evaluated HRQOL data in a predominately rural primary care population of GERD patients using the SF-36 and Psychological General Well-Being (PGWB) Index. Their findings were comparable to previous reports [7], [10], but they also found that quality of life was more impaired in patients reporting moderate and severe GERD symptoms than in patients reporting more mild symptoms. Even GERD patients without medical comorbidities such as diabetes or psychiatric disorders had impaired functioning and general well-being when compared with healthy controls. Dimenäs [11] demonstrated that untreated GERD patients had impaired psychological well-being (using the PGWB) when compared with patients with angina pectoris, mild heart failure, hypertension, or untreated duodenal ulcer. In a large previously published German study [12], using the Gastrointestinal Symptom Rating Scale (GSRS), the Quality of Life in Reflux and Dyspepsia (QOLRAD) questionnaire, the SF-36 as well as the Anxiety and Depression (HAD) scale, Madisch et al described the impact of GERD on HRQOL. Out of the complete sample, 70% of patients had moderate symptoms and approximately 68% suffered from disease-related symptoms more than 4 days a week. GERD affects significantly daily eating and drinking habits, functioning, and vitality, resulting in emotional distress and sleep disturbance. Even when GERD patients with psychiatric comorbidities were excluded, 8% of the patients were depressed and 25% were significantly anxious.

The timing of GERD symptoms affects HRQOL. Farup et al [13] evaluated the relationship of GERD symptom frequency and occurrence during the day using the SF-36. They concluded that the presence of nocturnal symptoms exacerbates the impact of GERD in all domains of the instrument. Moreover, the frequency and number of symptoms are inversely related with quality of life, with nocturnal symptoms significantly worsening HRQOL.

Symptom severity is not closely related to physiological or pathological extent of the reflux. Studies [14], [15] found that objective measurements of GERD such as 24 hour esophageal pH monitoring or esophageal manometry do not correlate with the severity of symptoms as reported by the patient. One study did report that symptom severity as measured by the GERD-HRQL did correlate with esophagitis score as independently assessed by upper endoscopy [15]. Eloubeidi and Provenzale [16] compared quality of life scores of patients with Barrett's esophagus, GERD without Barrett's esophagus and non-GERD controls. They found no difference between the GERD patients with and without Barrett's metaplasia, but both of these groups had significantly lower scores than non-GERD controls. Using the Gastrointestinal Quality of Life Index (GIQLI), others [17] showed that patients with Barrett's esophagus had a better quality of life before surgery when compared with GERD patients without Barrett's esophagus. This difference based on a less intensive symptom perception in patients with Barrett's esophagus. Others [18], [19] found that patient perceived quality of life did not seem to be affected by the presence or extent of esophagitis; but, rather, general well-being, daily activities and social functioning are impaired by symptoms. These studies demonstrated that GERD patients have a significant impairment of quality of life, and that this impairment is due to perceived symptoms severity and not to objective pathology.

The effect of medical treatment on quality-of-life in GERD patients

The primary goals of GERD treatment are symptomatic relief, decrease frequency of complications, and healing of esophagitis. From the patient's viewpoint, it is symptom relief which is of primary importance of GERD treatment. Although it is beyond the scope of this chapter to review all studies available, we will comment on a few of the most interesting. Prasad et al [20], using generic or disease-specific instruments or a combination of both, report a limited number of studies evaluating drug therapy in GERD patients. Table 1 presents several reports assessing HRQOL in the medical treatment of GERD.

Based on available evidence, one can conclude that proton pump inhibitors are superior to other antireflux medication, such H2 receptor antagonists. Nevertheless, the best strategy to manage GERD is still debatable. In 1997, Harris et al [21] published their findings using a decision analysis model comparing three different medical strategies for preventing esophagitis recurrence. Theses authors determined that the degree of quality of life impairment could be used to select the most efficient treatment concept: e.g., patients with poor quality of life should be treated with an initial therapy with proton pump inhibitors, whereas those with less quality of life impairment should receive H2 blockers first.

Mathias et al [22] performed a randomized, placebo-controlled trial of lansoprazole (15 mg and 30 mg, daily) and omeprazole (20 mg daily) in 1145 patients with acute erosive esophagitis. Using the SF-36, they found that all 3 treatment groups showed significant improvements in quality of life, although the differences between treatment groups was negligible.

McDougall et al [23] compared patients with heartburn and grade II–III esophagitis before and after treatment with omeprazole (20 mg daily) and to non-GERD control patients. The SF-36 domains of bodily pain, vitality, and social functioning were significantly lower in GERD patients than controls. After treatment, scores in 7 of the 8 domains measured by the SF-36 improved, but there was no significant difference in the scores of patients with and without healed esophagitis.

Table 1. Published studies on the effects of medical GERD treatment on quality of life

First author	Ref.	Type of study	Treatment	QoL instrument	Conclusion
Mathias	[22]	randomized, placebo-controlled trial	lansoprazole versus omeprazole	SF-36	all treatments improve QoL better than plazebo
Galmiche	[30]	3 arm randomized, placebo-controlled trial	omeprazole, cisapride, placebo	GSRS	omeprazole improves QoL more than cisapride
Watson	[24]	blinded crossover trial	omeprazole versus placebo	SF-36	omeprazole improves QoL in patients without esophagitis
McDougall	[23]	GERD patients with esophagitis grade II–III versus control	omeprazole	SF-36	omeprazole improves QoL in patients with/without healed esophagitis
Revicki	[29]	3 clinical trials, randomized, double-blind	omeprazole, ranitidine	PGWB, SF-36	both treatments improved QoL; medication that reduces GERD-related symptoms generally improves QoL
Mathias	[25]	3 arm clinical trials	lansoprazole versus ranitidine	SF-12	all treatments improved QoL in patients without esophagitis

QoL = Quality of Life

Watson et al [24], and Mathias et al [25] studied an interesting group of patients with GERD-like symptoms, but no esophagitis found by endoscopy. These patients were treated with placebo, omeprazole, lansoprazole, and ranitidine. In both reports, anti-reflux medication was able to improve HRQOL significantly despite no visible pre-treatment esophageal mucosal injury. Similarly, the effect of esomeprazole 40 mg on HRQOL was assessed by Lauritsen et al [26]. Based on the QOLRAD, esomeprazole resulted in improvements in all five domains of the used inventory and of symptoms.

Nevertheless, despite the potential of modern anti-reflux medication to control GERD-like symptoms and improved HRQOL, effective management requires patient compliance. Several factors are known to affect patient compliance with medical therapies [27] – one of these is the baseline impairment of HRQOL before treatment. Wilhelmsen et al [28] analyzed quality of life in patients with low-grade esophagitis during a 1 year follow-up with "on-demand" ranitidine therapy. They found that even though the number of reflux episodes did not change, patients experienced fever symptoms and improved quality-of-life.

However, an analysis of clinical trials [29], [30] has demonstrated that symptom improvement or resolution is directly associated with significant improvements in HRQOL. When treatment responders and non-responders are compared, in general, responders report significant improvements in HRQOL, often returning to general population levels.

Patient satisfaction is also an important outcome [31]. Even simple questions and Likert scales are useful for understanding patients' perspectives on treatments. Several studies have demonstrated high rates of satisfaction (70–94% satisfied) with antireflux medication [25], [32]–[34]. Comparing omeprazole and cimetidine, Bate et al [32] found that GERD patients with or without endoscopic esophagitis treated with omeprazole reported significantly higher levels of treatment satisfaction. Nelson et al [33] showed that patients treated with omeprazole, but later converted to lansoprazole, reported less treatment satisfaction. Sodorff and colleagues [34] presented the results of a hospital-based proton pump inhibitor (omeprazole versus lansoprazole) interchange program. As a result of their study, the authors concluded that patient-perceived outcomes such as satisfaction and expectations were not affected by this interchange program.

Satisfaction is an important outcome measure because not only is this affected by symptom improvement, but also affects treatment compliance and the willingness of the patient to continue treatment with a specific physician.

The effect of endoscopic treatment options on quality of life data

Recently there have been several instruments developed for the endoscopic treatment of GERD. This era was ushered in by Swain with the development of an endoscopic suturing device [35], leading to the development of the Endocinch® device [36]–[38] and subsequently other instruments. As all these devices are new, follow up has been relatively short. Table 2 lists

Table 2. Quality of life outcomes of endoscopic GERD treatments

Device (Ref.)	Instrument used	Outcome	Maximum follow-up
Endocinch [36]–[38]	GERD-HRQL	Initial results good, long-term high recurrence rate	2 years
Stretta [39], [40]	GERD-HRQL	Heartburn scores lower, most patients stay improved	2 years
Enteryx [41]	GERD-HRQL	Significant improvement, improvement in symptoms scores	12 months
N-Do [42]	GERD-HRQL	Sustained improvement in symptoms scores	12 months
Gatekeeper [43]	GERD-HRQL	Significant improvement in symptoms scores	6 months

these devices. The other instruments that have been have studied include the Stretta® radiofrequency device [39], [40], the Enteryx® biopolymer injections [41], the N-Do® gastric plicator [42] and the Gatekeeper® expandable prostheses [43].

The Endocinch® device has been the most thoroughly studied. Please see the chapter on endoscopic treatments for a more thorough description of the device. Mahmood et al [44], using the QOLRAD, presented the data of a one year prospective follow up. The performed procedure resulted in a significant improvement of emotional distress, sleep disturbances, food/drink problems, physical/social functioning and vitality compared with the baseline. Nevertheless, despite of symptom and quality of life improvement, 36% of well selected patients still suffered from symptoms and needed antireflux medication. In general, follow-up periods have ranged up to two years. The majority of clinical trials of the Endocinch® device have used the GERD-HRQL symptom severity questionnaire [36]–[38]. Initial results have been good, with 75% or more patients responding to the initial plication. Unfortunately, after several months many patients have recurrent symptoms. After two years only 20% of patients remain free of proton pump inhibitors. These are true recurrences with symptomatic patients also having abnormal 24-hour pH monitoring. Because of this the Endocinch®, in fact, has lost favor among gastroenterologists and surgeons.

The Stretta® device is based on radiofrequency energy transferred to the lower esophagus and gastric cardia. The mechanism of action has been debated [45] with evidence demonstrating that there is augmentation of the lower esophageal sphincter pressure, lowering of acid exposure as measured by 24-hour pH monitoring, and improved symptoms suggesting alleviation of acid reflux. However, others suggest that symptom relief is based on obliteration of the afferent vagal nerve fibers from the lower esophagus, which would inhibit pain perception. The longest follow-up has been for two years [40]. The initial clinical trials used the GERD-HRQL symptom severity questionnaire. The results showed that in patients who initially responded to treatment, overall heartburn symptom scores continue to be low. However, approximately 40% of patients will require medical therapy for recurrent symptoms. Richards et al [46] presented their first short term results comparing the Stretta procedure versus laparoscopic antireflux surgery. Six months after both procedures, using QOLRAD and SF-12, quality of life was significantly improved in both groups. Nevertheless, only 58% of the Stretta patients were off medication, whereas 97% of surgical patients were off proton pump inhibitors. Because of the favorable results, there is still enthusiasm among both surgeons and gastroenterologist for this device.

One of the newer devices available for treatment of reflux endoscopically is the Enteryx®. The substance is an ethylene vinyl alcohol copolymer which is dissolved in dimethyl sulfoxide, then directly injected into the muscle of the lower esophagus. The data of a prospective trail has been published using the GERD-HRQL symptom severity questionnaire [41]. It has shown that at 12 months 80% of evaluable patients were treatment responders with statistically significant improvement is the GERD-HRQL scores. Of the treatment responders, however, 12% continued to use proton pump inhibitors but at a lower dose. Heartburn and regurgitation symptom scores were significantly improved at 12 months as compared to baseline. In addition, there were also significant reductions in acid reflux as measured by 24-hours pH monitoring. Follow up, however has still been relatively short and long term outcomes are still lacking.

The N-Do® gastric plicator has also been recently developed to provide a full-thickness placation of the gastric cardia at the gastroesophageal junction. It is an improvement over the Endocinch® system as the Endocinch® only plicates gastric mucosa. A pilot study was published [42] which demonstrated that at 6 months the plication in seven patients were still intact. Using the GERD-HRQL symptom severity questionnaire patients reported that heartburn symptoms at 12 months were significantly reduced, and three of five evaluable patients were not taking anti-reflux medication. However, the numbers of patients treated, at least in published articles, is very small and follow-up is still quite short. Until more data is available this system can not be recommended for widespread use.

The Gatekeeper® system employs deployment of a expandable polyacrylonitrile based hydrogel prostheses into the esophageal submucosa to augment the lower esophageal sphincter pressure. The concept is quite similar to the Enteryx® system previously described, with the significant difference being that this is reversible and that the prosthesis can be removed. In a multi-center study published from Europe [43], using the GERD-HRQL symptom severity questionnaire patients had significant improvement in their symptom scores which was durable for six months. The total time the pH was less than four in these patients went from 9.1% to 6.1%. Therefore, this is another device, which deserves a more thorough evaluation and until that time should only be used in the setting of a clinical trial.

In conclusion, all these relatively new endoscopic procedures can be described as safe and more or less effective in a small and well selected group of patients. An improvement of symptoms and quality of life can be achieved as well as a reduction of antisecretory medication in the majority of the patients.

The effect of antireflux surgery on quality-of-life in GERD patients

In a recently published report by an EAES consensus group [47], the authors have highlighted the importance of quality of life evaluation in laparoscopic surgery. In addition, an evidence-based approach was undertaken to evaluate existing information about different areas of laparoscopic surgery and to appraise instruments used to give recommendations for their future use in surgery.

As with untreated GERD patients, patients who are referred for surgical therapy after failed medical therapy have significant impairments in quality of life. In addition to persistent symptoms, they are troubled by ineffective treatment, frustrated and/or anxious about their disease, suffer from impairments in everyday activities, including leisure activities, interpersonal and sexual relationships, and loss of endurance and strength [32]. Pope first discussed the relevance of quality of life in the assessment of antireflux surgery in 1992 [33]. Later, Glise et al [34] reported improvements in quality of life after laparoscopic antireflux surgery in a consecutive series of 40 patients. They used two instruments (the PGWB index, and the GSRS) to determine that antireflux surgery was better than untreated GERD patients and as good as, or even better than, optimal medical treatment. Since then, several reports have been published assessing the quality of life after antireflux surgery. Table 3 lists recent articles assessing quality of life after antireflux surgery.

In 1996, Hunter et al [35] published improved quality of life outcomes after their first 300 laparoscopic antireflux procedures using the SF-36. Another single unit report [32] of over 500 antireflux operations showed improved scores with the GIQLI within the first 5 years after surgery. Surgery lead to quality of life scores comparable to healthy controls. Bammer et al [36] published a 5 to 8 year follow-up after laparoscopic Nissen fundoplication. Using an *ad hoc* overall well-being score, they found patients scores improved significantly after antireflux surgery. As the most of studies have shown, laparoscopic antireflux surgery is able to improve quality of life in patients suffering from typical GERD-related symptoms. Using the GIQLI, Duffy et al [53] have shown that laparoscopic Nissen fundoplication is also able to improve HRQOL in GERD patients with atypical symptoms, similar to those with only typical symptoms.

Recently, a few publications have demonstrated similar results after laparoscopic redo fundoplication [37], [38]. In a prospective study of 30 patients undergoing laparoscopic redo fundoplication, Kamolz et al [37] used both the GIQLI and SF-36 to measure quality of life outcomes. They found significant improvements in quality of life using both instruments, which were comparable to healthy individuals within 1 year of surgery. This outcome was achieved in all patients independently of whether the primary intervention was performed laparoscopically or open. In a recent study from Khaitan et al [56], the authors showed by using the SF-36 and the QOLRAD, that patients undergoing redo-fundoplication achieved less good quality of life improvement than patients having primary intervention. Patient satisfaction and physical aspects were worse in the redo group up to 2 years after surgery. In contrast, mental components were similar between both groups.

As described before, several endoscopic techniques to treat GERD have been developed. There is only one study [57] describing experiences and quality of life changes of laparoscopic antireflux surgery after failed endoscopic gastroplication. The authors reported that surgical intervention is feasible and that quality of life improvement was achieved only in patients with typical symptoms. In addition, symptomatic outcome was similar to that with the de novo intervention despite of the fact that in some patients swallowing problems eventually persisted longer.

Using the SF-36, Khajanchee et al [58] showed improved quality of life scores in elderly patients. However, in comparison to younger patients, elderly patients improved less in 6 of the 8 domains of the SF-36. Their findings suggest that age *per se* should not be a contraindication for antireflux surgery. Others [55], [59] showed, using the GIQLI, that both laparoscopic fundoplication and refundoplication in the elderly are able to improve quality of life. One year after surgery, data were comparable to healthy controls.

Several authors have used quality of life assessments to compare the results of different surgical techniques. Blomqvist et al [60] and Velanovich [61] compared in a non-randomized fashion quality of life outcomes after laparoscopic and open antireflux surgery. Both studies concluded that laparoscopic surgery produces similar symptomatic outcomes as open surgery. In contrast, Nilsson et al [62] reported from results of a randomized trial comparing also laparoscopic versus open antireflux surgery. They concluded that PGWBI, diet and sleep improved postoperatively in both groups. There were only minor differences between both surgical groups, but in some aspects the outcome was better after open surgery.

Blomqvist et al [63] using the PGWB index and O'Boyle et al [64] using a visual analogue scale demonstrated that division of the short gastric vessels had no significant impact on surgical quality of life outcomes. However, these results have been disputed [65]. In an attempt to prevent recurrent hiatal hernia after laparoscopic antireflux surgery, another study [66] reported the use of a prosthetic mesh to reinforce the hiatal

Table 3. Published studies on the effects of surgical GERD treatment on quality of life

First author	Ref.	Type of study	Treatment	QoL instrument	Conclusion
Hunter	[51]	prospective, single arm	laparoscopic Nissen or Toupet fundoplication	SF-36, *ad hoc*	LARS improves QoL
Kamolz	[48]	prospective, single unit trial	laparoscopic fundoplication and refundoplication	GIQLI	both procedures improve QoL within 5 years
Kamolz	[55], [59]	prospective, single unit trial	laparoscopic fundoplication and refundoplication	GIQLI	both procedures improve QoL in the elderly patient
Khajanchee	[58]	prospective, non-randomized trial	LARS in the elderly versus younger patients	SF-36	LARS improves QoL in both groups of patients
Velanovich	[61]	prospective, non-randomized trial	laparoscopic and open antireflux surgery	SF-36, GERD-HRQL	LARS improves QoL better than open surgery
Blomqvist	[60]	prospective, non-randomized trial	laparoscopic and open antireflux surgery	PGWB	both procedures improve QoL
Blomqvist	[63]	prospective, randomized trial	LARS with/without division of short gastric vessels	PGWB, GSRS	both kind of procedures improve QoL without any differences
Fernando	[69]	prospective, non-randomized trial	laparoscopic Nissen and Toupet fundoplication	SF-36	both procedures improve QoL
Velanovich	[75]	retrospective review of a prospective database	laparoscopic and open antireflux procedures in GERD patients with / without psychiatric comorbidities	SF-36, GERD-HRQL	psychiatric comorbidities affect symptomatic and QoL outcomes

LARS = laparoscopic antireflux surgery
QoL = Quality of Life

crura. These authors conclude that use of a prosthetic mesh reduces the risk of a recurrent hiatal hernia without any negative impact on patients' quality of life as measure by the GIQLI, even though postoperative dysphagia was temporarily higher in these patients.

Quality-of-life instruments have also been used to compare the efficacy of laparoscopic Nissen (360 degree) fundoplication with that of laparoscopic Toupet (270 degree) fundoplication [67]–[70]. Zügel et al [70] showed in a retrospective analysis of 162 patients that both procedures had similar improvement of quality of life as measured by the GIQLI. Others have also reached a similar conclusion. However, other authors have reported that recurrent reflux is unacceptably high in patients undergoing the Toupet fundoplication [71]. It appears that this issue is still unsettled.

In a recent published study, Streets et al [72] showed that an excellent quality of life improvement after Nissen fundoplication primary depends on a successful elimination of GERD-related symptoms and not from the invasiveness of the surgical approach. Using the SF-36, the authors compared the quality of life outcome of the laparoscopic approach with the transthoracic Nissen fundoplication, showing that both procedures can achieve a comparable long-term outcome.

Finally, quality of life assessments can be used for a much more sensitive description of surgical outcomes. Several studies have shown that stress-related symptomatology in GERD patients [73], different comorbidities such as psychiatric disorders or chronic pain syndrome [74]–[77], dyspepsia or aerophagia [78], [79] are able to affect outcomes negatively. All these studies show that symptom relief of GERD is more complex than just correcting the pathophysiology of the disease. In this relation, latest results have shown that quality of life data can also be used to predict the outcome of antireflux surgery [80]. In a review of a prospectively gathered database, the author could show that the use of the generic SF-36 can preoperatively identify patients who were likely to be dissatisfied with antireflux surgery.

The same as for modern antireflux medication, primary as well as redo-fundoplication can result in a high degree of patient satisfaction (85–95% satisfied) as shown in several studies [56], [81] [84]. Rattner and Brooks [81] compared laparoscopic with open Nissen fundoplication. Despite of several benefits in the laparoscopic approach, patient satisfaction did not differ between both kind of procedures. The same as for primary antireflux surgery, as shown by Granderath et al [82], also laparoscopic refundoplication is able to achieve a high degree of patient satisfaction for a follow-up period of 3 to 5 years after surgical intervention. A very interesting result was reported from Klapow et al [83]. The authors presented the long-term results of laparoscopically performed Toupet fundoplication. Despite the fact that in a large percentage of the patients the symptomatic and objective physiologic outcome was unsatisfactory from medical view, the patient, themselves, were more satisfied, showing that an improvement, if not complete resolution of GERD-related symptoms can result in a relatively high degree of satisfaction. A comparable result was presented by Booth et al [84], showing that despite of surgical side-effects in about 20% of their patient, patients' satisfaction with surgical treatment was only rarely affected.

A comparison of medical versus surgical GERD treatment

Most studies dealing with direct comparison of medical and surgical treatment of GERD concerning quality of life have been non-randomized trials [48], [85]. Therefore, these results should be interpreted with caution. There are only a few randomized trials available [86], [87], with, in general, demonstrating equivalent results. Spechler et al [86], using the SF-36 and the Gastroesophageal Reflux Disease Activity Index (GRACI) concluded that there was no significant difference between the groups for any domain on the SF-36, except for bodily pain, which was significantly better in surgical patients. In contrast, Lundell et al [87] have used the PGWB and GSRS to compare both treatments. After 5 years of follow-up, no differences were found between the two groups. In both studies, antireflux surgery was performed by the open approach. A study, comparing laparoscopic antireflux surgery with antisecretory medication is under process.

Conclusion

Patients suffering from GERD have a wide spectrum of different symptoms. More importantly, how they perceive their symptoms and how these symptoms affect their lives is highly individualistic. It would be foolish to adopt a dogmatic policy of medical, endoscopic, or surgical treatment exclusively in this patient population. Both, gastroenterologists and surgeons have to be sensitive to how GERD affects each individual patient's quality of life before making treatment recommendations. From the patients' view [88], [89], improvement of symptoms and also quality of life are the leading expectations in surgical and medical treatment.

References

[1] Winkelstein A (1935) Peptic esophagitis. A new clinical entity. JAMA 104: 906–909

[2] Falk GW (2001) Gastroesophageal reflux disease and Barrett's esophagus. Endosc 33: 109–118

[3] Pace F, Bianchi Porro G (2004) Gastroesophageal reflux disease: a typical spectrum disease (a new conceptual framework is not needed). Am J Gastroenterol 99: 946–949

[4] WHO Constitution of the World Health Organization. In: Basic documents. Geneva, Switzerland: WHO, 1948

[5] Dent J, Brun J, Fendrick AM et al (1999) An evidence-based appraisal of reflux disease management – the Genval Workshop Report. Gut 44: S1–S16

[6] Dimenäs E, Glise H, Hallerbäck B et al (1995) Well-being and gastrointestinal symptoms among patients referred to endoscopy owing to suspected duodenal ulcer. Scand J Gastroenterol 30: 1046–1052

[7] Revicki DA, Wood M, Maton PN et al (1998) The impact of gastroesophageal reflux disease on health-related quality of life. Am J Med 104: 252–258

[8] Frank L, Kleinman L, Rentz A et al (2002) Health-related quality of life associated with irritable bowel syndrome: comparison with other chronic diseases. Clin Therapeut 24: 675–689

[9] Kaplan-Machlis B, Spielgler GE, Revicki DA (1999) Health-related quality of life in primary care patients with gastroesophageal reflux disease. Ann Pharmacother 33: 1032–1036

[10] Enck P, Dubois D, Marquis P (1999) Quality of life in patients with upper gastrointestinal symptoms: results from the domestic/international gastroenterology surveillance study (DIGEST). Scand J Gastroenterol 34 (Suppl): 48–54

[11] Dimenäs E (1993) Methodological aspects of evaluation of quality of life in upper gastrointestinal diseases. Scand J Gastroenterol 28 (Suppl): S18–S21

[12] Madisch A, Kulich KR, Malfertheiner P et al (2003) Impact of reflux disease on general and disease-related quality of life – evidence from a recent comparative methodological study in Germany. Z Gastroenterol 41: 1137–1143

[13] Farup C, Kleinman L, Sloan S et al (2001) The impact of nocturnal symptoms associated with gastroesophageal reflux disease on health-related quality of life. Arch Intern Med 161: 45–52

[14] Trus TL, Laycock WS, Branum GD et al (1997) Quality of life scores correlate poorly with subjective and objective measurements of gastroesophageal reflux. Presented at the 38th Annual Meeting of the Society for Surgery of the Alimentary Tract, Washington, DC, May

[15] Velanovich V, Karmy-Jones R (1998) Measuring gastroesophageal reflux disease: relationship between health-related quality-of-life scores and physiologic parameters. Am Surg 64: 649–653

[16] Eloubeidi MA, Provenzale D (2000) Health-related quality of life and severity of symptoms in patients with Barrett's esophagus and gastroesophageal reflux disease patients without Barrett's esophagus. Am J Gastroenterol 95: 1881–1887

[17] Kamolz T, Granderath FA, Pointner R (2003) Laparoscopic antireflux surgery. Disease-related quality of life assessment before and after surgery in GERD patients with and without Barrett's esophagus. Surg Endosc 17: 880–885

[18] Havelund T, Lind T, Wiklund I et al (1999) Quality of life in patients with heartburn but without esophagitis: effects of treatment with omeprazole. Am J Gastroenterol 94: 1782–1789

[19] Wiklund I, Bardhan KD, Müller-Lissner S et al (1998) Quality of life during acute and intermittent treatment of gastroesophageal reflux disease with omeprazole compared with ranitidine: results from a multi-center clinical trial. Ital J Gastroenterol Hepatol 30: 19–27

[20] Prasad M, Rentz A, Revicki DA (2003) The impact of treatment for gastro-oesophageal reflux disease on health-related quality of life. Pharmacoeconom 21: 769–790

[21] Harris RA, Kuppermann M, Richter JE (1997) Proton pump inhibitors or histamine-2 receptor antagonists for the prevention of recurrences of erosive reflux esophagitis: a cost-effectiveness analysis. Am J Gastroenterol 92: 2179–2187

[22] Mathias SD, Castell DO, Elkin EP et al (1996) Health-related quality of life of patients with acute erosive reflux esophagitis. Dig Dis Sci 41: 2123–2129

[23] McDougall NI, Collins JS, McFarland RJ et al (1998) The effect of treating reflux esophagitis with omepra-

zole on quality of life. Eur J Gastroenterol Hepatol 10: 451–454
[24] Watson RGP, Tham TCK, Johnston BT et al (1997) Double blind cross-over placebo controlled study of omeprazole in the treatment of patients with reflux symptoms and physiological levels of acid reflux – the "sensitive esophagus". Gut 40: 587–590
[25] Mathias SD, Colwell HH, Miller DP et al (2001) Health-related quality of life and quality days incrementally gained in symptomatic nonerosive GERD patients treated with lansoprazole or ranitidine. Dig Dis Sci 46: 2416–2423
[26] Lauritsen K, Junghard O, Eklund S et al (2002) Effect of esomeprazole 40 mg on healing, reflux symptoms, and quality of life in patients with reflux esophagitis. Abstract: DDW-AGA; 19–22 May 2002; San Franzisco (CA)
[27] Kamolz T (2002) An analysis of medical compliance in gastro-oesophageal reflux disease patients referred to pre-surgical examination. Dig Liver Dis 34: 183–189
[28] Wilhelmsen I, Hatlebakk JG, Olafsson S et al (1999) On demand therapy of reflux oesophagitis – a prospective study of symptoms, patient satisfaction and quality of life. Aliment Pharmacol Ther 13: 1035–1040
[29] Revicki DA, Crawley JA, Zodet MW et al (1999) Complete resolution of heartburn symptoms and health-related quality of life in patients with gastro-oesophageal reflux disease. Aliment Pharmacol Ther 13: 1621–1630
[30] Galmiche JP, Barthelmy P, Hemelin B (1997) Treating the symptoms of gastro-oesophageal reflux disease: a double-blind comparison of omeprazole and cisapride. Aliment Pharmacol Ther 11: 765–773
[31] Revicki DA (2004) Patient assessment of treatment satisfaction: methods and practical issues. Gut 53: S40–S44
[32] Bate CM, Green JR, Axon AT et al (1997) Omeprazole is more effective than cimetidine for the relief of all grades of gastro-oesophageal reflux disease-associated heartburn, irrespective of the presence or absence of endoscopic oesophagitis. Aliment Pharmacol Ther 11: 755–763
[33] Nelson WW, Vermeulen LC, Geurkink EA et al (2000) Clinical and humanistic outcomes in patients with gastroesophageal reflux disease converted from omeprazole to lansoprazole. Arch Intern Med 160: 2491–2506
[34] Sodorff MM, Galt KA, Galt MA et al (2002) Patient perceptions of a proton pump inhibitor therapeutic interchange program across the continuum of care. Pharmacother 22: 500–512
[35] Swain CP, Mills TN (1986) An endoscopic sewing machine. Gastrointest Endosc 32: 36–38
[36] Filipi CJ, Lehman GA, Rothstein RI et al (2001) Transoral, flexible endoscopic suturing for treatment of GERD: a multicenter trial. Gastrointest Endosc 53: 416–420
[37] Maple JT, Alexander JA, Gostout CJ et al (2001) Endoscopic gastroplasty for GERD: Not as good as billed? A single-center 6 month report. Am J Gastroenterol 96 (Suppl): 522
[38] Velanovich V, Ben-Menachem T, Goel S (2002) Case-control comparison of endoscopic gastroplication with lapraoscopic fundoplication in the management of gastroesophageal reflux disease. Surg Laparosc Endosc Percutan Tech 12: 219–223
[39] Corley DA, Katz P, Wo JM et al (2003) Improvement of gastroesophageal reflux symptoms after radiofrequency energy: a randomized, sham-controlled trail. Gastroenterol 125: 668–676
[40] Triadafilopoulous G (2004) Changes in GERD symptoms scores correlate with improvement in esophageal acute exposure after the Stretta procedure. Surg Endosc 18: 1038–1044
[41] Johnson DA, Ganz R, Aisenberg J et al (2003) Endoscopic implantation of Enteryx for treatment of GERD: 12-month results of a prospective trail. Am J Gastroenterol 98: 1921–1930
[42] Chuttani R, Sud R, Sachdev G et al (2003) A novel endoscopic full-thickness plication for the treatment of GERD: a pilot study. Endosc 58: 770–776
[43] Fockens P, Bruno MJ, Gabbrelli A et al (2004) Endoscopic augmentation of the lower esophageal sphincter for the treatment of gastroesophgeal reflux disease: a multicenter study of the Gatekeeper reflux repair system. Endosc 36: 682–689
[44] Mahmood Z, McMahon BP, Arfin Q et al (2003) Endocinch therapy for gastro-oesophageal reflux disease: a one year prospective follow up. Gut 52: 34–39
[45] Fuchs KH, Freys SM (2003) Endoscopic antireflux therapy. Surg Endosc 17: 1009–1016
[46] Richards WO, Houston HL, Torquati A et al (2003) Paradigm shift in the management of gastroesophageal reflux disease. Ann Surg 237: 638–647
[47] Korolija D, Sauerland S, Wood-Dauphinée S et al (2004) Evaluation of quality of life after laparoscopic surgery. Evidence-based guidelines of the EAES. Surg Endosc 18: 879–897
[48] Kamolz T, Granderath FA, Bammer T et al (2002) Mid- and long-term quality of life assessments after laparoscopic fundoplication and refundoplication: a

single unit review of more than 500 antireflux procedures. Dig Liver Dis 34: 470–476
[49] Pope II CE (1992) The quality of life following antireflux surgery. World J Surg 16: 355–358
[50] Glise H, Hallerbäck B, Johansson B (1995) Quality-of-life assessments in evaluation of laparoscopic Rosetti fundoplication. Surg Endosc 9: 183–189
[51] Hunter JG, Trus TL, Branum GD et al (1996) A physiologic approach to laparoscopic fundoplication for gastroesophageal reflux disease. Ann Surg 223: 673–687
[52] Bammer T, Hinder R, Klaus A et al (2001) Five to eight years outcome of the first laparoscopic Nissen fundoplications. J Gastrointest Surg 5: 42–48
[53] Duffy JP, Maggard M, Hiyama DT et al (2003) Laparoscopic Nissen fundoplication improves quality of life in patients with atypical symptoms of gastroesophageal reflux. Am Surg 69: 833–838
[54] Kamolz T, Bammer T, Pasiut M et al (2000) Health-related and disease-specific quality of life assessment after laparoscopic refundoplication. Chirurg 71: 707–711
[55] Kamolz T, Bammer T, Pasiut M et al (2002) Failed antireflux surgery: surgical outcome of laparoscopic refundoplication in the elderly. Hepato Gastroenterol 49: 865–868
[56] Khaitan L, Bhatt P, Richards W et al (2003) Comparison of patient satisfaction after redo and primary fundoplication. Surg Endosc 17: 1042–1045
[57] Velanovich V, Ben Menachem T (2002) Laparoscopic Nissen fundoplication after failed endoscopic gastroplication. J Laparoendosc Adv Surg Tech 12: 305–308
[58] Khajanchee YS, Urbach DR, Butler N et al (2002) Laparoscopic antireflux surgery in the elderly. Surgical outcome and effect on quality of life. Surg Endosc 16: 25–30
[59] Kamolz T, Bammer T, Granderath FA et al (2001) Quality of life and surgical outcome after laparoscopic surgery in the elderly gastroesophageal reflux disease patient. Scand J Gastroenterol 36: 116–120
[60] Blomqvist A, Lonroth H, Dalenbäck J et al (1996) Quality of life assessment after laparoscopic and open fundoplications. Results of a prospective, clinical study. Scand J Gastroenterol 31: 1052–1058
[61] Velanovich V (1996) Comparison of symptomatic and quality of life outcomes of laparoscopic versus open antireflux surgery. Surgery 126: 782–788
[62] Nilsson G, Larsson S, Johnsson F (2002) Randomized clinical trial of laparoscopic versus open fundoplication: evaluation of psychological well-being and changes in everyday life from a patients perspective. Scand J Gastroenterol 37: 385–391
[63] Blomqvist A, Dalenbäck J, Hagedorn C et al (2000) Impact of complete gastric fundus mobization on outcome after laparoscopic total fundoplication. J Gastrointest Surg 4: 493–500
[64] O'Boyle CJ, Watson DI, Jamieson GG et al (2002) Division of short gastric vessels at laparoscopic Nissen fundoplication: a prospective double-blind randomization trial with 5-year follow-up. Ann Surg 235: 165–170
[65] Soper N (2002) Fundoplication and the short gastric vessels: divide and conquer. Ann Surg 235: 171–173
[66] Kamolz T, Granderath FA, Bammer T et al (2002) Dysphagia and quality of life after laparoscopic Nissen fundoplication in patients with and without prostetic reinforcement of the hiatal crura. Surg Endosc 16: 572–577
[67] Kamolz T, Bammer T, Wykypiel H Jr et al (2000) Quality of life and surgical outcome after laparoscopic Nissen and Toupet fundoplication: one-year follow-up. Endosc 32: 363–368
[68] Kamolz T, Granderath FA, Bammer T et al (2002) Laparoscopic "floppy" Nissen fundoplication versus Toupet fundoplication: quality of life assessment of a 5 year follow-up (Part II). Endosc 34: 917–922
[69] Fernando HC, Luketich JD, Christie NA et al (2002) Outcomes of laparoscopic Toupet compared to laparoscopic Nissen fundoplication. Surg Endosc 16: 905–908
[70] Zügel N, Jung C, Bruer C et al (2002) A comparison of laparoscopic Toupet versus Nissen fundoplication in gastroesophageal reflux disease. Langenbeck's Arch Surg 386: 494–498
[71] Horvath KD, Jobe BA, Herron DM et al (1999) Laparoscopic Toupet fundoplication is an inadequate procedure for patients with severe reflux disease. J Gastrointest Surg 3: 583–591
[72] Streets CG, DeMeester SR, DeMeester TR et al (2002) Excellent quality of life after Nissen fundoplication depends on successful elimination of reflux symptoms and not from invasiveness of the surgical approach. Ann Thorac Surg 74: 1019–1025
[73] Kamolz T, Bammer T, Wykypiel H Jr et al (1999) Coping and personality in patients with or without stress-related symptoms of gastroesophageal reflux disease. Z Gastroenterol 37: 265–270
[74] Velanovich V, Karmy-Jones R (2001) Psychiatric disorders affect outcomes of antireflux operations for gastroesophageal reflux disease. Surg Endosc 15: 171–175
[75] Velanovich V (2003) The effect of chronic pain syndromes and psychoemotional disorders on symptomatic and quality of life outcomes of antireflux surgery. J Gastrointest Surg 7: 53–58

[76] Kamolz T, Bammer T, Granderath FA et al (2001) Laparoscopic antireflux surgery in gastro-oesophageal reflux disease patients with concomitant anxiety disorders. Dig Liver Dis 33: 659–664

[77] Kamolz T, Granderath FA, Pointner R (2002) Does major depression affect the outcome of laparoscopic antireflux surgery? Surg Endosc 16: 55–60

[78] Slim K, Bousquet J, Kwiatkowski F et al (2000) Quality of life before and after laparoscopic fundoplication. Am J Surg 180: 41–45

[79] Kamolz T, Bammer T, Granderath FA et al (2002) Comorbidity of aerophagia in GERD patients: outcome of laparoscopic antireflux surgery. Scand J Gastroenterol 37: 138–143

[80] Velanovich V (2004) Using quality of life measurements to predict patient satisfaction outcomes for antireflux surgery. Arch Surg 139: 621–626

[81] Rattner DW, Brooks DC (1995) Patient satisfaction following laparoscopic and open antireflux surgery. Arch Surg 130: 289–293

[82] Granderath FA, Kamolz T, Schweiger UM et al (2002) Long-term follow-up after laparoscopic refundoplication for failed antireflux surgery: quality of life, symptomatic outcome, and patient satisfaction. Gastrointest Surg 6: 812–818

[83] Klapow JC, Wilcox CM, Mallinger AP et al (2002) Characterization of long-term outcomes after Toupet fundoplication: symptoms, medication use, and health status. J Clin Gastroenterol 34: 509–515

[84] Booth MI, Jones L, Stratford J et al (2002) Results of laparoscopic Nissen fundoplication at 2–8 years after surgery. Br J Surg 89: 476–481

[85] Fernando HC, Schauer PR, Rosenblatt M et al (2002) Quality of life after antireflux surgery compared with nonoperative management for severe gastroesophageal reflux disease. J Am Coll Surg 194: 23–27

[86] Spechler SJ, Lee E, Ahnen D et al (2001) Long-term outcome of medical and surgical therapies for gastroesophageal reflux disease. JAMA 285: 2331–2338

[87] Lundell L, Miettinen P, Myrvold HE et al (2001) Continued (5-year) followup of a randomized clinical study comparing antireflux surgery and omeprazole in gastroesophageal reflux disease. J Am Coll Surg 192: 172–179

[88] Kamolz T, Pointner R (2002) Expectations of GERD patients in the outcome of laparoscopic antireflux surgery. Surg Laparosc Endosc Percutan Techn 12: 389–392

[89] Kamolz T, Pointner R (2004) What do heartburn sufferers expect from proton pump inhibitors when prescribed for the first time? Minerva Gastroenterol Dietol 50: (in press)

Chapter 27

THE PATIENTS' PERSPECTIVE

G. Nilsson

Department of Nursing, Faculty of Medicine, Lund University, Sweden

Introduction

This chapter will illuminate how symptoms of GERD, surgery and outcome interfere with patients' lives. Patients' narratives can help bridging the communication gap between patients and health professionals. The patient's view and priorities must be better understood [1].

To understand the illness experience

"Our ability to imagine the illness experience and to emphasize with those who are ill is severely limited" [2]. Novels describing patients' illness experiences have become invaluable sources for medical and health care professionals and students. An understanding of disease processes, treatments and outcomes is necessary for humane and effective care of patients [2]. Further, teaching of literature in medical schools has become widely accepted as a primary means to teach about the patients' experiences [3]. Likewise narrative medicine suggests that several dimensions of medical research, teaching and practice are imbued with narrative considerations and can be made more effective with narrative competence [3]. Narrative competence is the ability to acknowledge, absorb, interpret and act on the stories and plights of others [3]. A literature review involving patients as teachers showed that meeting real patients with firsthand experience of a condition, who have knowledge and teaching skills, offers learners important educational benefits [4]. Patients offer unique qualities that can improve communication, enhance the acquisition of skills and change attitudes towards patients by perceiving patients' experiences and expertise [4]. Patients' experiences are also useful to fellow patients. From on-going conversations with GERD-patients, it is obvious that patients not only request honest and clear information from health professionals but they also seek information from peers i.e. patients who have previously undergone antireflux surgery, and who will be able to report their experiences and outcomes after operation versus living with the disease before surgery. Describing the symptoms, the operation and the outcomes, i.e., daily life with illness, before and after surgical treatment, and illuminated from a patient perspective would be of importance. This will increase the understanding of living with chronic reflux disease, enhance information about the outcome of different treatments, e.g., surgery, from a patient perspective and constitute a foundation for decision-making about advantages or disadvantages. GERD-patients' experiences of illness and surgical treatment could promote an increase in information for future patients, next of kin and health professionals.

Well-being, health related quality of life, patient satisfaction

The traditional medical model, in which the primary focus is the diagnosis and treatment of symptoms and disease, has been the ruling health paradigm since the 15th century [5]. Thus, illness, not health, has been the primary concern of the health professions and the medical model has been the major influence upon health care providers for many generations [6]. This pattern has changed and the theoretical framework of health-related quality of life (HRQoL) is largely based on a multi-dimensional perspective of health as physical, psychological and social functioning and well-being along the lines of the WHO's (World Health Organization) definition of health: "a state of complete physical, mental and social well-being and not merely the absence of disease or infirmity" [7]. Ware (1987) has argued that five health concepts are inherent in this definition: physical health, mental health, social functioning, role functioning and general well-being [8].

In recent years more attention has been paid to aspects of well-being and HRQoL when evaluating surgical outcomes [9]. By examining how patients perceive and experience the impact on well-being and daily life both clinicians and patients should use this information to make well-informed decisions about treatment [1]. The patients must be in focus and important decisions regarding health care should incorporate the patient's own assessment of HRQoL [1]. A new health paradigm has emerged and a care-oriented model is replacing the cure-oriented traditional medical model of illness [6]. Health-related quality of life refers to the physical, psychological and social domains of health and are influenced by a person's experiences, beliefs, expectations and perceptions [10]. Therapeutic efforts focus today on improving patient functions as well as well-being and assessing patient health status as perceived by patients. "Although the objective dimension is important in defining a patient's degree of health, the patient's subjective perceptions and expectations translate that objective assessment into the actual quality of life experienced" [10]. Quality of life measures, per definition, represent the patient's view, it is and always will be subjective and should be so [1].

HRQoL is appropriate to clinical research since it highlights outcome measures important to clinical changes. HRQoL is increasingly used as an outcome in clinical trials and effectiveness research [11] and assessment of the patient's perceived situation might give valuable complementary information to the efficacity and functional variables traditionally used [12]. GERD has a substantial impact on the patient's well-being associated with heartburn, acid regurgitation and pain. Several researchers have reported that laparoscopic and open fundoplication reliably produce disease improvement in patients with GERD [13]–[15]. Especially in gastrointestinal surgery evaluation of quality of life data enables comparison of different therapy concepts and the efficacity of treatments should be measured not only with objective outcome criteria but also by evaluating patient satisfaction [16], [17]. Patients are concerned with their symptoms and how symptoms reflect daily living such as work, bending forward, eating and sleeping [1]. For example the patient may have to avoid favourite foods or regurgitations may wake the patient from sleep. We know that patient's self-assessment may differ substantially from the judgement of healthcare staff but it is the patient's perception that is the most significant [12], [16], [18], [19]. When interpreting research reports not only statistic significance is of importance; clinical significance of results obtained will enhance understanding of objective information such as functional status, symptoms and measurements assessed. To achieve a further comprehensive description of illness and outcome of treatments, narratives could be used to illuminate daily life to peers and professionals. Furthermore, from narratives objective measures could be clarified and explained and clinical matters of importance to patients might be highlighted. Clinical significance refers to the practical value or importance of the effect of an intervention, i.e., whether it makes any real difference to the patients in their functioning and everyday life [19]. Knowledge of patients' expectations of surgery due to the practical value of the effect of an operation could lead to improvement in satisfaction with surgery for future fellow patients. "After all, most patients who agree to undergo surgery do so because of troublesome symptoms and not because of objective signs, such as endoscopic findings or the result of 24-hour pH monitoring" [20].

Decision-making and patients participation

The Swedish Health and Medical Services Act is founded on a positive belief in the humans own ability to take responsibility for their health, make decisions about as well as having influence on their own care and treatments [21]. Several studies have addressed the question if patients want to participate in medical decision-making and the results of these studies have been mixed [22]. Decision-making is described in an Illness-Constellation Model by Morse and Johnson (1991) explaining that when the individuals no longer can manage their symptoms alone, a critical point is reached whereby the person transfers the responsibility for decision making to the physician [2]. When the sick person enters the medical system; choices become a medical prerogative. One of the factors that contribute to relinquishing of control on the part of the patient and at the same time feeling trust into a new situation is that "In the physician-patient relationship the physician is often viewed as expert and the patient as the follower of expert advice" [2]. However, there is a growing interest in providing information to support patients' participation in choosing treatments and decision-making [23]. To enable patients to join the decision-making process regarding their health, patient information should meet scientific standards [23]. Information should contain relevant, research based data in a form that is acceptable and useful to patients [24]. Patient partnership is on the agenda in England and is based on doctor's skills and patients seen as experts [25]. The doctor is well informed about diagnostic techniques, the causes of disease, prognosis, treatment options and preventive strategies but only the patient knows about the illness experience, social circumstances, habits and behaviour, attitudes to risk, values and preferences. Both types of knowledge are necessary to manage illness successfully and as partners they should be prepared to share information and take decisions jointly [25]. Patients require access to quality evidence based information to be able to take an active part in decisions about their health care [26]. Patient information that will support patients' involvement in treatment decisions must contain relevant research-based data [27]. In a study by Aronson et al (2001) they found that key elements to a successful outcome of laparoscopic antireflux surgery was their multidisciplinary approach to care delivery and a well-informed patient who understood the risks and benefits of the proposed surgery and the ways the patient could participate in his or her own recovery [28]. These nurses found that patients and their families benefited from the extensive education and psychological support provided by all members of the health care team, from the preoperative visit through the patient's follow-up phone call [28]. Kamolz and Pointner (2002) reported that the majority of patients with GERD, even if well informed about their disease, wanted to receive more information about GERD and its complications [29]. The same authors believe that subjective aspects of patients' expectations and perceptions such as symptoms, quality of life and satisfaction with surgery should be included as a standard in all future consensus reports [17]. Patients' expectations should be used for clarifying and discussing antireflux surgery-related issues with them before an intervention. Knowledge of patients' expectations should give the physicians a chance to reinforce or change the patients' expectations and ultimately improve the patients' satisfaction with surgery [17]. In a literature review by Frosch and Kaplan (1999), about patient participation in shared decision-making in clinical medicine, they concluded that shared decision-making is an important development in health care but more research is necessary in order to evaluate the most effective methods for engaging patients in decisions about their own health [22]. Patients who engaged in medical decision-making had a greater sense of personal control, lower levels of concern about their disease and were more satisfied with treatment [22]. To participate in decision-making involves access to information and knowledge from different aspects of treatments like subjective and objective outcome criteria. Furthermore, the patients need to comprehend the options and outcomes in order to consider and communicate the personal value they place on the benefits versus the harms [27].

Illuminating patients' illness experiences of GERD, surgery and outcome

In a qualitative study, patients with GERD were invited to talk openly about their experiences, thoughts, feelings and the consequences of living with their illness, going through surgery and the outcome [30]. Understanding patients' experiences should be in focus with clinical practice and might add another dimension to create more individulized treatments. Furthermore, combining quantitative and qualitative designs will lead to a more complete picture of the clinical topic researched. Below is a description of GERD, surgery and outcome from the patients' perspective.

The burden of illness

The patients described life with an always-present illness. The symptoms had started years before, often in their twenties or even earlier, and had eventually become worse and finally too hard to live with. They adjusted themselves to several restrictions in daily living and the number of restrictions increased over time and the burden of illness became heavier. From their point of view, they tried to live a normal life and considered themselves as healthy. They accepted their symptoms as inevitable and increased the medication in order to control their symptoms and to cure them. Different strategies were used, for example avoiding certain food and drinks, not carrying heavy things, sleeping with the head raised; instead of bending, they would go down on their knees when tying shoelaces, etc. They felt an inexpressible longing for food and drinks that they could not tolerate, e.g., fruit, vegetables, coffee and wine. One respondent, however, refused to change the diet and rather ate and drank what she liked and took the pain afterwards.

"Some get irritated and affected in not being able to eat what you want – but I eat what I want and drink what I want and then I have to take the smashes the hard way".
"...you had remedies; like Novalucol®, you ate it in large quantities, had a glass of water and then it (the pain) *was gone, then you had to take new ones after a while and you continued like that all the time".*
"I remember when I was teaching I had to pull out a drawer on the teacher's desk to put my foot on, I had to huddle up".
"When bending I always had acid regurgitations, the gullet was an open wound".
"Three days later after having had sausages for lunch, I could belch and have it back in my mouth and that was disgusting, you see".

The symptoms escalated over the years from mild to unbearable with corrosive damages in the throat. Many respondents said that stress added to their troubles of acid regurgitations, vomiting and pain. Daily difficulties were constantly burning pain, acid regurgitation and the contents from the stomach that rushed into their mouth. This became worse at night because when asleep they woke up with a full mouth and often were woken by coughing caused by stomach contents pouring into the windpipe, leading to feelings of annoyance and fear; what would happen if they did not wake up? In spite of disturbed sleep and even sleeping sitting in a chair, most respondents managed to go on and endured living with the worsened symptoms.

"I woke up more or less every night with my mouth full of stomach contents, you cough and then when you are asleep – it feels almost like you are suffocating".
"Lying sleepless at night – then of course you work poorly".
"At nights you had acid regurgitations in your mouth and nose. It rushed into the mouth, I had to sit and sleep in an armchair with a blanket".
"When I couldn't lie down but had to sit and sleep – then I went to the doctor".

All respondents had been taking medication for years and could not manage without it. They had started with mild drugs available without prescription and over the years passed on to the strongest ones after seeing a physician, often a general practitioner. They then recieved proton pump inhibitors or similar drugs, and mostly thought this medication was effective. Medication made the disease manageable but did not cure them. They could not cope without drugs; they always had to take their medication. However, in a previous study patients reported a weakening effect of the medication and some also stated that they had symptoms despite medication [31].

"Over-the – counter drugs did not help but it relieved and later I started with Losec®".
"In the beginning it was mostly Novalucol® or all these available without prescription but then I had Losec® for many years".
"You ate packages of medicine every week, nothing helped but you still hoped, it was hard, very hard".

The patients described themselves as hard working and very loyal to their places of work. They worked despite their symptoms, taking their medicine and were on sick leave only occasionally or never. Especially those who were self-employed described it as impossible to be sick – who would then run the business? However, their work was affected and hard to endure when it involved physical work such as bending or lifting. Furthermore, the illness had no visible signs and symptoms and that made it difficult for them to go on sick leave. They suffered mentally when collegues believed they tried to wangle or escape from their work. Stress and working too hard made the symptoms worse and aggravated the illness.

"You have to manage your work, you have to live..."
"You woke up at about 01.00 o'clock and then I couldn't sleep any more and then you are supposed to start working at 08.00 o'clock and that was hard. Then you had to swallow and swallow. . ."
"I personally felt it as a relief to have the operation, it was a document, an evidence to all who had not believed me that this was true, that I had not been lying and trying to avoid work".
"I was mentally distressed when the boss told me: You are only wangling, you are spending time at home sleeping!"

"As soon as I became stressed or was working too hard or eating something unsuitable...I vomited and got an awful pain in my stomach".
"I am self-employed and then you have no time to be ill".
"At the end when I didn't manage any longer, we sold the company".

Descriptions from the patients vary with respect to how their illness had influenced their family life. Some reported that the illness did not influence members of the family but only themselves, while others felt it was hard for the whole family and their chances of engaging in social life because of not being able to eat and drink normally. Patients also described how family members had or had had the same symptoms and they often compared themselves to them. They believed it might be hereditary.

"My family hasn't suffered...the children were already born when I had this and I had this all the time".
"I am tough, I never complain. Sure, they saw you were not feeling good, but you got used to it. You do that with pain and stuff like this, it's a part of life".
"The whole family was influenced and the work too, actually".
"My father has it and my twin sister".

The illness escalated and most patients described especially the nights as dreadful. When nights became unbearable, they were referred to a surgical department and the diagnosis of GERD was confirmed by different investigations (endoscopy, oesophageal manometry and 24-h pH monitoring). Some patients had suspected that they had a gastric ulcer because the symptoms got worse when they suffered from stress and because they took proton pump inhibitors. Patients felt relief given a diagnosis. To hear about surgery and to have an operation was seen with mixed feelings. For some it was a hard decision to have an operation but at the same time it was a way to get rid of their troubles. Some had been waiting for surgical technology to develop and an operation was the last option. Many had never had an operation before and felt that they were unaware of what it could mean. The patients saw it as something positive and felt trust in the operation and also saw it as important to try to get healthy. The operation to them was a means to get rid of the problem. However, two female patients expressed fearfulness of anaesthesia. One of these women had later experienced awareness during the operation but said very definitely that this had not left any traumatic implications: "if I should need another operation I wouldn't hesitate..."

"They measured how much acid I had during the nights...and they said you must have suffered a lot".
"He ran that tube into my throat, looked and said immediately – you are going to have an operation!"
"It was nothing that we decided over a day, just like that..."
"Not a bit worried, I have a calm personality, there were no problems at all" (about operation).
"I was worried not to wake up and see my kids again" (about anaesthesia).

The patients put their confidence in their physicians and they influenced the patients a great deal by inspiring feelings of trust and security. Most patients reported that the doctors encouraged and supported surgery, and they felt confident and secure when the doctor advised the operation. Some were urged by the doctor to have the operation because, as they were told, they were too young to be on medication for the rest of their lives. In a previous study [31], 70% of the patients said that the doctor/surgeon suggested the operation, when answering the question: Who proposed surgery? If the doctor was insecure or showed any doubt, then the patient was influenced likewise by these opinions.

"It felt as if I could only lie down and put my life in their hands and then it was all ready, that's what it felt like" (about the operation).
"He advised me to have this operation. Yes, I thought, if I could get rid of this problem, then it was OK".
"I was a little bit scared from the beginning because when we (patient and physician) *talked about operation, it was so complicated and I felt that the doctor did not want me to do the operation, I felt insecure..."*

After surgery the burden of illness was gone

The patients underwent either laparoscopic or open 360° fundoplication and their experiences of the outcome of the operation were overall positive independent of type of surgery. When the patients mentioned striking characteristics belonging to merely the laparoscopic or the open technique it will appear distinctly in the text below.

All patients described how their symptoms of the illness had disappeared after the operation. They had expected a good outcome but many regarded this as better than expected and they described a normal life, eating what they wanted, drinking coffee, sleeping the whole night through and no more medication. The feelings of being able to eat and drink what they wanted were tremendous, e.g. drinking red wine, coffee and eating green apples. Many patients described managing their work better after the operation and even saying that it had been an absolute requirement for being able to continue working. One respondent discovered cancer in her stomach a couple of years later, and that was like she said; only thanks to the fact of the absent reflux symptoms.

"I have not yet to this day, any problems concerning digestion and acidity of the stomach, regurgitations, heartburn, there are nothing of the kind, and no traces of the symptoms have come back. They have done it so good that I can even belch".
"You can't describe it, because I thought I would be better, but being totally out of symptoms, I never believed that".
"I am so happy that I made it, I sure am".
"What a relief – I have never felt so good in my stomach in my whole grown up life".
"All those symptoms are gone now with acid reflux and sleeping while sitting in a chair".
"The operation was a wonder. If I hadn't done it, I had been very bad today and I had probably not been working".
"If I had not been feeling so well after the antireflux surgery, I had never, never noticed the cancer. I had been dead by now!"

The postoperative period

The first postoperative period, all patients described pain when eating and drinking. However, patients with open surgery talked about pain related to the surgical technique i.e. the large wound and described the first days after operation as rather painful. They also felt great tiredness/weakness and had no energy. One patient's incision ruptured because he started working too soon, which he considered his own fault. Another considered that the incision was an obstacle to returning to work faster (he was a farmer). Two patients, one male and one female, did not like the scar for cosmetic reasons. The woman thought the scar was very ugly and disgusting (she was about forty-year-old and had just met a new man). Problems with the incision is reported in a previous study [32], other complaints were itching, tightness and infection.

"Those who had keyhole operation ran around while I walked bent over with a cushion on my stomach the first days" (open surgery).
"I bet myself to get well as soon as possible and only one week after the operation I was back at work helping out a little bit" (open surgery).
"Hell of a pain, I had an incision all over my belly...when I came home from the hospital, I was enormously tired" (open surgery).
"When looking back, I think the big problem was the wound" (open surgery).
"I was directly up and go, no troubles, only good, could eat directly on the second day and then I went home" (laparoscopy).

Side effects and complications of the operation

All respondents had side effects from the operation particularly eating difficulties and flatulence, but were bothered in varying degrees. After the operation, all had difficulties in eating related to a rapid feeling of fullness, and described a new technique for eating. They could not eat as quickly as they had used to do or take large bites of food. They had to chew very carefully and wash down their food with water otherwise the food got stuck. They also ate smaller portions. After about 6 months most patients described their eating habits as normal, but some said that they still did not take big bites of food and tried not to eat so fast.

"I had a little trouble in the beginning but that was because I took too big bites and that I ate as I used to, then I learned to eat less and to wash it down. Before I never drank until after the meal".
"It was hard to eat and swallow – you had to eat very, very little and often".

"I am eating normally now, everything. Yes, but if I am in a hurry, it can become like blocked. Then I have to lie down on the floor and it will disappear".

All respondents described problems with flatus or wind. These problems had not, like the eating problems, become normal. After five years, problems with wind still persisted. Many patients had severe bloating even before surgery but not to this extent. They described different ways of managing this related to their kind of work and social surroundings, and no problems if working outdoors or alone. As a consequence they avoided carbonated drinks and they chewed the food very, very carefully and ate slowly. A few could belch, and one patient described a new way of belching by moving his body in a certain way in order to force him to belch. He had learned this from changing positions in his job; he was a car mechanic. Being able to belch relieved many of the problems with the wind.

The wind was socially embarrassing and if they had to suppress it they got an awful pain in the stomach and in the chest. Several patients even described confusion with heart disease when they felt severe bloating, causing terrible tensions in their chest. When they were at home or had a "free" work situation they could neglect it but those who were surrounded by other people described the severe pain and even attacks of cramp as unbearable. Many described the smell as stinking and nauseous. They were satisfied that they could control passing flatus but wondered if this would become involuntarily when they got older.

In a previous study [31], patients' expectations and perceptions of the outcome of the operation before and after surgery were measured according to VAS (visual analog scale). Expectations of the operation preoperatively were significantly higher than perceptions of the operation after one month due to the most common side-effects of surgery i.e. dysphagia and flatulence as narrated by the patients.

Most patients were not able to vomit and some described fear of being sick with influenza. Many also described a rumbling and very noisy stomach. They described different strategies to control these new side effects, e.g. trying to avoid stress and not rushing about.

"I have big troubles with wind but in my job I can let off" (working as a farmer).

"When eating fast – you swallow air! You have to take your time".

"My stomach feels bloated, I put on a pair of trousers in the morning and think the clothes are fitting and by noon I have to unbutton".

"It is embarrassing when you go shopping, you turn around carefully to see if someone is near by, it smells very awful".

"They said you could get troubles with flatulence but that it would be to this extent, I hadn't even dreamt about. . .I wish I could belch when I am feeling as I was ready to burst".

"I was sea-sick and wanted to vomit but I couldn't, I can't vomit".

"If I work in my own speed it's OK but as soon as it becomes rush and stressful, it goes directly to my stomach".

Two complications of paralytic ileus were described, one with open surgery and one with laparoscopy. Both these patients had previously had their appendix removed. Another patient with open surgery described going acutely to the hospital because of feeling of sickness, gastroenteritis. One patient with laparoscopy had intestinal infection with heavy diarrhoea and described how this made him socially isolated since it was uncontrollable and made him hesitant about whether the operation had been worthwhile.

"One month afterwards I got ileuses and then I was enormously ill..., so I couldn't vomit and that is a disadvantage, not being able to vomit".

"The operation was very good but having these infected intestines...dependant on a lavatory all the time".

Sick leave

Some respondents described alertness and fast recovery and going back to work almost immediately, but some needed a longer recovery owing to open surgery combined with a manual job. Others who did manual labour, and independent of type of surgery, felt they needed a longer time to recover. Many patients also felt overstretched and needed a long time for recovery since their illness had bothered them for such a long time.

"...I needed to be on a long sick-leave because I worked as a cook and I had a very hard time" (female cook).
"I could not work as I had thought...I had to hire workers" (farmer).
"My work demanded lifting and I couldn't do that and then it was psychological too, feeling bad for may be 10 years before the operation and not taking care of yourself like you should have done. Then afterwards coming back and start taking care of yourself, psychological pain, like waking up to life again, and that taxed all my powers" (daycare centre).

Information and sharing experiences to future patients

Most patients were satisfied with the preoperative information they had received. They knew all about having to eat slowly, chewing carefully, washing down food with water and to avoiding carbonated drinks etc. Furthermore, they knew about probably not being able to belch and vomit, and increased bloating.

"Flatus, that is wind in the stomach, I have got that but they told me and warned me that this could happen, but I think that is personal side-effects".
"They told me about the wind and that I would have problems vomiting and with the wind. So I was a little prepared for that...and that there might be some side-effects afterwards. It didn't come as a surprise!".

They said, however, that it would have been good to get information from patients who had already had the operation, since it was hard to imagine the extent of the side effects, especially the increased bloating. Some told about how patients who were going to have an operation had phoned them and asked about their outcome. Some of those who had open surgery lacked information how to treat the incision. One respondent described how she massaged and softened the incision with an ointment but her daughter's physician had told her about that when her daughter was treated for burns.

All respondents emphasized the importance of having an operation and recommended it to other patients with the same troubles as they had had. They had recovered from GERD and they described a better quality of life afterwards. They rated their side-effects of very much less importance than the symptoms of GERD. Patients who had suffered from severe side-effects were more hesitant but admitted that it was a relief having no more illness symptoms. Although symptoms of flatulence and inability to belch were common, patients were satisfied with the operation. Satisfaction was primarily related to being free from reflux and burning pain. Findings of satisfaction, despite new symptoms, have been reported previously [32]–[35].

None of the patients in this qualitative study had taken any antireflux medication after surgery. They were well informed and knew that the outcome of an operation was very individual. One patient described before and after the operation as compared to hell and heaven. Another described the outcome as 98–99% health and 1–2% wind.

"If others have these troubles as I had, I absolutely think they should do this operation, but I don't know how it will turn out, perhaps everyone wont be as well as I am, it's very individual".
"I advise everyone with these symptoms, go for it, is it like this, so have the operation!".
"The operation was great but this other trouble..."
"No medication the day after the operation!"
"I ate a whole bottle of pills per week...no, I have not taken one pill since the operation. That's good – really you have to admit that".
"I am so happy that I had the operation".

Comments

Other GERD patients will probably recognize similar events and be able to refer to the above findings.

Another way for patients to describe the impact of GERD on their daily living is by using patient-completed tools, such as a simple screener [36]. There is such a tool for migraine illuminating how symptoms interfere with patients' lives by highlighting headache-related disability in daily life [37]. A corresponding tool might be useful for GERD patients.

References

[1] Glise H, Wiklund I (2002) Health-related quality of life and gastrointestinal disease. J Gastroenterol Hepatol 17 (Suppl): S72–S84
[2] Morse J, Johnson J (1991) The illness experience: dimensions of suffering. Newbury Park: Sage
[3] Charon R (2001) The patient-physician relationship. Narrative medicine: a model for empathy, reflection, profession, and trust. Jama 286: 1897–1902
[4] Wykurz G, Kelly D (2002) Developing the role of patients as teachers: literature review. BMJ 325: 818–821
[5] Allan JD, Hall BA (1988) Challenging the focus on technology: a critique of the medical model in a changing health care system. ANS Adv Nurs Sci 10: 22–34
[6] Hwu YJ, Coates VE, Boore JR (2001) The evolving concept of health in nursing research: 1988–1998. Patient Educ Couns 42: 105–114
[7] WHO. Primary health care. Report of the international conference of primary health care. Alma Ata, USSSR. Geneva 1978; 1: 6–12; 1978 Geneva 1978; 1: 6–12. Report No.: Geneva 1978; 1: 6–12
[8] Ware JE Jr (1987) Standards for validating health measures: definition and content. J Chronic Dis 40: 473–480
[9] Korolija D, Sauerland S, Wood-Dauphinee S et al (2004) Evaluation of quality of life after laparoscopic surgery: evidence-based guidelines of the European Association for Endoscopic Surgery. Surg Endosc 18: 879–897
[10] Testa MA, Simonson DC (1996) Assesment of quality-of-life outcomes. N Engl J Med 334: 835–840
[11] Wilson IB, Cleary PD (1995) Linking clinical variables with health-related quality of life. A conceptual model of patient outcomes. Jama 273: 59–65
[12] Dimenas E, Glise H, Hallerback B et al (1993) Quality of life in patients with upper gastrointestinal symptoms. An improved evaluation of treatment regimens? Scand J Gastroenterol 28: 681–687
[13] Laine S, Rantala A, Gullichsen R et al (1997) Laparoscopic vs conventional Nissen fundoplication. A prospective randomized study. Surg Endosc 11: 441–444
[14] Olsen MF, Josefson K, Dalenback J et al (1997) Respiratory function after laparoscopic and open fundoplication. Eur J Surg 163: 667–672
[15] Eshraghi N, Farahmand M, Soot SJ et al (1998) Comparison of outcomes of open versus laparoscopic Nissen fundoplication performed in a single practice. Am J Surg 175: 371–374
[16] Velanovich V (1999) Using quality-of-life instruments to assess surgical outcomes. Surgery 126: 1–4
[17] Kamolz T, Pointner R (2002) Expectations of patients with gastroesophageal reflux disease for the outcome of laparoscopic antireflux surgery. Surg Laparosc Endosc Percutan Tech 12: 389–392
[18] von Essen L, Sjoden PO (1991) Patient and staff perceptions of caring: review and replication. J Adv Nurs 16: 1363–1374
[19] Kazdin A (1998) Research design in clinical psychology. 3rd ed. Boston: Allyn and Bacon
[20] Sandbu R, Khamis H, Gustavsson S et al (2002) Long-term results of antireflux surgery indicate the need for a randomized clinical trial. Br J Surg 89: 225–230
[21] SFS 1982:763 [Code of statutes]. Health and Medical Services Act
[22] Frosch DL, Kaplan RM (1999) Shared decision making in clinical medicine: past research and future directions. Am J Prev Med 17: 285–294
[23] Coulter A (1998) Evidence based patient information. Is important, so there needs to be a national strategy to ensure it. BMJ 317: 225–226
[24] Coulter A, Entwistle V, Gilbert D (1999) Sharing decisions with patients: is the information good enough? BMJ 318: 318–322
[25] Coulter A (1999) Paternalism or partnership? Patients have grown up-and there's no going back. BMJ 319: 719–720
[26] Shepperd S, Charnock D, Gann B (1999) Helping patients access high quality health information. BMJ 319: 764–766
[27] O'Connor AM, Rostom A, Fiset V et al (1999) Decision aids for patients facing health treatment or screening decisions: systematic review. BMJ 319: 731–734
[28] Aronson BS, Yeakel S, Ferrer M et al (2001) Care of the laparoscopic Nissen fundoplication patient. Gastroenterol Nurs 24: 231–236; quiz 237–238
[29] Kamolz T (2002) Analysis of medical compliance in gastro-oesophageal reflux disease patients referred to pre-surgical examination. Dig Liver Dis 34: 183–189
[30] Nilsson G, Larsson S, Johnsson F et al (2002) Patients' experiences of illness, operation and outcome with reference to gastro-oesophageal reflux disease. J Adv Nurs 40: 307–315
[31] Nilsson G, Larsson S, Johnsson F (2002) Randomized clinical trial of laparoscopic versus open fundoplication: evaluation of psychological well-being and changes in everyday life from a patient perspective. Scand J Gastroenterol 37: 385–391
[32] Nilsson G, Wenner J, Larsson S et al (2004) Randomized clinical trial of laparoscopic versus open fundoplication for gastro-oesophageal reflux. Br J Surg 91: 552–559

[33] Rattner DW, Brooks DC (1995) Patient satisfaction following laparoscopic and open antireflux surgery. Arch Surg 130: 289–293; discussion 293–284
[34] Blomqvist A, Lonroth H, Dalenback J et al (1996) Quality of life assessment after laparoscopic and open fundoplications. Results of a prospective, clinical study. Scand J Gastroenterol 31: 1052–1058
[35] Klapow JC, Wilcox CM, Mallinger AP et al (2002) Characterization of long-term outcomes after Toupet fundoplication: symptoms, medication use, and health status. J Clin Gastroenterol 34: 509–515
[36] Wiklund I (2004) Review of the quality of life and burden of illness in gastroesophageal reflux disease. Dig Dis 22: 108–114
[37] Holmes WF, MacGregor EA, Sawyer JP et al (2001) Information about migraine disability influences physicians' perceptions of illness severity and treatment needs. Headache 41: 343–350

GASTROESOPHAGEAL REFLUX DISEASE: A PSYCHOLOGICAL PERSPECTIVE OF INTERACTION AND THERAPEUTIC IMPLICATIONS

T. Kamolz

Public Hospital of Zell am See, Zell am See, Austria

Introduction

Never before has the interaction between gastrointestinal disorders and psychosocial factors been analysed more intensively than in the past two decades. Heartburn suffers represent a heterogeneous group of patients with considerable symptom overlap. The biopsychosocial model of diseases is a remarkable step forward in the process of understanding more about GERD and GERD-like diseases. As shown, several psychological and social aspects have potentially important roles in the presentation and symptom perception of GERD. A primary causative role for these psychological factors remains unproven. However, factors such as stress and coping strategies, personality traits or psychiatric comorbidities interact through recognized psychophysiologic or behavioural mechanism to affect the clinical presentation of GERD. Recognizing these possible levels of interaction has significant implications for those who want to understand the development and the sensitivity of GERD-related symptoms as well as diagnostics and selection of optimal treatment.

Gastroesophageal reflux disease (GERD) is a very common chronic condition, particularly frequent in primary care setting, with a high economic burden on Western society, and represents the most common disease of the upper gastrointestinal tract. Approximately 40% of the adult Western population suffer from GERD-related symptoms monthly. Persistent untreated GERD can lead to esophageal strictures, premalignant Barrett's esophagus, and a potential risk of adenocarcinoma of the esophagus [1], [2].

The primary symptoms of GERD are heartburn, epigastric pain or regurgitation, but it may also be associated with extraesophageal manifestations, such as asthma, chest pain and ortolaryngologic disorders. However, more accurate anamnesis raises an additional spectrum of untypical symptoms which can be linked to GERD [3], [4]. Nevertheless, a symptom is how a person perceives and interprets a stimulus. Therefore, GERD symptoms and the perceived severity are more than the simple pathological reflux of gastric contents back into the esophagus. The purpose of this chapter is to analyse the relationship between GERD and possible psychological aspects such as stress or patients' personality.

A psychological perspective

In daily practice, significant discrepancies occur between endoscopic severity of GERD, and the patient's symptom experience and quality of life impairment. These discrepancies cannot be explained by simple morphologic findings, and usually are considered to be related to psychological factors according to a bio-psycho-social model of disease. Recent advances in the understanding of the interaction between psychological factors and the brain-gut axis, provide a challenging opportunity for all to establish a more comprehensive understanding of GERD. A bio-psycho-social model integrates the various physical and psychosocial factors that contribute to the patient's illness and offers a comprehensive and effective approach for the diagnosis and a multidisciplinary management of GERD.

Since the end of the 1970's, an increased number of studies have been performed in order to establish potential relations between the symptoms and causal factors of GERD on the one side, and psycho-physiological, as well as other psychologically relevant aspects on the other. Recent studies have shown, that up to 60% of patients with GERD-related symptoms noticed an increase in complaints under conditions of stress [5], [6]. On the basis of pH monitoring of reflux patients, it could be established that less than 20% of the objective reflux episodes accompany subjective reflux symptoms, as seen from the patients point of view [7]. Contrary to this, complaints without objective results are perceived [8] whereby a slight correlation between acid exposure in the esophagus and symptom perception is acknowledge [9].

In recent years, numerous studies in this context have been performed in order to link possible psychophysiological factors such as psychological stress or personality aspects with reflux-associated processes. It must be noted that the majority of these studies proceeded under laboratory conditions and therefore did not take into consideration everyday stress situations, or partly were conducted with healthy individuals. In addition, some of the physiological stressors performed produced highly individual threshold values with respect to their perception, despite defined physical properties and well standardised research practices in relation to the sampling. Furthermore, the intensity of mental stressors depends from motivation as well as the intellectual potential and pre-experiences or expectational attitude are sample dependent. As a consequence of this, some results are under controversial discussion.

The impact of psychological stress on esophageal manometry

In the 1920th [10], [11] the first known tests with respect to changes in motility of the distal esophagus and laboratory induced stress had already been conducted by Jacobson. Approximately 40 years later, Rubin et al [12] conclude that non-propulsive contractions in the distal esophagus can be induced in 5 healthy individuals through burdensome questioning. An other survey [13] investigated the effects of the "cold-pressor-task", noise disturbance of 100 dB and cognitive problem solving exercises on esophagal manometric values in 25 healthy individuals. A short-lived rise in pressure at the lower esophageal sphincter, followed by relaxation and changes in esophageal motility occurred under both physiological and cognitive stress conditions. Additionally, Ayres et al [14] found comparable results in patients with irritable colon, as did Anderson et al [15] in 19 patients with non-cardiac chest pain. A significant rise in amplitude of esophagus contraction occurred under a variety of stress conditions, whereby cognitive problem solving exercises proved to be more burdensome that noise disturbance. Other investigations [16], [17] proved that stress is accompanied by a postprandial slowing of sphincter relaxation or gives rise to intensified contraction of the hiatal crura whereby, in principle, a rise in sphincter pressure and reduced reflux occurs. From these results it is possible to infer, that different stress conditions lead to changes in esophagus motility and changes to the lower sphincter, and can thus be partly linked to reflux events. However, changes as a result of long-term stress on the function of the gastroesophageal junction have not been shown.

Psychological stress and pH-monitoring

Several investigations into possible relations between laboratory stress and pH monitoring produced negative results. Bradley et al [6] found no relation between distinct experimental stressors and objective parameters such as the number of reflux episodes, duration of the longest reflux phase or the total acid value of the test phase in 17 reflux patients. Whereas, other physiological parameters such as heart rate and blood pressure rose significantly, providing evidence as to the stressful nature of the test phase. In contrast to the above, patients with subjective links between stress and their reflux symptoms, a significant rise in exclusively subjectively perceived complaints experienced under test conditions. Others [18] achieved partly comparable results in healthy subjects, during the course of their investigations into postprandial reflux. Likewise, Sonnenberg et al [19] found no association of any sort between noise disturbance and acid secretion in the stomach, blood supply to the mucosa in healthy subjects.

Nevertheless, Holtman et al [20] reported interesting findings: the authors investigated the effect of mental stress on the gastric acid secretion with respect to personality traits. The trait "impulsiveness" was found to be a relevant one in healthy subjects. People with highly pronounced "impulsiveness" exhibited a significant rise in acid, whilst the acid values fell in people with less pronounced "impulsiveness". These results lead to the conclusion that stress evokes only limited changes in acid secretion. A change would most likely take place in the subgroup of GERD patients with a subjective interaction between stress and perceived symptoms and within the confines of emotion and a defined personality structure. A further moderating variable could be "fear" [21], [22]. This increases in times of stress and leads via the neuronal level, centrally, to a sensitising of physiological processes and thereby to increased symptom and pain perception. That such an event could eventually form the basis for sensitive esophagus or NERD (non-esophagitis reflux disease) in patients, is at the very least, under debate and the subject of current studies. Fundamentally, it is known that patients suffering from endoscopic negative reflux disease display a comparable symptom spectrum and with corresponding intensity, as well as identical disease profile to patients with an erosive disease [23].

Personality traits and symptom perception

As mentioned above, beside impulsiveness and fear, it seems that other characteristics such as social withdrawal, depression or somatisation can also be associated with changes in motility and gastric acid secretion [21], [22], [24]–[26].

Own results [27] on 100 reflux patients support the view that besides partly significant differences in personality, differences in the stress management strategies of routine daily life exist between stress sensitive and unspecified stress reflux patients. Stress sensitive patients favour an intensely active stress management; frequently show aggressive tendencies and are more likely to forego social support respectively display less tendency of flight when under stress. As far as their personality structure is concerned, they perceive themselves as highly achievement orientated, experience at the same time a greater number of physical complaints and tend toward psychosomatic misperceptions. Moreover, a part from more numerous and more stressful reflux symptoms, stress specific reflux patients report further gastrointestinal symptoms. These, despite successful surgical therapy performed in the light of intensifies or displaced symptoms, nevertheless come to the forefront. Significant differences with respect to the time of day (upright versus supine refluxers) at which events occur could also be confirmed. Over 90% stress sensitive GERD patients can be described as daytime refluxers. Differences in objective parameters (DeMeester Score, esophageal manometry) have not been found. Velanovich et al [28] came to similar conclusions. The authors found no or only slight correlation between the pressure on the lower esophageal sphincter, results from pH monitoring, the degree of GERD and quality of life. Significant links were only found between the number of perceived complaints and quality of life.

Wright et al (under submission) report the data of an experimental investigation, examining whether exposure to psychological stress may produce an increase in objective reflux episodes or modify subjective perceptions of symptoms. The used experimental stressor induced a significant increase in cortisol and state anxiety, but was not associated with any increase in reflux episodes. However, the experimental group was unable to exactly identify their level of symptom severity. The authors conclude that their findings are relevant because they indicate that perception of anxiety or exposure to stress clearly affects the personal ability to interpret accurately the severity of perceived symptoms. Therefore, it might be possible if patients under antireflux medication, when they become stressed they may still perceive themselves to be experiencing reflux symptoms, even if medication was physiologically successful.

The results of a longitudinal study concerning to life stress on chronic symptoms of heartburn have been published by Naliboff et al [29]. In a group of 60 patients with current heartburn symptoms, the authors evaluated the presence of stressful life events retrospectively over a period of 6 months and prospectively for 4 months. In addition, symptom severity, quality of life, anxiety and depression as well as vital exhaustion were measured. Based on the results, they concluded that symptom severity appears to be most responsive to major life events and that vital exhaustion in relation to sustained stress may represents the psychophysiological symptom complex most closely associated with heartburn exacerbation. In contrast, affective and subjective stress ratings were not strongly related to heartburn severity. But depression showed a strong relation to heartburn medication use and anxiety to impaired quality of life. The authors finally suspected that potential mechanisms for these results include an increased level and frequency of esophageal acid exposure, an inhibition of gastric emptying or a stress-induced hypersensitivity of the esophagus.

On the basis of these reports, it does not seem to be a question of a "psycho-physiological" disease, as was previously thought, even if GERD-related symptoms are significantly more present in patients with psychiatric comorbidities [24], [30]. However, it is certain that GERD, that is, the perception of GERD symptoms as a result of psychological stress, a particular type of personality structure can be influenced in some of the patients. This knowledge should therefore be incorporated in the process of medical diagnosis and therapy of at least this element of patients.

NERD and "functional heartburn"

On the basis of current research, it has to be assumed, however, that NERD is fundamentally not the question of a pure psychological phenomenon. Quigley [31] offers a detailed review of non erosive reflux disease. Cohen and Snape [32] present a plausible hypothetical model of potential psycho-physiological and cognitive interactions between excitatory and inhibitory neurohumeral substances with stress and their effect on the distal sphincter. Few neuro-physiological studies of the gastroesophageal junction [33], [34] describe nervous reflux and stimulation processes which are responsible for the perception of pain, vomiting or false sensations and which can at least, be indirectly linked to reflux events. Kellow et al [35] or Drossman et al [36] present reviews about fundamental principles of neuro-gastroenterology with respect to physiology and symptom perception.

In 1991, Pustorino et al [37] compared more than 60 patients with GERD-related symptoms, with or without endoscopic evidence of esophagitis, using the Middlesex Hospital Questionnaire to analyse personality traits and manometric findings. The authors did not found any significant differences in psychological traits or manometric data between patients with or without esophagitis, but significant differences between both groups and controls. Neurotic traits were significantly more pronounced in GERD-like patients than in healthy controls or patients without any digestive disorder. In addition, the authors found a close relation between psychological traits and manometric data. Therefore, they concluded that psychological aspects play a role in the pathogenic process of GERD, even if other aspects may be necessary to develop an esophagitis.

In approximately 40% of NERD patients no evidence for a pathological acid burden on the distal esophagus has been found using pH monitoring. Despite existing parallels to GERD or NERD, the disease profile is described as "functional heartburn" and according to the "Rome II Consensus Report" is categorised under functional esophagus disorders [38]. As per definition, the diagnosis "functional heartburn" is given when primary symptoms (heartburn or chest pain) appear for a period of 12 weeks (within the previous 12 months) and without any pathological explanation such as GERD, achalasia or esophageal motility disorders. Contrary to patients with GERD, there is a significantly stronger link between acid exposure (whether low or normal) in the distal esophagus and the timely perception of symptoms in patients diagnosed with "functional heartburn" [39]. The real cause in unclear, however, hypersensitivity of the receptors in the esophagus to intraluminal stimuli is primarily suspected [39], [40] (hypersensitive esophagus). Shi et al [41] experimentally showed (intra esophageal balloon distention test) that mechanical stimuli lead to symptoms significantly earlier in these patients than in other individuals. Mixed reflux, as a further factor is also discussed [42]. Principally, psychological factors are also discussed alongside the various possible physiological explanations. In contrast to other functional gastrointestinal disorders very few studies exist [22], [43], [44] which concentrate exclusively on possible links between psychological factors and "functional heartburn", rather, it is more than likely the case that partly highly controversial results exist. The most probable potential factors are stress or fear. Treatment is per se identical with all GERD but with limited success of common antireflux medication [45]. Furthermore, the prescribing of antidepressive medication or pain modulators in low doses are also under discussion.

Is there a possible link between psychological aspects and Barrett's esophagus or carcinoma?

In general, gastroesophageal reflux disease is a risk factor for adenocarcinoma of the esophagus, and incidence has significantly increased during the past 20 years. Adenocarcinoma may develop from Barrett esophagus which is associated with chronic reflux. Certain factors associated with Barrett's esophagus also hold for esophageal adenocarcinoma: greater severity of reflux symptoms, specific pattern of symptoms (particularly nocturnal), longer duration of symptoms, white race, and male gender or a high body mass index [46], [47]. However, the distribution of these factors over the time and also genders does not match the pattern of adenocarcinoma occurrence well.

It is known that psychological aspects are associated with an impaired immune function and an increased susceptibility to cancer [48], [49]. In this relation, less is known about a possible link between psychological aspects and GERD complications. Based on a MEDLINE research, only 2 studies were found in this relation: In a case report, Dessureault et al [50] reported from the association of Barrett's esophagus and invasive squamous cell carcinoma of the distal esophagus in a young woman with a history of self-induced psychogenic vomiting. This report illustrated the complicated associations between human behavior and pathogenic mechanisms involved in carcinogenesis.

Jansson et al [51] published the results of a nationwide Swedish population-based case-control study. Aim of the study was to evaluate and analyse if stressful psychosocial working conditions might be involved in the etiology of esophageal cancer. The authors hypothesized that eventually work-related stress could decrease the sphincter pressure of the lower esophageal sphincter, thereby promoting reflux, and finally esophageal or gastric cardia adenocarcinoma, respectively that work-related stressors could impair the immune system leading to cancer. As a result of their study, they did not found any associations between job strain and cancer risk, but a moderately strong association between having a covert coping style when treated unfairly at work and developing a tumor. In addition, they analysed that subjects reporting from low work place satisfaction have an almost 3-fold increased risk of an esophageal adenocarcinoma which might be explained by an increased occurrence of reflux secondary to stress response. Nevertheless, the authors concluded that these findings must be interpreted cautiously and that further investigations are needed.

The impact of psychological factors on medical treatment concepts

From the medical point of view, there are two fundamentally different treatment concepts, which can each be followed when indications are clearly defined. In the present chapter, the potential option of endoscopic treatment procedures has been excluded. Generally, the aim of any GERD therapy, besides the achievement of a disease free state, and thereby an improvement in patients quality of life as seen from the patients point of view, is the healing of esophagitis, the prevention of the development of progressive disease and also prevention with respect to the development of a potential Barretts' esophagus. This fundamental aim of therapy can be achieved with the use of antazida, prokinetics, H2 antagonists and/or proton pump inhibitors. The signal to discuss surgical therapy is only given if suffering is particularly high and quality of life is severely impaired; if complications of GERD have arisen; if a causal functional defect is evident and lastly, if general health of the patient is good enough to withstand an operation [2].

Accompanying medical therapy, patients are in most cases obliged to initiate particular behavioural changes in order to achieve a further improvement in the disease profile [52]. However, no prospective randomized studies exist, which unequivocally and wholly support the efficacy of these theoretical improvement measures. Here, it is primarily a question of behaviour related measures of everyday habits, and a consequence of this is the emergence of the first possible psychologically oriented interventions. It is common known that it is not always easy, despite medical advice, to effect behavioral change or the abandonment of daily rituals (e.g., weight reduction, eating behaviour, stress management). This is often only achievable through appropriate psychological intervention.

Independently from the medical treatment option, the patients' view and expectations in a therapy becomes an important factor in relation to compliance and therefore also for efficacy. Own data [53] show, that patients expectations in a PPI therapy are as follows: The leading expectations have been: (1) an improvement (61%) or elimination (33%) of perceived symptoms; (2) healing of esophagitis (50%); (3) in 46% of the patients a return to normal daily life and in 44% an improvement of quality of life respectively. A number of 36% expected no further therapy following this initial treatment, 34% no side-effects of PPI treatment, and only 4% had no real expectations in a prescribed antireflux medication. The same as for medical treatment, an improvement of symptoms is the leading expectation of patients in a possible antireflux operation [54]. In contrast, none of the surgical patients expect an elimination of all perceived symptoms. This result is in relation to previous findings suggesting that even if not all symptoms are eliminated, patients satisfaction with treatment can be high and quality of life may be improved [55], [56].

Nevertheless, GERD is a chronic condition and the majority of the patients' need a life-long medication to treat their symptoms. In this relation it has to be stated that a long-term use of drug therapy is always a question of patients expectations and compliance, even if a "on demand" therapy is under debate. As previously shown [57], approximately 25% of GERD patients referred to pre-surgical examination are not compliant in relation to medical prescriptions, and about 40% are just partly compliant. The reasons for being non-compliant are, in general, a rejection of any kind of medication use, less information about GERD, low severity of GERD, but also an aspect of patients' personality which also affects quality of surgical outcome. In general, next to medical compliance also the aspect of health care seeking has to be seen in relation to patients' personality. As shown by Johnston et al [58], health care seeking in heartburn suffers is in relation to factors such as increased phobia, obsessionality, somatization, and less social support when compared with heartburn suffers who had never sought medical help. Therefore, aspects such as health care seeking or compliance with prescribed medication are associated with psychological and social factors.

Interventions from a psychological view

Several studies have been conducted from a psychological point of view. These investigated the effect of biofeedback on the lower esophageal sphincter pressure and on reflux symptoms [59]–[61]. Due to the high technological cost involved, most of these were single case studies. Gordon et al [61] used biofeedback to alter the resting pressure of the lower esophageal sphincter from 2.7 mmHg to 8.7 mmHg in only 10 sittings in a patient who had been suffering from GERD-related symptoms for 8 years. At the same time, reflux symptoms and also the number of single reflux events were significantly reduced. The effect of hypnosis induced deep relaxation on gastric acid secretion was investigated and a reduction in the latter was evident [62]. This technique is nevertheless concerned with a selective method which presupposes a special choice of patient and is therefore of only limited application.

Only one systematically applied investigation was concerned with the effect of progressive muscle relaxation (originally by Jacobson) on reflux events. This relaxation technique is easy to learn, efficient and is successfully practised in phobia therapy, stress management or on patients with gastrointestinal disorders. McDonald-Haile et al [63] were able to show that progressive muscle relaxation, leads to a reduction in subjective symptoms, as well as to an objectively lower acid exposition in the esophagus. Additionally, an anxiolytic effect was also achieved. Unclear, however, is the exact mode of operation of this relaxation on reflux events. According to the authors, in the context of perceptional changes, not only is it possible to directly influence the gastroesophageal junction and the hiatal crura, it is also possible to influence these areas via an anxiolytic change in the form of a moderation process.

In contrast to medical therapy, surgical intervention studies substantiate the effect of psychological factors on the subjective quality of the results [64], [65]. Personality traits seem to play an essential role in the subjective assessment of stress on postoperatively essential adaptation processes (e.g., eating behavior) as well as in the subjective assessment of dysphagia and satisfaction with surgery. As previously shown [65], the subjective degree of swallowing problems after laparoscopic antireflux surgery is predictable by patients personality in relation to the possibility to cope with a postoperative situation. The used construct "locus of control" showed that patients with an increased believe in luck or fate respectively a low degree of personal abilities suffered from a significantly higher degree of subjective dysphagia but without any objective evidence.

Also in respect to patients' personality, using the same construct as described before, the initial degree of compliance with former antireflux medication seems to be a good predictor of surgical outcome. Own data [66] have shown that surgically treated patients with former non-compliance with medication are eventually limited good candidates for surgery. In contrast to compliant patients, these group of patients significantly suffered from higher a degree of dysphagia and other so called surgical side-effects (e.g., gas-related problems), needed postoperatively more additional medical intervention including redo-surgery, and quality of life improvement or patients' satisfaction was comparable negatively affected. In relation to these findings, initial results of an existing intervention study substantiate with respect to this the positive effect of an additional, psychological intervention on surgical patients [67].

The effect of psychiatric comorbidities on treatment

Finally, an essential aspect should be pointed out: It is certain that a not inconsiderable number of psychiatric disorders can appear as comorbidity to gastrointestinal diseases [68]–[70]. As Avidan et al [30] have show, GERD-related symptoms significantly occur more frequently in patients with than without a diagnosed psychiatric disorder. The reflux symptoms are not associated with any specific type of psychotropic medication, type of psychiatric disorder, the lifestyle did not influence the presence of reflux symptoms and, in general, may reflect a reduced threshold for or distorted perception of symptoms. In this respect, prevalence between 5% and 20% are put forward according to disorder profile. Depression and panic disorders are in the forefront [71]. The literature alludes to possible associations with the emergence of panic disorder where there are existing functional esophageal disorders, just as there can be with GERD [72], [73]. In this relation, Stanghellini [74] has shown that the most notable factors for the development of upper gastrointestinal symptoms, including GERD-related symptoms, were found to be various indicators of psychological stress and psychiatric disorders.

Behavioural techniques exist in the treatment of panic disorders with GERD symptoms. Own results, also, surprisingly substantiate a positive effect of laproscopic antireflux surgery in GERD patients with comorbidity of a panic disorder. In this way, the elimination of anxiety disorders in one third of these patients was achieved within the first few postoperative months [75]. In contrast, other psychiatric comorbidities in GERD patients are able to affect surgical outcome negatively [76]–[78]. As previously published [78], GERD patients with major depression as a comorbidity, when treated with laparoscopic Nissen fundoplication, show a significant lower quality of life improvement and a higher degree of swallowing problems or postoperative adaptation problems in comparison to patients who underwent a Toupet fundoplication. The authors concluded that eventually a Toupet fundoplication, independently from manometric findings, could be beneficial in such a group of patients with psychiatric comorbidities to improve subjective surgical outcome. However, further investigations in this field are needed and could be helpful for all, gastroenterologists as well as surgeons, to find an optimal procedure resulting in a high level of patients satisfaction and quality of life improvement. In conclusion, GERD patients with psychiatric disorders are rarely satisfied with the results of antireflux surgery. Moreover, these patients demonstrated less symptomatic relief than patients without psychiatric disorders. These results suggest that even patients who might otherwise be candidates for antireflux surgery may have a poor symptomatic outcome, if they also have psychiatric comorbidities. Antireflux surgery in these patients should be approached with great trepidation!

Conclusion

Gastroesophageal reflux disease (GERD) can be traced back to disorders of the gastroesophageal junction. But several psychological factors and psychiatric disorders interact through recognized psychophysiologic or behavioural mechanisms to affect the clinical presentation and treatment outcome. Even if many aspects are still unknown, the following is conceivable: that well defined personality factors moderate the effect of stress on the gastroesophageal junction, just as they can influence the perception and assessment of symptoms. Additionally, psychiatric disorders as comorbidities can also accompany GERD. For this reason, it is necessary to consider if an extension of hitherto psychological interventions could be helpful in patients with a subjective link between reflux and stress on an emotional personality related level, or in patients with attendant psychiatric disorders. This broadening relates both to the conservative use of antireflux medication and to surgical therapy, since a postoperative shift in symptoms can occur. The effectiveness of psychological interventions in several gastrointestinal patient groups could already be shown in the past. Whereas evidence for their effectiveness in patients suffering with GERD is partly still outstanding and should be investigated in the future especially as several individual promising starts have been made.

References

[1] Armstrong D (1994) Reflux disease and Barrett's oesophagus. Endoscopy 26: 9–19

[2] Dent J, Brun J, Fendrick AM et al (1999) An evidence-based appraisal of reflux disease management – the Genval Workshop report. Gut 44: 1–16

[3] Klauser AG, Schindlbeck NE, Müller-Lissner SA (1990) Symptoms in gastro-oesophageal reflux disease. Lancet 335: 205–208

[4] Heading RC, Castell DO (2003) Clinical spectrum and diagnosis of gastroesophageal reflux disease. In: The esophagus (Castell DO, Richter JE, eds). Philadelphia: Lippincott, pp 381–388

[5] A Gallup survey on heartburn across America (1988) The gallup organisation. New York: Princeton

[6] Bradley A, Richter JE, Pulliam TJ et al (1993) The relationship between stress and symptoms of gastro-esophageal reflux: the influence of psychological factors. Am J Gastroenterol 88: 11–19

[7] Baldi F, Ferrarini P, Longanesi A et al (1989) Acid gastroesophagael reflux and symptom occurence. Analysis of some factors influencing their association. Dig Dis Sci 34: 1890–1893

[8] Johnson DA, Winters C, Spurling TJ et al (1987) Esophageal acid sensitivity in Barrett's esophagus. J Clin Gastroenterol 9: 23–27

[9] Singh S, Richter JE, Bradley LA, Haile JM (1993) The symptom index: differential usefulness in suspected acid-related complaints of heartburn and chest pain. Dig Dis Sci 38: 1402–1408

[10] Jacobson E (1925) Voluntary relaxation of the esophagus. Am J Physiol 72: 387–392

[11] Jacobson E (1927) Spastic esophagus and mucous colitis. Arch Int Med 39: 433–438

[12] Rubin J, Nagler R, Spiro HM, Pilot ML (1962) Measuring the effect of emotions on esophageal motility. Psychosom Med 24: 170–176

[13] Young LD, Richter JE, Anderson KO et al (1987) The effects of psychological and environmental stressors on peristaltic esophageal contractions in healthy volunteers. Psychophysiology 24: 132–141

[14] Ayres RCS, Robertson DAF, Naylor K, Smith CL (1989) Stress and oesophageal motility in normal subjects and patients with irretable bowel syndrome. Gut 30: 1540–1543

[15] Anderson KO, Dalton CB, Bradley LA, Richter JE (1989) Stress induces alterations of esophageal pressures in healthy and non-cardiac chest pain patients. Dig Dis Sci 34: 83–91

[16] Penagini R, Bartesaghi B, Bianchi PA (1992) Effect of cold stress on postprandial lower esophageal sphincter competence and gastroesophageal reflux in healthy subjects. Dig Dis Sci 37: 1200–1205

[17] Mittal RK, Stewart WR, Ramahi M et al (1992) Psychological stress increases tonic and phasic activity of the crural diaphragm and impairs relaxation of the lower esophageal sphincter. Gastroenterol 102: A487

[18] Cook IJ, Collins SM (1986) Does acute emotional stress influence frequency or duration of gastroesophageal reflux in human subjects? Gastroenterol 90: A1380

[19] Sonnenberg A, Donga M, Erckenbrecht JF, Wienbeck M (1984) The effect of mental stress induced by noise on gastric acid secretion and mucosal blood flow. Scand J Gastroenterol 19: 45–48

[20] Holtman G, Kriebel R, Singer MV (1990) Mental stress and gastric acid secretion: do personality traits influence the response? Dig Dis Sci 35: 998–1007

[21] Baker LH, Lieberman D, Oehlke M (1995) Psychological distress in patients with gastroesophageal reflux disease. Am J Gastroenterol 90: 1797–3

[22] Johnston BT, Lewis SA, Collins SA et al (1995) Acid perception in gastro-oesophageal reflux disease is dependent on psychosocial factors. Scand J Gastroenterol 30: 1–5

[23] Tew S, Jamieson GG, Pilowsky I, Myers J (1997) The illness behavior of patients with gastroesophageal reflux disease with and without endoscopic esophagitis. Dis Esophagus 10: 9–15

[24] Nielzen S, Pettersson KI, Regnell G, Svenson R (1986) The role of psychiatric factors in symptoms of hiatus hernia or gastric reflux. Acta Psychiatr Scand 73: 214–220

[25] Clouse RE, Lustman PJ (1983) Psychiatric illness and contraction abnormalities of the esophagus. N Engl J Med 309: 1337–1342

[26] Feldman M, Walker P, Goldschmiedt M, Cannon D (1992) Role of affect and personality in acid secretion and serum gastrin concentration. Gastroenterol 102: 175–180

[27] Kamolz T, Bammer T, Wykypiel H Jr, Pointner R (1999) Streßverarbeitung und Persönlichkeitsstruktur

bei Patienten mit und ohne streßassoziierter Symptomatik der gastroösophagealen Refluxkrankheit. Z Gastroenterol 37: 265–270
[28] Velanovich V, Karmy-Jones R (1998) Measurement gastroesophageal reflux disease: relationship between health-related quality of life score and physiologic parameters. Am Surg 64: 649–653
[29] Naliboff BD, Mayer M, Fass R et al (2004) The effect of life stress on symptoms of heartburn. Psychosom Med 66: 426–434
[30] Avidan B, Sonnenberg A, Giblovich H, Sontag SJ (2001) Reflux symptoms are associated with psychiatric disease. Aliment Pharmacol Ther 15: 1907–1912
[31] Quigley EM (2001) Non-erosive reflux disease: Part of the spectrum of gastro-oesophageal reflux disease, a component of functional dispepsia, or both? Eur J Gastroenterol Hepatol 13: S13–S18
[32] Cohen S, Snape WJ Jr (81977) The role of psychophysiological factors in disorders of oesophageal function. Clin Gastroenterol 6: 569–579
[33] Goyal RK, Skarupta JN, Saha JK (1992) Properties of esophageal mechanosensitive receptors. In: Advances in the innervation of the gastrointestinal tract (Holle GE, Wood JD, eds). Elsevier, pp 523–537
[34] Grundy D (1992) Extrinsic reflex pathways in the upper gastrointestinal tract and their central processing. In: Advances in the innervation of the gastrointestinal tract (Holle GE, Wood JD, eds). Elsevier, pp 539–546
[35] Kellow JE, Delvaux M, Azpiroz F et al (1999) Principles of applied neurogastroenterology: physiology/ motility-sensation. Gut 45: 17–24
[36] Drossman DA, Creed FH, Olden KW et al (1999) Psychosocial aspects of functional gastrointestinal disorders. Gut 45: 25–30
[37] Pustorino S, Guerrisi O, Calipari G et al (1991) Psycho-emotional distress and gastroesophageal reflux syndrome. Minerva Gastroenterol Dietol 37: 1–9
[38] Clouse RE, Richter JE, Heading RC et al (1999) Functional esophageal disorders. Gut 45 (Suppl 11): 31–36
[39] Janssens JP, Vantrappen G (1992) Irritable esophagus. Am J Med 92: 27–32
[40] Trimble KC, Pryde A, Heading RC (1995) Lowered oesophageal sensory thresholds in patients with symptomatic but not excess gastro-oesophageal reflux disease: evidence for a spectrum of visceral sensitivity in GORD. Gut 37: 7–12
[41] Shi G, Tatum RP, Joehl RJ, Kahrilas PJ (1999) Esophageal sensitivity and symptom perception in gastroesophageal reflux disease. Curr Gastroenterol Rep 1: 214–219
[42] Vaezi MF, Richter JE (1999) Importance of duodeno-gastro-esophageal reflux in the medical outpatient practice. Hepatogastroenterol 46: 40–47
[43] Norton GR, Norton PJ, Asmundson GJ et al (1999) Neurotic butterflies in my stomach: the role of anxiety, anxiety sensitivity and depression in functional gastrointestinal disorders. J Psychosom Res 47: 233–240
[44] Johnston BT, Lewis SA, Love AH (1995) Stress, personality and social support in gastro-oesophageal reflux disease. J Psychosom Res 39: 221–226
[45] Fass R, Tougas G (2002) Functional heartburn: the stimulus, the pain, and the brain. Gut 51: 885–892
[46] Chang JT, Katzka DA (2004) Gastroesophageal reflux disease, Barrett esophagus, and esophageal adenocarcinoma. Arch Intern Med 164: 1482–1488
[47] Shaheen N, Ransohoff DF (2002) Gastroesophageal reflux, Barrett esophagus, and esophageal cancer: scientific review. JAMA 287: 1972–1981
[48] Garssen B (2002) Psycho-oncology and cancer: linking psychosocial factors with cancer development. Ann Oncol 13: S171–S175
[49] Kiecolt-Glaser JK, Robles TF, Heffner KL et al (2002) Psycho-oncology and cancer: psychoneuroimmunology and cancer. Ann Oncol 13: S165–S169
[50] Dessureault S, Coppola D, Weitzner M et al (2002) Barrett's esophagus and squamous cell carcinoma in a patient with psychogenic vomiting. Int J Gastrointest Cancer 32: 57–61
[51] Jansson C, Johansson ALV, Jeding K et al (2004) Psychosocial working conditions and the risk of esophageal and gastric cardia cancers. Europ J Epidemiol 19: 631–641
[52] Meining A, Classen M (2000) The role of diet and lifestyle measures in the pathogenesis and treatment of gastroesophageal reflux disease. Am J Gastroenterol 95: 2692–2697
[53] Kamolz T, Pointner R (2004) What do heartburn suffers expect from proton pump inhibitors when prescribed for the first time? Minerva Gastroenterol Dietol 50: in press
[54] Kamolz T, Pointner R (2002) Expectations of GERD patients in the outcome of laparoscopic antireflux surgery. Surg Laparosc Endosc Percutan Techn 12: 389–392
[55] Contini S, Bertelé A, Nervi G et al (2002) Quality of life for patients with gastroesophageal reflux disease 2 years after laparoscopic fundoplication. Surg Endosc 16: 1555–1560
[56] Klapow JC, Wilcox M, Malinger AP et al (2002) Characterization of long-term outcomes after Toupet fundoplication. J Clin gastroenterol 34: 509–515

[57] Kamolz T (2002) Analysis of medical compliance in gastro-oesophageal reflux disease patients referred to pre-surgical examination. Digest Liver Dis 34: 183–189
[58] Johnston BT, Gunning J, Lewis SA (1996) Health care seeking by heartburn suffers is associated with psychosocial factors. Am J Gastroenterol 91: 2500–2504
[59] Schuster MM (1983) Disorders of the esophagus: application of psychophysiological methods in treatment. In: Psychophysiology of the gastrointestinal tract (Hözl R, Whitehead WE, eds). New York: Plenum, pp 33–42
[60] Shay SS, Johnson LF, Wong RKH et al (1986) Rumination, heartburn, and daytime gastroesophageal reflux: a case study with mechanism defined and successfully treated with biofeedback therapy. J Clin Gastroenterol 8: 115–126
[61] Gordon A, Gordon E, Berelowitz M et al (1983) Biofeedback improvement of lower esophageal sphincter pressures and reflux symptoms. J Clin Gastroenterol 5: 235–237
[62] Klein KB, Speigel D (1989) Modulation of gastric acid secretion by hypnosis. Gastroenterol 96: 1383–1387
[63] McDonald-Haile J, Bradley LA, Baily MA et al (1994) Relaxation training reduces symptom reports and acid exposure in patients with gastroesophageal reflux disease. Gastroenterol 107: 61–69
[64] Watson DI, Chan ASL, Myers JC, Jamieson GG (1997) Illness behavior influences the outcome of laparoscopic antireflux surgery. J Am Coll Surg 184: 44–48
[65] Kamolz T, Bammer T, Pointner R (2000) Predictability of dysphagia after laparoscopic Nissen fundoplication. Am J Gastroenterol 95: 408–414
[66] Kamolz T, Granderath FA, Pointner R (2003) The outcome of laparoscopic antireflux surgery in relation to patients' subjective degree of compliance with former antireflux medication. Surg Laparosc Endosc Percutan Tech 13: 155–160
[67] Kamolz T, Granderath FA, Bammer T et al (2001) Psychological intervention influences the outcome of laparoscopic antireflux surgery in patients with stress-related symptoms of gastroesophageal reflux disease. Scand J Gastroenterol 36: 800–805
[68] Walker EA, Katon WJ, Jemelka RP, Roy-Bryne PP (1992) Comorbidity of gastrointestinal complaints, depression, and anxiety in the Epidemiologic Catchment Area (ECA) Study. Am J Med 92: 26–30
[69] Hochstrasser B, Angst J (1996) The Zürich Study: XXII. Epidemiology of gastrointestinal complaints and comorbidity with anxiety and depression. Eur Arch Psychiatry Clin Neurosci 246: 261–272
[70] Mayer EA, Craske M, Naliboff BD (2001) Depression, anxiety, and the gastrointestinal system. J Clin Psychiatry 62: S28–S37
[71] Lydiard RB, Greenwald S, Weissman MM et al (1994) Panic disorder and gastrointestinal symptoms: findings from the NIMH Epidemiologic Catchment Area project. Am J Psychiatry 151: 64–70
[72] Wiklund I, Butler-Wheelhouse P (1996) Psychosocial factors and their role in symptomatic gastroesophageal reflux disease and functional dyspepsia. Scand J Gastroenterol 220: S94–S100
[73] Locke GR 3rd, Weaver AL, Melton LJ 3rd, Talley NJ (2004) Psychosocial factors are linked to functional gastrointestinal disorders: a population based nested case-control study. Am J Gastroenterol 99: 350–357
[74] Stanghellini V (1999) Relationship between upper gastrointestinal symptoms and lifestyle, psychosocial factors and comorbidity in the general population: results from the Domestic/International gastroenterology Surveillance Study (DIGEST). Scand J Gastroenterol 231: 29–37
[75] Kamolz T, Bammer T, Granderath FA, Pointner R (2001) Laparoscopic antireflux surgery in GERD patients with concomitant anxiety disorders. Dig Liver Dis 33: 659–664
[76] Velanovich V (2003) The effect of chronic pain syndromes and psychoemotional disorders on symptomatic and quality of life outcomes of antireflux surgery. J Gastrointest Surg 7: 53–58
[77] Velanovich V, Karmy-Jones R (2001) Psychiatric disorders affect outcomes of antireflux operations for gastroesophageal reflux disease. Surg Endosc 15: 171–175
[78] Kamolz T, Granderath FA, Pointner R (2003) Does major depression affect the outcome of laparoscopic antireflux surgery. Surg Endosc 17: 55–60

Chapter 29

ECONOMIC ANALYSES OF GERD

N. Vakil and N. Guda

University of Wisconsin Medical School, Milwaukee, MI, USA

Introduction

GERD is a chronic disorder in the majority of cases and frequently requires prolonged therapy. The symptoms of reflux disease have a profound effect on quality of life and work performance making GERD an expensive disease for society to manage. Health related expenditures are generally described as **direct costs** (the costs of providing and obtaining treatment) and the **indirect costs** (other costs due to the disease such as time lost from work that are not related to the provision of health care). When competitive management strategies are compared, the cost of each strategy must be balanced against its effectiveness. When new treatments become available the cost often increases and the benefit of improved therapeutic response can be assessed by cost-effectiveness studies. A new therapeutic intervention that increases therapeutic efficacy but costs less than standard therapy is the ideal new treatment. While this is the goal of new therapeutic interventions, most innovations in medicine increase both cost and effectiveness and the trade-off between the increased cost and improved effectiveness must be determined by cost-effectiveness studies. There are three general approaches to the management of any chronic disease: (1) Reduce costs regardless of outcome, (2) Improve outcomes regardless of cost, and (3) Maximize outcomes within the constraints of available resources. Cost-effectiveness studies help to optimize clinical outcomes within the constraints of available resources.

The cost of reflux disease to society

Reflux disease is an important economic problem in most western countries. The economic ramifications of the disease are becoming increasingly apparent. Levin et al [1] reported the cost of managing reflux disease in a managed care setting (Kaiser Permanente of Northern California). They calculated the GERD related costs in a cohort of patients with acid related disorders. With adjustment of the data to determine the costs attributable to GERD, the total cost of managing GERD was $471 per person with pharmacy costs accounting for $156 of this amount and outpatient costs accounting for $279. Inpatient costs were small at $35/per person. In the first 6 months after the diagnosis, outpatient costs remain the highest component cost of GERD management accounting for a large proportion of the adjusted costs ($246 out of a total of $289). These data suggest that pharmacy costs account for a small proportion of the total costs of acute or chronic management of the disease. A cost of illness study by Lair showed that drugs only accounted for approximately 50% of total direct costs of GERD treatment [2]. A study from Sweden recently evaluated the direct and indirect costs of GERD [3]. The total cost to Swedish society of dyspepsia, PUD and GERD in 1997 was $US424 million, or $US63 per adult. Direct costs totaled $US258 million (61%) while indirect costs totaled $US166 million (39%). The highest proportions of costs were due to drugs and sick leave, these being 37 and 34%, respectively. A Swiss study found that the mean direct medical costs of GERD were dominated by medication costs, were 185 Swiss Francs per patient-year (95% CI: CHF 140–230) and the cost of managing GERD accounted for 0.5% of Switzerland's total health care expenditures [4]. GERD has also been shown to cause significant work loss through time off work and reduced productivity while at work, and also to reduce productivity during regular daily activities [5]. The indirect costs of the disease need to be considered in economic assessments of GERD. In a recent US study, 30% of heartburn sufferers reported reduced productivity. Over 48% of respondents with severe symptoms reported reduced productivity, compared with 40% and 12% of respondents with moderate and mild symptoms, respectively [6]. Patients value symptom relief and are willing to pay for relief. In willingness to pay studies, patients with GERD were willing to pay up to US $182 to obtain complete relief in a short period of time without side effects. Patients with less severe GERD symptoms were willing to pay more to avoid side effects ($58 vs $38). Older patients were less willing to pay for better relief than younger patients [7]. Another study assessed patients willingness to pay for a given reduction in the risk of having a relapse of heartburn while on treatment with an acid suppressant [8]. The authors showed that patients were willing to take on significant out of pocket expenses ($US 60–90 over a 1–3 month period). In summary, these data suggest that GERD is a significant burden to patients and society in terms of cost. Untreated GERD is associated with loss of productivity and the long-term management of this disease is also associated with significant cost. Patients value symptom relief and are willing to pay for complete symptom relief.

The cost of different treatment strategies for GERD

Different treatment modalities for GERD have been reviewed elsewhere in this book. This section will deal only with the economic implications of management decisions and treatment strategies.

Proton pump inhibitors and H_2-receptor antagonists

A number of economic models that have compared the costs of H2 receptor antagonist therapy to proton pump inhibitor therapy in erosive esophagitis in the acute and long-term management of erosive GERD. These studies balance the higher efficacy with proton pump inhibitors and their higher cost with the lower costs of H2 receptor antagonists and their lower efficacy. Most of these studies have suggested that a proton pump inhibitor based strategy is cost-effective compared to H2 receptor antagonists [9]–[17]. Recent studies have compared the costs of generic proton pump inhibitors to generic H2 receptor antagonists, which are now widely available. Goreee et al [18] used the cost of generic ranitidine in Canada in their base case analysis comparing ranitidine to omeprazole. In this model, maintenance therapy with PPI did have better clinical outcomes but was not the dominant strategy in economic terms. With the availability of generic and over the counter omeprazole in the United States, this model deserves re-evaluation because the lower costs of over the counter omeprazole were not considered in the original publication. In an economic model based on clinical trials comparing esomeprazole and omeprazole for the treatment of acute erosive GERD, the cost-effectiveness of esomeprazole 40 mg and omeprazole 20 mg over an 8-week period was compared [19]. The esomepraole strategy was found to be dominant over the omeprazole strategy. Time with GERD (defined as the time with endoscopic evidence of erosions) was 2.9 weeks in the esomeprazole group and 3.6 weeks in the omeprazole group. Zagari et al [20] used a decision analytic model and estimated the one-year direct cost of treating patients with proton pump inhibitors ($1192) was lower than the total cost for a branded H2 RA ($1495) and comparable to a generic H2 RA ($1152).

Step-up vs step down therapy for uninvestigated heartburn

Sonnenberg et al examined a systematic approach to the management of GERD in the Veterans Administration system in the USA. They assessed a step-wise strategy beginning with a generic H2 RA. Failures with this strategy would be treated with a higher dose of H2 RA therapy and failures to the latter treated with proton pump inhibitors (step-up therapy) [21]. This economic model suggested that an average of $916 could be saved per patient every 5 years by using a step-up strategy. Clinical data from the same group suggests that a step-up strategy may be effective in clinical practice [22]. In contrast, data from a clinical trial in primary care suggest that neither step-up or step-down therapy provided optimal control of heartburn over a 20 week period [23]. Results from a recent multi-center, randomized, open-labeled study with economic end-points provides some interesting results. Patients with symptoms of GERD (uninvestigated) in primary care practices in West Virginia were evaluated. 268 patients were randomized to omeprazole 20 mg once a day or ranitidine 150 mg (brand-name) bid for up to 6 months. At 6 months, there was no significant difference in total costs between the groups but symptoms were better controlled in the omeprazole group [24]. This study showed that while the initial acquisition costs of proton-pump inhibitor therapy may be higher, the overall costs may be similar because of the poorer efficacy in the H2 RA group. Another recent study evaluated the cost of step-wise management strategies employed by managed care organizations [25]. This was a prospective randomized economic trial in 4 large managed care organizations. 685 patients with GERD were randomized to omeprazole 20 mg or ranitidine 150 mg bid for 4 weeks. Additional 4-week therapy was given to patients as required. Investigations and office visits were determined over the 16-week period by usual practice. Omeprazole was more effective in controlling symptoms in these patients. Patients spent more money for over-the-counter heartburn remedies in the ranitidine group compared to patients treated with omeprazole. As most pharmacy data systems do not capture information on over the counter medications, many economic evaluations fail to adequately account for the costs associated with inadequate therapy. Failures of therapy can be expensive and need more careful consideration in future studies.

Discontinuous maintenance therapy: on demand and intermittent therapy

Studies in primary care settings have shown that many patients with GERD do not take medications on a regular basis and frequently take maintenance medication for GERD on an as-needed basis [26]. While continuous maintenance medical therapy has been the standard recommendation for patients with GERD, recent studies suggest that patients with non-erosive reflux disease may be managed with therapy that is intermittent (i.e., taken in short courses of 1–2 weeks when symptoms occur) or on-demand (medication is taken when the patient experiences symptoms). Intermittent therapy may be patient-driven or physician-driven, i.e., patients may choose to initiate a short course of therapy or the physician may make the determination based on the patient's symptoms.

In a recent study, 677 patients with endoscopy negative or mild-moderate erosive GERD in primary care were randomized to ranitidine 150 mg bid, low-dose omeprazole (10 mg) or standard dose omeprazole (20 mg) for 2 weeks [27]. If they had symptom relief they continued with the maintenance phase of the study where they received 2-week courses of intermittent therapy with the regimen that had worked in the first instance. At the end of one year of maintenance therapy approximately half the patients did not require treatment for at least 6 months of the study period despite satisfactory control of symptoms. A cost analysis based on this study found no difference between the cost of the omeprazole arm and the ranitidine arm using cost data from a number of European countries that were part of the trial. These data suggest that on a cost basis, there is little to be gained from a step-up approach in patients with endoscopy negative reflux disease [28]. This study demonstrated that the use of short intermittent courses of therapy in patients with mild erosive reflux disease or non-erosive reflux disease is cost-effective.

On-demand therapy is particularly interesting in non-erosive reflux disease because the main focus is on symptom relief as there is no discernable mucosal injury. In one study, 424 patients with endoscopy negative reflux disease were randomized to placebo or PPI (omeprazole 20 mg or omeprazole 10 mg) on demand [29]. At 6 months follow-up, 29% of patients had failed on demand therapy and needed daily maintenance therapy. However 83% of patients randomized to on-demand therapy with omeprazole 20 mg a day were satisfactorily maintained over the 6-month time frame. The mean number of omeprazole capsules used per day was 0.43, suggesting that the total medication use was reduced by approximately 50%. In another recent study of esomeprazole therapy, 320 patients with endoscopy negative reflux disease who had complete symptom resolution after 4 weeks of therapy with either esomeprazole 20 mg or omeprazole 20 mg were randomized to receive esomeprazole 20 mg on-demand or placebo on-demand for 6 months [30]. Medication intake was measured using electronic chips embedded in the caps of the medication containers. On average, esomeprazole was taken once every three days and 86% of patients were managed with on-demand therapy compared to 49% in the placebo group. These data suggest that on-demand therapy is effective and can substantially reduce the costs of maintenance therapy. A recent study however challenges these notions. A prospective, open, randomized multicentre study with parallel group design was conducted in 155 general practice clinics, and included 1357 endoscopically uninvestigated patients with symptoms suggestive of gastro-oesophageal reflux disease [31]. The aim of the study was to assess the differences in direct medical costs between a patient-controlled on-demand treatment strategy with esomeprazole, 20 mg daily, and general practitioner-controlled intermittent treatment strategies with esomeprazole, 40 mg daily, for either 2 or 4 weeks. The mean direct medical costs were 182, 221 and 195 euros for patient-controlled on-demand treatment and 2 weeks and 4 weeks of general practitioner-controlled intermittent treatment, respectively, showing no statistically significant difference. The comparable mean total costs were 211, 344 and 300 euros, i.e., significantly lower for patients treated on-demand compared with either of the general practitioner-controlled intermittent treatment strategies. On-demand therapy may therefore not decrease total management costs for GERD but may be less expensive than intermittent therapy which requires repeated physician contact.

Fundoplication as an alternative to maintenance therapy

(a) Early models with limited long term follow-up data

Laparoscopic fundoplication has been recommended on cost-effectiveness grounds as an alternative to long-term medical therapy. Viljakka et al evaluated the lifetime costs of managing GERD in Finland [32]. The medical regimens were ranitidine (150 or 300 mg/day), omeprazole (20 or 40 mg/day), and lansoprazole (30 mg/day), with costs calculated for total life expectancy after diagnosis and for one-third of that time. Costs for open or laparoscopic surgery (Nissen fundoplication) included pre- and post-operative investigations, sick leave, and calculated financial loss due to fatal outcome. The cost of open or laparoscopic operation was less than that of lifelong daily treatment with proton pump inhibitors or ranitidine, 300 mg daily. This model did not take into account the cost of managing complications of surgery and did not include the cost of recurrence after surgery. In a cost analysis from the Netherlands, Van den Boom et al concluded that laparoscopic surgery was less expensive than medical therapy and suggested that the two methods of maintenance became equal at 1.4 years [33]. Huedebert et al originally published a model that suggested that laparoscopic fundoplication and omeprazole therapy became equal at 10 years based on US data [34]. In the light of recent data on long term outcomes with surgical therapy the model required revision because the original model did not include the costs of failed therapy and complications [35]. The repeat analysis showed that medical therapy is associated with total costs of $8,798 and 4.59 quality-adjusted life-years, whereas the surgical strategy is more expensive ($10,475) and less effective (4.55 quality-adjusted life-years). The results were robust to most one-way sensitivity analyses. The authors concluded that long-term medical therapy with proton pump inhibitors is the preferred strategy for patients with gastroesophageal reflux disease and severe esophagitis. This study highlights the importance of using primary, patient-derived data rather than expert opinion. Two recent studies from routine care highlight the problems with assuming a perfect outcome with surgery. In routine practice Vakil et al demonstrated that outcomes were poorer in routine practice than in expert surgical centers [36]. Over 3 years of follow-up, 32% of patients after fundoplication were taking medications on a regular basis for treatment of heartburn, 11% required esophageal dilation for dysphagia, and 7% had repeat surgical procedures. The costs of these interventions have not been considered in the economic models reported to date. These data suggest that the cost-effectiveness studies available to date are based on limited data on long-term outcome and may need revision as more data as the long-term outcomes of laparoscopic fundoplication in routine practice become available.

(b) Open fundoplication compared with medical therapy

A carefully conducted multicenter randomized trial evaluated the cost-effectiveness of open fundoplication vs medical therapy. After initial treatment of refluxoesophagitis with omeprazole to control symptoms and to heal esophagitis, 154 patients were randomised to continue treatment with omeprazole (20 or 40 mg daily) and 144 patients to have an open antireflux operation. The costs were assessed over five years from randomisation. Five year direct medical costs per patient with omeprazole were significantly lower than for those having anti-reflux surgery. When indirect costs (loss of production due to GERD related sick leave) were also included, the cost of surgical treatment increased substantially and exceeded the cost of medical treatment further.

Endoscopic therapy for reflux disease

There is only one cost-effectiveness analysis evaluating medical therapy compared to endoscopic therapy for GERD [37]. As the long-term outcomes are poorly characterized with all of these therapies, the assumptions are open to question. The baseline probabilities in the model were an annual endotherapy failure rate of 20%, a partial failure rate of 10%, and a complication rate of 1%. Pharmacotherapy was the least costly approach, irrespective of time, if the daily cost of a proton pump inhibitor was less than $140 a month or if endotherapy costed more than $3400. Current PPI costs in the USA are well below $100/month. This model does not consider the long-term savings with endotherapy or the cost of complications of endoscopic therapy. Further studies of endoscopic therapy are necessary before appropriate cost-effectiveness studies can be performed.

References

[1] Levin TR, Schmittdiel JA, Kunz K, Henning JM, Henke CJ, Colby CJ, Selby JV (1997) Costs of acid reflux disorders to a health maintenance organization. Am J Med 103: 520–528

[2] Lair TJ, Fu Q, Anderson DR, Crawley JA (1998) Utilisation and expenditures in the treatment of patients with gastroesophageal reflux disease. Dis Manage Health Outcome 4(6): 325–336

[3] Agreus L, Borgquist L (2002) The cost of gastro-oesophageal reflux disease, dyspepsia and peptic ulcer disease in Sweden. Pharmacoeconomics 20(5): 347–355

[4] Schwenkglenks M, Marbet UA, Szucs TD (2004) Epidemiology and costs of gastroesophageal reflux disease in Switzerland: a population-based study. Soz Praventivmed 49(1): 51–61

[5] Wahlqvist P et al (1999) Measuring lost productivity in patients with gastro-oesophageal reflux disease using a productivity questionnaire (WPAI-GORD). Medical Decision Making 19: 532–536

[6] Dean BB, Crawley JA, Schmitt CM, Wong J, Ofman JJ (2003) The burden of illness of gastro-oesophageal reflux disease: impact on work productivity. Aliment Pharmacol Ther 17(10): 1309–1317

[7] Kleinman L, McIntosh E, Ryan M, Schmier J, Crawley J, Locke GR 3rd, De Lissovoy G (2002) Willingness to pay for complete symptom relief of gastroesophageal reflux disease. Arch Intern Med 162(12): 1361–1366

[8] Kartman B, Stålhammar NO, Johannesson M (1996) Valuation of health changes with the contingent valuation method: a test of scope and question order effects. Health Economics 5: 531–541

[9] Hillman AL, Bloom BS, Fendrick AM, Schwartz JS (1992) Cost and quality effects of alternative treatments for persistent GERD. Arch Int Med 152: 1467–1472

[10] Glise H (1995) Quality of life and cost of therapy in reflux disease. Scand J Gastroenterol 210 (Suppl): 38–42

[11] Bate CM et al (1997) Omeprazole is more effective than cimetidine for the relief of all grades of gastro-oesophageal reflux disease-associated heartburn, irrespective of the presence or absence of endoscopic oesophagitis. Aliment Pharmacol Ther 11: 755–763

[12] Bate CM, Richardson PDI (1994) Cost-effectiveness of omeprazole in the management of gastroesophageal reflux disease in clinical practice. Br J Med Econ 7: 81–97

[13] Bate CM, Richardson PDI (1992) Symptomatic assessment and cost effectiveness of treatment for reflux oesophagitis: comparisons of omeprazole and histamine H2-receptor antagonists. Br J Med Econ 2: 37–48

[14] Bloom B et al (1995) Omeprazole or ranitidine plus metoclopramide for patients with severe erosive esophagitis: a cost-effectiveness analysis. Pharmacoeconomics 8(4): 343–349

[15] Lindberg G (1994) Omeprazole vs ranitidine in reflux oesophagitis. Pharmacoeconomics 5: 27–34

[16] Ofman JJ et al (2000) Cost effectiveness of rabeprazole versus generic ranitidine for symptom resolution in patients with erosive esophagitis. Am J Managed Care 6(8): 905–916

[17] Phillips C, Moore A (1997) Trial and error-an expensive luxury: economic analysis of effectiveness of proton pump inhibitors and histamine anatgonists in treating reflux disease. Br J Med Econ 11: 55–63

[18] Goeree R, O'Brien B, Hunt R, Blackhouse G, Willan A, Watson J (1999) Economic evaluation of long term management strategies for erosive oesophagitis. Pharmacoeconomics 16: 679–697

[19] Wahlquist P (2000) In Finland, Sweden and the UK, esomeprazole is cost-effective compared with omeprazole for the acute treatment of patients with reflux esophagitis. Value in Health 3: 360
[20] Zagari M, Villa KF, Freston JW (1995) Proton pump inhibitors versus H2 receptor antagonists for the treatment of erosive gastroesophageal reflux disease. A cost-comparative study. Am J Managed Care 1: 247–255
[21] Sonnenberg A, Indaomi J, Becker L (1999) Economic analysis of step-wise treatment of gastro-esophageal reflux disease. Ailment Pharmacol Ther 13: 1003–1013
[22] Inadomi JM, Jamal R, Murata GH, Hoffman RM, Lavezo LA, Virgil JM, Swanson KM, Sonnenberg A (2001) Step-down management of gastro-esophageal reflux disease. Gastroenterology 121: 1095–1100
[23] Howden CW, Henning JM, Huang B, Lukasik N, Freston JW (2001) Management of heartburn in a large, randomized, community-based study: comparison of 4 therapeutic strategies. Am J Gastroenterol 96: 1704–1710
[24] Kaplan-Machitz B, Spiegler GE, Zodet MW, Revicki DA (2000) Effectiveness and costs of omeprazole vs ranitidine for treatment of symptomatic gastroesophageal reflux disease in primary clinics in West Virginia. Arch Fam Med 9: 624–630
[25] Crawley JA, Andersson T, Joshua-Gotlib S, Levine D (1999) Are patients carrying the burden of managed care cost control measures. Am J Gastroenterol 94: 2750
[26] Hungin P, Rubin G, O'Flanagan H (1999) Long-term prescribing of proton pump inhibitors in general practice. Br J Gen Practice 49: 451–453
[27] Bardhan KD, Muller-Lissner S, Bigard M, Bianchi Porro G, Ponce J, Hosie J, Scott M, Weir D, Gillon K, Peacock R, Fulton C (1999) Symptomatic gastroesophageal reflux disease: double blind controlled study of intermittent treatment with omeprazole or ranitidine. BMJ 318: 502–507
[28] Stalhammer NO, Carlsson J, Peacock R, Muller-Lissner S, Bigard MA, Porro GB, Ponce J, Hosie J, Scott M, Weir D, Fulton C, Gillon K, Bardhan K (1999) Cost-effectiveness of Omeprazole and ranitidine in Intermittent treatment of symptomatic GERD. Pharmacocconomics 16: 485–497
[29] Lind T, Havelund T, Lundell L, Glise H, Lauritsen K, Pederson S, Anker-Hansen, Stubberod A, Eriksson G, Carlsson R, Junghard O (1999) On demand therapy with omeprazole for the long-term management of patients with heartburn without esophagitis – a placebo-controlled randomized trial. Aliment Pharmacol Ther 13: 907–914
[30] Talley N, Lauritsen K, Tunturi-Hihnala H, Lind T, Moum B, Bang C et al (2001) Esomeprazole 20 mg maintains symptom control in endoscopy-negative GERD: a randomized placebo-controlled trial of on-demand therapy for 6 months. Aliment Pharmacol Ther 15: 347–354
[31] Meineche-Schmidt V, Juhl HH, Ostergaard JE, Luckow A, Hvenegaard A (2004) Costs and efficacy of three different esomeprazole treatment strategies for long-term management of gastro-oesophageal reflux symptoms in primary care. Aliment Pharmacol Ther 19(8): 907–915
[32] Viljakka M, Nevalainen J, Isolauri J (1997) Lifetime costs of surgical versus medical treatment of severe gastro-oesophageal reflux disease in Finland. Scand J Gastroenterol 32(8): 766–772
[33] Van Den Boom G, Go PM, Hameeteman W, Dallemagne B, Ament AJ (1996) Cost effectiveness of medical versus surgical treatment in patients with severe or refractory gastroesophageal reflux disease in the Netherlands. Scand J Gastroenterol 31(1): 1–9
[34] Heudebert GR, Marks R, Wilcox CM, Centor RM (1997) Choice of long-term strategy for the management of patients with severe esophagitis: a cost-utility analysis. Gastroenterology 112(4): 1078–1086
[35] Spechler SJ, Lee E, Ahnen D, Goyal RK, Hirano I, Ramirez F et al (2001) Long-term outcome of medical and surgical therapies for gastroesophageal reflux disease: follow-up of a randomized controlled trial. JAMA 285(18): 2331–2338
[36] Vakil N, Shaw M, Kirby R (2003) Clinical effectiveness of laparoscopic fundoplication in a U.S. community. Am J Med 114(1): 1–5
[37] Harewood GC, Gostout CJ (2003) Cost analysis of endoscopic antireflux procedures: endoluminal plication vs. radiofrequency coagulation vs. treatment with a proton pump inhibitor. Gastrointest Endosc 58(4): 493–499

Springer and the Environment